Manual of Allergy and Clinical Immunology for Otolaryngologists

Manual of Allergy and Clinical Immunology for Otolaryngologists

David L. Rosenstreich, MD
Marvin P. Fried, MD, FACS
Gabriele S. de Vos, MD, MSc
Alexis H. Jackman, MD, FACS

Plural Publishing Inc.

PLURAL PUBLISHING
INC.

5521 Ruffin Road
San Diego, CA 92123

e-mail: info@pluralpublishing.com
Website: http://www.pluralpublishing.com

Typeset in 10½/13 Palatino by Flanagan's Publishing Services, Inc.
Printed in Korea by Four Colour Print Group

NOTICE TO THE READER
Care has been taken to confirm the accuracy of the indications, procedures, drug dosages, and diagnosis and remediation protocols presented in this book and to ensure that they conform to the practices of the general medical and health services communities. However, the authors, editors, and publisher are not responsible for errors or omissions or for any consequences from application of the information in this book and make no warranty, expressed or implied, with respect to the currency, completeness, or accuracy of the contents of the publication. The diagnostic and remediation protocols and the medications described do not necessarily have specific approval by the Food and Drug administration for use in the disorders and/or diseases and dosages for which they are recommended. Application of this information in a particular situation remains the professional responsibility of the practitioner. Because standards of practice and usage change, it is the responsibility of the practitioner to keep abreast of revised recommendations, dosages, and procedures.

We would like to thank Dr. Estelle Levetin, PhD, Faculty of Biological Science, University of Tulsa, for her generous donation of the pollen grain pictures for the front cover.

Library of Congress Cataloging-in-Publication Data

Manual of allergy and clinical immunology for otolaryngologists / [edited by] David L. Rosenstreich, Marvin P. Fried, Gabriele S. de Vos, Alexis H. Jackman.
p. ; cm.
Includes bibliographical references and index.
ISBN 978-1-59756-623-0 (alk. paper)—ISBN 1-59756-623-3 (alk. paper)
I. Rosenstreich, David L., editor. II. Fried, Marvin P., editor. III. De Vos, Gabriele S., editor. IV. Jackman, Alexis H., editor.
[DNLM: 1. Immune System Diseases—Handbooks. 2. Hypersensitivity—Handbooks. WD 301]
RF46.5
617.5'1079—dc23

2015015165

Contents

Foreword

The fields of allergy, immunology, and otolaryngology are inextricably linked. Immunologic dysregulation is recognized to be the underpinning of a wide variety of diseases of the head and neck, and on a daily basis the practicing otolaryngologist must draw upon principles of allergy and immunology in the diagnosis and treatment of patients. For example, it is a rare patient presenting with a sinonasal complaint in whom consideration of allergic etiologies is not relevant. The otolaryngologist must also have a strong understanding of autoimmune illnesses to recognize the unique array of potential head and neck manifestations associated with autoimmune disease. Equally important, a deeper understanding of immunopathology may be the key to unlocking the mechanisms of major diseases ranging from chronic rhinosinusitis to head and neck cancer. Thus, it is imperative for the otolaryngologist to master principles of allergy and immunology in order to provide optimal patient care.

The body of knowledge encompassed by allergy and immunology is rapidly evolving and expanding, posing a great challenge for otolaryngologists seeking to keep up with diagnostic and treatment advances in the field. This splendid textbook offers a comprehensive, multidisciplinary encapsulation of contemporary allergy and immunology for the otolaryngologist. Drs. Rosenstreich, Fried, de Vos, and Jackman have assembled an illustrious group of authors who have managed to distill the essentials of allergy and immunology for the otolaryngologist without sacrificing scientific content or detail. The reader will appreciate clear elucidation of basic science concepts and the practical translation of basic science principles to the clinical management of otolaryngologic illnesses. Diagnostic and treatment guidelines are presented with a comprehensive and pragmatic approach. This book is essential reading for all otolaryngologists, from trainees looking to grasp the breadth of overlap between otolaryngology and allergy/immunology, to seasoned otolaryngologists seeking to update their fund of knowledge with the latest developments in immunophysiology and clinical treatment. The knowledge gained from this expertly edited volume will benefit our patients tremendously.

—Peter H. Hwang, MD
Professor and Chief
Division of Rhinology and Endoscopic Skull Base Surgery
Department of Otolaryngology-Head & Neck Surgery
Stanford University School of Medicine

Preface

The modern practice of otorhinolaryngology (ORL) is multifaceted. Intrinsic to the understanding of the myriad disorders that affect the head and neck is the interaction with the environment and the body's response to it. Allergy and immunology are the basis of so many of these interactions that in order to care for these patients, understanding of these relationships is critical.

There is a paucity of information on the broad range of allergic topics that specifically focus on the head and neck and the practice of ORL. Certainly sections of current textbooks cover the topic superficially, and scientific papers are exceptionally detailed. The editors of this textbook sought to create in one source the information needed by otorhinolaryngologists to care for their patients. We were fortunate to obtain collaboration of some of the foremost experts in the field, mostly in the specialties of allergy and immunology. The authors responded to our request to specifically address the head and neck and yet cover the broader issues where appropriate.

We are pleased with their efforts and feel that this book offers an up-to-date resource that is exceptionally unique and not available anywhere else. We are certain that you will agree.

Contributors

Marcella R. Aquino, MD, FACAAI, FAAAAI
Assistant Professor of Clinical Medicine
SUNY at Stonybrook
Winthrop University Hospital
Mineola, New York
Chapter 10

Jonathan A. Bernstein, MD
Professor of Medicine
Department of Internal Medicine, Division of Immunology/Allergy
University of Cincinnati College of Medicine
Cincinnati, Ohio
Chapter 12

Irene Blanco, MD, MS
Assistant Professor of Clinical Medicine
Montefiore Medical Center
Bronx, New York
Chapter 13

Larry Borish, MD
Professor of Medicine and Microbiology
University of Virginia Health System
Charlottesville, Virginia
Chapter 18

Marco D. Caversaccio, MD
Chairman and Director
Department of Otolaryngology-Head and Neck Surgery
University Hospital
Bern, Switzerland
Chapter 8

Melanie Chong, MD
Department of Allergy and Immunology
Winthrop University Hospital
Mineola, New York
Chapter 10

Antonella Cianferoni, MD, PhD
Assistant Professor of Pediatrics
Perelman School of Medicine
University of Pennsylvania
Department of Pediatrics
Allergy and Immunology Division
The Children's Hospital of Philadelphia
Philadelphia, Pennsylvania
Chapter 11

Jasmeen S. Dara, MD, MS
Assistant Professor of Pediatrics
Divisions of Allergy & Immunology and Pediatric Infectious Diseases
Albert Einstein College of Medicine and Montefiore Medical Center
Bronx, New York
Chapter 16

Mark Davis-Lorton, MD, FAAAAI, FACAAI
Director of Clinical Immunology
Division of Rheumatology, Immunology and Allergy
Winthrop University Hospital
Mineola, New York
Chapter 7

Ma. Lourdes B. de Asis, MD, MPH, FAAAI
Allergy & Asthma Consultants of Rockland & Bergen
West Nyack, New York
Chapter 17

Gabriele S. de Vos, MD, MSc
Division Chief Allergy & Immunology
Department of Medicine
Jacobi Medical Center
Assistant Professor
Department of Medicine
Albert Einstein College of Medicine
Bronx, New York
Chapters 3 and 9

Anthony E. J. Dubois, MD, PhD
Professor of Pediatric Allergy
Department of Pediatric Pulmonology & Pediatric Allergy

Beatrix Children's Hospital, University Medical Center Groningen
Groningen Research Institute for Asthma & COPD, University of Groningen
Groningen, Netherlands
Chapter 4

Judd H. Fastenberg, MD
Resident, Department of Otolaryngology-Head and Neck Surgery
Montefiore Medical Center
Albert Einstein College of Medicine
Bronx, New York
Chapter 5

Denisa E. Ferastraoaru, MD
Assistant Professor
Division of Allergy and Immunology, Department of Medicine
Monefiore Medical Center
Albert Einstein College of Medicine
Bronx, New York
Chapters 1 and 2

Luz Fonacier, MD
Professor of Clinical Medicine
State University of New York at Stony Brook
Stony Brook, New York
Head of Allergy & Training Program Director
Winthrop University Hospital
Mineola, New York
Chapters 7 and 10

Marvin P. Fried, MD, FACS
Professor of Otolaryngology-Head and Neck Surgery
University Chairman
Albert Einstein College of Medicine
Montefiore Medical Center
Bronx, New York

Marianne Frieri, MD, PhD, FACAAI, FAAAAI
Chief of Allergy Immunology
Nassau University Medical Center
East Meadow, New York
Department of Medicine
Professor of Medicine and Pathology
State University of New York at Stony Brook
Stony Brook, New York
Chapter 9

Tatyana Gavrilova, MD
Assistant Professor
Albert Einstein College of Medicine
Attending Physician
Division of Allergy & Immunology (Pediatrics)
Montefiore Medical Center
Bronx, New York
Chapter 15

Laura M. Gober, MD
Attending Physician, Division of Allergy and Immunology
The Children's Hospital of Philadelphia
Philadelphia, Pennsylvania
Chapter 11

Harris Goldstein, MD
Associate Dean for Scientific Resources
Director, Einstein-Montefiore Center for AIDS Research
Professor of Pediatrics and Microbiology & Immunology
Albert Einstein College of Medicine
Bronx, New York
Chapter 1

Jennifer Guttman, MD
Internal Medicine Resident
Montefiore Medical Center
Albert Einstein College of Medicine
Bronx, New York
Chapter 13

Missak Haigentz, Jr., MD
Associate Professor of Clinical Medicine and Otorhinolaryngology-Head and Neck Surgery
Albert Einstein College of Medicine
Montefiore Medical Center
Bronx, New York
Chapter 14

Alexis H. Jackman, MD, FACS
Department of Otorhinolaryngology
Albert Einstein College of Medicine
Montefiore Medical Center

Bronx, New York
Chapter 5

Sunit P. Jariwala, MD
Assistant Professor
Department of Medicine (Allergy/Immunology)
Albert Einstein College of Medicine
Montefiore Medical Center
Bronx, New York
Chapter 6

Joseph E. Jones, MS
Senior Medical Science Liaison
Therma Fisher Scientific
Powell, Ohio
Chapter 3

Gerard H. Koppelman, MD, PhD
Professor of Pediatric Pulmonology
Department of Pediatric Pulmonology & Pediatric Allergy
Beatrix Children's Hospital, University Medical Center Groningen
Groningen Research Institute for Asthma & COPD, University of Groningen
Groningen, Netherlands
Chapter 4

Thomas J. Ow, MD, MS, FACS
Assistant Professor
Department of Otorhinolaryngology-Head and Neck Surgery and
Department of Pathology
Montefiore Medical Center and Albert Einstein College of Medicine
Bronx, New York
Chapter 14

Werner J. Pichler, MD
ADR-AC GmbH
Holligenstrasse 91
3008 Bern
Switzerland
Chapter 8

Juliane A. Pichler, MD
Department of Otolaryngology
University Hospital
Bern, Switzerland
Chapter 8

Manish Ramesh, MBBS, PhD
Assistant Professor
Division of Allergy and Immunology, Department of Medicine
Montefiore Medical Center
Bronx, New York
Chapter 2

Deepa Rastogi, MBBS, MS
Joseph S. Blume Faculty Scholar in Pediatric Development
Albert Einstein College of Medicine
Children's Hospital at Montefiore
Bronx, New York
Chapter 6

William R. Reisacher, MD, FACS, FAAOA
Associate Professor of Otolaryngology
Department of Otolaryngology-Head and Neck Surgery
Weill Cornell Medical College/New York Presbyterian Hospital
New York, New York
Chapter 17

David L. Rosenstreich, MD
Chief, Division of Allergy and Immunology, Department of Medicine
Professor, Departments of Medicine, Microbiology and Immunology and Otolaryngology
Albert Einstein College of Medicine
Montefiore Medical Center
Bronx, New York
Chapter 2

Anna Rossovsky Smith, MD
Asthma and Allergic Disease Center
University of Virginia Health System
Charlottesville, Virginia
Chapter 18

Arye Rubinstein, MD
Chief, Division of Allergy and Immunology, Department of Pediatrics
Professor, Microbiology and Immunology Albert Einstein College of Medicine
Bronx, New York
Chapters 15 and 16

Kristin Schmidlin, MD
Allergy & Immunology Fellow
Division of Immunology, Allergy, & Rheumatology
University of Cincinnati–College of Medicine
Cincinnati, Ohio
Chapter 12

Jenny Shliozberg, MD
Associate Professor
Department of Pediatrics
Albert Einstein College of Medicine
Bronx, New York
Chapter 16

Sumita Sinha, MD
Assistant Professor, Division of Pulmonary Medicine
Montefiore Medical Center
Albert Einstein College of Medicine
Bronx, New York
Chapter 6

Jonathan M. Spergel, MD, PhD
Chief, Allergy Section
The Children's Hospital of Philadelphia
Professor of Pediatrics
Perelman School of Medicine at University of Pennsylvania
Philadelphia, Pennsylvania
Chapter 11

Ryan Steele, DO, MS
Fellow
Allergy and Immunology
Winthrop University Hospital
Mineola, New York
Chapter 10

Clement E. Tagoe, MB, ChB, PhD
Associate Professor of Clinical Medicine
Albert Einstein College of Medicine
Montefiore Medical Center
Bronx, New York
Chapter 13

Robert Tamayev, MD, PhD
Internal Medicine Resident
Montefiore Medical Center
Bronx, New York
Chapter 1

C. Doriene van Ginkel, BSc, MD/PhD Student
Department of Pediatric Pulmonology & Pediatric Allergy
Beatrix Children's Hospital, University Medical Center Groningen
Groningen Research Institute for Asthma & COPD, University of Groningen
Groningen, Netherlands
Chapter 4

Sincerest thanks to my wonderful wife Vicki; my children and their spouses, Jonathan, Peter and Molly, and Rebecca and Jed; and my precious grandchildren, Riley, Avner, Tory, Penelope, Lucien and Izidore, for their deeply appreciated love and support throughout the years.

—DLR

Thank you to my amazing wife Rita, and family Jaimie and Brian, Karen and Dan; Noah, Sam, Evie, Kaela, and Jayda for their unending love and support.

—MPF

I deeply thank my husband Kujtim Balidemaj for his invaluable support and encouragement to complete this book, and my children Nora and Ema for their patience and endurance. In addition, I thank all my mentors, colleagues, and friends for their many years of support that made this work possible.

—GSDV

Heartfelt thanks to my husband, Patrick, and my son, Mac, for their love and support, to my parents for their gift of an education, and to my patients who challenge and inspire me.

—AHJ

1

Fundamentals of Immunity

Denisa E. Ferastraoaru, Robert Tamayev, and Harris Goldstein

OVERVIEW OF IMMUNITY

The discipline of Immunology is focused on studying the function of the immune system, including the mechanisms utilized by our body to defend itself against different types of infections and malfunctions that result in immunological disorders. Since we are constantly exposed to innumerable microorganisms (normal microflora or pathogenic ones), our immune system has to identify foreign pathogens from self and prevent them from causing disease. This process is generally termed the *immune response*.

There have been numerous advances in our current understanding of how the immune system functions through its immune responses. Given the complexity of this subject, we can only provide in this chapter a basic introduction to the main components and functions of the immune system. We highlight the most common terms used in immunology and how the immune system is involved in the pathophysiology of ear, nose, and throat disorders.

One of the main functions of the immune response is to identify the microorganisms that threaten the human body, by recognizing any molecule or part of a molecule that is present in potentially harmful or foreign substances. These foreign molecules are termed *antigens* (*anti*body *gen*erators)[1] and are usually proteins or polysaccharides, and less frequently lipids, and can be endogenous or exogenous. Specific cells use a variety of mechanisms to take up or bind the antigens and to degrade them once captured.

Highly specialized structures expressed by lymphocytes recognize antigens, and these lymphocytes along with a number of other cells, effector molecule and enzymes, constitute the immune system. The immune system is considered to have 2 basic types of defense mechanisms. The adaptive immune response consists of responses that develop during the lifetime of an individual in response to exposure to new antigens. Its main function is to protect against infections by producing antibodies and forming memory cells. The innate immune response is present from birth and consists of a number of different components, including physical barriers (skin, mucous membranes, and low gastric pH), enzymes, and cells that act nonspecifically against infectious organisms.[2,3]

> There are 2 types of immune responses that work closely together: adaptive and innate.

THE INNATE IMMUNE SYSTEM

The innate immune system, the nonspecific portion of the immune response, is primed to respond immediately to and provide host defenses against microorganisms. It is capable of mounting a rapid response against any pathogenic invader that infiltrates the skin and mucous membranes, and to initiate signals that recruit and activate a subsequent adaptive immune response. The innate and adaptive immune responses work in close conjunction.

> Innate and adaptive immune responses work closely together.

The innate immune system consists of fixed barriers such as the skin, which prevents entry of a pathogen into the body, and epithelial and mucosal layers that possess different factors that prevent pathogen invasion (eg, cytocidal molecules such as defensins, or cells with beating cilia that clear exterior pathogens). In addition, environmental conditions, such as the acidity of the stomach, and resident normal flora of the gastrointestinal and urogenital tracts prevent unrestricted entrance of pathogens into the bloodstream.[4]

The innate system relies on a limited number of genetically encoded receptors (pattern recognition receptors, PRRs) that recognize structural motifs common to bacterial or viral pathogens (pathogen-associated molecular patterns, PAMPs).[2] Other distinct receptors recognize molecules expressed normally by cells of the body ("self" molecules). Identification of these self molecules delivers an inhibitory signal to immune cells that prevents activation of the immune response against host tissues. Natural killer (NK) cells are another type of protective cell that kills abnormal cells that have downregulated their molecular histocompatibility complex (MHC) class I proteins due to pathogen infection or neoplastic transformation.[5]

> Skin, mucosa, stomach acidity, NK cells, complement system, toll-like receptors (TLRs), and chemokines are all components of the innate immune system.

Components of the Innate Immune System

Cells of the Innate Immune System

Phagocytes. Phagocytic cells (neutrophils and macrophages) are 2 of the major cellular components of the innate immune system. Their main function is to identify and kill pathogens that enter the body through a process called *phagocytosis*. Through this process, bacteria and other foreign substances are ingested after PAMPs on the pathogen surface are recognized by PRRs or after pathogens have been opsonized by specific molecules (such as C3 molecules of the complement or immunoglobulin G). The foreign particle is trapped in a phagocytic vesicle (phagosome) inside the phagocytic cell. The phagosome then fuses with a lysosome forming a phagolysosome where the foreign substances are degraded by different enzymatic processes[4] (Figure 1–1).

An important mechanism by which phagocytes kill ingested bacteria is through the release of bacteriolytic enzymes that break down the pathogen. This activity is augmented by a respiratory burst, where the cells utilize different enzymes (NADPH [nicotine adenine dinucleotide phosphate] oxidase, myeloperoxidase, and nitric oxide) to produce bactericidal-free oxygen radicals. Lack of NADPH oxidase results in chronic granulomatous disease, an X-linked recessive disorder characterized by recurrent infections with catalase positive organisms such as *Staphylococcus aureus*. Although the phagocytes of these patients can ingest the pathogen, they cannot kill it, leading to chronic infection and abscess formation (reviewed in Chapter 15).

> Lack of NADPH oxidase results in chronic granulomatous disease (CGD), characterized by infections with catalase-positive organisms (eg, *S aureus*).

An alternative mechanism for attacking an endocytosed pathogen is by producing small molecules such as defensins, bacteriocidal peptides that perforate bacterial cell walls, and lactoferrin, which decreases iron stores available to pathogens thereby slowing their growth.

In addition, phagocytes send out other signals, either through immunologic proteins or peptides (cytokines and chemokines), or through cell-surface receptors that initiate activation of the adaptive immune response.

Neutrophils. Neutrophils play a crucial role in the innate inflammatory response and are the first circulating cells to migrate toward the site of infection. Neutrophils are produced and mature in the bone marrow and then are released into the bloodstream.

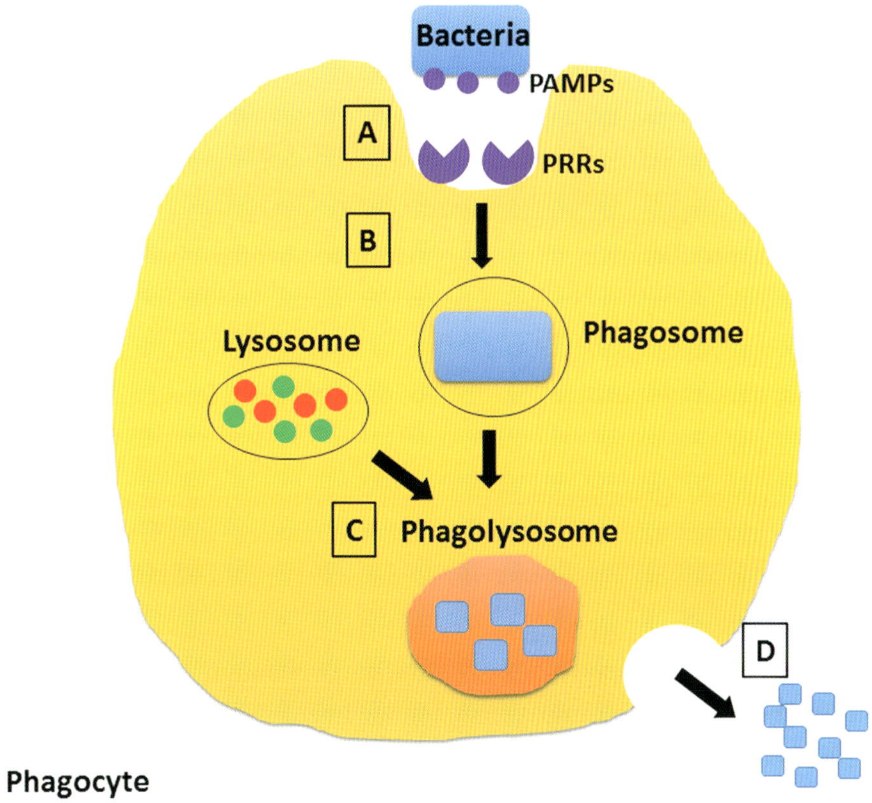

Figure 1-1. The process of phagocytosis. A. PAMPs on the surface of bacteria are recognized by PRRs on the surface of phagocytes. B. The bacteria are internalized in the phagosome. C. The phagosome fuses with a lysosome (which contains different bactericidal enzymes) forming the phagolysosome where the bacteria are lysed. D. The lysed bacterial particles are removed through the process of exocytosis.

They are the main phagocytic population in the body and are found in great numbers in the bloodstream and in infected areas.

Activation of neutrophils involves the detection of PAMPs through PRRs which stimulates activation of the nuclear factor (NF)-kB pathway. This initiates activation of different effector cell functions including degranulation, the oxidative burst, and mediators production.[6]

Neutrophils have surface receptors for immunoglobulin G (IgG) and the C3b component of the complement system, which enable them to identify their targets after they have been opsonized by these molecules. Neutrophils target binding causes internalization of the pathogen followed by the release of bactericidal enzymes and bacterial death.

The main cytocidal mediators produced by neutrophils include serine proteases, reactive oxygen species, defensins, and cytokines:

- Serine proteases (neutrophil elastase and proteinase 3) are found in neutrophil granules. Their main function is to degrade and kill phagocytosed pathogens.[7]
- Reactive oxygen species (superoxide, hydrogen peroxide, and hydroxyl radical) are generated by the actions of different enzymes such as NADPH oxidase, superoxide dismutase, and myeloperoxidase. They also kill phagocytosed pathogens.

- Defensins are small peptides that exert their antimicrobial activity through increasing microbe cell membrane permeability.[8]
- Cytokines are proinflammatory, anti-inflammatory, and/or growth inducers. Neutrophils produce a diverse repertoire of cytokines. Cytokine production is increased by inflammatory stimuli such as the Gram-negative bacterial cell wall lipopolysaccharide (LPS) and the lipoteichoic acids of the Gram-positive bacterial cell walls.[9]

After neutrophil activation, digestion and killing of the engulfed microorganisms, the neutrophils die through the process of programmed cell death (apoptosis) or via necrosis. Apoptosis is induced by cellular enzymes (caspases) which lead to nuclear collapse, cytosolic vacuolization, and cell shrinkage. Necrosis is the process where the neutrophil bursts and releases its contents. This cycle of formation and death of neutrophils is a very important homeostatic mechanism for maintaining the correct amount of neutrophils in the blood, enabling them to exert their functions but also allowing for the eventual resolution of the inflammatory process.[10]

Macrophages. Macrophages develop from the differentiation of blood-derived monocytes. This differentiation process takes place in most tissues, especially in those where pathogens are likely to enter such as the skin and gastrointestinal and respiratory tracts.

Macrophage cell surface receptors recognize danger signals (eg, bacterial LPS) that trigger activating signals resulting in a proinflammatory response that kills phagocytosed intracellular pathogens.

Macrophage activation also leads to release of cytokines such as interleukin (IL)-1, -12, and TNF (tumor necrosis factor) which stimulate the adaptive immune response. One of these cytokine functions is to induce the differentiation of T helper (T_H) 1 cells. In addition to phagocytosis and stimulation of T_H1 cell differentiation, macrophages can act as antigen-presenting cells (APCs) and present processed peptides to T cells.

Similar to neutrophils, macrophages secrete a variety of pro-inflammatory and cytocidal molecules including enzymes, growth factors, lipid mediators (leukotrienes and prostaglandins), and reactive oxygen species.[11]

Dendritic Cells. Dendritic cells (DCs) are the most important APCs in the body. Their cell surface is characterized by long membrane projections called dendrites, which give the cell its name. The DCs develop in the bone marrow, circulate in the blood, and then migrate into different peripheral tissues such as the skin (Langerhans cells) and the mucosa of the upper and lower airways and gastrointestinal tract. They remain in the tissues in an inactive state until they bind antigen. Once they encounter an antigen, they upregulate specific surface receptors and become mature DCs. They then migrate into draining lymph nodes where they activate B and T cells by presenting the bound processed antigen.

The APCs such as dendritic cells can take up antigens through different processes, including endocytosis, macropinocytosis, or phagocytosis.

Endocytosis is a receptor-mediated process in which cell membrane clathrin-coated pits bind antigens forming clathrin-coated vesicles.[12] In the process of macropinocytosis, the invagination of the membrane forms a pocket that develops into a vesicle filled with a large amount of fluid and diverse pathogens or antigens.[13] This vesicle then fuses with a lysosome resulting in antigen digestion and processing (Figure 1–2).

As described earlier in the chapter, through the process of phagocytosis the foreign substances are opsonized by C3 or IgG, ingested by the phagocytic cells, and processed with the use of different enzymes leading to their removal.

Through these 3 processes, extracellular allergens are processed and bound to MHC class II molecules for subsequent presentation to $CD4^+$ T cells. The details of antigen presentation and T-cell activation are discussed later in this chapter.

Natural Killer (NK) Cells. Natural killer (NK) cells are effector cells of the innate immune system whose role is to identify and mark for death, cells that are infected with viruses or tumor cells that attempt to evade killing by effector ($CD8^+$) T cells.

The NK cells are derived from bone marrow stem cells and circulate in the blood. They have both

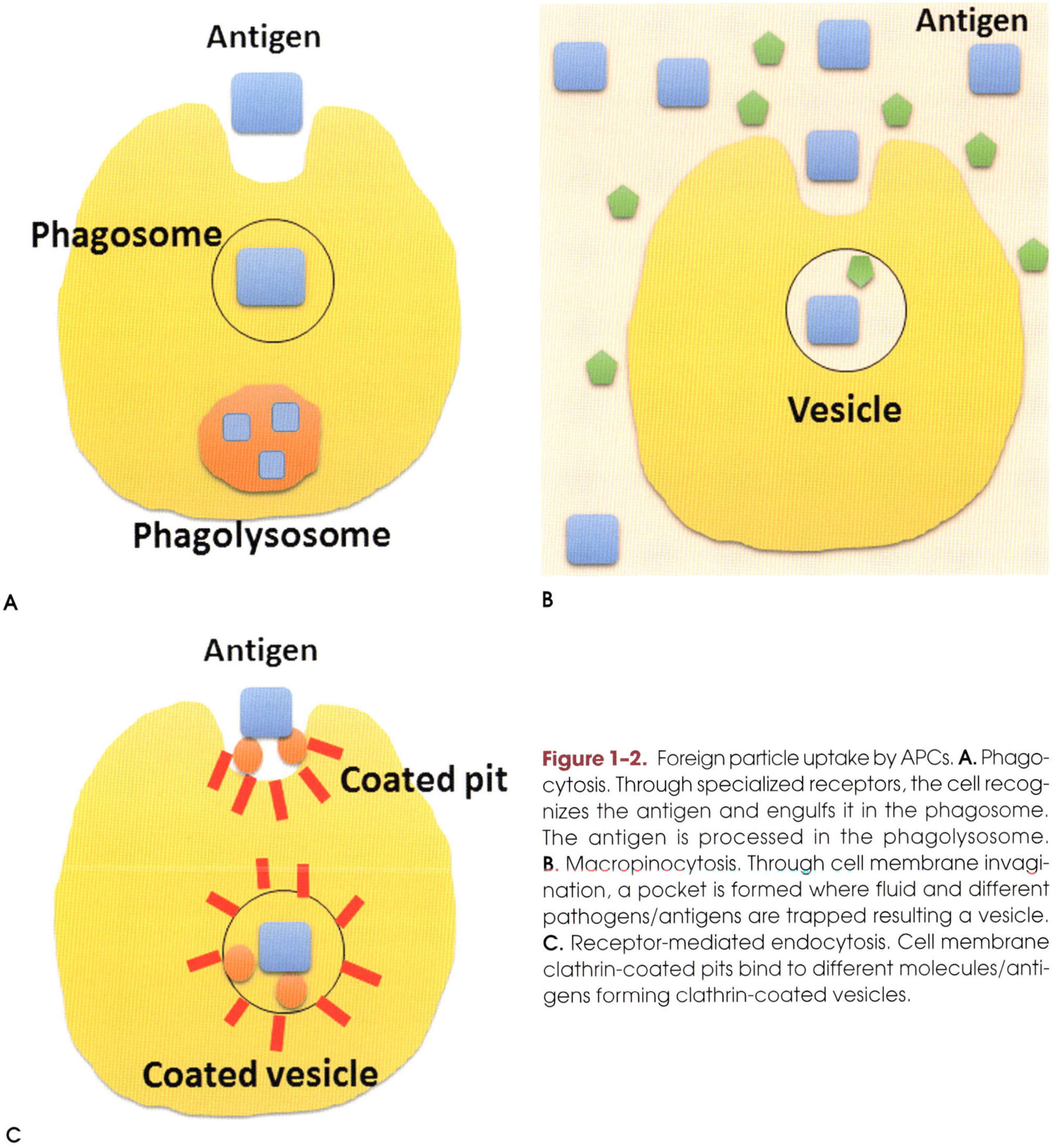

Figure 1–2. Foreign particle uptake by APCs. **A.** Phagocytosis. Through specialized receptors, the cell recognizes the antigen and engulfs it in the phagosome. The antigen is processed in the phagolysosome. **B.** Macropinocytosis. Through cell membrane invagination, a pocket is formed where fluid and different pathogens/antigens are trapped resulting a vesicle. **C.** Receptor-mediated endocytosis. Cell membrane clathrin-coated pits bind to different molecules/antigens forming clathrin-coated vesicles.

cell surface-activating receptors (that activate the NK cells when they bind to target cells) and inhibitory receptors (that transmit an inhibitory signal if the NK cells bind to a cell which has MHC class I molecules on its surface). The NK cells identify potential targets by evaluating target cell class I MHC expression using special receptors (killer immunoglobulin-like receptors, KIRs).

If the potential target cells are normal and not malignant or infected, and have normal MHC class

I molecule expression, NK cell cytotoxic activity is inhibited. If, however, the cell is infected or malignant and consequently expresses low levels of MHC class I molecules, the inhibitory signal is reduced, and the NK cell cytotoxic pathway is activated. The NK cells kill target cells by releasing small cytocidal molecules (granzymes or perforins). They also express Fas ligand, which binds to the Fas receptor on the target cell, inducing target cell apoptosis.[14,15]

The NK cells also produce the cytokine interferon gamma (IFN-γ), which is capable of killing virus-infected cells.

> The NK cells kill virus-infected cells and neoplastic cells.

Lymphocytes. Lymphocytes play a pivotal role in the normal function of the immune system. Their major function is to generate adaptive immune responses after exposure to pathogens, but they also play an important role in the innate immune response. Lymphocytes can be found in the mucosa of the airways or gastrointestinal system and produce some early cytokines that help initiate adaptive immune functions.

Lymphocyte types and their function in adaptive immunity are discussed in more detail later in this chapter.

Recognition Strategies of the Innate Immune System

Toll-Like Receptors (TLRs). For the process of phagocytosis to take place, phagocytes have to first recognize their targets. This is accomplished through toll-like receptors (TLRs), membrane proteins found on the surface of phagocytic cells, B lymphocytes, and epithelial cells. These receptors, of which 10 are currently described in humans, recognize specific pathogen antigens termed PAMPs. Different PAMPs include endotoxins and peptidoglycans on bacteria, mannans in the cell wall of yeast, and single- or double-stranded RNA of viruses. Once a TLR binds to a PAMP, downstream signals lead to activation of specific genes resulting in the release of cytokines, reactive oxygen species, chemokines, selectins, and other innate immune mediators, all of which play a role in the inflammatory response.[16]

Each TLR is a dimeric protein that recognizes a distinct microbial product. For example, TLR5 recognizes flagellin, TLR4 recognizes LPS, and TLR7 recognizes intracellular RNA (Table 1–1). Once the

Table 1–1. Toll-Like Receptors (TLRs) and Their Ligands

TLR	Ligands	Cellular Location
TLR1	Soluble bacterial factors and tri-acyl peptides	Extracellular
TLR2	Carbohydrates, zymosan, viral proteins	Extracellular and intracellular
TLR3	Viral dsRNA and ssRNA	Intracellular
TLR4	Lipopolysaccharide	Extracellular and intracellular
TLR5	Flagellae	Extracellular
TLR6	Mycoplasma lipopeptides	Extracellular and intracellular
TLR7	ssRNA (influenza, HIV)	Extracellular and intracellular
TLR8	ssRNA	Extracellular and intracellular
TLR9	DNA (unmethylated cytosine and guanine sequences CpG)	Intracellular
TLR10	Unknown	Intracellular

TLRs recognize the microbial product, an activating signal is transmitted, and nuclear factor kB is activated resulting in production of proinflammatory cytokines, maturation of dendritic cells, and activation of other immunologic responses.[17]

> Phagocytes recognize PAMPs through TLRs. This binding leads to activation of different signals and recruitment of a number of other immune cells.

Damage-Associated Molecular Patterns (DAMPs). Damage-associated molecular patterns (DAMPs) are common metabolic products resulting from the cell lysis and tissue damage that occur during the process of inflammation and infection. The most well characterized of these are uric acid, heat shock proteins, extracellular DNA or RNA, and different endogenous molecules ("alarmins").[18] Alarmins are cell-derived molecules that can activate APCs and are potent mediators of inflammation, and are an important link between innate and adaptive immune responses. Examples of alarmins are enzymes such as HMG1, S100A8, A100A9, or S100A12 and molecules such as cathelidicins.[1] The DAMPs are recognized by specialized receptors on the cells of the innate immune system, and their binding stimulates signals that initiate inflammation.

The Complement System

The complement system includes a number of immunologically active serum proteins (C1-C9, factors B, D, H, I) that become sequentially activated through enzymatic cleavage. Each cleavage product then activates the next protein in a cascading sequence, leading to the production of immunostimulatory and cytocidal molecules and a rapid response against invading pathogens. The complement proteins are synthesized in the liver and circulate in the blood in an inactive state.

There are 3 separate pathways by which the complement system can be activated: the classical pathway, the lectin pathway, and the alternative pathway. All 3 pathways converge at the step where one component, complement factor 3 (C3) is cleaved into 2 active fragments, C3a and C3b, which then leads to the formation of the membrane attack complex (MAC).

> The complement system is part of the innate immune system and consists of 3 distinct activation/effector pathways: classical, alternative, and lectin.

The Classical Pathway. In the classical pathway, an antibody, usually IgG or IgM, binds to an antigen or a pathogen forming immune complexes that activate the complement cascade.

The first molecule of the classical pathway is C1 which is composed of 3 components: C1q (which can bind IgG or IgM), C1r, and C1s. Once the immunoglobulin binds the C1q, C1r is activated, resulting in activation of C1s which becomes an enzyme that cleaves the next component, C4, into 2 active fragments, a larger fragment (C4b) that continues the complement cascade, and a smaller fragment (C4a). The next protein that binds to the generated, enzymatically active C1C4b complex is C2, which is also cleaved into a larger and a smaller fragment. The C4bC2b complex then cleaves C3 into 2 fragments, C3b and C3a. The cascade continues with the cleavage of C5 to C5a, which is capable of recruiting neutrophils, and C5b which is part of the MAC. The MAC is formed by C5b-C9 molecules and directly lyses bacteria by creating holes in the cell membranes of bacteria[19,20] (Figure 1–3). The absence of the late components of complement such as a deficiency in factor C8, leads to a lack of a MAC. Patients with these deficiencies are not able to eradicate encapsulated organisms such as *Neisseria meningitides* and are at increased risk for developing diseases such as meningococcal meningitis. Patients with deficiencies of early complement components (eg, C2 or C3 immunodeficiency) are also at risk for developing recurrent bacterial infections.

In addition to their cytocidal activities, activated complement components possess other immunological properties. C3a is an anaphylatoxin that stimulates the release of histamine from mast cells and has the capacity to recruit other cells such as phagocytes at the site of inflammation. C3b combines with IgG bound to pathogens to facilitate pathogen opsonization.

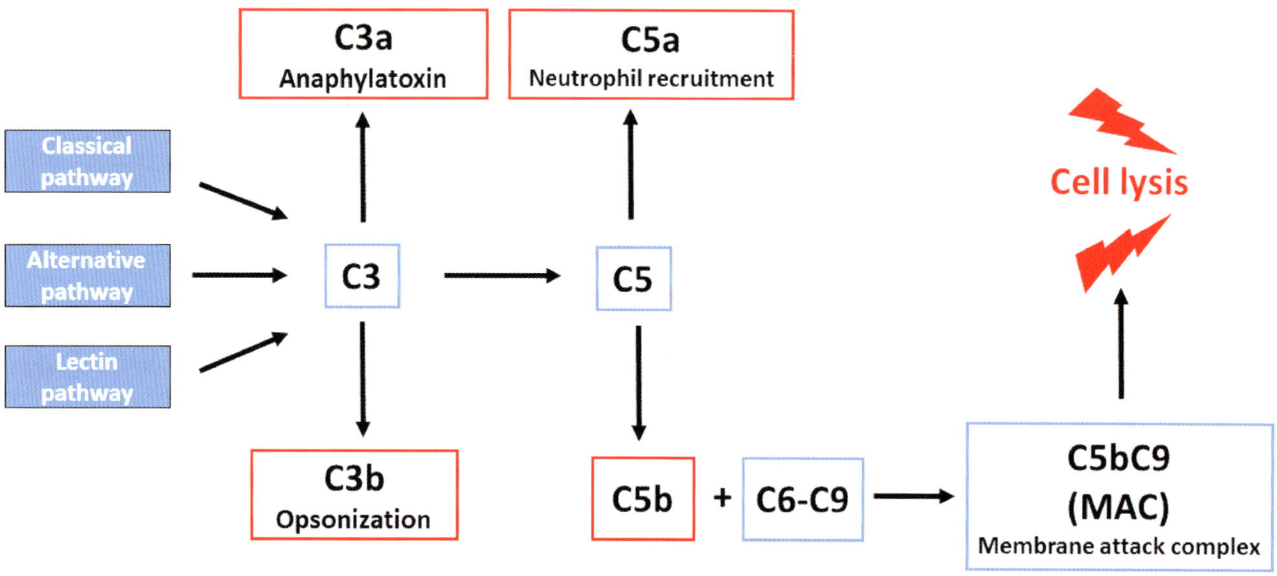

Figure 1–3. Complement cascade. The 3 complement pathways (classical, alternative, and lectin) converge on the cleavage of C3 to C3a. C3a is an anaphylatoxin that stimulates histamine release from mast cells. C3b promotes pathogen opsonization. C5a is a neutrophil chemoattractant. C5b together with C6-C9 is part of MAC. MAC forms holes in the cell membrane causing cell lysis.

> The complement components, C5b-C9, form the MAC. Deficiency in any of the MAC components causes susceptibility to meningococcal infections.

Hereditary angioedema (HAE) is due to a deficiency of a complement cascade regulatory protein, C1 esterase inhibitor. It is an autosomal dominant disorder that may lead to recurrent angioedema, which is not mediated by histamine. Diagnosis is made by low levels and/or decreased function of C1 esterase inhibitor. The role of the C1 esterase inhibitor is to inactivate the protease activity of C1 (which normally leads to further complement cascade activation) and to regulate the kinin system. If C1 inhibitor is deficient, increased amounts of active components of complement and bradykinin are produced. Bradykinin produces vasodilation with increased permeability resulting in quick and sudden swelling of the face, tongue, and airways, which can result in death from severe edema of the airways preventing proper airflow to the lungs. Because of the uncontrolled activation of the complement cascade and consumption of early complement components, patients with C1 esterase inhibitor deficiency usually have low serum levels of C4 and sometimes C1 (reviewed in Chapter 7).[21,22]

The Lectin Pathway. In the lectin pathway, the complement cascade can be activated by binding of a serum mannose-binding lectin (MBL) to pathogen-specific molecules such as mannose or other bacteria-specific carbohydrate residues. This pathway does not require immunoglobulin to be activated. The MBL binds to residues on the bacterial surface and induces cleavage of C4 and C2, which then together cleave and activate C3 (see Figure 1–3). The activated C3 then initiates the rest of the cascade which continues through the activation of C9. Both low and elevated levels of mannose-binding lectin are associated with different infectious and autoimmune processes.[23,24]

The Alternative Pathway. The alternative pathway consists of a number of proteins distinct from the classical complement components that can also initiate activation of C3 (see Figure 1–3). These proteins include factors B, D, I, and properdin. In the alternative pathway, C3 is first activated by binding to the surface of pathogens (C3 activation is normally inhibited on the cell surface of humans). C3 then binds factor B which is a protein similar to C2 of the classical pathway. Factor B is cleaved by factor D into the fragments, Bb and Ba. The C3bBb is the C3 convertase of the alternative pathway, and this complex can bind and cleave another C3 molecule. The activated C3 then initiates the rest of the cascade, which continues through the activation of C9. The C3bBb complex is unstable and requires another factor, properdin, for stabilization.

Factor I inactivates C3b and C4b. Its deficiency leads to low C3 levels and has been associated with recurrent bacterial infections.[25]

THE INFLAMMATORY RESPONSE

The inflammatory response plays a crucial role in eliminating pathogens. It is readily recognized clinically by the appearance of redness, swelling, heat, and pain which are the result of vasodilation and the action of many mediators and cells (prostaglandins, leukotrienes, and the complement system). Sinusitis is a good example of an inflammatory reaction.

If a pathogen invades the host through the nostrils, the immune system responds by producing cytokines, including interleukin (IL)-1 and tumor necrosis factor (TNF)-α that recruit neutrophils and macrophages. Increased levels of kinin, IL-1, IL-6, and IL-8 have been detected in the nasal secretions of patients with acute viral rhinosinusitis.[26]

Neutrophils initially migrate out of the blood vessels and enter the nasal mucosa through a series of distinct steps. The process begins with "rolling," where the neutrophil adheres to the vessel wall with the help of endothelial cell surface molecules (selectins). The next step is neutrophil adhesion to the blood vessel through the interaction between neutrophil cell surface proteins (intercellular adhesion molecules, ICAMs) and endothelial cell surface proteins (integrins). The adherent neutrophils then transmigrate through the vessel into the interstitial space and begin phagocytosing the pathogens and releasing different mediators at the site of the injury. If the neutrophils cannot completely eliminate the pathogen, local APCs bind and internalize the pathogen antigens and present them to T cells. The T cells can mount a strong response and eliminate the pathogen (Figure 1–4).

However, if the pathogen is resistant to immune elimination, it will lead to chronic sinusitis characterized by chronic inflammation. Nasal tissue samples taken from patients with chronic rhinosinusitis have increased levels of leukotrienes C_4, D_4, and E_4 and increased levels of eosinophilic inflammatory products.[27]

Cytokines

The process of identifying and clearing an invading pathogen requires the production of cytokines, small soluble molecules with multiple immunological activities, including initiating and maintaining an inflammatory reaction or acting as mediators between cells.

The term *cytokine* is a general name used to describe this large group of molecules, but there are different commonly used terms to describe specific cytokines: interleukins are cytokines that act as mediators between different type of leukocytes; lymphokines are cytokines produced by lymphocytes once they are activated; and monokines are cytokines produced by phagocytic cells.

Specific cytokines are used clinically as biological response modifiers for the treatment of different disorders including asthma, rheumatoid arthritis, and malignancy.

During the process of infection/inflammation, monokines are released after phagocytic cells recognize the pathogen by its binding to TLRs. The cytokines IL-1, TNF-α, and IL-6 are secreted by macrophages after exposure to a TLR-binding pathogen. These cytokines trigger an inflammatory response by recruiting other inflammatory components such as neutrophils and NK cells and also initiate activation of the adaptive immune response.[28]

Cytokines can also enter the circulation and produce effector functions at sites distal from the site of inflammation. They can stimulate the hypothalamus to induce fever. Fever increases the metabolic rate, which promotes immune reactivity and simultaneously decreases the replicative capacity of pathogens. Once an infection is cleared, inhibitory cytokines such as IL-10 are secreted, which help deactivate macrophages.

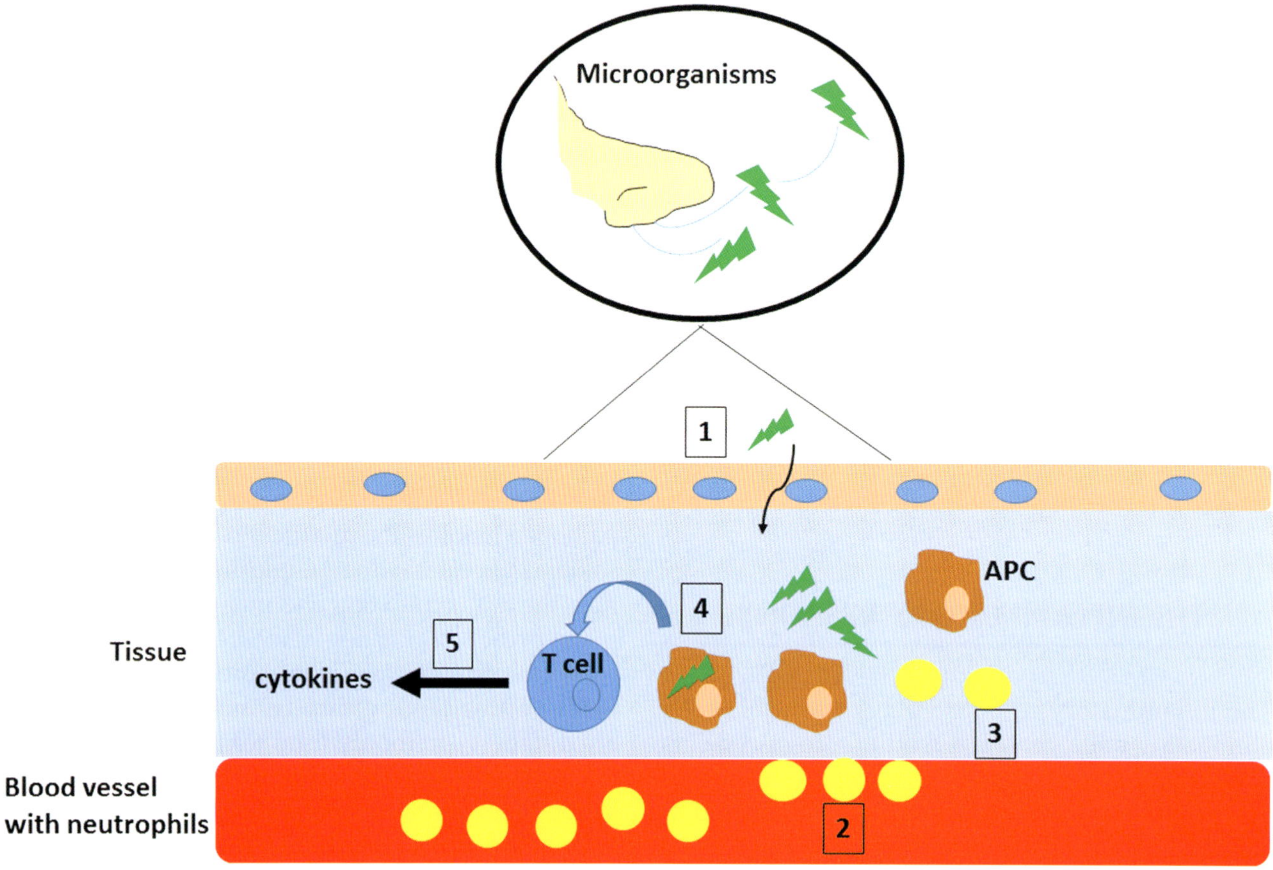

Figure 1–4. The inflammatory process in sinusitis. 1. Microorganisms enter the nasal/sinus mucosa. 2. Neutrophils are recruited to the site of inflammation from the bloodstream. The neutrophils roll and then adhere to the blood vessel to enter the mucosa. This process is mediated by the interactions of integrins, selectins, and other adhesion molecules. 3. Through diapedesis, the neutrophils enter the tissue and phagocytize the microorganisms. 4. If neutrophils cannot kill the pathogens, the local APCs ingest the microorganisms, process their proteins into peptides, and present them to T cells. 5. T cells become activated and release different cytokines that drive an infection-clearing immune response. If the pathogens are not killed, this will lead to chronic inflammation and persistent chronic symptoms.

Interferons are another class of cytokines produced by the innate immune system; they have antiviral and immunostimulatory activities. Interferons are secreted by injured and virally infected cells and may be triggered by activation of TLRs that recognize viral motifs such as double-stranded RNA. Their role is to protect the infected cells, to inhibit virus replication, and to activate both NK cells and cytotoxic T cells which are virucidal.[4] Table 1–2 lists the most important cytokines, their biological effects, and how different diseases are treated by using or blocking these molecules.

THE ADAPTIVE IMMUNE SYSTEM

Unlike the innate immune system, humans are not born with a "ready to act" adaptive immune system. The adaptive immune response is highly specific and is the result of exposure to specific activating pathogens.

Adaptive immune responses can be both antibody and cell mediated, which are mediated by B and T cells, respectively. The fundamental process underlying the development of an effective adaptive

Table 1-2. The Most Common Cytokines and Their Main Functions

Type of Cytokine	Produced by	Effect	Comments
IL-1	Macrophages, monocytes, dendritic cells, endothelial cells	Stimulates proliferation of B and T cells; increases synthesis of prostaglandins; increases production of acute phase reactants in liver; produces fever	Anti-IL-1 medications (eg, anakinra) are used in inflammatory conditions, ranging from rheumatoid arthritis to autoinflammatory syndromes.
IL-2	T cells	Activates T cells	Two anti-IL-2 receptor monoclonal antibodies (daclizumab and basiliximab) are used for prevention of rejection in renal transplant.
IL-3	T cells	Stimulates proliferation of hematopoietic stem cells	
IL-4	T_H2 cells and mast cells	Stimulates activation and proliferation of macrophages, B cells, T cells, and plasma cells, and promotes IgE production	Anti-IL-4 therapy (dupilumab) is studied as an asthma treatment.
IL-5	T_H2 cells	Activates eosinophils	Anti-IL-5 (mepolizumab) therapy was used in trials for asthma treatment and eosinophilic esophagitis.
IL-6	Macrophages and T cells	Increases production of acute phase reactants in liver	Anti-IL-6 drugs (sirukumab) can be utilized in rheumatoid arthritis.
IL-7	Stromal cells in bone marrow	Stimulates proliferation of hematopoietic stem cells into lymphoid progenitors	
IL-8	Macrophages, endothelial cell, and T cells	Involved in chemotaxis of leukocytes	
IL-10	Macrophages and T_{reg} cells	Activates B cells; inhibits T_H1 responses and macrophages	Recombinant IL-10 can be tried in patients with inflammatory bowel syndrome.
IL-12	Macrophages	Activates T cells and NK cells	IL-12 use may have future therapeutic roles against melanoma.
TNF-α (tumor necrosis factor)	Macrophages, monocytes, dendritic cells, endothelial cells, and T cells	Induces expression of cellular adhesion molecules and activates T cells; increases production of acute phase reactants in liver; plays a role in granuloma formation	Anti-TNF medications (eg, infliximab) are used in rheumatoid arthritis, ankylosing spondylitis, psoriatic arthritis, inflammatory bowel syndrome
TGF-β (transforming growth factor)	Macrophages and T cells	Stimulates proliferation of T cells and macrophages; induces apoptosis; stimulates T_{reg} differentiation; together with IL-6 stimulates T_H17 differentiation	

continues

Table 1–2. *continued*

Type of Cytokine	Produced by	Effect	Comments
INF-γ (interferon gamma)	T_H1 cells	Activates macrophages, T cells, B cells, and NK cells	Peg-interferon is used against Hepatitis B and C.
IL-13	T_H2 cells	Activates B cells; inhibits macrophages and the inflammatory response	Anti-IL-13 (lebrikizumab) therapy may be a possible therapy in asthma patients.
IL-15	Macrophages	Activates T cells and NK cells	Current trials are attempting to use IL-15 in renal cell carcinoma and melanoma to stimulate cytotoxic T cells.

immune response involves the clonal expansion of antigen-specific T or B lymphocytes.

When these responses are induced by an infection, immunity develops naturally; when the immune responses are induced through vaccination, immunity is artificially acquired. In most cases, the adaptive immune response results in immunological memory, which confers lifelong protective immunity, preventing reinfection by the same pathogen.

Cells of the immune system are located in both primary and secondary lymphoid organs.

> Primary lymphoid organs: bone marrow and thymus. Secondary lymphoid organs: lymph nodes, tonsils, adenoids, and spleen.

Primary Lymphoid Organs

The primary lymphoid organs include the bone marrow and thymus, which are the respective sites of B and T cell maturation.

The bone marrow is the major hematopoietic organ and is the place where all blood cell types except mature T cells are formed (red blood cells, platelets, B cells, NK cells, granulocytes, and immature lymphocytes). Maturation of T cells takes place in the thymus, but the initial production of T cells comes from bone marrow-derived stem cells.

The proliferation and maturation of precursor cells in the bone marrow are stimulated by specific cytokines (colony stimulating factors, CSFs). The thymus is the site of maturation of T cells. It consists of 2 lobes and is situated partly in the thorax and partly in the neck. Each lobe has numerous lobules formed by small follicles. Each follicle is divided into a cortical and medullar area with different functions in T cell development.

The thymic cortex is the site where T-cell receptor gene rearrangement takes place. After being processed in the thymic cortex, T-cells that already have a T-cell receptor and have undergone positive selection migrate to the thymic medulla. In the thymic medulla, T cells are exposed to the products of the *AIRE* (autoimmune regulator) gene expressed on the thymic medullary epithelium. Autoreactive T cells are removed in the thymic medulla.[29] These processes are described in more detail later in the chapter.

Genetic mutations resulting in the loss of thymic function are responsible for the DiGeorge syndrome, characterized by immunodeficiency and increased susceptibility to infection.

Secondary Lymphoid Organs

The secondary lymphoid organs, such as the lymph nodes, spleen, tonsils, adenoids, and Peyer patches are the tissues where the naïve B cells and T cells recognize antigens, become activated, proliferate, and mature into effector cells. The secondary lymphoid organs are also the main locations where the innate and adaptive immune systems interact.

The APCs (macrophages, monocytes, dendritic cells), which are cellular components of the innate immune system, ingest pathogens, process the fragments into antigenic peptides, and present them to the T cells in the secondary lymphoid organs, initiating the adaptive immune response.

> Secondary lymphoid organs include lymph nodes, spleen, and mucosa-associated lymphoid tissue (MALT).

Lymph nodes are located at vascular junctions where the afferent lymphatic vessels bring antigens, naïve lymphocytes (that have not yet encountered antigen) and antigen-presenting cells. The site where the cells and antigens enter the lymph node is called high endothelial venule (HEV) which consists of a specialized endothelium that contains different adhesion molecules and produces chemokines (eg, CCL19 and CCL21 that allow the interaction between lymphocytes and the HEV, resulting in transmigration of T cells into the lymph node paracortical regions).[30]

Each lymph node is covered by a capsule and is divided into a cortical region and medulla. The medulla contains plasma cells, B and T cells, and macrophages. The cortex consists mainly of B cells that reside in primary follicles. Once the B cells are activated, they form germinal centers and the primary follicle then becomes a secondary follicle. There is also a paracortical area that contains mostly T cells that lies between the cortical region and medulla. The lymphocytes leave the lymph nodes via efferent lymphatic vessels and return to the bloodstream.[31]

A large secondary lymphoid organ, MALT, is found throughout the respiratory, gastrointestinal, and reproductive organ linings. Lymphocytes reside in these tissues and circulate between the lymphatic system and the bloodstream. When they encounter a pathogen, they clonally expand and mediate mucosal immunity. Part of the MALT are the adenoids, lingual tonsils, and palatine tonsils, which together make up Waldeyer ring.

The tonsils and adenoids are composed of the crypt epithelium, the extrafollicular area, the mantle zone of the lymphoid follicles, and the follicular germinal centers. The resting B cells reside in primary follicles, and once they become activated after encountering antigen, they form collections of activated B lymphocytes (germinal centers). Maturation of B cells leads to generation of immunoglobulins that play a crucial role in the defense against pathogens in the upper airways.[32]

In contrast to lymph nodes, tonsils and adenoids do not have afferent lymphatics, which can bring in APCs; instead APCs are contained in the crypt epithelium.

Cells of the Adaptive Immune Response

B Lymphocytes

The B lymphocytes (B cells) are a subpopulation of lymphocytes that mature in the bone marrow. These cells were termed B cells because they were initially identified in the Bursa of Fabricius in chicks. In the bone marrow, B cells precursors undergo a process of antigen-independent development and immunoglobulin gene rearrangement. During this process, B cells express B-cell receptors (BCRs) on their surface which is essential for their further maturation.

The main function of B cells is to synthesize antibodies, but they also have the ability to take up protein antigens, process them, and present constituent peptides to T cells in order to recruit their help to facilitate antibody production. The B cells can therefore function as APCs and share this capacity with other immune cells such as dendritic cells.

> B cells produce antibodies and present antigens to T cells.

Immunoglobulins. There are 5 different classes of immunoglobulins (isotypes): IgG, IgM, IgA, IgE, and IgD. The general structure of immunoglobulins is illustrated using the IgG antibody molecule.

The immunoglobulin molecule is a Y-shaped glycoprotein composed of 2 identical light chains (L) (either kappa or lambda variants), and 2 identical heavy chains (H) linked together by disulfide bonds. Each chain contains a variable region (V_L or V_H) that forms 2 antigen-binding sites (paratopes). They also contain one or more constant region domains (C_L,

C_H). The heavy chain type determines the antibody isotype and contains isotype-specific Fc regions that contribute to the functional activity of the isotype.

The Fc portion of the C_H confers different isotype-specific effector functions to the Ig molecule: (1) enabling IgG to bind to IgG-specific FcRγ receptors expressed on the surface of phagocytic cells and facilitate their capacity to ingest pathogens coated with IgG; (2) enabling IgE to bind to IgE-specific FcRε receptors expressed on the surface of eosinophils, mast cells; and (3) enabling immunoglobulins to bind to different cells and complement components.

Some isotypes such as IgG and IgA have a flexible domain where the arms of the antibody molecule form a Y (the hinge region) (Figure 1–5).

> There are 5 classes of immunoglobulins: IgG, IgA, IgM, IgE, and IgD.

Formation of both heavy and light chains is directed by gene rearrangement, a process in which the segments of genomic DNA are rearranged and joined together in a special fashion (Figure 1–6).

The V domain of the light chain is encoded by 2 segments: the V (variable) gene segment and the J (joining) gene segment. The C domain of the light chain is encoded at a considerable distance away from the sequence encoding the V region. Through splicing of the RNA, the C gene encoding the C region of the light chain comes close to the VJ segment.

The formation of the heavy chain is similar to the light chain. The V region of the heavy chain is encoded by 3 segments: the D (diversity) gene segment, the V (variable) gene segment, and the J (joining) gene segment. The first step is joining of the D and J gene segments and then addition of the V gene segment. The C region of the heavy chain is brought closer to the VDJ segment through splicing of the RNA.

The heavy chain is the first chain that is formed through the process of immunoglobulin gene rearrangement. This process is directed by a complex of enzymes (V [D] J recombinase). The most impor-

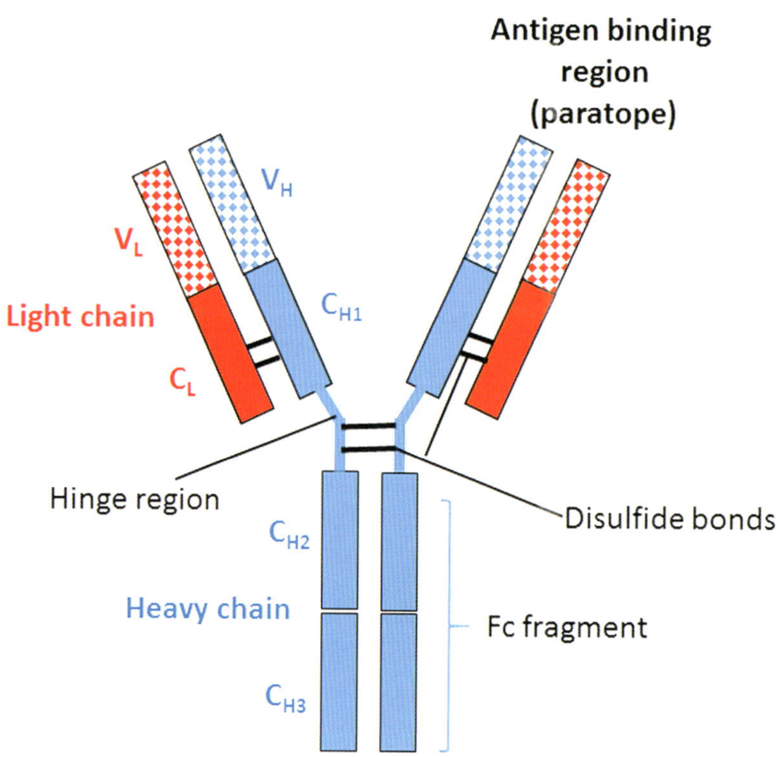

Figure 1–5. The immunoglobulin molecule.

tant enzymes involved are the products of recombination-activating genes (RAGs) named RAG-1 and RAG-2 which are expressed only in developing lymphocytes.[33] Other enzymes involved are found in many other cells and are mainly involved in the process of DNA repair.

Lack of enzymes involved in the process of V(D)J recombination results in severe combined immunodeficiency (SCID) characterized by low number and function of B and T cells due to a block of lymphocyte development at the gene-rearrangement stage.

The process of producing different isotypes is termed *immunoglobulin class switching* or *isotype switching*. During this process, the variable region of the antibody heavy chain and the entire light chain remains the same, but the constant region of the heavy chain is changed. There are 9 constant region genes in the immunoglobulin loci which encode different heavy chains sequences providing the functional characteristics for each antibody isotype and subclass: μ (IgM); δ (IgD); γ_1, γ_2, γ_3, and γ_4 (IgG1, IgG2, IgG3, and IgG4); α_1 and α_2 (IgA1 and IgA2); and ε (IgE).

Class switching is a biological mechanism that involves genetic recombination mediated by different enzymes. Naïve B cells (which did not encounter their specific antigen) produce both IgM and IgD through alternate splicing of mRNA transcripts encoding both constant regions. In order to produce other isotypes following activation of the naïve B cells, the class switch recombination has to take place. The activity of a series of enzymes such as activation-induced cytidine deaminase (AID), uracil DNA glycosylase, and apyrimidic/apurinic

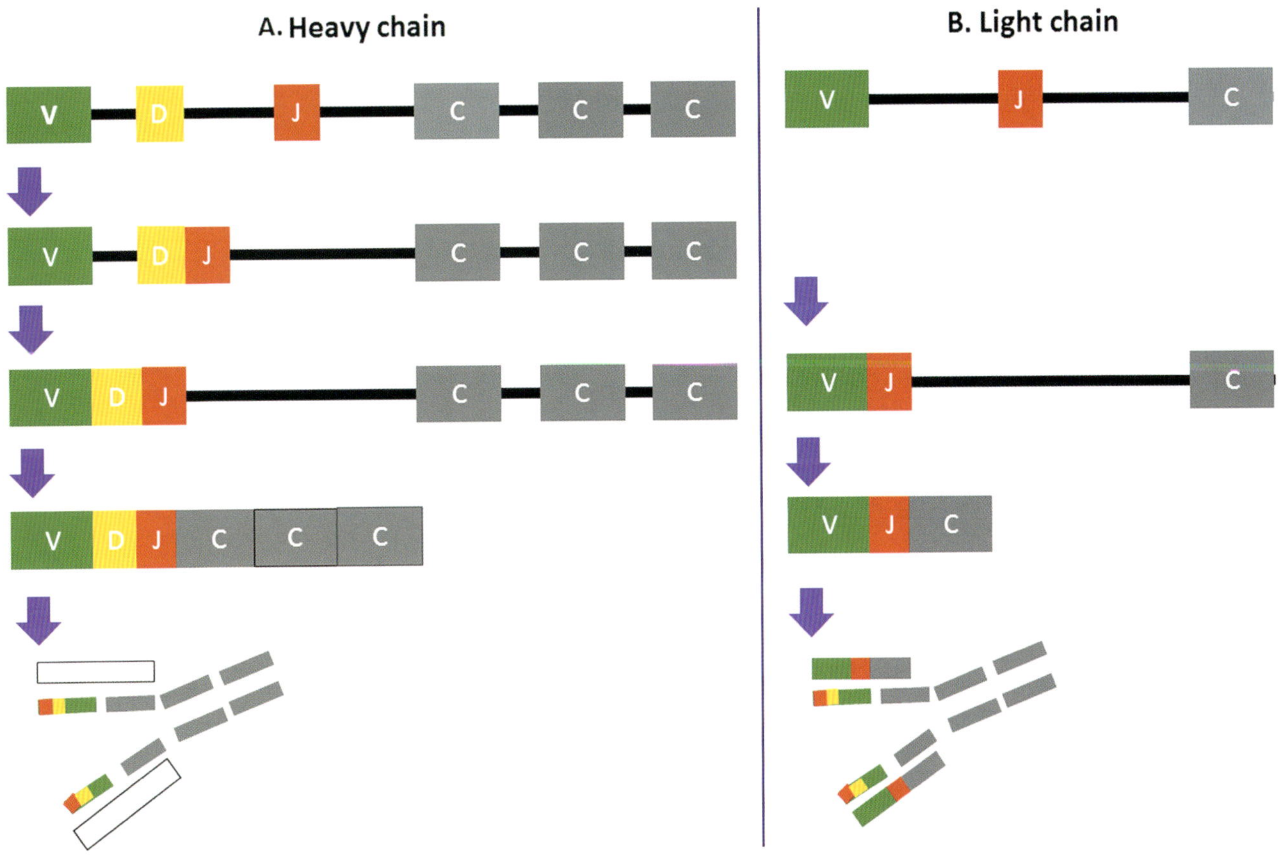

Figure 1-6. Immunoglobulin gene rearrangement. **A.** Heavy chain gene rearrangement: the D and J gene segments join, then the V gene segment joints the DJ sequence. The C region exons come together and join the VDJ sequence. **B.** Light chain rearrangement: the V and J gene segments join together. The C gene segment joins the VJ sequence.

(AP)-endonucleases is required.[34] Deficiencies of these enzymes lead to deficient production of IgG and IgA with normal production of IgM, resulting in recurrent infections.

> Deficiency of enzymes involved in antibody class switching leads to deficient IgG and IgA levels resulting in recurrent infections. IgM levels remain normal.

Immunoglobulins have 3 main functions. Besides binding to and neutralizing antigens (eg, antitoxins), immunoglobulins facilitate the removal of microorganisms by macrophages. This process is termed *opsonization* and involves coating of the pathogen by immunoglobulins which then bind to Fc receptors on the phagocyte surface, followed by ingestion and destruction by the phagocytes. Another important function of antibodies is to activate the complement system, a component of the innate immune response that helps eliminate pathogens by various mechanisms (Table 1–3).

> Immunoglobulin functions include antigen neutralization, pathogen opsonization, and complement activation.

Specific Functions of Immunoglobulins Depend on the Isotype. For example, IgA plays a critical role in mucosal immunity.[35] IgA has 2 subclasses (IgA1 and IgA2) and exists in a dimeric form that is called secretory IgA (sIgA). The dimeric form is composed of 2 molecules of IgA joined by J chain (Figure 1–7). Secretory IgA plays an important role in defending the mucous membranes of the upper respiratory airways from common infections. sIgA neutralizes viruses and bacterial surface antigens, favoring their uptake and destruction by macrophages.[36] Moreover, sIgA blocks the adhesion of bacteria by acting on bacterial M proteins,[37] but once the infection is established, a bacterial IgA1 protease can degrade the sIgA, compromising the nasal mucosal immune barrier, which might represent the first event in the pathogenesis of inflammatory respiratory disease.[38]

Table 1–3. Antibody Isotypes and Their Main Characteristics

Isotype	Characteristics	Major Functions	Additional Features
IgM	First antibody produced in an immune response	The best activator of the complement cascade	J chain binds 5 molecules of IgM, forming a pentamer with 10 binding sites, greatly increasing its avidity for antigen (Figure 1–7)
IgG	Second type of antibody produced in an immune response 4 subclasses: IgG1, IgG2, IgG3, IgG4	Neutralizes antigens, opsonization, activates complement	Always monomeric; it is the only class of Ig transferred through placenta; maternal IgG protects the newborn up to 6 months of age
IgA	Found in mucosal tissues, including the respiratory and gastrointestinal tract; 2 subclasses: IgA1, IgA2	Protects epithelial surfaces from infectious agents and enteric toxins; binds antigen, preventing allergic reactions	J chain binds 2 molecules of IgA together forming a dimer (see Figure 1–7); transferred through breast milk
IgE	Present in low levels in the blood; mainly bound to mast cells and basophils	Involved in allergic responses (triggers mast cell activation) and defense against parasites	IgE is the major antibody effector of allergies and can be elevated in the blood of these patients
IgD	Functions as an antigen receptor on mature B cells	Can activate basophils and mast cells	Coexpressed with IgM by alternate splicing of the mRNA transcript

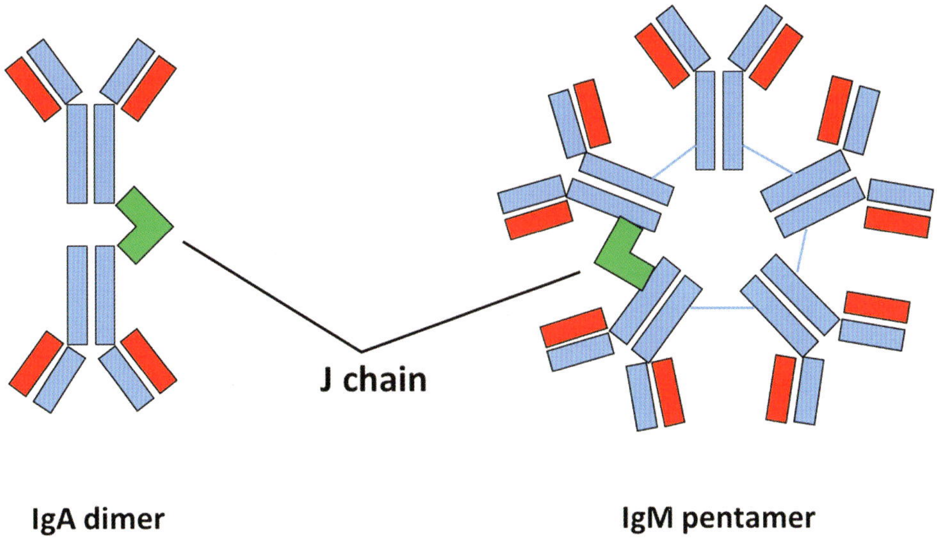

Figure 1-7. IgA immunoglobulins can form dimers, and IgM immunoglobulins can form pentamers. The molecules are joined by the J chain.

Individuals with decreased or absent IgA levels but normal levels of other immunoglobulins, (selective IgA deficiency), can present with frequent infections, particularly in the respiratory, gastrointestinal, and genitourinary tracts. When suspected, the diagnosis can be confirmed by laboratory measurement of the IgA level in the blood.

> IgA defends the mucosa of the respiratory, gastrointestinal, and urogenital tracts, and selective IgA deficiency can result in recurrent respiratory or gastrointestinal infections.

IgM is a strong complement activator due to its pentameric structure (see Figure 1–7). This structure is composed of 5 molecules of IgM joined together by J chain via disulfide bonds. IgM is not an effective opsonin, but by activating the complement and releasing its C3b component, it contributes greatly to opsonization. Each molecule of immunoglobulin has 2 antigen-binding sites; therefore, the pentameric structure has a much higher avidity for antigen through its 10 antigen-binding sites.

In some cases, patients have decreased levels of immunoglobulins along with poor antibody responses to vaccination. This fails to protect them against common microorganisms leading to increased susceptibility to infections in the lung, sinuses, and ears. These patients often have an immunodeficiency termed *common variable immunodeficiency* (CVID) that is due to malfunction of genes associated with B-cell development and function. CVID is characterized by recurrent infections involving the upper and lower respiratory systems, gastrointestinal tract, skin, and ear. Infections respond to antibiotics but recur upon their discontinuation. The treatment is to replenish the immunoglobulins intravenously (every 3–4 weeks) or subcutaneously (weekly). (See Chapter 15.)

> Low IgG levels are present in CVID and result in recurrent respiratory infections.

T Lymphocytes

T lymphocytes (T cells) are the most abundant white blood cells produced in the bone marrow, but their final stage of development is in the thymus, which is why they are termed *T cells*.[39] An effective immune system requires T-cell activation.

Unlike B cells, T cells do not produce antibodies, but they play a major role in activating B cells to produce immunoglobulins. T cells contain specialized cell surface receptors (T-cell receptors, TCRs) that recognize fragments of antigens on the surfaces of infected or neoplastic cells, or on APCs. Following activation by antigen, T cells produce different molecules (interleukins or cytokines) that have role in activating and/or killing specific cells. This effector limb of the immune system is called *cell-mediated immunity*.

> T cells activate B cells and produce chemokines that attract and/or activate other cells.

Once T cells have completed their development in the thymus, they recirculate as naïve T cells between the bloodstream and peripheral lymphoid organs until they encounter the antigen specific for their TCR. Naïve T cells differentiate into effector T cells once they bind to their specific antigen and become mature T cells with new functions capable of more effective antigen recognition and removal.

> T cells encounter antigens and become activated in lymph nodes, adenoids, and tonsils.

Naïve T cells interact with specific antigens in the peripheral lymphoid organs. To enter these lymphatic organs, T lymphocytes cross the endothelial cells of the high endothelial venules (HEVs) through the processes of rolling, activation, adhesion, and diapedesis. Different integrins (eg, LFA-1; leukocyte functional antigen-1), selectins (eg, L selectin), adhesion molecules (eg, ICAMs, intercellular adhesion molecules), and chemokines are involved in recruiting lymphocytes into the lymph nodes. The process of migration of T cells into lymphatic tissue is necessary because naive T cells do not efficiently recognize antigens at sites of infection. Instead, pathogens are taken up by APCs and transported to the lymphoid tissues for presentation to T cells. In the lymphoid organs, mature APCs such as dendritic cells, present the antigen to the T lymphocytes, resulting in T-cell activation.[40,41]

Interaction Between T Cells and Antigen-Presenting Cells. T cells cannot recognize a soluble antigen. The antigen has to be first broken down into smaller peptide fragments and then bound to carrier self-molecules such as MHC molecules on the surface of APCs. Functionally different T cells are distinguished by their cluster of differentiation (CD) cell surface markers. The 2 major types of T cells are $CD4^+$ or $CD8^+$. Peripheral T cells do not express both CD4 and CD8 simultaneously.

$CD8^+$ T cells recognize peptides presented by MHC class I molecules, while CD4 T cells recognize peptides presented by MHC class II molecules.[42]

> $CD8^+$ T cells recognize pathogens presented by MHC I. $CD4^+$ T cells recognize pathogens presented by MHC II.

The major histocompatibility complex encodes a set of cell surface molecules that primarily mediate interactions between T cells and APCs but also determines the compatibility between a donor and the recipient of organ transplants.

In order for a T cell to become activated, the MHC on the APC has to present the antigenic peptide as a MHC:peptide complex, which then binds to the T cell surface receptor (TCR).

> TCR on T cells recognizes the MHC:peptide complex which along with other costimulatory molecules, activates the T cells.

Similarly to immunoglobulins, most TCRs are composed of an α and a β chain, and each chain has an antigen-recognizing variable (V) and a constant (C) region. The TCR is associated on the membrane with other surface markers such as CD4 or CD8 and CD3, and other costimulatory molecules (CD28). After antigen binding, the TCR transmits an activation signal into the T lymphocyte[43] (Figure 1–8).

The molecular process of TCR formation is similar to that which occurs for immunoglobulins and requires gene rearrangements in which the same enzymes (RAG-1, RAG-2) are involved. Since TCRs are critical for T-cell activation and antigen removal, deficiencies of enzymes involved in production of TCRs will result in SCID in which T and B cell

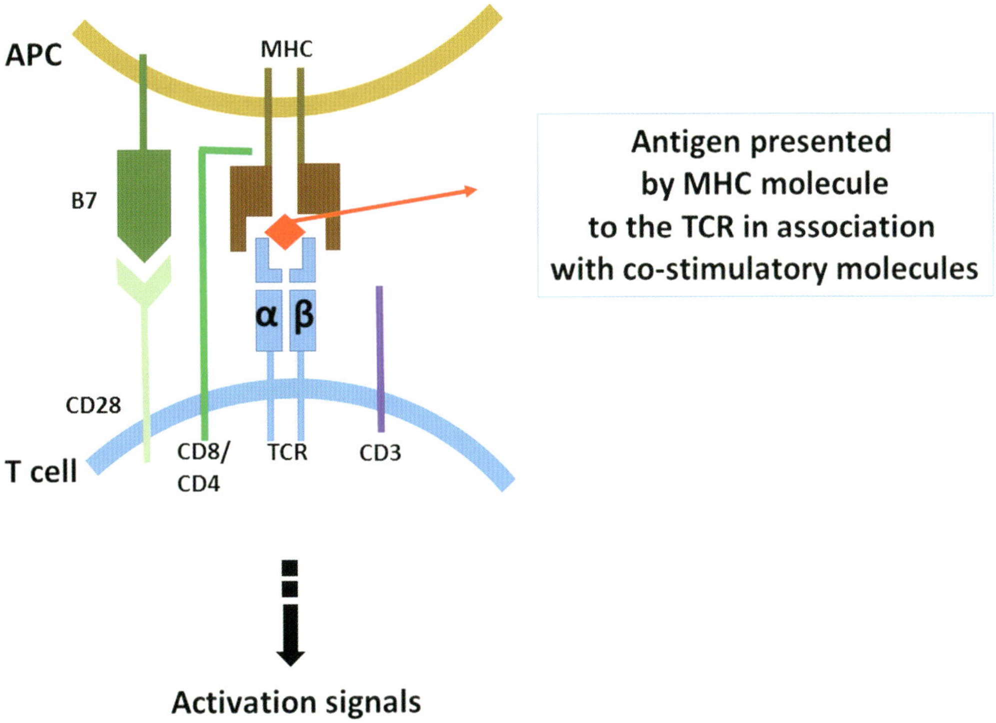

Figure 1–8. Interaction between T cells and APCs. The APC presents the antigen to the T lymphocyte using the MHC molecule. The TCR recognizes the antigen and in conjunction with CD8 (if the T cell is a CD8+ T cell) or CD4 (if the T cell is a CD4+ T cell), CD3 and costimulatory molecules (CD28; B7) transmit activation signals into the T cell.

functions are severely compromised. SCID patients develop severe infections leading to death in early infancy.

> Deficiency of enzymes involved in TCR formation results in SCID, leading to severe infections and death in early infancy.

Types of T Cells and Their Main Functions: T Helper Cells and Cytotoxic T Cells. $CD4^+$ T cells are known as helper T cells (T_H) because their main function is to help the activation of other immune cells. They are essential in B-cell activation and isotype switching. The main types of $CD4^+$ effector subsets are T_H1, T_H2, T_H17, regulatory T cells (T_{Reg}), and T follicular helper cells (T_{FH}) (Table 1–4).

T_H1 cells activate macrophages to kill intracellular bacteria (eg, mycobacteria) by producing different cytokines such as interferon γ (IFN- γ). They are also essential for B cell antibody (IgG) production.

T_H2 cells help to control parasitic infections by producing cytokines that recruit and activate eosinophils, such as interleukin 4 (IL-4), IL-5, and IL-13. Cytokines produced by T_H2 cells are involved in IgE class switching which is also important for defense against parasitic infections, but is also the main class of antibody involved in the allergic response.

T_H17 cells secrete IL-17 which stimulates recruitment of neutrophils to sites of infection protecting against extracellular bacterial and fungal infections. T_{FH} have important role in stimulating B cells and class switching. T_{Reg} cells suppress T-cell activity and help prevent the development of autoimmune disorders.

$CD8^+$ T cells differentiate into cytotoxic T cells which are specialized to kill cells infected with intracellular pathogens, such as viruses. Upon recognition

Table 1–4. Main Types of T Helper Cells and Their Functions

T Helper Cell Type	Cytokines Produced	Function
T_H1	IFN-γ, IL-2	Activates macrophages enabling them to destroy intracellular bacteria; has anti-inflammatory role; induces production of opsonizing antibodies
T_H2	IL-4, IL-5, IL-13	Provides defense against parasitic infections; stimulates IgE class switching
T_H17	IL-17	Recruits neutrophils to fight against extracellular bacteria and fungi
T_{FH}	IFN-γ, IL-4, IL-5	Stimulates immunoglobulin class switching
T_{Reg}	IL-10	Suppresses T-cell activity and prevents development of autoimmunity

of the antigen on the surface of infected cells, cytotoxic T cells release cytotoxic granules containing preformed cytotoxic proteins and inject them into the cytosol of the target cell inducing cell death or apoptosis. The cytotoxic proteins include perforin, granzymes, and granulysin. Perforin facilitates entry of other cytotoxic proteins into the cytosol of the target cell, triggering apoptosis through activation of different enzymes[44] (Figure 1–9).

> $CD8^+$ cells release cytotoxic proteins leading to cell death (apoptosis).

Interaction Between T Cells and B Cells. Antibody responses to most antigens require a complex interaction between APCs, T cells, and B cells. The surface immunoglobulins that serve as B-cell receptors (BCR) on naïve B lymphocytes recognize a specific soluble antigen which is internalized by the B cell and degraded into small peptides that are presented with the help of MHC class II molecule to $CD4^+$ helper T cells. When the activated $CD4^+$ T helper cell recognizes and binds to the peptide:MHC II complex on the surface of B cells, it induces the B cells to proliferate, class-switch, and differentiate into plasma cells and produce specific antibodies. The interaction between B and T cells is mediated by the binding between the CD40 ligand on T cells and CD40 on the B cells (and other costimulatory molecule pairs) and by the direct release of cytokines. This process occurs in the secondary lymphoid organs to which helper T cells and B cells migrate[45] (Figure 1–10).

> The BCRs on B cells recognize the antigen. The antigen is presented through MHC II to T_H cells. T_H cells are activated and stimulate B cells to produce antibodies.

Other Cell Types

Eosinophils are white blood cells that are important effectors in defense against parasites. They are also involved with other inflammatory processes, especially allergic reactions. Eosinophils were originally named because of their ability to be stained with a red dye, eosin.

Eosinophils develop and mature from hematopoietic progenitor cells in the bone marrow under the influence of IL-5 and IL-3 and are then released into the circulation. The vast majority of eosinophils are located in the tissues where they are involved in T_H2-mediated reactions.

Once activated, eosinophils release some preformed proinflammatory mediators which are stored in their granules, and also newly synthesize other mediator molecules. One major component of the specific eosinophil granule is the major basic protein (MBP) which is cytotoxic for parasites. High levels of MBP are also found in the bronchial tissues of asthmatic patients. Other important preformed

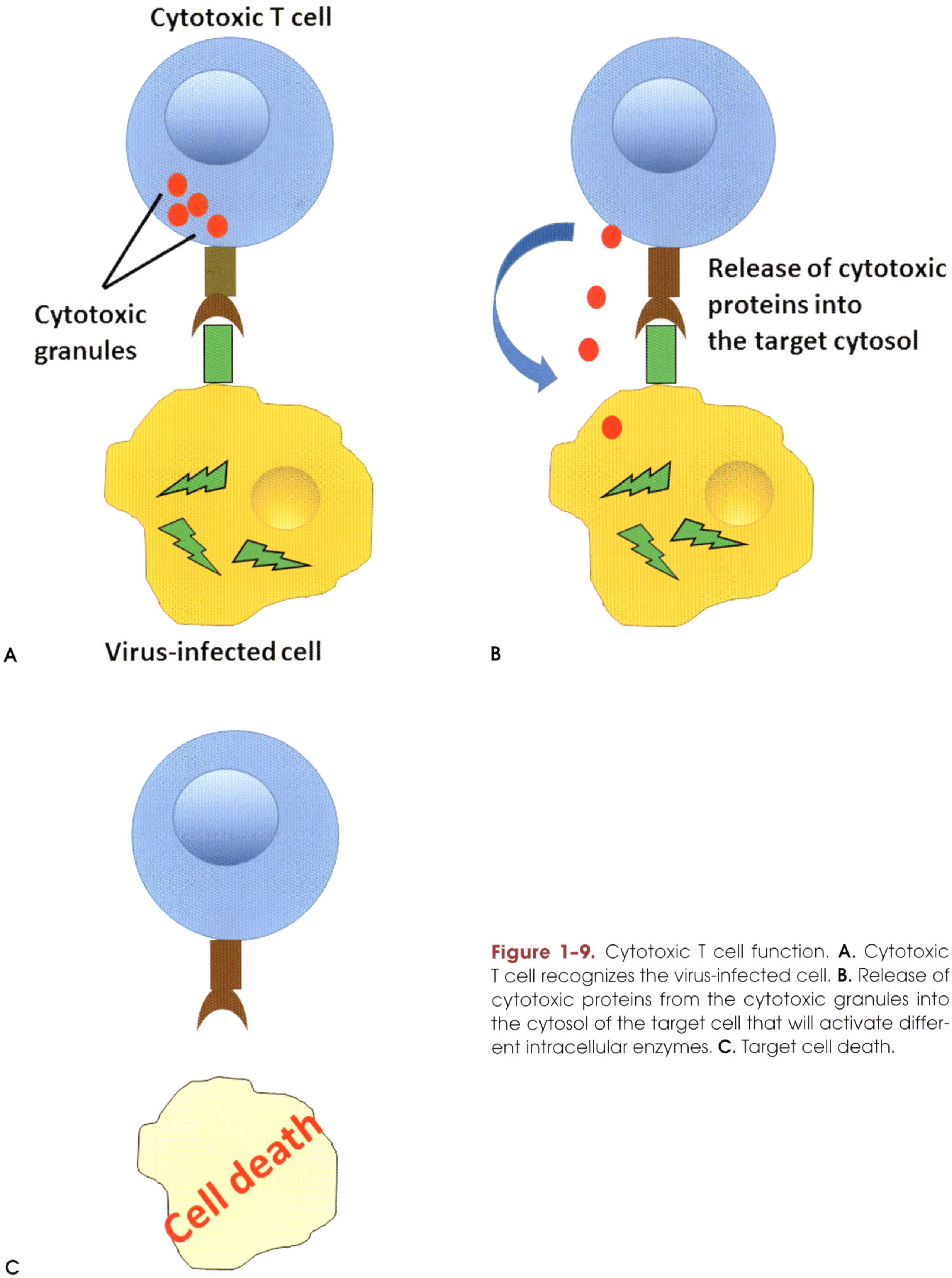

Figure 1-9. Cytotoxic T cell function. **A.** Cytotoxic T cell recognizes the virus-infected cell. **B.** Release of cytotoxic proteins from the cytotoxic granules into the cytosol of the target cell that will activate different intracellular enzymes. **C.** Target cell death.

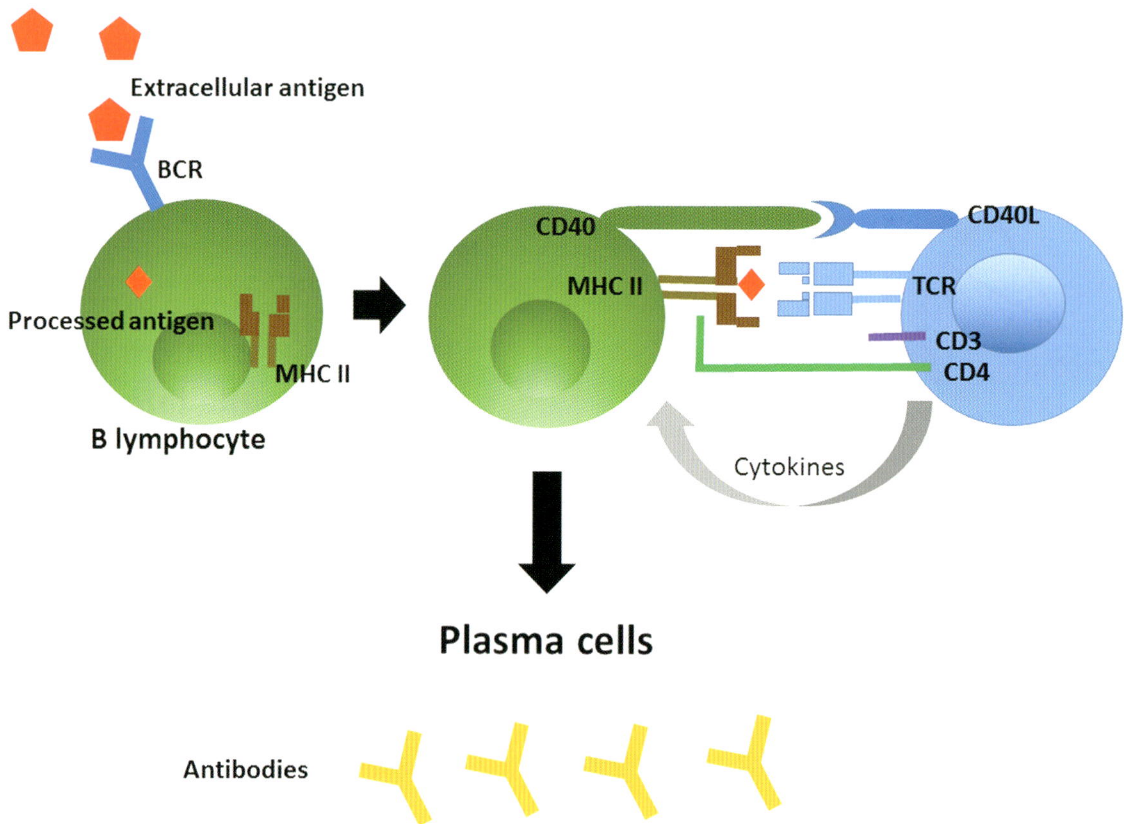

Figure 1-10. Interaction between B and T cells. The extracellular antigen is bound to a BCR (immunoglobulin) on the surface of naïve B cells. The antigen is then internalized, processed, and reexpressed on the surface of B cells coupled to MHC II molecules. The processed antigen is presented to antigen-specific $CD4^{+}$ T cells. The TCR recognizes the presented peptide and activates the T cells, simulating them to express CD40L and to release cytokines. The interaction between CD40 (on B cells) and CD40L (on T cells), along with the interaction with other costimulatory molecules, together with the action of secreted cytokines, stimulates the B cells to undergo class switching from IgM and start producing another immunoglobulin isotype. The B cell then differentiates into a specific antibody-producing plasma cell.

cytotoxic mediators that are rapidly released or produced after eosinophil activation and degranulation include eosinophilic cationic protein (ECP), eosinophil peroxidase (EPO), and a number of different cytokines.[46,47]

Basophils develop in the bone marrow from the same hematopoietic progenitor cells as eosinophils, under the influence of IL-3. From the bone marrow, they are released in the circulation where they represent less than 1% of all leukocytes. They have similar functions, receptors, and activities as mast cells. After activation, basophils release their preformed mediators and also synthesize mediators and cytokines. Histamine is the major preformed mediator stored in basophils granules. Basophils play an important role in host defense, particularly against parasites.

Mast cells arise from pluripotent bone marrow hematopoietic stem cells and then circulate in the blood. They then migrate into tissues where they mature under the influence of stem cell factor (SCF). Mast cells play a central role in the pathogenesis of allergic reactions, and in host defense against different pathogens. IgE possesses the unusual ability of being able to bind to high-affinity receptors for IgE (FcεRI) on the surface of mast cells while still monomeric (ie, without first complexing to antigen). Mast cells bind IgE molecules with many different specificities and remain quiescent until a specific antigen cross-links 2 adjacent bound IgE molecules. Once activated, mast cells release preformed mediators or synthesize new molecules. Histamine is the most important mediator found in mast cell granules, and it plays a central role in bronchoconstriction, increase in mucosal secretions, and action on endothelial cells. Mediator release results in edema, erythema, skin itching, rhinorrhea, bronchospasm, nausea and vomiting, hypotension, and abdominal cramps. Mast cells can also be activated by the binding of complement-derived anaphylatoxins (C3a or C5a).

AUTOIMMUNITY AND TOLERANCE

Autoimmune responses affect about 5% of the population and involve the development of antibodies against self-antigens (autoantibodies) which can damage self-tissues causing a variety of autoimmune diseases. Manifestations of autoimmune diseases differ depending on the tissues targeted by the autoantibodies, their severity, and the type of damage caused.

The immune system has mechanisms to distinguish self-antigens from non-self-antigens, preventing the development of autoimmunity. This is accomplished by removing during their early stages of development, those B and T cells which have high affinity for self-molecules, inducing self-tolerance. However, some self-reactive lymphocytes are not eliminated and may subsequently trigger autoimmunity. Depending on the site where the tolerance develops, it can be divided into 2 stages, central or peripheral tolerance.

Central Tolerance

Central tolerance is achieved at the sites of T and B cell maturation and requires acquisition of antigen specificity in the thymus and bone marrow, respectively. The lymphocytes are exposed to different self-antigens during maturation, and if they strongly recognize them, they are destroyed by the process of apoptosis (negative selection).

Positive selection of T cells refers to the process by which some, only mildly self-reactive immature T cells, differentiate into $CD4^+$ $CD8^+$ (double positive) cells and migrate deeper into the thymic cortex. Double-positive T cells undergo further negative selection. Those cells that strongly recognize self-peptide are eliminated by apoptosis.

Central tolerance is very effective because the lymphocytes are exposed to multiple self-antigens during their formation, particularly the T cells in the thymus. A single transcription factor, AIRE (autoimmune regulator), is responsible for the expression of many genes that encode different peripheral self-antigens in the thymus, which are then presented to immature T cells. Mutations in the *AIRE* gene that encode AIRE transcriptional factors prevent expression of peripheral antigens in the thymus and lead to the inability to eliminate autoreactive lymphocytes. An *AIRE* gene defect causes APECED (autoimmune polyendocrinopathy-candidiasis-ectodermal dystrophy) also known as APS-1 (autoimmune polyglandular syndrome -1) that is associated with multiple autoimmune symptoms.[48]

> Central tolerance is directed by the *AIRE* gene. Mutation in *AIRE* leads to an autoimmune condition (APECED).

Peripheral Tolerance

As described above, immature lymphocytes with a high affinity for self-molecules are deleted at their site of formation in the central lymphoid organs. The mature lymphocytes that arrive in the periphery possess only a lower affinity for self-antigens. They do not respond to these self-antigens and are functionally self-ignorant. Interestingly, such "ignorant cells" can increase their affinity for self-antigens upon exposure to different costimulatory factors such as infections. This is possible because some infectious agents express epitopes similarly to self-antigens leading to autoreactivity against self-molecules. The immune system has other mechanisms that complement central tolerance and are capable of destroying self-reactive lymphocytes.

Once such self-reactive lymphocytes are present in the periphery, other regulatory T cells (T_{Reg} cells) have the capacity to suppress them. If T_{Reg} cells encounter the self-antigen in the periphery, they secrete inhibitory cytokines such as IL-10 and TGF-β that act on the nearby autoreactive T cells. T_{Reg} cells express CD4 and CD25 on their surface, and express the transcription factor, FoxP3. Patients with mutations in the gene expressing FoxP3 or patients with defective $CD4^+$ $CD25^+$ T_{Reg} cells, develop autoimmune syndromes such as systemic lupus erythematosus, diabetes, or multiple sclerosis).[49]

> Peripheral tolerance is directed by $T_{Reg.}$ cells.

Autoimmunity may arise spontaneously in genetically susceptible individuals exposed to certain environmental factors where the elimination mechanisms described above are not sufficient to fight against autoantibody production. Consequently, autoimmune cells initiate a process that results in a chronic inflammatory state characterized by tissue destruction due to accumulation of inflammatory cells and the release of various inflammatory mediators.

An example of autoimmune disease with nasal involvement is granulomatosis with polyangiitis, formerly known as Wegener granulomatosis. Patients with this autoimmune disorder produce antineutrophil cytoplasmic antibodies (ANCAs) directed against proteinase 3, an enzyme found in neutrophils. Binding of ANCA leads to neutrophil activation, endothelial adherence, and degranulation causing endothelial cell damage.

Autoimmune disorders are treated by immunosuppressive therapy with anti-inflammatory drugs such as corticosteroids that inhibit different arms of the immune system. However, these drugs have various adverse effects that complicate the administration of immunosuppressive therapy.

Otolaryngologists may encounter patients with different diseases who are being treated with immunosuppressive medications. Moreover, otolaryngologists may prescribe corticosteroids for various conditions. A list of the most commonly used immunosuppressive medications, their mechanisms of action, indications, and most frequent adverse effects is shown in Table 1–5.

ROLE OF VACCINES IN EAR, NOSE, AND THROAT PATHOLOGY

Introduction

The goal of vaccination is to create an immunological response against a pathogen that has been

Table 1–5. The Most Common Immunosuppressive Medications Encountered by Otolaryngologists, Their Mechanisms of Action, Indications, and Side Effects

Type of Medication	Mechanism of Action	Indications	Adverse Effects
Corticosteroids	Suppress cell-mediated and humoral immunity by inhibiting genes coding IL-1, IL-2, IL-3, IL-4, and IL-5	Used for treatment of inflammation, autoimmune disorders, including autoimmune sensorineural hearing loss	Risk of infections, cataract, osteoporosis, elevated blood glucose (if long-term treatment)
Cyclophosphamide	Induces cells apoptosis through its metabolites	Autoimmune disorders including systemic lupus erythematosus, Wegener granulomatosis, cancer	Pancytopenia, hemorrhagic cystitis
Methotrexate	Inhibits synthesis of DNA, RNA; inhibits T-cell activation	Autoimmune disorders including rheumatoid arthritis, Behcet disease	Myelosuppression, pulmonary toxicity, hepatotoxicity
Azathioprine	Prevents clonal expansion of lymphocytes	To prevent transplant rejection	
Cyclosporine/ tacrolimus	Inhibits lymphokine production and interleukin release, leading to a reduced function of effector T cells	To prevent transplant rejection	Cyclosporine—nephrotoxic

killed, weakened, or rendered nonvirulent. Once a response is achieved, the immune system is able to establish immunological memory and to mount a quick response if an actual infection occurs.

There are numerous types of vaccines. Killed vaccines are the safest since the pathogen is completely deactivated; however, they sometimes do not sufficiently stimulate an immune response (eg, Pertussis and some influenza vaccines). Attenuated live vaccines induce a more potent immunological response because the organism in the vaccine is able to replicate inducing a greater activation of the immune system. Although the attenuated pathogen can replicate, it is unable to cause disease because the organism is significantly weakened, enabling the innate immune system or primary response to clear it before it causes disease. As a result, these vaccines are safe and highly immunogenic (eg, measles-mumps-rubella [MMR], oral polio vaccine, smallpox vaccine, some influenza vaccines). Attenuated live vaccines usually are not used in immunodeficient patients or pregnant women because their compromised immune system may not be able to control the replication of the attenuated pathogen.

Polysaccharide Vaccines

Until recently, *Haemophilus influenzae* was the most common causative bacterial agent for epiglottitis and sinus infections. However, widespread immunization with the *H. influenzae* type B (Hib) vaccine has dramatically decreased *H. influenzae* type B infections, and now patients only present with infection by nontypable *H. influenzae* (NTHI) for which the vaccine-induced antibodies are not effective.

> Hib vaccine has almost eradicated Hib epiglottitis and sinusitis.

Many of the bacteria responsible for invasive bacterial disease in childhood have a polysaccharide capsule conferring a survival advantage to these bacteria. Hib has a polyribosyl ribitol phosphate (PRP) capsule and antibodies against PRP protect those at risk for Hib. Therefore, administration of purified PRP was thought to confer immunity. Studies show that when given in the first 2 years of life, immunization with PRP induces low titers of antibodies and are not protective.[50] This is due to the fact that although PRP is recognized by B-cell receptors, it cannot be presented to T cells, therefore T helper cells are not recruited to induce a potent antibody response. Since epiglottitis was very common in young children, another modality of conferring immunity against Hib was pursued.

It was known from prior studies that bacterial polysaccharides conjugated to proteins enhance the capacity of the polysaccharide to induce an antibody response. In this way, the carrier protein is presented to the T cells by MHC class II molecules expressed by B cells providing T cells help to drive B cell maturation, IgG production, and memory B cell production. As a result, bacterial polysaccharides conjugated to proteins are more immunogenic than polysaccharides alone.[51] The current vaccination against Hib starts at 2 months of age and uses a conjugated polysaccharide Hib vaccine.

Normally, most children begin to make stronger immune responses to encapsulated bacteria around 2 years of age. Children and adults who fail to develop the immune response to the polysaccharide coating bacteria but otherwise have normal antibody levels, have a specific antibody deficiency. This can be assessed by immunization with a *S. pneumoniae* polysaccharide vaccine and then measuring the antibody titers after 1 month. If they do not mount adequate titers and have recurrent ear infections, upper and lower respiratory tract infections, these patients might benefit from immunoglobulin replacement therapy.

> Failure to produce antibodies against polysaccharide bacterial capsule can lead to respiratory infections due to specific antibody deficiency.

REFERENCES

1. Klaus S, Axel U. Paul Ehrlich's magic bullet concept: 100 years of progress. *Nature Rev Cancer*. 2008; 8(6): 473–480.
2. Janeway CA Jr, Medzhitov R. Innate immune recognition. *Annu Rev Immunol*. 2002;20:197.
3. K. Murphy. *Janeway's Immunobiology* (8th ed.). New York, NY: Garland Science; 2011.
4. Turvey SE, Broide DH. Innate immunity. *J Allergy Clin Immunol*. 2010;125(suppl 2):S24–S32.

5. Joncker NT, Raulet DH. Regulation of NK cell responsiveness to achieve self-tolerance and maximal responses to diseased target cells. *Immunol Rev*. 2008; 224:85–97.
6. Bainton DF, Ullyot JL, Farquhar MG. The development of neutrophilic polymorphonuclear leukocytes in human bone marrow. *J Exp Med*. 1971;134(4):907–934.
7. Pham CT. Neutrophil serine proteases: specific regulators of inflammation. *Nat Rev Immunol*. 2006;Jul 6(7):541–550.
8. Segal AW. How neutrophils kill microbes. *Annu Rev Immunol*. 2005;23:197–223.
9. Hattar K, Grandel U, Moeller A, et al. Lipoteichoic acid (LTA) from *Staphylococcus aureus* stimulates human neutrophil cytokine release by a CD14-dependent, toll-like-receptor-independent mechanism: autocrine role of tumor necrosis factor-[alpha] in mediating LTA-induced interleukin-8 generation. *Crit Care Med*. 2006;Mar 34(3): 835–841.
10. Scheel-Toellner D, Wang KQ, Webb PR, et al. Early events in spontaneous neutrophil apoptosis. *Biochem Soc Trans*. 2004;32(pt 3):461–464.
11. Mosser DM, Edwards JP. Exploring the full spectrum of macrophage activation. *Nat Rev Immunol*. 2008;8(12): 958–969
12. Platt C, Ma J, Chalouni C, Ebersold M, Bou-Reslan H, Carano R. Mature dendritic cells use endocytic receptors to capture and present antigens. *Proc Natl Acad Sci USA*. 2010;107(9):4287–4292.
13. Sallusto F, Cella M, Danieli C, Lanzavecchia A. Dendritic cells use macropinocytosis and the mannose receptor to concentrate macromolecules in the major histocompatibility complex class II compartment: downregulation by cytokines and bacterial products. *J Exp Med*. 1995; 182(2):389–400.
14. Warren HS, Smyth MJ. NK cells and apoptosis. *Immunol Cell Biol*. 1999;77(1):64–75
15. Terabe M, Berzofsky JA.The immunoregulatory role of type I and type II NKT cells in cancer and other diseases. *Cancer Immunol Immunother*. 2014;63(3):199–213.
16. Takeda K, Akira S. Toll-like receptors in innate immunity. *Int Immunol*. 2005;17(1):1–14.
17. Turvey SE, Broide DH. Innate immunity. *J Allergy Clin Immunol*. 2010;125(suppl 2):S24–S32.
18. Chan JK, Roth J, Oppenheim JJ, Tracey KJ, Vogl T, Feldmann M, Horwood N, Nanchahal J. Alarmins: awaiting a clinical response. *J Clin Invest*. 2012;122(8):2711–2719.
19. Frank MM. Complement disorders and hereditary angioedema. *J Allergy Clin Immunol*. 2010;125(2, suppl 2): S262–S271.
20. Abbas AK, Lichtman AH, Pillai S. *Cellular and Molecular Immunology*. Philadelphia, PA: Elsevier/Saunders. 7th ed.; 2012.
21. Zuraw BL. Clinical practice. Hereditary angioedema. *N Engl J Med*. 2008;359(10):1027–1036.
22. Bork K, Meng G, Staubach P, Hardt J. Hereditary angioedema: new findings concerning symptoms, affected organs, and course. *Am J Med*. 2006;119(3):267–274.
23. Bouwman LH, Roep BO, Roos A. Mannose-binding lectin: clinical implications for infection, transplantation, and autoimmunity. *Hum Immunol*. 2006;67(4-5): 247–256.
24. Petersen SV, Thiel S, Jensenius JC. The mannan-binding lectin pathway of complement activation: biology and disease association. *Mol Immunol*. 2001;38 (2–3): 133–149.
25. Nilsson SC, Sim RB, Lea SM, Fremeaux-Bacchi V, Blom AM. Complement factor I in health and disease. *Mol Immunol*. 2011;48(14):1611–1620.
26. Röseler S, Holtappels G, Wagenmann M, Bachert C. Elevated levels of interleukins IL-1 beta, IL-6 and IL-8 in naturally acquired viral rhinitis. *Eur Arch Otorhinolaryngol*. 1995;252(suppl 1):S61–S63.
27. Pérez-Novo CA, Claeys C, Van Cauwenberge P, Bachert C. Expression of eicosanoid receptors subtypes and eosinophilic inflammation: implication on chronic rhinosinusitis. *Respir Res*. 2006;7:75.
28. Dinarello CA. Proinflammatory cytokines. *Chest*. 2000; 118(2):503–508.
29. Miller, JF. The discovery of thymus function and of thymus-derived lymphocytes. *Immunol Rev*. 2002;185(1): 7–14.
30. Ruddle NH, Akirav EM. Secondary lymphoid organs: responding to genetic and environmental cues in ontogeny and the immune response. *J Immunol*. 2009;183(4): 2205–2212.
31. Garside P, Ingulli E, Merica RR, Johnson JG, Noelle RJ, Jenkins MK. Visualization of specific B and T lymphocyte interactions in the lymph node. *Science*. 1998;281(5373):96–99.
32. Brandtzaeg P. Immunology of tonsils and adenoids: everything the ENT surgeon needs to know. *Int J Pediatr Otorhinolaryngol*. 2003;67(suppl 1):S69–S76.
33. Borghesi L, Milcarek C. From B cell to plasma cell: regulation of V(D)J recombination and antibody secretion. *Immunol Res*. 2006;36(1–3):27–32.
34. Durandy A. Activation-induced cytidine deaminase: a dual role in class-switch recombination and somatic hypermutation. *Eur J Immunol*. 2003;33(8):2069–2073.
35. Underdown B, Schiff J. Immunoglobulin A: strategic defense initiative at the mucosal surface. *Annu Rev Immunol*. 1984;4(1):389–417.
36. Bellussi L, Cambi J, Passali D. Functional maturation of nasal mucosa: role of secretory immunoglobulin A (SIgA). *Multidiscip Respir Med*. 2013;8(1):46.
37. Kurono Y, Fujiyoshi T, Mogi G. Secretory IgA and bacterial adherence to nasal mucosal cells. *Ann Otol Rhinol Laryngol*. 1989;98:273–277.
38. Gilian M, Reinholdt J, Mortensen SB, Sorensen CH. Perturbation of mucosal immune defence mechanisms by bacterial IgA proteases. *Bull Eur Physiopathol Respir*. 1983; 19(2):99–104.
39. Schwarz BA, Bhandoola A .Trafficking from the bone marrow to the thymus: a prerequisite for thymopoiesis. *Immunol Rev*. 2006;209:47–57.

40. Park EJ, Peixoto A, Imai Y, Goodarzi A. Distinct roles for LFA-1 affinity regulation during T-cell adhesion, diapedesis, and interstitial migration in lymph nodes. *Blood*. 2010;115(8):1572–1581.
41. Faveeuw C, Di Mauro ME, Price AA, Ager A. Roles of alpha(4) integrins/VCAM-1 and LFA-1/ICAM-1 in the binding and transendothelial migration of T lymphocytes and T lymphoblasts across high endothelial venules. *Int Immunol*. 2000;12(3):241–251.
42. Viret C, Wong FS, Janeway CA. Designing and maintaining the mature TCR repertoire: the continuum of self-peptide:self-MHC complex recognition. *Immunity*. 1999;10:559.
43. Krogsgaard M. How T cells "see" antigen. *Nat Immunol*. 2005;6:239–245.
44. Groscurth P, Filgueira L. Killing mechanisms of cytotoxic T lymphocytes. *Physiology*. 1998;13(1):17–21.
45. Parker D. T cell-dependent B cell activation. *Annu Rev Immunol*. 1993;11(1):331–360.
46. Stone KD, Prussin C, Metcalfe DD. IgE, mast cells, basophils, and eosinophils. *J Allergy Clin Immunol*. 2010;125: S73–S80.
47. Hogan S, Rosenberg H, Moqbel R, et al. Eosinophils: biological properties and role in health and disease. *Clin Exp Allergy*. 2008;38(5):709–750.
48. Gallo V, Giardino G, Capalbo D, et al. Alterations of the autoimmune regulator transcription factor and failure of central tolerance: APECED as a model. *Expert Rev Clin Immunol*. 2013;9(1):43–51.
49. Itoh M, Takahashi T, Sakaguchi N, et al. Thymus and autoimmunity: production of $CD25^+CD4^+$ naturally anergic and suppressive T cells as a key function of the thymus in maintaining immunologic self-tolerance. *J Immunol*. 1999;162:5317–5326.
50. Peltola H, Kayhty H, Sivonen A, Makela H. *Haemophilus influenzae* type b capsular polysaccharide vaccine in children, a double-blind field study of 100000 vaccines 3 months to 5 years of age in Finland. *Pediatrics*. 1977;60:730.
51. Hougs L, Juul L, Ditzel HJ, Heilmann C, Svejgaard A, Barington T. The first dose of a *Haemophilus influenzae* type b conjugate vaccine reactivates memory B cells: evidence for extensive clonal selection, intraclonal affinity maturation, and multiple isotype switches to IgA2. *J Immunol*. 1999;162:224.

2

Immunological Hypersensitivity Reactions

Denisa E. Ferastraoaru, Manish Ramesh, and David L. Rosenstreich

INTRODUCTION

Hypersensitivity reactions are characterized by amplified immune responses to antigens following a second contact with that particular antigen. All immunologically mediated responses that occur in our body were classified into 4 types by Gell and Coombs in 1963.[1] This classification depends upon the cells and mediators involved, and the latency and severity of the reaction. Type I, II, and III hypersensitivity reactions are antibody mediated and are characterized by the action of different classes of antibodies that interact with the allergen, resulting in effector cell activation and tissue injury. Type IV reactions are mediated by T cells (Table 2–1).

> There are 4 major types of hypersensitivity reactions: types I, II, and III are antibody mediated; type IV is mediated by T cells.

A further classification of type IV delayed hypersensitivity reactions was made by Pichler in 2003 which depends on the cells that are recruited upon T-cell activation and subsequent release of different cytokines and chemokines: monocytes (type IVa), eosinophils (type IVb), or neutrophils (type IVd). Type IVc delayed hypersensitivity reactions are mediated by either $CD4^+$ or $CD8^+$ T cells that seem to participate in all type IV reactions.[2]

Clinically, it is sometimes difficult to differentiate between the 4 categories of hypersensitivity reactions because they can overlap significantly.

TYPE I HYPERSENSITIVITY-IMMEDIATE (ALLERGIC) HYPERSENSITIVITY

Type I hypersensitivity reactions are immediate-type allergic reactions and are mediated primarily by IgE antibodies. Allergic rhinoconjunctivitis, allergic asthma, atopic dermatitis, anaphylaxis, and some drug allergies are examples of type I responses. Immediate type hypersensitivity involves mast cell or basophil degranulation after allergens bind cell surface-specific IgE antibodies. Mast cell and basophil mediators released after their activation produce the symptoms.[3] Once specific IgE molecules are produced, the individual is sensitized to that antigen. The predisposition to become IgE-sensitized to otherwise innocuous, environmental allergens is termed *atopy*, and such individuals are referred to as *atopic*.

> Type I reactions are IgE mediated. Examples of type I reactions include allergic rhinoconjunctivitis, allergic asthma, atopic dermatitis, anaphylaxis, and some drug allergies.

Epidemiology

The prevalence of atopic diseases has increased significantly over the last few decades, especially in industrialized societies. In the United States, asthma prevalence increased from 7% in 2001 to 8.4% in 2010, when 25.7 million persons had asthma[4] with

Table 2–1. Classification of Hypersensitivity Reactions and Their Main Characteristics

Type of Hypersensitivity Reaction	Mediators	Effector Mechanism	Examples	Comments
Type I (immediate)	IgE	Mast cell/basophil activation	Allergic rhinoconjunctivitis, allergic asthma, atopic dermatitis, anaphylaxis, some drug allergies	The response occurs rapidly, within seconds–minutes.
Type II (cytotoxic)	IgG, IgM	Complement activation; phagocytosis	Autoimmune thrombocytopenia, autoimmune hemolytic anemia, Graves' disease	Antibodies bind self-antigens or neoantigens on target cells leading to their destruction by phagocytosis or complement activation
Type III (immune complex disease)	IgG	Immune complex formation	Arthus reaction, serum sickness, systemic lupus erythematosus, rheumatoid arthritis	Antibodies form immune complexes with soluble antigens that deposit in vessels and tissues resulting in local or systemic inflammation
Type IV (delayed reaction; cell mediated)				
IVa	T_H1 cells activate monocytes/ macrophage	Release of different inflammatory mediators; effector T cells	Allergic contact dermatitis, tuberculin testing	Occurs in 24 to 72 h
IVb	T_H2 cells activate eosinophils		Chronic asthma, chronic allergic rhinoconjunctivitis	
IVc	Cytotoxic T cells		Contact dermatitis, maculopapular and bullous rash	
IVd	T cells activate neutrophils		Behcet disease, acute generalized exanthematous pustulosis (AGEP)	

higher rates in females and African Americans.[5] In children, up to 90% of asthma cases are thought to be allergic in nature, compared with 50% to 70% in adults.[6] It is estimated that allergic rhinitis is the most prevalent allergic disease[7] and worldwide it affects between 10% and 30% of the population.[8] In 2012, food and skin allergies were reported in 5.6% and 10% of children, respectively, over the previous 12 months.[9]

Hygiene Hypothesis

Over the past decades there has been a significant increase in the prevalence of allergic diseases, especially in the developed world. There is a considerably lower prevalence in developing countries and in the rural areas of more developed countries.[10,11] It was postulated that a lack of childhood infections in developed countries, due to improved hygiene and use of antibiotics, might be altering immune homeostasis, resulting in increased atopy. Consistent with this hypothesis is the finding that children who lived on farms, especially those who drank unpasteurized milk, had a lower prevalence of asthma and atopy. This was thought to be due in part to exposure to a wider range of microorganisms.[12,13] Similarly, there is an inverse correlation between hay fever prevalence and the number of siblings in a family, presumably because of increased exposure to infections.[14] The theory that exposure to certain infections and microorganisms early in life protects against allergic diseases is referred to as the *hygiene hypothesis*.

> The hygiene hypothesis is the theory that early life exposure to certain infections and microorganisms protects against developing allergic disorders.

Gut and airway microbial colonizations and their role in establishing immune system homeostasis have been extensively studied in the last decades. Starting in utero, the fetus is exposed to diverse microbial organisms from the maternal oral and gut microbiome[15] which stimulate the fetal immune system; this process continues intrapartum (especially with a vaginal delivery) and postnatally.[16] Decreased bacterial diversity of the infant's intestinal flora is associated with an increased risk of allergic rhinitis and eosinophilia,[17] allergic sensitization, and food allergy.[18] Both the gastrointestinal and airway microbiomes appear to play a role in this antiallergic effect.[19]

Several mechanisms have been proposed as explanations for the immunological phenomena underlying the hygiene hypothesis. A lack of microbial burden in early childhood redirects the T_H1 immunity toward a T_H2 phenotype, predisposing to allergic disorders.[20]

It is noteworthy that heavy, chronic parasitic infections, which induce a T_H2 response, are also protective against allergic disorders.[21–23] When exposed to parasitic antigens, lymphocytes from chronically parasite infected children produce large amounts of IL-10, an immunosuppressive cytokine. IL-10 is produced by T_{Reg} cells and controls the balance between T_H2 allergic response[24] and T_H1, T_H17 autoimmune/autoinflammatory responses.[25] Taken together, these findings suggest that the immunological changes underlying the hygiene hypothesis involves the generation of more effective immunoregulation mediated by T_{Reg} cells and IL-10. Interestingly, the relationship between parasites (especially helminths) and inflammatory diseases is not strictly limited to allergic disorders but also applies to autoimmunity.[26]

In addition to microbiome changes, the worldwide increase in atopy increase is probably due to other factors, including genetic predisposition, dietary changes,[27] and the presence of increased exposure to allergy-promoting adjuvants related to urbanization, such as air pollution and tobacco smoke[28] (Figure 2–1).

Pathogenic Mechanisms

IgE antibodies directed against the allergen are produced by plasma cells derived from B cells after class switching induced by T_H2 cell-mediated help (as described in Chapter 1). Type I hypersensitivity reactions can be triggered by many different types of allergens, but the mechanism of this response can be illustrated by using inhaled allergens as an example (Figure 2–2). Immediate hypersensitivity begins with a sensitization phase. The inhaled antigen binds to antigen-specific immunoglobulin molecules expressed on the surface of B cells (B-cell receptors, BCRs) or is taken up by other antigen-presenting cells (APCs) and is then presented to specific $CD4^+$ T_H2 cells in the secondary lymphoid organs. Once $CD4^+$ T_H2 cells are activated, they can activate B cells. This process involves a CD40/CD40L interaction and secretion of cytokines including IL-4, resulting in IgE class switching and differentiation of B cells into plasma cells. Plasma cells produce specific immunoglobulin E (sIgE) antibodies for that

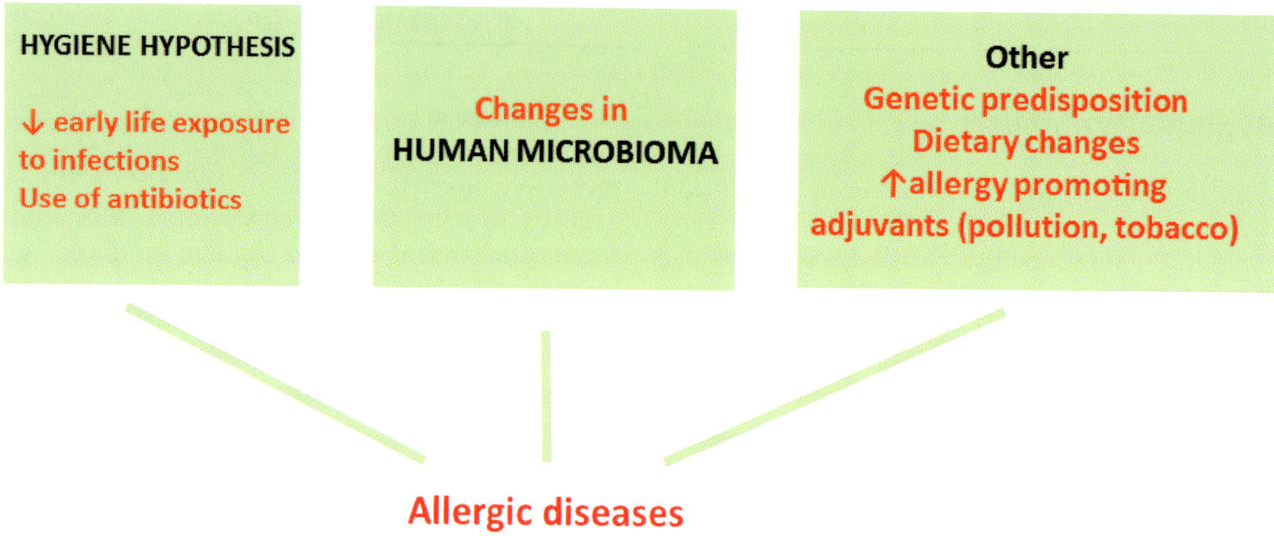

Figure 2-1. Decreased early life exposure to infections, use of antibiotics, changes in the human microbiome, genetic predisposition, dietary changes, and increased exposure to allergy promoting adjuvants are all associated with an increased risk of developing allergic disorders.

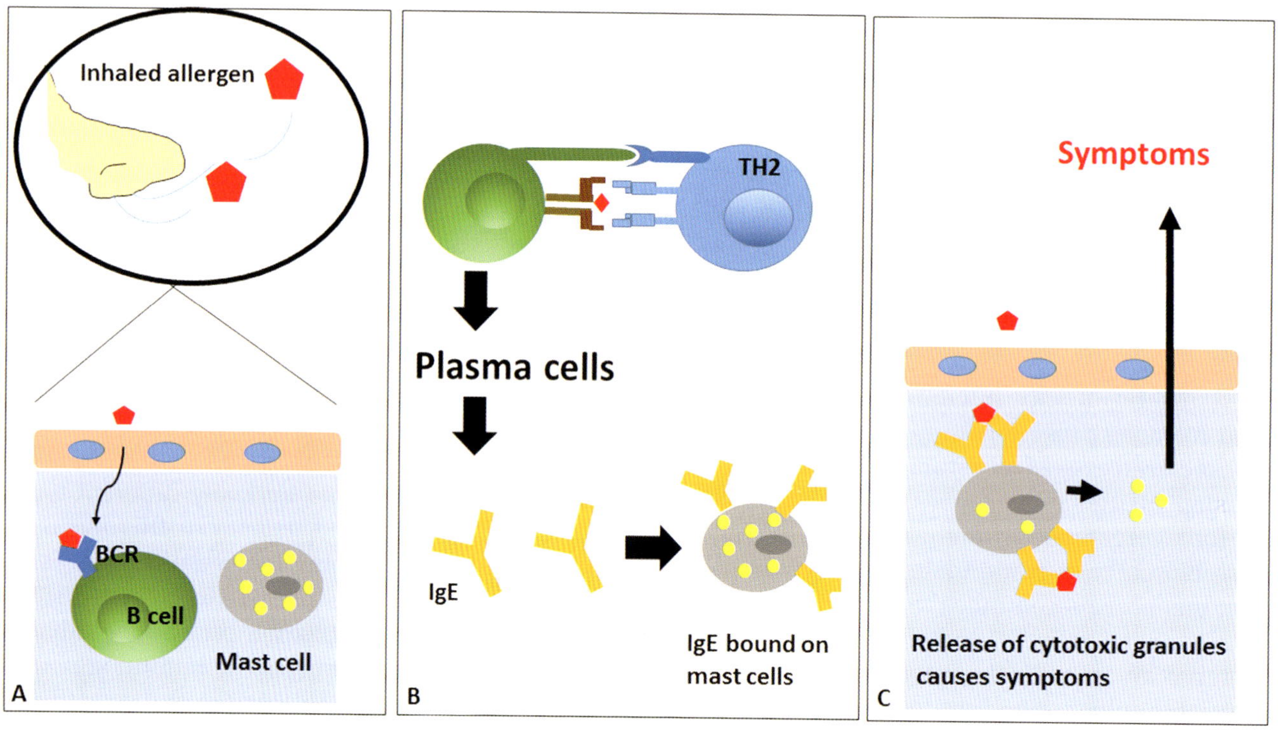

Figure 2-2. Type I hypersensitivity reaction to an inhaled allergen. **A.** The inhaled allergen is taken up by B cells (after binding to B-cell receptor—BCR) or other APCs; in this example the allergen is recognized by the B cells. **B.** Once the allergen is processed by APCs, it is presented to naïve T cells in secondary lymphoid organs which become T_H2 cells. Through different signals (involving recognition by TCR of peptide: MHC II complex, CD40-CD40L interaction) the B cells differentiate into plasma cells and following exposure to IL-4, produce specific IgE through the process of class switching. The allergen-specific IgE bind to receptors on local mast cells, basophils and eosinophils. **C.** On subsequent exposure to the same allergen, the IgE bound on the surface of mast cells and eosinophils bind the allergen, triggering mast cell and eosinophil activation and the release of their granules, which are responsible for clinical allergic symptoms.

particular allergen. Monomeric, sIgE binds through its Fc portion to specific high-affinity IgE receptors (FcεRI) on the surface of mast cells, basophils, or activated eosinophils. Once bound to the FcεRI, the sIgE allergen-binding site remains exposed and available for future interactions with allergen. This initial stage of IgE formation may occur without producing clinical symptoms.

The second phase of immediate hypersensitivity is the effector phase. On subsequent exposure to the same allergen, the mast cell-bound sIgE recognizes the allergen and binds it. The allergen cross-links 2 adjacent FcεRI-bound sIgE molecules inducing mast cell activation. Upon activation, these cells release their granular content which contains a wide variety of biologically active substances such as histamine and tryptase, which cause tissue inflammation and allergic symptoms (sneezing, nasal and eye pruritis, and wheezing).[29] High-affinity FcεRIs are also present on basophils and eosinophils, and these cells can also be activated after binding allergen.

> At the first interaction with the allergen, B cells produce IgE that binds to mast cells. On subsequent exposure, the allergen cross-links 2 adjacent IgE molecules on the mast cell surface, causing activation and the release of different mediators responsible for allergic symptomatology.

Immediate hypersensitivity effector stage reactions consist of 2 phases. The process just described occurs within 1 hour and is termed the *early phase.*

The second phase ("late phase") of immediate hypersensitivity reactions occurs when allergen is present in larger amounts and persists in the body. Symptoms appear 2 to 10 hours after the initial exposure and depend on the site where the allergen has accumulated and the inflammatory reaction is taking place. These can include local swelling, nasal congestion, and bronchoconstriction. Continued production of early phase mediators also contributes to late-phase symptoms. By the sixth hour after initial allergen exposure, there is an accumulation at the reaction site of neutrophils, basophils, and eosinophils. These release their granular proteins and produce increased amounts of different proinflammatory mediators including vascular endothelial growth factor (VEGF); the cytokines IL-4, IL-5, IL-6, and IL-8; and leukotrienes.[30] An example of a late-phase reaction in type I hypersensitivity is the local edema that can appear in some patients a few hours after skin testing[31] or the secondary, delayed airway obstruction that occurs after a single allergen exposure in asthmatic patients. Symptoms of late-phase reaction usually begin to wane by 24 hours, and are still present at 48 to 72 hours in less than 50% of individuals.[30]

Immunoglobulin E

Immunoglobulin E (IgE) is the primary recognition/effector molecule of immediate hypersensitivity reactions. It has 2 important properties that distinguish it from other types of immunoglobulins.

First, unlike other immunoglobulins, which are produced primarily in the peripheral lymphoid organs (spleen and lymph nodes), most IgE is produced locally, in tissues where allergen is deposited, such as the nasal, bronchial, and gastrointestinal mucosa.

Second, IgE can bind to its receptor without having to first complex with an antigen (ie, while still monomeric). Because of these properties, after secretion from the plasma cell IgE diffuses passively through the tissue until it encounters an unoccupied mast cell FcεRI where it binds and remains bound for a long period of time (cell-bound IgE has a half-life of weeks to months).[32]

Immunoglobulin E usually escapes into the circulation only if all of the local mast cell FcεRIs are occupied. Because most of the IgE in the body is primarily bound to effector cells in tissues, IgE has the lowest serum concentration among all 5 immunoglobulin classes.[33] Because of this low serum concentration, IgE was not definitively identified and purified until 1967,[34] much later than the other 4 classes of immunoglobulins.

The structure of IgE is similar to other immunoglobulins: a monomer formed by 2 light chains (κ or λ light chains) with their variable and constant regions and 2 heavy chains (ε heavy chains) with 4 constant regions and 1 variable region. The Fc portion of the IgE binds to specific IgE receptors on the cell surface (Figure 2–3). IgE is heavier than the other

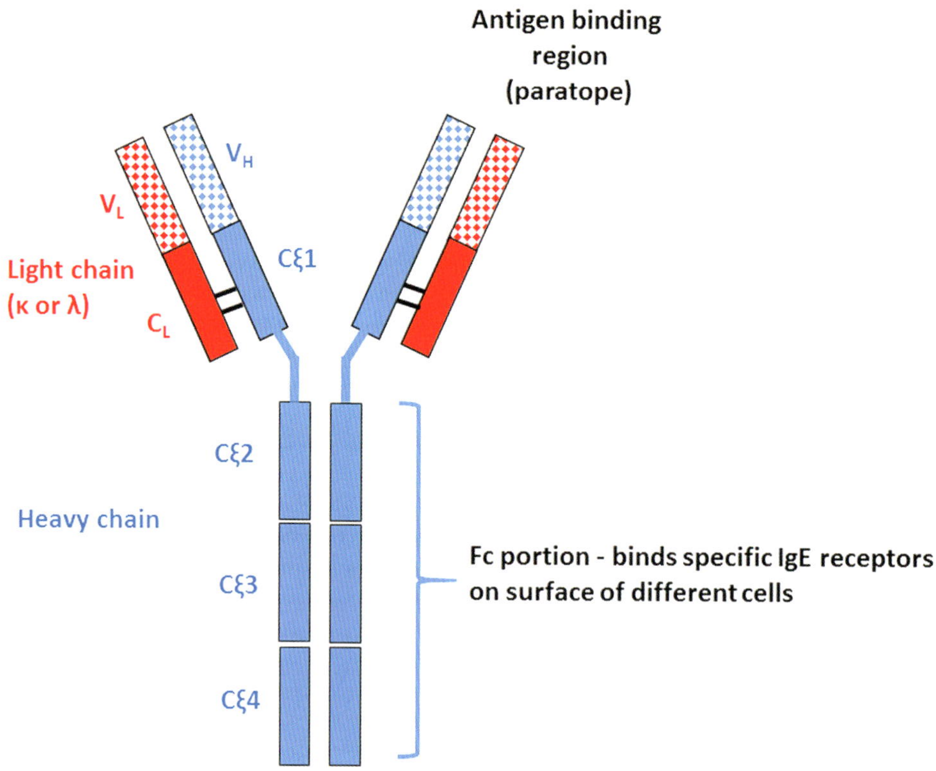

Figure 2–3. The structure of immunoglobulin E. (V_L, variable region of the light chain; C_L, constant region of the light chain; V_H, variable region of the heavy chain; Cε1–4, constant regions of the heavy chain. Cε2, 3, 4 form the Fc portion of the IgE which binds the IgE receptors. The paratope is formed by the variable regions of both light and heavy chains and binds the antigen.

immunoglobulins because it contains an extra common region domain (CH4). This domain is necessary for IgE binding to its receptor and is also heat labile.

> Most IgE remains bound to the surface of tissue-dwelling mast cells. As a result, it has the lowest serum concentration of all the immunoglobulin classes.

IgE Receptors. Immunoglobulin E binds to 2 types of cell surface receptors, the high-affinity receptor (FcεRI) and the low-affinity receptor (FcεRII).

The high-affinity receptor is present only on mast cells, basophils, eosinophils, and dendritic cells (APCs). It is a tetramer ($\alpha\beta\gamma_2$) on mast cells, basophils, and eosinophils, and a trimer ($\alpha\gamma_2$) on APCs. The α portion of this receptor binds the Fc region of the IgE.[35] Once the allergen binds to the cell surface bound IgE, the high-affinity receptor sends downstream signals through the β chain, resulting in cell degranulation and the subsequent release of the mediators and cytokines involved in allergic inflammation.

The low-affinity IgE receptor is present on many different cell types and is identical to the CD23 antigen. It is thought to be important in the regulation of IgE levels and controlling B cell growth and differentiation.[36] Its soluble form can prevent binding of IgE to FcεRI[37] and theoretically can represent a therapeutic approach for treatment of type I hypersensitivity reactions. However, experimental removal or reduction of CD23 antigen does not diminish immediate hypersensitivity reactions, indicating that this receptor is not essential for this type of hypersensitivity.

> IgE binds to the high-affinity receptor (FcεRI) and the low-affinity receptor (FcεRII) on the surface of cells.

Regulation of Allergic Immunity: Cytokines. As defined earlier in the chapter, the excessive production of IgE in response to allergens is a hallmark of the atopic state. The class switching from IgM to IgE requires the help of the T_H2 cytokines, IL-4 and IL-13. In contrast, other T_H1 cytokines such as interferon γ (IFN γ), IL-12, IL-18, and IL-21 are inhibitors of IgE class switching.[38,39]

> IL-4 and IL-13 are involved in IgE class switching. IFN-γ and IL-21 are inhibitors of IgE class switching.

Interleukin-4 is produced by T_H2 lymphocytes, mast cells, and eosinophils. In mast cells and eosinophils the IL-4 is found in their granules from where it can be easily released during the allergic response.[40] Besides its main function of inducing class switching from IgM to the IgE isotype, IL-4 induces the expression of adhesion molecules (VCAM-1) on endothelial cells that allow the adhesion of T cells, basophils, and eosinophils, enhancing the development of allergic reactions.[41] Experimental exposure of sinonasal epithelium to either IL-4 or IL-13 causes alterations of intercellular junctions with increased permeability, and resultant edema, nasal discharge, and environmental reactivity.[42] In contrast, it is known that immunotherapy in patients with perennial rhinitis results in significantly decreased levels of serum IL-4.[43]

Interleukin-13 has many of the same properties as IL-4, including the ability to induce IgE class switching and increased expression of endothelial cell adhesion molecules. In addition, IL-13 stimulates excessive mucus production and makes the airways hyperreactive in asthmatic patients[44] and is elevated in the serum of patients with chronic rhinosinusitis and nasal polyps.[45]

Interferon-γ is produced by T_H1 cells and suppresses the IL-4 induction of germline epsilon transcripts as well as switch recombination to epsilon,[46] resulting in diminished IgE class switching and diminished expression of IgE receptors.[29] Studies show that IFN-γ levels increase in patients receiving immunotherapy, and it is associated with improvement of both symptoms and medication use.[47,48] Interferon-γ promotes IgG production by B cells in these patients which is associated with a reduced inflammatory response to allergens.[49]

Mast Cells, Basophils, and Eosinophils

Mast Cells. Mast cells are involved in many different pathophysiologic processes[50] but are essential for IgE-mediated allergic reactions.[51] They are derived from pluripotent hematopoietic stem cells of the bone marrow, circulate in the blood as mononuclear cells, and then migrate into tissues where they undergo maturation and terminal differentiation. They contain 2 distinct cell surface markers: FcεRI and CD 117 (c-kit). CD 117 is a receptor tyrosine kinase that binds the stem cell factor (SCF) and plays an important role in mast cell activation, differentiation, and survival. After activation, mast cells can immediately release granule-associated mediators and produce lipid-derived substances such as leukotrienes that induce immediate and late-phase allergic inflammation.[52]

Mast cells are divided into 2 phenotypes based on their neutral protease content: MC_{TC} and MC_T. The MC_{TC} contain tryptase, chymase, carboxypeptidase, and cathepsin G and are found mostly in the skin and bronchial, gastrointestinal, and nasal mucosa. The MC_T subset is located primarily in the alveolar walls and in gastrointestinal and airway epithelium, and these cells contain only tryptase as their neutral protease (Table 2–2).[53] Human mast cells are also heterogeneous with respect to cytokine content. Bronchial and nasal mucosa biopsies in patients with allergic asthma and nasal allergies found that IL-4 was distributed among both mast cell phenotypes, but it was expressed preferentially by the MC_{TC} subset.[54]

> MC_{TC} contain tryptase and chymase and are found in skin, bronchial, gastrointestinal, and nasal mucosa. MC_T contain tryptase and are found in the alveolar walls and in gastrointestinal and airway epithelium.

Table 2–2. Mast Cell Subtypes, Their Neutral Protease Content, and Tissue Location

Mast Cell Subtype	Neutral Protease	Location
MC_{TC}	Tryptase, chymase, carboxypeptidase, cathepsin G	Skin, bronchial, gastrointestinal, and nasal mucosa
MC_{T}	Tryptase	Alveolar walls, gastrointestinal and airways epithelium

The granules of mast cells contain preformed mediators that are released once the mast cell is activated, but mast cells can also synthesize new potent allergic mediators such as eicosanoids (eg, thromboxane, prostaglandin D2, leukotriene C4, and leukotriene D4). Preformed substances include histamine, proteoglycans (mainly heparin), and serine proteases such as tryptase or chymase. Heparin stabilizes the β-tryptase tetramer and once released from this complex, it can function as an anticoagulant and promoter of fibroblast activation.[29]

Physiological Effects of Histamine and Leukotrienes. Histamine is synthesized by the action of histidine decarboxylase which removes a carboxyl group from L-histidine. Once histamine is formed, it is either degraded immediately by different enzymes, or is stored as a preformed mediator in mast cells, eosinophils, and basophils. After exposure to an appropriate allergen, these cells are activated and release histamine. Histamine acts by binding to 4 different histamine receptors (H1R, H2R, H3R, and H4R). Histamine is also involved in the recruitment of other cells to the site of the allergic inflammation.

> Histamine is one of the most important mediators of the allergic inflammatory response.

The H1 histamine receptors are found in the central nervous system, smooth muscles, and vascular endothelial cells. Histamine acts on bronchial smooth muscle to induce bronchoconstriction; causes retraction of endothelial cells and resultant leakage of serum out of the blood vessels; causes vasodilation of terminal arterioles; and causes itching. The effects of histamine on nasal mucosa are well documented and include sneezing (due to neural stimulation), increased mucus secretion, and nasal congestion due to vasodilation and increased capillary permeability.[55] The latter effects produce increased turbinate volume, which reduces nasal airflow and increases nasal airway resistance.[56] Histamine H1-receptor antagonists are used to treat allergic symptoms and prevent nasal itching, rhinorrhea, and sneezing.

The H2 histamine receptors are found mainly on parietal cells of the gastric mucosa and are involved in stimulation of acid secretion, but are also found on vascular smooth muscle cells, nasal mucosa, and submucosal glands in the nose. Histamine action on H2 histamine receptors can potentially increase nasal airway swelling and produce rhinorrhea.[57] The combination of H1 and H2 receptor activation can worsen these symptoms.

The H3 histamine receptors are found in the central and peripheral nervous systems and in the nasal submucosal glands, so H3 activation can also stimulate mucous secretion. Animal models suggest that blocking the H3 histamine receptor enhances the decongestant effect of an H1 antihistamine.[58]

The H4 histamine receptors are located on eosinophils, mast cells, basophils, nasal mucosa (nerves), lung, and colon. When histamine binds to these receptors it influences the chemotaxis and action of eosinophils and mast cells. Theoretically, stimulation of H4 histamine receptor could increase the inflammatory activity seen in allergic rhinitis.[59]

Cysteinyl leukotrienes (CysLTs) are lipid-derived mediators and include leukotriene C4 (LTC_4), LTD_4, and LTE_4, which are released primarily by mast cells, basophils, eosinophils, and monocytes. They bind to type 1 and type 2 cysLT-receptors.

> CysLTs include LTC4, LTD4, and LTE4 and are synthesized from arachidonic acid.

Unlike histamine, cysLTs are not stored in cytoplasmic granules but are newly synthesized from arachidonic acid after cellular activation. The CysLTs are produced in large amounts in allergic inflammatory conditions such as asthma and allergic rhinitis. Levels of cysLTs are elevated in patients with symptomatic allergic rhinitis and symptoms correlate with increased cysLT levels.[60] They stimulate mucous glands, producing rhinorrhea, and LTD4 is 5000-fold more potent than histamine in inducing nasal congestion in patients with allergic rhinitis.[61] The CysLTs also enhance production of other inflammatory mediators, further potentiating the allergic response.

Elevated levels of cysLTs are found in patients with aspirin-exacerbated respiratory disease (AERD), a disease characterized by nasal polyposis, chronic rhinosinusitis, asthma, and aspirin sensitivity. Aspirin desensitization improves their respiratory symptoms, along with shrinkage of nasal polyps and improvement in the sense of smell. Addition of aspirin decreases the likelihood of additional surgical intervention over a 2-year period.[62]

Blocking the $cysLT_1$ receptors with medications such as montelukast or zafirlukast can reduce the inflammation mediated by cysLTs, and these medications are useful in the treatment of allergic rhinitis and asthma.[63]

Basophils. Basophils represent about 1% of the circulating white blood cells but are responsible for most of the histamine release by blood cells during an IgE-mediated reaction.[64]

Basophils develop from bone marrow pluripotent stem cells under the influence of IL-3 and are released into the circulation where they survive only for a few days. Similar to mast cells, basophils are able to bind monomeric IgE with high affinity through the FcεRI. Once basophils are activated, they release preformed mediators stored in cytoplasmic granules and synthesize new inflammatory mediators in the same manner as mast cells. Both mast cells and basophils produce large amounts of IL-4 and IL-13 (which are 2 critical T_H2 cytokines in the pathogenesis of allergic responses), but tryptase levels are lower in basophils than in mast cells.

Basophils also produce cysLTs similarly to mast cells, but unlike mast cells, do not produce the arachidonic acid metabolite, prostaglandin D2.[35] Besides their involvement in allergic inflammatory response, basophils along with eosinophils are important contributors to antiparasite immunity.

Eosinophils. Eosinophils are a subtype of white blood cells derived from bone marrow pluripotent stem cells under the influence of IL-3, IL-5, and GM-CSF. They were named *eosinophils* because their granules stain red with acidic dyes such as eosin. They play a prominent role in both allergic reactions and inflammatory responses against helminthic parasites. Once they are released from the bone marrow and enter the blood, the eosinophil's half-life is only 8 to 18 hours, but in the tissues they can live up to 5 days.[65]

> Eosinophils and basophils are involved in both allergic reactions and antiparasite immunity.

Some eosinophil-derived mediators are preformed and stored in granules, while others are newly synthesized after activation. The mediators found in eosinophil granules include major basic protein (MBP), eosinophil cationic protein (ECP), Charcot-Leyden crystals (a lysophospholipase enzyme), and eosinophil peroxidase (EPX). Human MBP is cytotoxic to helminths and certain bacteria, but most importantly in terms of hypersensitivity diseases, is also able to damage upper respiratory epithelium.[66]

Eosinophils produce a number of different cytokines, including IL-4, which is present in increased amounts in the epithelial airways of patients with allergic diseases, and TGF-β1 which contributes to the histopathology of nasal polyps.[67] Eosinophils are very strong producers of cysLTs which contribute to their allergy-promoting effects.

Charcot-Leyden crystals are characteristic of eosinophils, although they are not unique to these cells. They are able to bind to the cell surface carbohydrates of microorganisms and are typically found at the sites of eosinophil accumulation, such as the sputum of asthmatic patients,[68] the "allergic mucin" of patients with fungal sinusitis[69] or in allergic rhinitis.[70]

Allergens

The understanding of hypersensitivity reactions is incomplete without an understanding of the allergens involved. Allergenicity, or the ability of an antigen to generate an allergic response, is not determined by any single biochemical or structural characteristic. The term *allergen* is used both to describe a macromolecular or cellular structure such as birch pollen, or to describe an individual allergenic protein (eg, Bet v 1 protein of birch). Individual proteins are also called *allergen components*. Allergens have been classified into major and minor. Major allergens are responsible for allergic sensitization in the majority of studied subjects. This is population dependent and arbitrary. Allergens can be classified on the basis of the anatomical site of the allergic reaction or on the mode of exposure (eg, aeroallergens, contact allergens, or food allergens). Allergenic substances can also be classified on the basis of their biochemical characteristics (eg, proteins, glycans), function (seed storage proteins; actin-associated muscle proteins), or cross-reactivity (eg, Bet v 1 homologs).

The biochemical nature of allergenic substances is somewhat restricted by the type of hypersensitivity reaction they provoke. With few exceptions, allergens involved in type I hypersensitivity are large molecules such proteins or glycans, or sometimes in the case of drugs, are haptens (small molecules that are incomplete antigens but bind to self-proteins to form complete allergens). The majority of allergens in type IV hypersensitivity reactions are small molecules or even individual elements (eg, metals). This section will focus on clinically important allergens involved in type I reactions. Our understanding of allergic diseases has been greatly enhanced by our understanding of the nature of individual allergens.

Allergen Nomenclature. The nomenclature of naturally occurring allergens involved in IgE-mediated allergies is maintained by the World Health Organization (WHO) and the International Union of Immunological Societies (IUIS) Allergen Nomenclature Sub-Committee. Allergens are named by the first 3 letters of the genus followed by a single letter from the species name and a number[71–73] (Figure 2–4). The cat major allergen, Fel d 1 derives its name from *Felis domesticus*. Allergens from a single species with greater than 67% homology are called *isoallergens* and are designated by 2 numbers following a decimal point (eg, the ragweed allergens Amb a 1.01 and Amb a 1.02). Polymorphic variants of the same protein (typically with >90% sequence identity) are called *isoforms* and are designated by 2 additional numbers.[71]

Allergen Structure and Biology. Although no single biochemical characteristic (linear or spatial structure, amino acid composition, glycosylation) has been found to confer allergenicity, allergens are restricted in their distribution to certain protein families. Even though the protein family (Pfam) database (release 26.0 http://pfam.xfam.org/) describes 13672 protein families, only 186 families contain described allergens (AllFam database http://www.meduniwien.ac.at/allergens/allfam/).[74] Only 20 families of protein contain 80% of all the currently described food allergens. Some recurrent themes include muscle proteins and actin binding proteins (tropomysin, profilins), storage proteins, and proteins with hydrophobic domains (lipid transfer proteins, Lipocalins). However, the reason why only some proteins are allergenic is not well understood. Table 2–3 lists the most common and significant allergenic protein families.

Aeroallergens

Pollen Allergens. Pollen allergies are caused by wind-pollinated (anemophilus) plants that produce large amounts of airborne pollen. Pollen yields per flower cluster (catkin) vary from 1.25 million pollen grains for oak trees to 6 million grains per catkin for birch trees. The estimated yield per birch tree in a season is over 5 billion pollen grains[75] Several species among plants are responsible for most pollen allergies, and these pollens have been characterized at the

Bet v 1.0103

$$= \frac{\text{Bet}}{3\ letters\ of Genus}\ \frac{\text{v}}{1\ letter\ of\ Species}\ \frac{1}{Allergen\ number} \cdot \frac{01}{Isoallergen}\ \frac{03}{Isoform}$$

Figure 2–4. Allergen nomenclature.

Table 2-3. Allergen Families

Allergen	Description	Allergen	Source
Plant Derived			
Prolamin superfamily[82]	Proline- and glutamine-rich storage proteins that have a conserved pattern of 6 or 8 cysteine residues that form intramolecular disulfide bonds; the disulfide bonds confer a degree of stability to heat, pH, and proteolysis[21]; this makes them potent food allergens		
2S Albumin	Group of seed storage proteins from a diverse group of dicot plants; major food allergens in several nuts; there is limited cross-reactivity across the group	Ara h 2	Major peanut allergen
		Ara h 6	Peanut
		Jug r 1	Walnut
		Cor a 8	Hazelnut
		Pru du 3	Almond
Nonspecific lipid transfer proteins (nsLTP)	Proteins characterized by a hydrophobic core; found in the epidermal layer of fruits and are major allergens in rosacea fruits[21]	Mal d 3	Apple
		Pru p 3	Peach
		Tri a 14	Wheat
Cereal prolamins	Wheat gliadins belong to this group and are important inducers of exercise-induced anaphylaxis	ω-gliadin/ Tri a 19	Wheat
Soybean hydrophobic protein	Similar to nsLTP; major allergen in soy	Gly m 1	Soy
Profilin	Ubiquitous actin-binding proteins that are highly conserved across plant species; found in pollens, plant foods, and latex and are responsible for the wide cross-reactivity between these allergens[22]; usually minor allergens (only 10%–20% patients sensitized) except in soy (50% sensitized)	Amb a 8	Ragweed pollen
		Art v 4	Mugwort pollen
		Bet v 2	Birch pollen
		Phl p 12	Timothy grass pollen
		Hev b 8	Latex
		Mus a 1	Banana
		Man i 3	Mango
		Pru du 4	Almond
PR10	Function of these proteins is not well understood, but they are widely distributed in pollen, seeds, and fruits; they are major inhalant allergens for birch and related trees; cross-reactive with fruit proteins and is the most common cause of pollen-food syndrome	Bet v 1	Birch
		Fag s 1	Beech
		Dau c 1	Carrot
		Mal d 1	Apple
		Fra a 1	Strawberry
		Ara h 8	Peanut
		Gly m 4	Soy
Cupin superfamily	Seed storage proteins that are major allergens in nuts, seeds, and legumes		
7S Globulin (vicillin)		Ana o 1	Cashew
		Ara h 1	Peanut
		Jug r 2	Walnut
		Ses i 3	Sesame
		Len c 1	Lentil

continues

Table 2–3. *continued*

Allergen	Description	Allergen	Source
11S Globulin (Legumin)		Ana o 2	Cashew
		Ara h 3	Peanut
		Ses i 6	Sesame
Expansins	Major grass pollen allergens; widely distributed in plants but are only significant causes of allergies to grass	Phl p 1	Timothy grass
Class I chitinase/Hevein like	The chief importance of this group of proteins is that they are the cause of latex-fruit syndrome	Hev b 6	Latex
		Pers a 1	Avocado
		Mus a 2	Banana
Animal Allergens			
Lipocalins	This group includes several very important inhalant and ingested allergens; these proteins transport small hydrophobic molecules, such as lipids and steroid hormones; they have low sequence similarity but share tertiary structure	Bos d 5 (beta lactoglobulin)	Cow's milk
		Can f 1	Dog
		Can f 2	Dog
		Fel d 4	Cat
Tropomyosin	Invertebrate tropomyosin that is highly conserved and widely distributed; responsible for cross-sensitization to various inhalant and ingested allergens	Bla g 7	Cockroach
		Chi o 1	Snow crab
		Der p 10	Dust mite
		Pen a 1	Shrimp
		Ani s 3	Anisakis nematode
Parvalbumins	Calcium-binding muscle proteins; major allergens in fish		
Serum albumin	Minor allergens in several species; highly cross-reactive; responsible for cat-pork syndrome		

structural and molecular levels. The chief tree pollen allergens in North America belong to the angiosperm families, Fagales (birch, alder, beech, and oak), Lamiales (ash, olive, and privet), and the some gymnosperms (cedar, juniper, and cypress). The principal allergens in angiosperm pollens are PR-10 (Bet v 1 related proteins), profilins, nsLTPs, Ole e 1-like proteins, and minor allergens such as polcalcins and isoflavone reductase (see Table 2–3). PR-10 proteins and profilins are widely distributed and highly cross-reactive.

Angiosperm Tree Pollen. Angiosperm trees and weeds belong to a larger class of tricolpates, all characterized by pollen grains that have 3 colpi or grooves and includes a large number of allergenic species (Figure 2–5A). Whereas cross-reactivity among members of the same family or subfamily commonly occurs, cross-reactivity across families is seen less often. Prominent exceptions to this are the beech (Fagaceae), birch (Betulaceae), and oak (Quercus) families. These pollens are among the most important contributors to springtime allergies, particularly in the Northeastern United States and in Scandinavian countries. Other members include alders and hornbeams. The major cross-reacting allergens in these species are pathogenesis-related protein group 10 (PR-10) proteins (group 1 allergens). The prototypical protein of this group is Bet v 1, the major allergen of birch pollen. PR-10 proteins from pollens, fruits, nuts, and vegetables

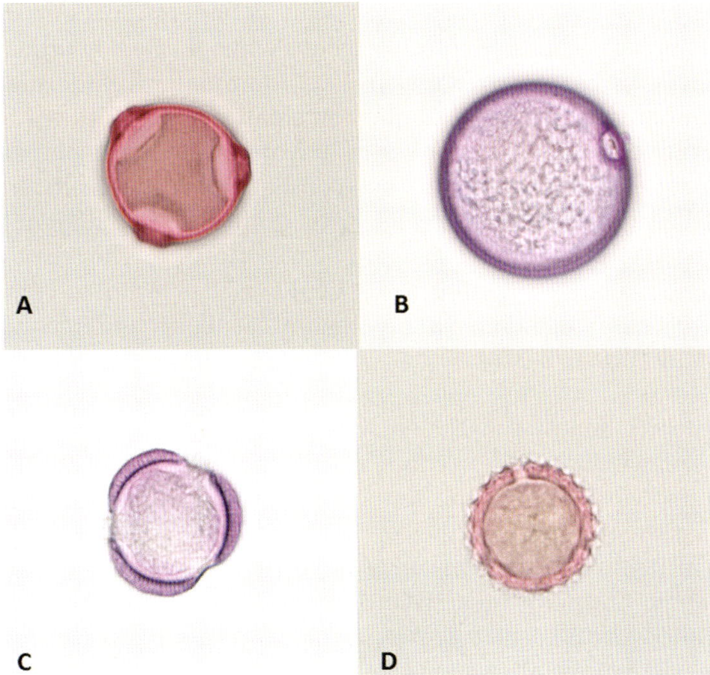

Figure 2–5. Microscopic view of pollen grains. **A.** Birch pollen, an example of tricolpate tree pollen. **B.** Monoporate grass pollen. **C.** Mugwort (*Artemisia*) pollen **D.** Spiny appearance of ragweed pollen. Images courtesy of Estelle Levetin, PhD, Biological Science, University of Tulsa.

show extensive cross-reactivity and are responsible for most cases of Pollen-Food syndrome. Profilins (group 2 allergens) are of lesser importance but also show extensive cross-reactivity.

Maple and Box elder pollens produce large amounts of pollen grains that have a prominent tricolpate structure, giving them a characteristic "beach ball" appearance on microscopy. There is extensive cross-reactivity within this family. Other families that include allergenically important trees include Salicaceae (Aspens, Poplars, and Cottonwoods), Rosales (Elms), and Oleaceae (Olives, Ash, and Privet). Olives are a key cause of pollen allergies in the Mediterranean region. Group 1 allergens (Ole e 1) are major allergens from Oleaceae. This protein shows homology to group 11 grass pollen allergens and soybean-trypsin inhibitor though the clinical significance of this homology is unclear.

Weed Pollens. Most clinically significant weeds belong to the following families: Amaranthecae (amaranths and chenopods); Polygonaceae (docks and sorrels); Asteraceae (ragweed and *Artemesia*); and Urticaceae (nettles and pellitory). On microscopy, amaranth-chenopod pollens are periporate, giving them a characteristic "golf ball appearance." In contrast, ragweed pollens have a "spiny appearance" (Figure 2–5D). Amaranths and ragweeds are extensively cross-reactive. The major allergen in ragweed is Amb a 1 (previously known as Antigen E or AgE). Ragweed extracts are often quantified using the concentration of AgE or Amb a 1. Cross-reactivity among other weeds is less consistent. Consequently, weed extracts for allergen immunotherapy should include all locally relevant species. Profilins (eg, Art v 4) from Mugwort (*Artemisia*) pollen (Figure 2–5C) frequently cross-react with vegetables and spices of the Apiaceae family (eg, celery, carrot, anise, and caraway) causing pollen-food syndromes such as Mugwort-Celery-Spice syndrome.

Grass Pollen. Most relevant allergenic grasses belong to the family Poaceae and its 3 subfamilies Pooideae, Panicoideae, and Chloridoideae. Northern grasses (Timothy, Kentucky Blue, fescue, ryegrass, orchard, and sweet vernal) belong to Pooideae and are characterized by extensive cross-reactivity due to a high degree of homology of allergen groups 1, two-thirds, and 5. This extensive cross-reactivity enables sublingual immunotherapy with a single species (timothy) to effectively treat grass pollen allergy. The southern grasses (Bahia and Johnson grass [Panicoideae] and Bermuda [Chloridoideae]) have limited cross-reactivity with northern grasses since they lack group 2 and 5 allergens. On microscopy, all grass pollen have a similar smooth, single-pore (monoporate) structure (Figure 2–5B).

Conifers. Allergenic conifers (gymnosperms) belong to the family Cupressaceae, which includes cedars, junipers, and cypress trees. Most patients are sensitized to Group 1 and 2 allergens. Both families of allergens are involved in pectin metabolism and show extensive homology and cross-reactivity among species. Group 1 allergens are pectate lyases, and group 2 allergens are polymethylgalacturonases. Conifers share minor antigens such as profilins with angiosperms, but these are rarely clinically relevant.[75]

Allergens From Animal Sources

Mammalian Allergens. Mammalian allergens include common household indoor allergens (pets) and occupational allergens (laboratory animals). Pet sensitization is associated with more severe asthma.[76] The major mammalian allergens are epidermal proteins or secreted proteins, from saliva, sweat, urine, or milk. With the exception of the cat, major mammalian allergens tend to be lipocalins. Most lipocalins do not show sequence homology or cross-reactivity even within the same species.[77] A clinically significant exception to this are the dog (Can f 2) and cat (Fel d 4) allergens that show clinical cross-reactivity though they have little sequence homology. This may be important for cat and dog cosensitization. Can f 2 also shares a high degree of sequence homology with other allergens, including mouse (Mus m 1), rat (Rat n 1), horse (Equ c 1), and cow (Bos d 1). Other common allergens include serum proteins such as albumins and immunoglobulin molecules. Serum albumins are usually minor allergens but have a high degree of sequence homology and cross-reactivity. For example, cat Fel d 2 cross-reacts with several mammalian albumins and is responsible for the Cat-Pork syndrome, where some cat-allergic patients have food-allergic reactions when they eat mammalian meats such as pork.

Mammalian epidermal allergens are present on small size particles (<1 to 20 μm). About 15% to 20% of pet allergen is on particles <5 μm in size and consequently can remain airborne for extended periods of time.[74,75,78,79] Rodent allergens have a similar distribution.[74,78] This may explain the immediate oculonasal symptoms commonly experienced by many cat allergy sufferers when they enter buildings where cats reside. This small size also allows these respirable particles access to the smallest airways, triggering asthma symptoms. On the other hand, a surprising protective effect of early life exposure to cat allergen has been observed in several studies.[80,81]

Cat allergen can transfer easily on clothing, and levels are measureable in most homes and public places, even where there are no cats residing.[79,82,83] Due to this property, cat allergen has been described as being "sticky." This may be important for the sensitization of individuals who have never lived in cat-containing households. The major cat allergen is Fel d 1 which is a secretoglobin secreted from salivary, sebaceous, and anal glands. Fel d 2 (cat albumin) is an important allergen in only a minority of patients. Other cat allergens include Fel d3 (cystatin), Fel d 4 (lipocalin), Fel d 5 (IgA), and Fel d 6 (IgM).

The major dog allergens are Can f 1 and Can f 2, which are lipocalins with little sequence homology. A little over half of all subjects are sensitized to Can f 1. Other dog allergens include Can f 3 (serum albumin), Can f 4 (lipid-binding odorant-carrying protein), Can f 5 (prostatic kallikrein), and Can f 6 (lipocalin). Like cat allergens, dog allergens accumulate in house dust, are airborne, and transfer readily on clothing.

Unlike cat and dog allergens, which are epithelial, the major allergens of mouse and rat are secreted in the urine. Over 80% of mouse and rat allergic subjects are Mus m 1 or Rat n 1 sensitized, respectively. Both of these proteins are lipocalins that show sequence homology to each other. These allergens remain suspended in the air as small (<7 μm), respirable particles, and are widely dispersed. Perhaps as a result of this easy dispersibility, inner-city studies have documented mouse allergen in up to 95% of households.[84] The National Cooperative Inner City Asthma Study (NCICAS) demonstrated a correlation between mouse allergen levels, mouse IgE antibodies, asthma biomarkers, and declining lung function in asthmatic adolescents.[81,85]

Dust Mite Allergen. Dust mites are microscopic, sightless arachnids. The most common species in North America are *Dermatophagoides pteronyssinus* and *Dermatophagoides farinae*. *D. pteronyssinus* has a worldwide distribution. In Southern states such as Florida and the Caribbean, the tropical mite, *B. tropicalis*, is an important allergen. These mites feed on host skin scales and other material. They harvest moisture from the atmosphere and their survival depends on the presence of a high relative humidity (>50%). They thrive in a narrow temperature range (65°F to 80°F). This property can be exploited for dust mite control, and mites are killed by exposure to temperatures above 140°F (standard clothing dryer appliance). Several dust mite allergens have been described that are grouped by homology. Group 1 allergens (Der p 1 and Der f 1) are part of the peritrophic membrane, a matrix secreted around food that partitions indigestible food particles from nutrients. The peritrophic membrane is excreted with the fecal pellets, which are ideally sized (10 to 35 μm) to serve as aeroallergens (Figure 2–6). As a result, whole culture extracts (mites + feces) have a substantially higher concentration of group 1 dust mite allergens than pure mite bodies. Group 2 allergens are somatic antigens with a high degree of sequence homology. Der p 10 is a tropomyosin "pan-allergen" that cross-reacts with cockroach and crustacean tropomyosins. Dust mite allergen is usually found on particles 10 μm or larger. As a result, undisturbed mite allergen is seldom airborne. However, mite allergen that has settled on bedding is in close proximity to sleeping individuals. Unlike pet allergens, where a protective effect has been noted with early exposure, exposure to high levels of allergen at 1 year of age is associated with an increased risk of asthma development and lower age of onset of symptoms.[86] Several studies have highlighted the association between dust mite sensitization and asthma or rhinitis. High levels of dust mite IgE correlate with a greater severity of atopic dermatitis.

Dust mite extracts for testing and immunotherapy can be manufactured from mites or cultures. In the United States, the US Food and Drug Administration (FDA) has standardized *D. pteronyssinus* and *D. farinae* extracts and requires that these be derived from isolated mites. In Europe both the mite body and mite culture extracts are available. Unlike mite body extracts, which contain nearly equal amounts of group 1 and group 2 allergens, culture extracts, which include fecal pellets, have a relative abundance of group 2 allergens. In the United States, dust mite allergens are standardized using an intradermal

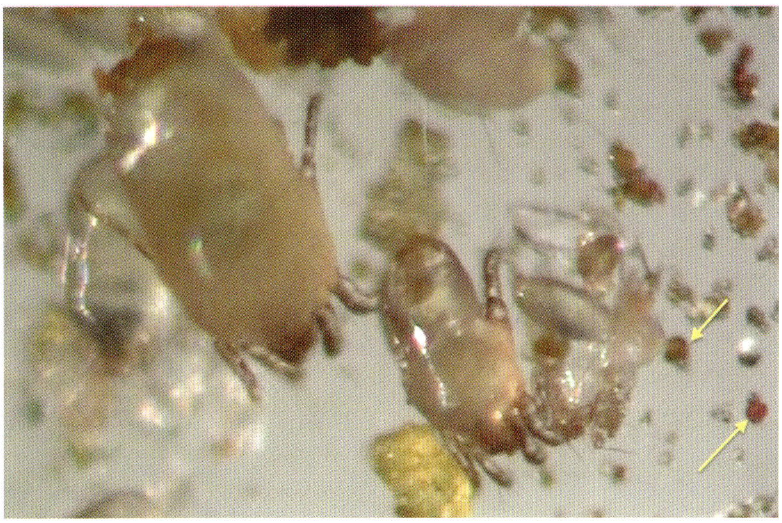

Figure 2–6. Dust mites and mite feces. Arrows point to mite fecal particles. Reprinted with permission from Jeffrey Miller, MD. Copyright © Mission: Allergy, Inc.

human bioassay, and standards are maintained at the Center for Biologics Evaluation and Research (CBER).

Cockroach Allergen. The 2 major species of cockroach found in the United States are the German cockroach (*Blattella germanica*) and the American cockroach (*Periplaneta americana*). Cockroach is a particularly important allergen in inner-city asthma. Cockroach-sensitized asthmatic children exposed to high levels of roach allergen had significantly higher morbidity.[87] The German cockroach is found worldwide and is the dominant species in North America. The principal cockroach allergens are Bla g 1, Bla g 2, and Bla g 4. Most subjects are sensitized to Bla g 2, a species-specific allergen. Bla g 1 cross-reacts with Per a 1, the dominant allergen in the American cockroach. The allergens are somatic allergens but are also found in fecal matter. Fecal matter may be a more important source of airborne allergen.

Fungal Allergens. Fungi are ubiquitous eukaryotes that are usually saprophytic organisms. They have complex life cycles involving a sexual and an asexual reproductive cycle. They are morphologically characterized by their hyphal structure and by the shape and structure of their spores, which either develop in sacs called *asci* (Ascomycota) or *sporangia* (Zygomycota). Modern techniques of speciation involve a polymerase chain reaction (PCR)-based method that sequences the internal transcribed spacer (ITS) of ribosomal RNA. Allergies can develop to the spores or the hyphal antigens and can often be triggered by submicron-sized particles. Due to their complex lifestyle, source material for making allergen extracts is important and hyphal cultures may not contain spore-derived allergens. Some allergens such as heat shock proteins, enolases, aldehyde dehydrogenases, and thioredoxins are shared across species. They may be the major or minor allergen depending on the species. However, many species possess species-specific allergens. The functions of some of the major allergens such as Alt a 1 from Alternaria and Cla h 1 from Cladosporium are not known.

Food Allergens

Over 90% of anaphylactic food allergies are caused by 8 foods: milk, egg, peanut, tree nuts, wheat, soy, fish, and shellfish. The relative clinical importance of specific allergens can vary based on dietary practices. Buckwheat is a common allergen in Japan where it is commonly used in the production of foods such as soba noodles, but not an important food allergen in the United States. Allergens can be classified as type 1 allergens—heat-stable allergens associated with anaphylactic reaction and gastrointestinal sensitization—and type 2 allergens—heat-labile allergens usually associated with oral allergy syndrome and primary respiratory sensitization. Most type 1 allergens are high protein–content foods that are introduced early in life. Type 2 allergens in contrast tend to be fruits and vegetables.

Milk. There are 2 major classes of proteins in milk: caseins and whey proteins. Caseins constitute 70% to 80% the total protein content of milk by weight and are more likely to be clinically relevant allergens compared to whey proteins. Whey proteins include β-lactoglobulin, α-lactalbumin, immunoglobulins, bovine serum albumin (BSA), and small amounts of various other proteins. Whey proteins (particularly BSA) are probably the cause of beef cross-reactivity observed in about 10% of milk allergic individuals. Beta-lactoglobulin and α-lactalbumin are thermolabile and after 60 minutes of extensive heating are virtually undetectable.[88] Caseins are not destroyed by heat but do undergo conformational changes. What distinguishes baked milk-reactive individuals from baked milk-tolerant individuals is the ability of their IgEs to bind linear epitopes and to recognize extensively heated caseins.[84,88] Mammalian milk such as goat milk extensively cross-reacts with cow's milk and hence is a poor substitute in cow's milk allergy.[89]

Egg. Over 20 allergenic proteins have been identified in chicken eggs. However, the chief allergens are ovomucoid (OVM) (Gal d 1), ovalbumin (OVA) (Gal d 2), ovotransferrin (Gal d 3), and lysozyme (Gal d 4). Ovomucoid is the most allergenic protein, and this may be due, at least in part, to its heat stability.[90] The presence of antibody against sequential epitopes is associated with persistent allergy and like milk, may be one of the distinguishing characteristics between baked egg-tolerant and baked egg-sensitive individuals, although this has not been demonstrated conclusively.[84,86,88,90]

Peanut. Peanut is the most common food allergy in school-age children. The major allergens are Ara h 1, Ara h 2, and Ara h 3. Ara h 1, 2, and 3 are seed storage proteins belonging to the vicillin, conglutinin, and glycinin families. Ara h 4 and Ara h 6 appear to be isoforms of Ara h 3 and Ara h 2, respectively. Ara h 8 is a PR 10 protein that is commonly found to be elevated in patients with birch pollinosis and is a common cause of positive peanut skin tests in patients without clinical allergic symptoms. Ara h 5 is a profilin. Allergic responses to several other proteins have been described in peanut.

Immune responses against Ara h 2 are associated with a greater likelihood of being associated with clinical allergy and with increased severity of allergic reactions.[87,91] Ara h 2 is 100 times more allergenically potent than Ara 1 and Ara h3, by basophil activation and allergy skin tests.[92] This may be due to the heat and pepsin stability of Ara h 2 that results from its many disulfide bridges. Ara h 1 antibodies have been found in over 80% of peanut allergic patients. Ara h 1 is a glycosylated protein that has been shown to stimulate Th2 skewed immune responses in dendritic cells via the receptor DC-SIGN.[93]

Tree Nuts. As a group, tree nuts are a prominent cause of food allergies and anaphylaxis, particularly in children. The rate of resolution of these allergies is low (probably <5%). Walnuts and cashews are the most common causes of tree nut allergies.[94] Other nuts, including almonds, pecans, pistachios, hazelnuts, brazil nuts, macadamia nuts, and pine nuts, are less frequent causes of allergic reactions. There is a high degree of cross-reactivity between walnuts and pecans and cashews and pistachios, respectively. The principal allergens in tree nuts are vicillins, 2S albumins, and lipid transfer protein (Table 2–4). Hazelnuts have high levels of a PR 10 protein Cor a 1 which leads to frequent positive tests and oral allergy syndrome in some patients with birch pollinosis.

Table 2-4. Tree Nut Allergens

Type of Nut	Allergen Type: LTP	Storage Proteins	Profilin	PR10
Peanut	Ara h 9	Ara h 1 Ara h 2 Ara h 3 Ara h 6 Ara h 7	Ara h 5	Ara h 8
Walnut	Jug r 3	Jug r 1 Jug r 2 Jug r 4		
Pecan		Car i 1		
Cashew		Ana o 1 Ana o 2 Ana o 3		
Pistachio		Pis v 1 Pis v 2 Pis v 3		
Almond	Pru du 3	Pru du 6	Pru du 4	
Hazelnut	Cor a 8	Cor a 9 Cor a 11	Cor a 2	Cor a 1
Brazil nut				
Soy	Gly m 1	Gly m 5 Gly m 6	Gly m 3	Gly m 4

Wheat and Other Grains. Cereal grains like wheat contain several allergenically important proteins. The globulin and glutenins are major wheat allergens (eg, Tri a 20, Tri a 26), and omega-5 gliadin (Tri a 19) is an important cause of food-dependent exercise-induced anaphylaxis.[95] Alpha-amylase inhibitors (AAIs) and α-amylase/trypsin inhibitors (AATIs) such as Tri a 15 (monomeric alpha amylase inhibitor are involved in respiratory allergies (occupational asthma in bakers) and food allergic reactions, while lipid transfer proteins are involved in allergic reactions to wheat- and barley-derived beers. Cross-reactivity is present between wheat, barley, and rye. AAIs and AATIs have been identified in barley and rye as well, and profilins are ubiquitous in all the grains.

Soy. Soy is ubiquitous in processed foods. It has gained importance as an alternative source of a high-quality protein and as a food substitute for milk and egg allergic children. The soybean, also known as edamame, can be processed into a flour, milk, and curd (tofu). Various soy derivatives are also found in processed foods. Soy lecithin, which is protein free, is commonly used as an emulsifier and is not allergenic. The major soy allergens are the lipid transfer protein, Gly m 1, and seed storage proteins of the cupin family, Gly m 5 and Gly m 6. In addition, Gly m 1 has been implicated as a cause of occupational asthma from exposure to soy hulls. Gly m 2 is also important for aeroallergies. Gly m 3, a profilin, and Gly m 4, a Bet v 1–related protein, are labile components that may be important causes of pollen-food syndrome.

Fruits and Vegetables. The labile allergens, PR10 and profilins, are the most common fruit and vegetable allergens. The major allergens from *Rosaceae* species (eg, apple [Mal d 1], cherry [Pru av 1], apricot [Pru ar 1], and pear [Pyr c 1]) and *Apiaceae* species (carrot [Dau c 1], celery [Api g 1]) are all PR10 proteins. Anaphylactic reactions due to *Rosaceae* fruits are caused by LTP antigen (Pru p 3 in peach and Mal d 3 in apple).

Fish. The major allergen in bony fish is parvalbumin (eg, Gal c 1 in cod fish). Cross-reactivity among fish is common. Many patients who react to fish are able to tolerate extensively cooked tuna and salmon in canned form. This may be because of a 100-fold lower parvalbumin content in the muscle of fish such as tuna and salmon compared to fish like carp.[92,96] Other allergens that have been identified in fish include the fish proteins, enolase and aldolase. Some patients who react to tropical fish are sensitized to unique allergens other than parvalbumin. Allergy to the fish nematode, *Anisakis* can develop in some individuals and lead to a history of inconsistent fish allergic reactions.[97] There is cross-reactivity between *Anisakis* and other invertebrate allergens.

Shellfish. Shellfish are a major cause of food allergic reactions in US adults, affecting up to 2.3% of the population.[98] It is the most common cause of new onset anaphylactic food allergies in adults. There are 2 major groups of shellfish that are consumed worldwide—crustaceans (shrimp, crab, lobster, crayfish) and mollusks (clams, scallops, squid, octopus, mussels, and oysters). Tropomyosin is the major allergen in adults with crustacean allergy. It widely cross-reacts with tropomyosins in other invertebrates, including dust mites and cockroaches.[95,99] Myosin light chain is another major allergen that has been identified in shellfish allergies, and in some shellfish-allergic children, the sarcoplasmic calcium-binding protein has been identified as a major allergen.[100]

Carbohydrate Allergens (α-Gal)

Immunoglobulin E (IgE) antibodies to the galactose-α-1,3-galactose (α-Gal) moiety are now recognized as the basis of a unique delayed allergic reaction to certain mammalian meats, as well as some respiratory allergies (cats and dogs). This carbohydrate moiety is widely present in nonhuman primates. The pathogenesis of this unique allergy involves being bitten by the lone star tick (*Amblyomma americanum*). The exact mechanism of the induction of an IgE response to α-Gal after the tick bite is not well understood.[101] Mammalian meat allergic reactions usually occur about 6 hours after the ingestion of the allergen. Interestingly, this sugar is also found on the monoclonal antibody Cetuximab, and similar anaphylactic reactions to this biologic agent have been described in post tick bite α-Gal sensitized individuals.

Protective Role of Immediate Hypersensitivity

Immunoglobulin (IgE)-mediated hypersensitivity is not only involved in generating typical allergic reactions. Its major function is to protect the body against pathogens like worms, insects, and parasites that are too large to be eliminated by the other types of immunity (antibodies or effector cells). Frequent observations of elevated serum IgE levels in helminth-infected patients were one of the initial clues that IgE may help defend against parasites. The role of IgE in antiparasite immunity has been extensively studied using mice made IgE deficient by gene targeting, who develop impaired antischistosomal immunity.[102] In addition, IgE antibodies are required for the elimination of helminthic worms such as *Trichinella* from the intestine.[103]

It is known that IgE-mediated hypersensitivity requires exposure to certain antigens to which the cells involved in the allergic immune response were previously sensitized. However, in addition to this antigen-dependent mechanism of allergic reactions, antigen-independent effects of IgE have been described regarding mast cell biology, including activation, migration, adhesion, and production of mast cell mediators.[104] These mechanisms are not fully understood, but studies investigating IgE-mast cell interaction show that in the absence of a specific antigen, IgE can serve as a mast cell growth factor or can trigger cytokine production by mast cells through signaling via FcεRI.[105]

New physiological IgE roles, not clearly defined yet, have been proposed during the last years. One of them is possible involvement of IgE in fighting against certain neoplasms. This has been observed with IgE monoclonal antibody against mouse mammary tumor virus,[106] colorectal adenorcarcinoma,[107] and ovarian carcinoma,[108] where it inhibited tumor growth.

Diagnosis of Immediate Hypersensitivity

Extensive evidence has defined the role of T_H2 cells in atopic individuals by producing IL-4 (which leads to IgE synthesis) and IL-5 (resulting in recruitment and maturation of eosinophils), and elevated IgE levels are found in patients with a variety of allergic diseases. Diagnostic tests for allergic diseases have been developed based on these immune mechanisms. Methods for diagnosing type I hypersensitivity reactions are discussed in more detail in Chapter 3.

The test of choice is the skin test, which involves the appearance of a wheal-and-flare reaction at the site of skin puncture with an allergen.

Another diagnostic test is the measurement of allergen-specific IgE levels in the serum. The diagnostic value of measuring serum-specific IgE is comparable to skin testing, especially for environmental and food allergens, and is the test of choice in infants and in patients with severe allergic reactions in whom skin testing would expose them to unnecessary risks. The levels of specific IgE do not exactly correlate with disease severity but indicate the probability of developing an allergic reaction when exposed to the tested allergen.

> Type I reactions are diagnosed by skin testing or by measurement of allergen-specific serum IgE levels.

Nasal challenges with specific allergens are rarely performed but represent an important diagnostic tool especially in the diagnosis of patients with local allergic rhinitis. These patients develop nasal symptoms after exposure to an environmental allergen, but their skin tests are negative and the serum-specific IgE levels are normal. The immunologic phenotype of these patients is characterized by local nasal production of specific IgE, and they have a T_H2 nasal cellular response to aeroallergens.[109,110]

> Nasal challenges can be performed if skin testing and specific IgE levels are negative, but there is a strong suspicion for allergic rhinitis.

Treatment

There are essentially 3 treatments for most allergic problems: environmental control, medications, and allergic immunotherapy.

Environmental Control

Introduction. All allergic disorders are caused by exposure to external allergens. It is therefore intuitive that avoidance or elimination of exposures to these agents should reduce allergy symptoms and reverse allergic inflammation. There is evidence that this is the case, and as a result, environmental control measures should be a part of the treatment regimen for all patients with allergic disease.[111] Most measures are directed toward controlling the indoor environment, but there are some measures for reducing exposure to outdoor allergens such as pollens that can be helpful as well. For indoor allergen avoidance, it is difficult for patients to completely control everything in the home. It is therefore useful to focus on the sleep environment, which is where most individuals spend the most amount of time in a recumbent position, exposed to the most allergens. It is also useful to institute allergen elimination measures for any other areas in the home where patients are exposed to obvious allergens (ie, recreation rooms with carpets where children lie on the floor, or damp, moldy basement rooms where adult patients exercise or have a study) and for places outside the home where specific allergen exposures exist such as work sites or schools (dust, animals or fumes). In general, it is helpful to try and minimize exposure to as many potential allergens as possible rather than limit elimination measures only to those allergens to which the patient has documented sensitization, since no type of allergy testing has a positive predictive value of 100%, and even in individuals who are not currently sensitized, continued exposure to allergen increases the risk of future sensitization. Studies have shown that the most effective environmental control regimens are those that involve elimination of all allergens, while those that focus on single allergens have not been as successful.[112]

General Indoor Environmental Control Measures. The objective of these measures is to minimize exposure to the most common indoor allergens (dust mites, pet dander, feathers, mold spores, and other allergens in dust such as cockroach and mouse). A simple and useful scheme for reducing bedroom allergen exposure is shown in Table 2–5.

Animals and Pets. Step 1 is to try a reduce exposure to mammalian pets. The major source of most mammalian allergens is shed skin proteins ("dander"). Most patients are unwilling or unable to get rid of their pets, so the most reasonable and practical approach is to keep pets out of the bedroom at all times. Once the pet stays out of the bedroom, thorough washing/cleaning of all the bedding and upholstered furniture is necessary to eliminate residual pet allergen (dander). It is also useful to cover the bed with some type of spread during the day that is removed at night in case the pet does get into the room. There is no good evidence that frequent washing of pets is useful in significantly reducing allergen in the home.[113] Similarly, there is no evidence that any type of cat or dog is significantly less allergenic despite commercial claims to the contrary.[114] It should be noted that this advice about pet elimination only holds for the treatment of already sensitized patients. In contrast, there is evidence that exposure to some household pets during the first year of life is protective against the development of asthma.[115]

Feathers. Step 2 is to remove any feather- or down-containing bedding (pillows, comforters, or mattress pillow tops). Alternatively, it is possible to encase these items with allergen-impermeable covers (discussed below). The allergenic potential of feather or down bedding is surprisingly controversial, but there are reports suggesting an association with asthma[116] and with more serious respiratory disorders such as hypersensitivity pneumonitis ("feather duvet lung").[117] It has been our experience that removal or covering of these items can be very helpful in some patients and is easy to do.

Forced Air Ventilation. Most dust particles are heavy and do not remain in the ambient air for very long. However, if there is any form of forced air ventilation in the home (heating or central air conditioning), dust particles remain suspended and become more of a problem for allergic patients. In addition, allergens such as dust and mold spores collect in forced air ductwork and contribute to patients' allergic exposures. Because of this, allergic patients should try to avoid living in homes with forced air ventilation. If this is not possible, then it is important that the air be filtered as well as possible (Step 3). For most patients who have access, this can be done by inserting disposable filters (eg, Filtrete®) into the forced air unit. These filters are available in most hardware stores and come in various efficiencies of particle removal. In general, patients should use the highest efficiency filters that they can afford, and the filters should be changed every 3 months if the forced air units are in frequent use. More permanent, central high-efficiency particulate aggregate (HEPA) purification units are also available.

Humidifiers. Step 4 is to reduce humidity in the bedroom. Constant humidification of bedroom air fosters the growth of dust mites and mold spores.[118] If the home is centrally humidified, the humidity should be set below 50%. Continuous use of free-standing bedroom humidifiers or other sources of

Table 2-5. General Instructions for Reducing Allergen Exposure in the Sleep Environment

The Allergen-Free Bedroom	
All surroundings of the dust-sensitive patient should be as free as possible from any dust. This is the single most important step in treatment of asthma and allergies. Do as much as you can, since anything you do will be helpful.	
Step 1. Pets	Remove any furry or feathered animals from the bedroom, permanently. No pets should ever be in the bedroom, even when the patient is not there.
Step 2. Bedding	Discard any feather (or down) pillows or quilts. Use hypoallergenic (polyester) pillows and washable blankets. Blankets should be washed immediately and then frequently to keep them dust free.
Step 3. Heating and air conditioning	Forced air ventilation is very bad for patients. Buy filter material (Vent-gard or equivalent) and install in the bedroom air inlet vent, so that all the air that enters the room is filtered. Wash or change this filter every month.
Step 4. Humidifiers	Do not regularly use humidifiers of any kind. Increased humidity increases the growth of dust mites and molds and will make you worse. The most effective way to keep your air passages comfortable during the night is to keep the bedroom very cold (55°F–60°F).
Step 5. Allergen impermeable covers	The patient's bed must have special allergy covers that completely encase any pillows, the mattress, and the box spring. Do this even on new bedding.
Step 6. Rugs	Remove any rugs and carpets. All rugs trap dust whether they are wool or synthetics. Hardwood or vinyl floors are preferable, but a washable throw rug can be used. If it is impossible to remove carpeting, vigorous vacuuming must be performed daily.
Step 7. Vacuum cleaners	Vacuum cleaners blow a lot of fine dust out the back. Purchase special allergen-proof vacuum cleaner bags. HEPA vacuum cleaners work well but are very expensive.
Step 8. HEPA air purifiers	HEPA room air purifiers are very useful when there are allergens floating in the air in your bedroom, such as pet dander, mold spores, or cigarette smoke, or if there is forced air ventilation. They can run all the time, but only when the door and windows are closed.
Step 9. General cleanup and other dust collectors	Remove all upholstered furniture, drapes, old books and newspapers, and stuffed animals. Wooden or metal chairs and plain light curtains can be used. Clean the woodwork and floors to remove all traces of dust.
Step 10. Regular cleaning	The room must be cleaned daily and given a thorough and complete cleaning once a week. Clean the floors, furniture, tops of doors, window frames, sills, etc, with a damp cloth. Air the room thoroughly but keep the door of this room closed as much as possible. Remember, the cleaner the room, the better the patient will feel.

humidity (pots of water on the steam radiators) should be avoided. Dryness of the nasal mucosa at night comes from high ambient temperatures, and patients can avoid this problem by keeping the bedroom as cold as tolerable at night.

Bedding Covers. Step 5 is to encase the pillows, mattress, and box spring in allergen-impermeable covers. This will reduce patient exposure to dust mites, dust mite feces, and any other allergens that settle onto or into the bedding.[119] Anything that is not encased should be washed weekly. Washing in hot water and/or drying in a clothing dryer is usually sufficient to kill any dust mites and destroy most allergens.[120] Encasings that are made of tightly woven cotton (pore size <6 μm) are the most effective and are available from many allergy supply companies. These should be washed several times/

year to remove any settled dust. Plastic covers are much less expensive but are not as comfortable as the woven cotton covers. They also need to be wiped down frequently. However, if cost is an issue, plastic covers are better than no covers at all.

Rugs and Carpets. Step 6 is to remove carpeting from the bedroom. All forms of carpeting (wool, synthetic, shag, or flat) act as dust and allergen reservoirs and should be removed. Hard floors of some type (wood, tile, or vinyl) are preferable. If the carpeting cannot be removed, it is important to vacuum it frequently to try and remove residual dust, although this will be only partially successful. Similarly, other potential dust collectors should be removed from the bedroom (upholstered furniture or heavy, nonwashable drapes). Vacuuming is best done with a special vacuum cleaner that contains a built-in HEPA filter[121] (Step 7). Vacuuming with an ordinary vacuum cleaner does not trap small allergenic particles, and vacuuming will spread these in the air.

Air Purifiers. Step 8 is to install a HEPA air purifier in the room if airborne allergens are present. Most dust particles are heavy and quickly settle out, so a HEPA air purifier is usually not necessary to remove these. However, other allergens, such as pet danders and mold spores, are contained on smaller particles that remain airborne, and HEPA air purifiers are useful for removing these. There is some evidence that HEPA air purifiers are helpful in certain situations.[122] In general, most HEPA air purifiers are made to clean the air in a single room and need to be matched to the size of the room. In order to be useful, the doors and windows need to be closed when the purifier is in operation. They can be purchased commercially from many different sources including department and appliance stores, websites, and allergy supply companies.

General Cleaning and Removal of Dust Collectors. The last steps (9 and 10) include removal of dust collectors and other allergen sources (old newspapers, stuffed animals) and performing regular cleaning of the room to keep dust accumulation to a minimum. Generally, it is helpful to limit a child to one favorite stuffed animal that can be washed regularly in hot water.

Mold Spore Elimination. Mold spore exposure in a home, especially in a sleep environment, can cause serious respiratory problems even in non-mold-allergic patients, so it is important to identify any mold exposure problem and remediate it.[123] Obvious signs of mold growth include surface stains, surface dampness, and musty or moldy odors. Frequently, patients will not be aware of a mold problem, but visitors will remark on a moldy odor or will comment that they experience symptoms (cough or sneeze) after entering the patient's home. Molds only grow indoors where there is source of moisture, so identifying and removing the source is essential. Typical water sources in apartments include leaky pipes, leaks from apartments or the roof above the patient, and leaks from steam radiators or air conditioners. One serious problem for patients who live in brick apartment buildings is that with age, the mortar between the bricks cracks and allows water intrusion into the apartments when it rains. Fixing this problem requires a great deal of effort and involves replacing all the old mortar in the outer walls ("re-pointing the bricks"). This is typically done by the building owner and is usually not under the control of the patient, but if it is not done, water will continue to enter the apartment and mold growth will continue. Obvious mold growth and stains can be removed by washing with a dilute bleach solution, but unless the underlying water intrusion problem is corrected, the molds will continue to grow and will remain a health problem.

Vermin Elimination. The most common allergenic vermin in homes include cockroaches and mice. Cockroach allergen exposure is a known cause of asthma morbidity.[124,125] However, most patients are not aware that cockroach allergen becomes part of the dust in a home and that it is not necessary to see living cockroaches in order to have allergic problems from cockroaches. Eradication of cockroach allergen involves a combination of pest control measures and the dust elimination measures described previously. For allergic patients, integrated pest management that uses multiple different elimination measures is safer and more effective than simply relying on insecticides and is the recommended procedure.[126]

Mice can also be a significant cause of allergic problems, in part because they normally excrete an allergenic protein in their urine that becomes widely distributed throughout homes.[127] Integrated pest management measures should be instituted to eliminate mice, but in many cases professional extermination may be necessary.[128]

More recently, in some areas of the United States, home infestation with Asian ladybugs and brown marmorated stink bugs has become a problem, and these often cause allergic problems for patients.[129,130] Their eradication usually requires professional extermination.

Pollen Avoidance. For patients who are highly allergic to pollen and experience significant symptoms during pollination seasons, there are a number of simple measures that can be taken that reduce pollen exposure and help reduce symptoms (Table 2–6).

Table 2-6. Pollen Avoidance Measures

Monitor pollen counts and minimize outdoor exposure when pollen counts are very high.
Stay indoors on dry, windy days.
Avoid outdoor activity like running in the early morning when pollen counts are highest.
Keep doors and windows closed during pollen season and try to use air conditioning in the home.
Do not hang laundry outside since pollen sticks to these items.
Drive with car windows closed and use air conditioning.
Avoid mowing the lawn or raking leaves, which stirs up pollen and molds.
Wear a dust mask when performing outdoor activities such as gardening.
After being outside, remove external clothing items that may be covered with pollen and hang them near the front entrance to the house.
Shower and wash hair after being outside.

Medications

Antihistamine Therapy. The term *antihistamine* used in the medical literature is generally reserved for medications that inhibit the effects of histamine on H_1-histamine receptors. All antihistamines act as inverse agonists that combine with and stabilize the inactive form of the H_1-receptor, shifting the equilibrium toward the inactive state.[131]

Antihistamines have a number of clinical indications, ranging from allergic conditions such as rhinitis, dermatitis, conjunctivitis, drug allergies to nonallergic conditions such as motion sickness, vertigo, and insomnia.[132] Antihistamines are the most common treatment used in allergic diseases and can be administered orally, intramuscularly, intravenously intranasally, or as ophthalmic preparations.

> H1 antihistamine therapy is the most common treatment used in allergic diseases.

H1 antihistamines are generally categorized as first- or second-generation drugs. First-generation H1 antihistamines (eg, diphenhydramine, hydroxyzine, and chlorpheniramine) are lipophilic substances that can easily cross the blood-brain barrier resulting in sedation and drowsiness with cognitive impairment. They are also competitive inhibitors of muscarinic receptors and have significant anticholinergic effects (eg, dry mouth, drying nasal secretions, blurry vision, urinary retention, and tachycardia).

> First-generation H1 antihistamines are sedating because they easily cross the blood-brain barrier due to their lipophilic structure.

Second-generation H1 antihistamines (eg, loratadine, desloratadine, fexofenadine, cetirizine, and levocetirizine) have higher specificity for binding H1 receptors, do not cross the blood-brain barrier, and are relatively nonsedating. It is important to understand that several of the second-generation agents are not completely free of sedative effects when given at higher doses. Compared with first-generation agents, they also have a lower binding affinity for muscarinic receptors and have less anticholinergic side effects.[133]

In addition to their antiallergic effects, antihistamines also have some anti-inflammatory properties and can inhibit mast cell activation and mediator release, inhibit expression of adhesion molecules and eosinophil chemotaxis.[134] Due to these properties, antihistamines can also decrease nasal obstruction, an effect that is mostly seen with the second-generation drugs.[135] Most antihistamines are metabolized in the liver by cytochrome P450, except cetirizine and levocetirizine which are renally excreted. Fexofenadine is secreted into the biliary tract without any metabolic change and is then eliminated through the intestine. Understanding of their metabolism helps determine which medications to use in patients with severe liver or kidney dysfunction and can prevent harmful drug interactions, especially when medications metabolized in the liver by cytochrome P450 are given concomitantly.

In patients with allergic rhinoconjunctivitis, antihistamines relieve nasal and conjunctival itching, rhinorrhea, and nasal congestion and improve quality of life.[136] Topical intranasal and ophthalmic medications have a more rapid onset of action than orally administered antihistamines, but usually require administration several times a day.

Other histamine receptor antagonists such as ranitidine act primarily on H2 receptors. The combination of H1 and H2 antihistamine medications significantly relieves rhinorrhea and diminishes allergen-induced reduction of nasal blood flow.[137]

Glucocorticoids. Glucocorticoids are widely used to treat a variety of allergic diseases because they are potent inhibitors of inflammation. The anti-inflammatory effects are exerted through the complex glucocorticoid/glucocorticoid receptor which enters the nucleus and modulates the transcription of a variety of genes including cytokines, enzymes, and adhesion molecules.[138] Glucocorticoids can be administered by different routes, including orally, intramuscularly, intravenously, inhaled, topically as nasal or ophthalmic solutions, or as creams/ointments/lotions.

> Corticosteroids are potent inhibitors of inflammation that act by modulating the transcription of a variety of genes coding inflammatory substances.

Glucocorticoids have a role in treatment of the late phase of the type I hypersensitivity reactions but are less effective in treating the early phase. They are widely used to treat bronchial asthma, where different mechanisms of action help reverse the pathologic processes. For example, glucocorticoids relieve bronchospasm, decrease mucosal edema, and reduce bronchial secretions. Because glucocorticoids produce eosinopenia, they reduce the amounts of different inflammatory and cytotoxic mediators such as major basic protein that are released from eosinophils.[139]

In patients with allergic rhinitis, intranasal corticosteroids are accepted as safe and effective first-line therapy. Several intranasal corticosteroids are available, and all are efficacious in treating the acute symptoms or as prophylaxis for allergic rhinitis, providing almost complete prevention of late-phase symptoms. Intranasal corticosteroids relieve nasal congestion, rhinorrhea, itching, and sneezing.[140]

Antileukotriene Therapy. There are 2 classes of medications in this category: leukotriene receptor antagonists (montelukast and zafirlukast) and a 5-lipoxygenase inhibitor (zileuton).

Studies show that leukotriene receptor antagonists are similar to oral H1 receptor blockers in terms of efficacy in patients with allergic rhinitis, but inferior to intranasal corticosteroids. Combinations of leukotriene receptor antagonist and antihistamine are also inferior to nasal corticosteroids.[141]

Antileukotriene therapy is recommended as an alternative treatment to low-dose inhaled glucocorticosteroids in patients with moderately severe asthma and as a complementary treatment in patients with more severe asthma. Also these medications can be used in chronic cough, as therapy for episodes of wheezing caused by viral infections,[142] in aspirin-exacerbated respiratory disease,[143] or in nasal polyposis.[144]

Epinephrine. Epinephrine is a sympathomimetic agent having both alpha- and beta-adrenergic effects and is the emergency, life-saving medical treatment for anaphylaxis. Through its action on α1-adrenergic receptors, it decreases mucosal edema and produces vasoconstriction with a subsequent increase in peripheral resistance. Epinephrine produces bronchodilation and decreases mediator release from mast cells and basophils by direct action on β2-adrenergic receptors. Side effects of epinephrine are common but tend to be relatively mild and transient and include tremor, tachycardia, anxiety, and pallor. In rare cases, epinephrine can produce pulmonary edema, arrhythmias, or myocardial infarction. These complications occur primarily because of problems with incorrect dose, route, or inappropriate dilution. The dose of epinephrine is 0.01 mg/kg at 1:1000 dilution administered intramuscularly or subcutaneously or at 1:10 000 if administered intravenously. The dose can be repeated every 5 to 20 minutes if the patient does not have good clinical response.[145] Despite the known side effect of epinephrine, there are no contraindications to using epinephrine in emergency situations.

> Epinephrine is the treatment of choice in anaphylaxis. Autoinjectors with epinephrine are prescribed to those patients at risk.

Anti-IgE Therapy. Since type I hypersensitivity reactions are characterized by elevated IgE levels, therapeutic targeting to lower serum IgE can be done using an IgG monoclonal antibody to IgE (omalizumab). Currently, omalizumab is approved to treat allergic asthma and chronic idiopathic urticaria, but it is also effective for treating allergic rhinitis and nasal polyposis.[146,147] It specifically binds to plasma IgE, preventing it from binding to FcεRI on the mast cell or eosinophil surfaces. In addition, over the long term, omalizumab downregulates the FcεRI receptors, decreasing the responsiveness of these cells to allergen-mediated degranulation.[148]

> Omalizumab is a monoclonal antibody that binds free IgE and inhibits its binding to mast cells.

Immunotherapy and Desensitization

Allergen-specific T_H1 cells are capable of downregulating the T_H2 response through production of inhibitory IFN-γ. This mechanism has been extensively researched as a possible treatment in patients with allergies.

Immunotherapy ("allergy shots") is the treatment of choice for patients with allergic rhinitis in which symptoms are not controlled with medications and environmental control measures. It consists of administration of injections of increasing amounts of aeroallergen to which the patient was found to have a type I hypersensitivity reaction (by skin testing or in vitro detection of specific IgE levels). As a result, the patient is able to tolerate exposure to the administered allergen with fewer symptoms. The immunologic changes that occur during immunotherapy include shifting of the T_H2 immune response to a T_H1 phenotype, resulting in decreased IgE levels and an increase in allergen-specific IgG antibodies, a decrease of allergen-specific histamine release and an increase in T_{Reg} cells.[149] (Reviewed in Chapter 17.)

> Allergy shots allow the allergic patient to tolerate exposure to the administered allergen with fewer symptoms.

Unlike allergic immunotherapy, which induces a relatively permanent form of immunologic tolerance, desensitization refers to the procedure that produces a temporary ability to tolerate an allergen to which a patient is sensitive. Desensitization is used most frequently for drug allergies and is a procedure that specifically reduces reactivity to a specific drug to which a patient is allergic and allows the patient to receive the medication safely. The patient is given very small doses of the required medication with the doses being gradually increased until the full medication dose is reached. During this procedure, the patient's mast cells slowly degranulate in a step-wise fashion. At the end of the procedure, when the patient has been exposed to the drug at a full therapeutic dose, the drug-specific mast cells have depleted their entire granular content and the patient no longer reacts to the culprit drug. Once the desensitization is completed, some of the drug needs to be taken daily in order to prevent the drug-specific mast cells from re-forming their granules and again being capable of mediating an allergic reaction to that drug. The desensitization is not permanent, and once the medication is stopped for a longer period of time (usually 24 hours), the patient has to undergo the same desensitization protocol if the same medication is again necessary.[150–153] Desensitization can also be done for non-IgE–mediated reaction such as aspirin allergy in aspirin-exacerbated respiratory disease or for delayed reactions to drugs such as allopurinol, but the mechanisms by which these treatments work are not well understood (reviewed in Chapter 8).

Drug desensitization allows the patient with IgE-mediated reaction to receive that medication safely.

TYPE II HYPERSENSITIVITY REACTIONS

Pathogenetic Mechanisms

Type II hypersensitivity reactions are cytotoxic reactions mediated by IgG or IgM antibodies that are directed against the individual's own cells or tissues. The antibody binding to the cell activates the complement system causing destruction of the targeted cells.

Common Clinical Manifestations

Typical type II reactions are transfusion reactions from incompatible blood (from anti-ABO IgM or IgG) or hemolytic disease of newborn infants (Rh+) born to Rh– mothers (from anti-Rh IgG) (Figure 2–7).

Granulomatosis with polyangiitis (Wegener granulomatosis) is also a type of cytotoxic hypersensitivity reaction. It is characterized by severe, granulomatous inflammation of the small-medium vessels in the nose, lungs, and kidneys. The initiating event in this condition is the production of antineutrophil cytotoplasmic antibodies (ANCAs) against the leukocyte enzyme, proteinase-3. ANCA binding to neutrophils induces their activation and the subsequent development of necrotizing inflammation of blood vessel walls or vasculitis. Vasculitis and granuloma formation (predominantly in the respiratory tract) are both found in Wegener granulomatosis.[154]

Wegener granulomatosis is an example of type II hypersensitivity reaction.

Type II hypersensitivity reactions can result in drug-induced hemolytic anemia (quinidine or penicillin), thrombocytopenia (heparin, quinidine, or vancomycin) or granulocytopenia (many different drugs).[155] Other examples of type II hypersensitivity reactions include systemic lupus erythematosus (autoantibodies may induce type II reactions resulting in depletion of red blood cells, platelets, and leukocytes), Goodpasture syndrome (autoantibodies against both glomerular and pulmonary basement membranes cause acute glomerulonephritis and a hemorrhagic form of pneumonitis) and idiopathic thrombocytopenic purpura (ITP) (antiplatelet autoantibodies)[156] (Table 2–7).

Type II hypersensitivity reactions can be confirmed by both nonspecific laboratory tests (complete blood cell count, sedimentation rate or

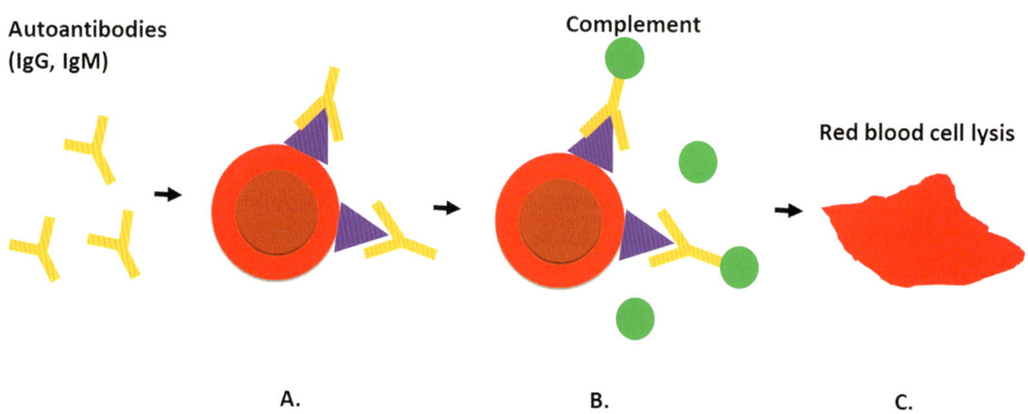

Figure 2–7. Type II hypersensitivity reaction (red blood cell lysis). **A.** Autoantibodies (IgG or IgM) recognize self red blood cells antigens and bind to them. **B.** Antigen-antibody complex formation leads to activation of complement. **C.** After complement is activated pores are formed in the red blood cell membrane which then lyses.

Table 2-7. Common Examples of Type II Hypersensitivity Reactions

Examples of Type II Hypersensitivity Reactions	Antibodies
Transfusion reactions from incompatible blood	Anti-ABO IgM or IgG
Hemolytic disease of newborn infants (Rh+) born to Rh– mothers	Anti-Rh IgG
Systemic lupus erythematosus	Autoantibodies against red blood cells, platelets, leukocytes
Goodpasture syndrome	Autoantibodies against glomerular and pulmonary basement membranes (linear pattern on immunofluorescence)
Idiopathic thrombocytopenic purpura (ITP)	Antiplatelet autoantibodies
Myasthenia gravis:	Acetylcholine receptor antibody
Graves' disease	Anti-TSH receptor antibody
Pernicious anemia	Antiparietal cell antibody

C-reactive protein level, the presence of nuclear/cytoplasmic autoantibodies, serum complement levels) and specific laboratory tests (direct and indirect Coombs tests for drug-induced hemolytic anemia).

Treatment

Primary treatment is discontinuation of the offending drug if the symptoms are the result of administration of a medication. Treatment with corticosteroids or other immunosuppressive medications may be warranted in some patients, depending on the severity of the disease.

TYPE III HYPERSENSITIVITY REACTIONS

Pathogenetic Mechanisms

Type III hypersensitivity reactions are caused by the deposition of soluble immune complexes in different tissues, which cause immune-mediated damage, mainly through complement activation. The immune complexes are formed by either IgM or IgG bound to antigen. Type III reactions develop over a period of hours and may occur locally or systemically (as described below).

> Type III hypersensitivity reactions are mediated by IgG or IgM-antigen immune complexes.

The development of a type III hypersensitivity reaction depends on the route of antigen entry, the ratio of the antigen/antibody, the size of the immune complexes, and the class of antibody involved. Based on the antigen-antibody ratio, the precipitation of immune complexes occurs in 3 zones: the equivalence zone (characterized by equal amount of antibody and antigen) and the zones of antibody or antigen excess characterized by formation of small and soluble immune complexes that can deposit in different tissues resulting in their damage.[31] Large immune complexes are rapidly cleared by the mononuclear phagocytic system, while small immune complexes continue to circulate and can cause tissue injury.[157] Type III hypersensitivity reactions develop in clinical situations where small, soluble immune complexes form (usually in the zone of antibody excess).

Common Clinical Manifestations

Experimentally, a type III reaction will develop if an antigen is injected into the skin in a host that has high levels of existing IgG antibodies to that antigen. An inflammatory reaction develops at the injection site after 4 to 6 hours, giving the appearance of a positive skin test. The delay is due to the time it takes for antibody-antigen complexes to form, complement activation to occur with generation of chemotactic fragments (eg, C5a) and the subsequent influx of neutrophils. This is classically referred to as an Arthus reaction after the immunologist Maurice Arthus who first described the reaction.

The classical example of a systemic type III reaction is what would occur in the pre-antibiotic era after treating pneumonia with heterologous, antipneumococcal horse serum. Initially patients would improve from the antibacterial effects of the serum. However, after 7 to 10 days, patients would become febrile and develop disseminated arthritis, an urticarial rash, lymphadenopathy, and sometimes renal abnormalities ("serum sickness"). Serum sickness developed after the patient began to make antibodies to the injected horse serum, and antigen (horse serum) levels dropped low enough so that amount of anti-horse serum IgG exceeded the amounts of antigen (zone of antibody excess). Soluble antigen-antibody complexes would form in the blood, deposit in the tissues, and initiate the complement/neutrophil-mediated inflammatory reaction in the tissues[12] (Figures 2–8 and 2–9).

Type III reactions that develop in response to other types of antigens, that are similar to the serum sickness reaction described above, are referred to as serum sickness–like reactions. The antigen can be a foreign protein, a viral or bacterial protein, a drug, or a self-antigen that is recognized by the immune system as being non-self (autoimmunity). Systemic lupus erythematosus is the good example of a type III hypersensitivity reaction. In this disease, autoantibodies react with DNA released from cells and form immune complexes that are deposited in different tissues such as the kidney (glomerulonephritis), blood vessels (vasculitis), joints (arthritis), and serosal membranes (pericarditis and pleuritis). The most common causes of type III reactions are drug reactions, although patients treated with anti-snake-venom sera are liable to develop this type of reaction (Table 2–8).

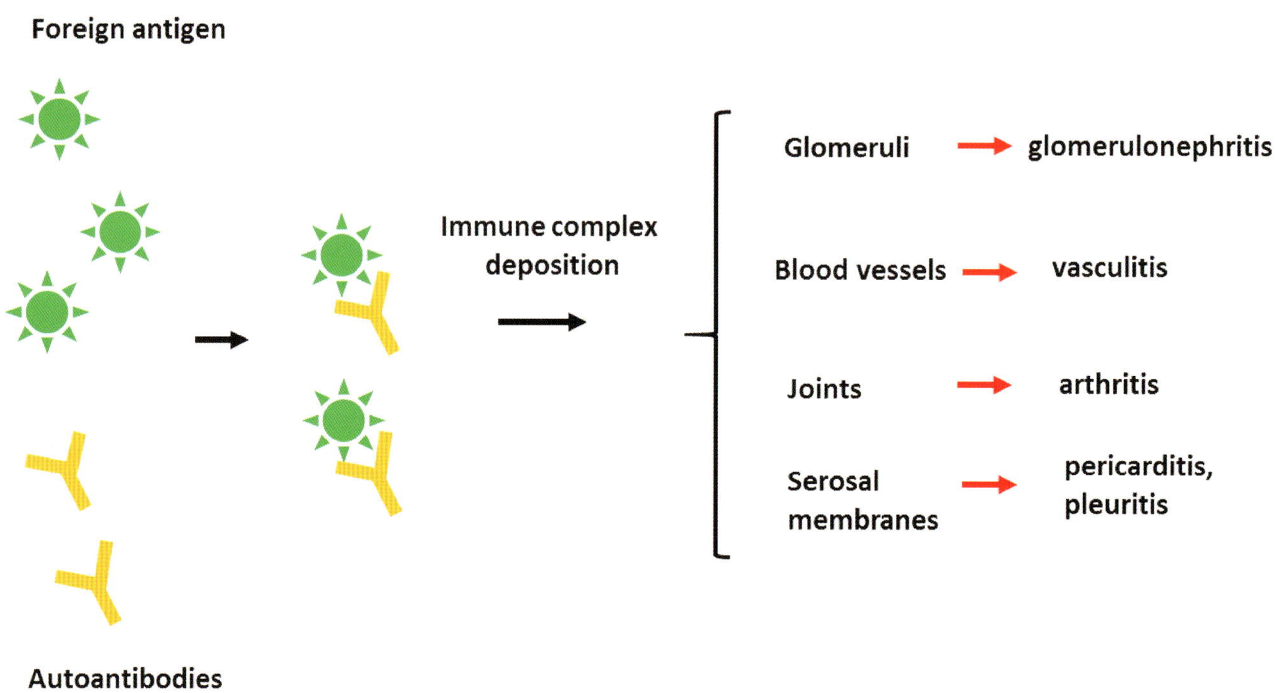

Figure 2–8. Type III hypersensitivity reaction. Foreign antigen binds autoantibodies forming immune complexes that deposit in different organs resulting local and systemic inflammation.

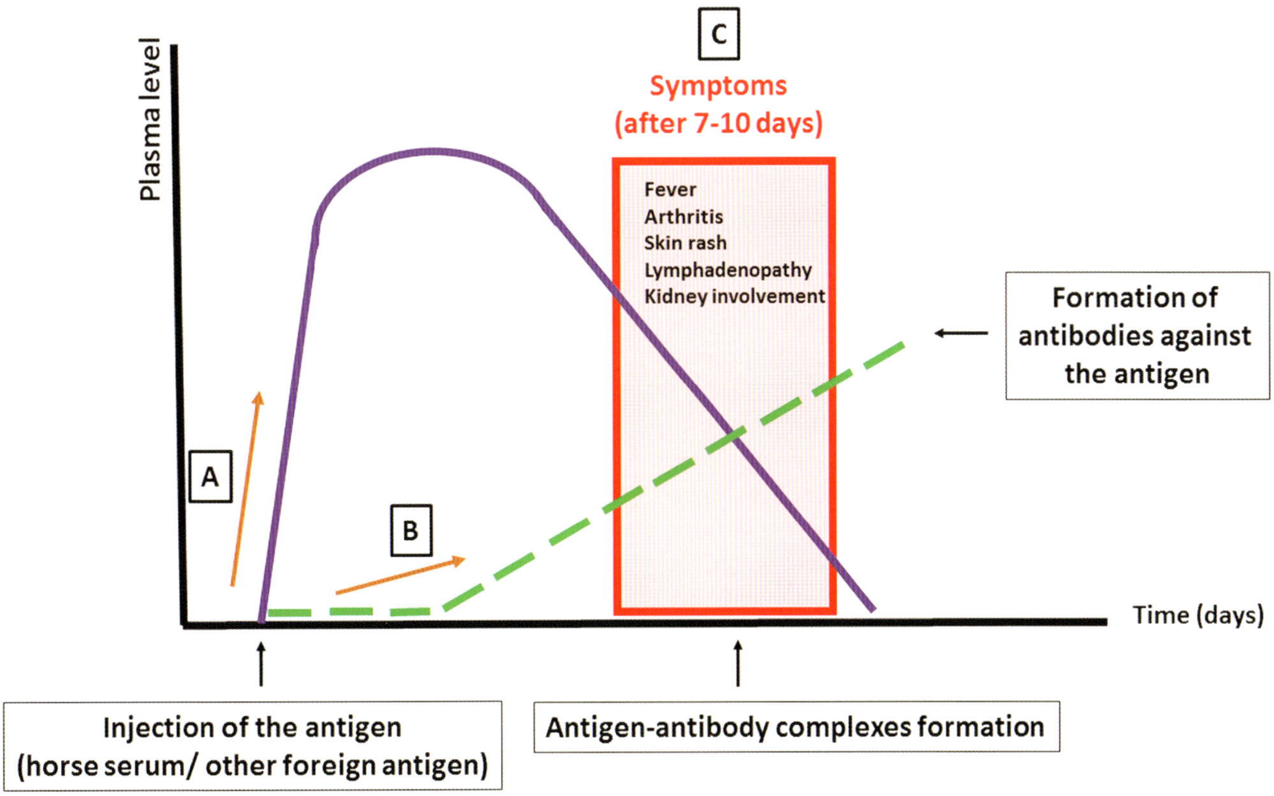

Figure 2-9. Development of serum sickness. A. The antigen is injected (horse serum in the classical serum-sickness or other foreign antigen in serum sickness-like reactions). B. Formation of antibodies against the injected antigen. C. After 7 to 10 days, once the plasma levels of antibodies are higher than the antigen plasma levels, soluble antigen-antibody complexes are deposited in different organs and patients become symptomatic.

Table 2-8. Common Examples of Type III Hypersensitivity Reactions

Examples of Type III Hypersensitivity Reactions
Serum sickness
Arthus reaction
Drug reaction
Immune complex glomerulonephritis
Systemic lupus erythematosus
Rheumatoid arthritis

Similar to type II hypersensitivity reactions, the diagnosis of type III hypersensitivity reactions can be made with nonspecific and specific laboratory tests.

Treatment

In order to reduce the inflammation, corticosteroids or other immunosuppressant medications are used. If the reaction is thought to be medication induced, the culprit drug should be stopped.

TYPE IV HYPERSENSITIVITY REACTIONS

Pathogenetic Mechanisms

Type IV hypersensitivity reactions are cell mediated and antibody independent and are subclassified into 4 types depending on the cells involved and the cytokines produced: IVa, IVb, IVc, and IVd.

Type IVa

Type IVa reactions are mediated by T_H1 cells. For this reaction to take place, the T_H1 cells must have already been exposed to the antigen. On a subsequent exposure, T_H1 cells recognize the antigen presented by APCs in the lymph nodes, from where $T_H1$cells migrate to the site of antigen deposition (skin or mucosa) and release cytokines and chemokines. This results in recruitment of mononuclear cells and other cells to the location of the antigen and stimulation of local inflammation. This type of response is termed *delayed-type hypersensitivity*, because the symptoms appear after 24 to 72 hours, the time required for previously sensitized T_H1 to travel from the lymph nodes to the skin or mucosa and recruit inflammatory cells.[2] Examples of type IVa hypersensitivity reactions include tuberculin (PPD) skin tests and allergic contact dermatitis (Figure 2–10).

Delayed-type hypersensitivity reactions have been seen in response to inhaled nasal corticosteroids and can present as nasal pruritus, pruritic eruptions around the nostrils, or local angioedema.[158]

> Type IVa hypersensitivity reactions are mediated by T_H1 cells.

Type IVb Reactions

Type IVb reactions are mediated by T_H2 cells, which secrete IL-4, IL-5, and IL-13 leading to B-cell activation with subsequent IgE production and eosinophilic inflammation. This type of hypersensitivity is similar to the late phase of the type I immediate reaction and is characteristic of chronic allergic disorders (chronic allergic asthma, chronic rhinoconjunctivitis) and medication hypersensitivity reactions.[2]

> Type IVb hypersensitivity reactions are mediated by T_H2 cells.

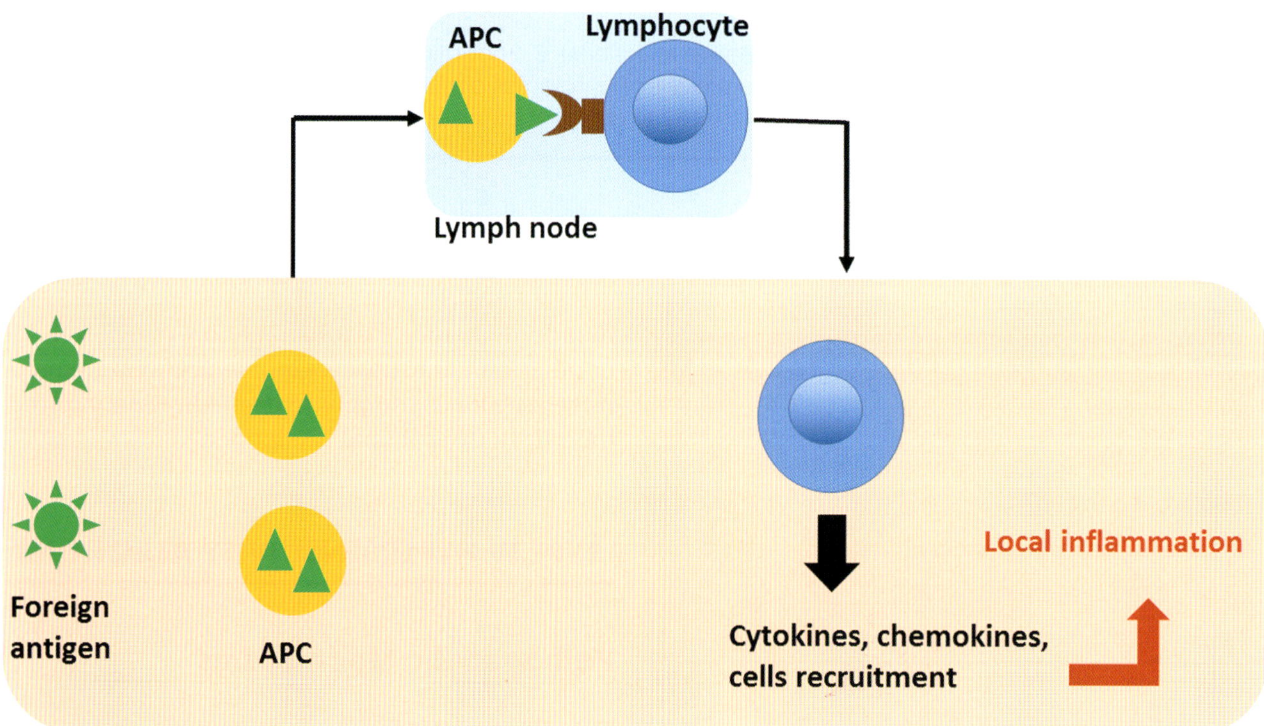

Figure 2–10. Type IVa hypersensitivity reaction in the skin. The foreign antigen is taken by the local antigen-presenting cells (APCs). APCs process the antigen and present it in the lymph nodes to previously sensitized T_H1 cells. The activated lymphocytes migrate to the skin where they release different cytokines and chemokines, producing cell recruitment and local inflammation.

Type IVc

Type IVc hypersensitivity reactions occur mostly in drug-induced skin rashes where cytotoxic T cells play a major role. These cells migrate into the tissues and kill keratinocytes causing disorders such as bullous skin reactions like Stevens-Johnson syndrome and toxic epidermal necrolysis (reviewed in Chapter 8).[159,160]

> Type IVc hypersensitivity reactions are mediated by cytotoxic T cells.

Type IVd

Type IVd reactions are characterized by sterile neutrophilic inflammation promoted by different cytokines released by T cells. The prototype for this reaction is acute generalized exanthematous pustulosis (AGEP) which is a rare, acute pustular skin eruption associated with certain medications intake (eg, ampicillin, hydroxychloroquine, carbamazepine, diltiazem). (Reviewed in Chapter 8.)[161,162]

> Type IVd hypersensitivity reactions are characterized by neutrophilic inflammation.

Treatment

The treatment for type IV hypersensitivity reactions depends on the type of reaction. Type IVa reactions are easily resolved through trigger avoidance and the use of topical steroids. The management of type IVb reactions is the same as for type I immediate reactions and consists of antihistamines, steroids, leukotrienes modulators, and immunotherapy to prevent/treat allergic symptoms. In types IVc and IVd, the mainstay of treatment is removing the offending medication and sometimes may require administration of corticosteroids.

REFERENCES

1. Gell PGH, Coombs RRA, eds. *Clinical Aspects of Immunology*. Oxford, UK: Blackwell; 1963.
2. Pichler WJ. Delayed drug hypersensitivity reactions. *Ann Intern Med*. 2003 Oct 21;139(8):683–693.
3. Busse WW. Mechanisms and advances in allergic diseases. *J Allergy Clin Immunol*. 2000;105:S593–S598.
4. Akinbami LJ, Moorman JE, Bailey C, et al. *Trends in Asthma Prevalence, Health Care Use, and Mortality in the United States, 2001–2010*. Hyattsville, MD: National Center for Health Statistics; May 2012.
5. Centers for Disease Control and Prevention. *National Health Interview Survey Raw Data, 1997–2011*. Hyattsville, MD: National Center for Health Statistics.
6. Akinbami LJ, Moorman, JE, Bailey C, et al. *Trends in Asthma Prevalence, Health Care Use and Mortality: United States, 2001–2010*. Hyattsville, MD: National Center for Health Statistics; 2012:1–6.
7. Schoenwetter WF. Allergic rhinitis: epidemiology and natural history. *Allergy Asthma Proc*. Jan–Feb 2000;21(1):1–6.
8. Pawankar R, Walkter Canonica G, Holgate ST, Lockey RF. *White Book on Allergy. Executive Summary*. Geneva, Switzerland: World Health Organization; 2011–2012.
9. Bloom B, Jones LI, Freeman G. Summary health statistics for US children: National Health Interview Survey, 2012. National Center for Health Statistics. *Vital Health Stat*. 2013;10(258).
10. Von Ehrenstein OS, Von Mutius E, Illi S, Baumann L, Böhm O, von Kries R. Reduced risk of hay fever and asthma among children of farmers. *Clin Exp Allergy*. 2000 Feb;30(2):187–193.
11. Yemaneberhan H, Bekele Z, Venn A, Lewis S, Parry E, Britton J. Prevalence of wheeze and asthma and relation to atopy in urban and rural Ethiopia. *Lancet*. 1997 Jul 12; 350(9071):85–90.
12. Ege MJ, Mayer M, Normand AC, et al. Exposure to environmental microorganisms and childhood asthma. *N Engl J Med*. 2011;364(8):701–709.
13. Perkin MR, Strachan DP. Which aspects of the farming lifestyle explain the inverse association with childhood allergy? *J Allergy Clin Immunol*. 2006 Jun;117(6):1374–1381.
14. Strachan DP. Hay fever, hygiene, and household size. *BMJ*. 1989 Nov 18;299(6710):1259–1260.
15. Funkhouser LJ, Bordenstein SR. Mom knows best: the universality of maternal microbial transmission. *PLoS Biol*. 2013;11.
16. Weiss ST, Litonjua AA. Vitamin D, the gut microbiome, and the hygiene hypothesis. How does asthma begin? *Am J Respir Crit Care Med*. 2015 Mar 1;191(5):492–493.
17. Bisgaard H, Li N, Bonnelykke K, et al. Reduced diversity of the intestinal microbiota during infancy is associated with increased risk of allergic disease at school age. *J Allergy Clin Immunol*. 2011 Sep;128(3):646–652.e1–e5.
18. Azad MB, Konya T, Guttman DS, et al; CHILD Study Investigators. Infant gut microbiota and food sensitization: associations in the first year of life. *Clin Exp Allergy*. 2015 Mar;45(3):632–643.
19. Huang YJ, Boushey HA. The microbiome in asthma. *J Allergy Clin Immunol*. 2015 Jan;135(1):25–30.
20. Matricardi PM, Bonini S. High microbial turnover rate preventing atopy: a solution to inconsistencies impinging

on the hygiene hypothesis? *Clin Exp Allergy*. 2000 Nov; 30(11):1506–1510.
21. van den Biggelaar AH, van Ree R, Rodrigues LC, et al. Decreased atopy in children infected with *Schistosoma haematobium*: a role for parasite-induced interleukin-10. *Lancet*. 2000 Nov 18;356(9243):1723–1727.
22. Nyan OA, Walraven GE, Banya WA, et al. Atopy, intestinal helminth infection and total serum IgE in rural and urban adult Gambian communities. *Clin Exp Allergy*. 2001 Nov;31(11):1672–1678.
23. Scrivener S, Yemaneberhan H, Zebenigus M, et al. Independent effects of intestinal parasite infection and domestic allergen exposure on risk of wheeze in Ethiopia: a nested case-control study. *Lancet*. 2001 Nov 3; 358(9292):1493–1499.
24. Akdis M, Verhagen J, Taylor A. Immune responses in healthy and allergic individuals are characterized by a fine balance between allergen-specific T regulatory 1 and T helper 2 cells. *J Exp Med*. 2004;199:1567–1575.
25. Kim JM, Rasmussen JP, Rudensky AY. Regulatory T cells prevent catastrophic autoimmunity throughout the lifespan of mice. *Nat Immunol*. 2007;8:191–197.
26. Capron M. Effect of parasite infection on allergic disease. *Allergy*. 2011 Jul;66 (suppl 95):16–18.
27. Devereux G. The increase in the prevalence of asthma and allergy: food for thought. *Nat Rev Immunol*. 2006;6: 869–874.
28. Marsland BJ. Influences of the microbiome on the early origins of allergic asthma. *Ann Am Thorac Soc*. 2013 Dec; 10(suppl):S165–S169.
29. von Bubnoff D, Geiger E, Bieber T. Antigen-presenting cells in allergy. *J Allergy Clin Immunol*. Sep 2001; 108(3):329–339.
30. Zweiman B, Moskovitz AR, von ALlmen C. Comparison of inflammatory events during developing immunoglobulin E-mediated late-phase reactions and delayed-hypersensitivity reactions. *Clin Diagn Lab Immunol*. 1998 Jul;5(4):574–577.
31. Murphy K, Travers P, Walport M. *Janeway's Immunobiology*. 7th ed. New York, NY: Garland Science; 2008.
32. Achatz G, Lamers M, Crameri R. Membrane bound IgE: the key receptor to restrict high IgE levels. *Open Immunol J*. 2008;1;25–32.
33. Smith P, Ownby DR. Clinical significance of IgE. In: Adkinson N, Bochner BS, Busse WW, Holgate ST, Lemanske RF, Simons FER, eds. *Middleton's Allergy: Principles and Practice*. 7th ed. St Louis, MO: Mosby Elsevier; 2009.
34. Galli Lantz CS. Allergy. In: Paul WE, ed. *Fundamental Immunology*. 4th ed. Philadelphia, PA: Lippincott-Raven; 1999:1127–1129.
35. Stone KD, Prussin C, Metcalfe DD. IgE, mast cells, basophils, and eosinophils. *J Allergy Clin Immunol*. 2010; 125(2, suppl 2):S73–S80.
36. Kikutani H, Yokota A, Uchibayashi N, et al. Structure and function of Fc epsilon receptor II (Fc epsilon RII/ CD23): a point of contact between the effector phase of allergy and B cell differentiation. *Ciba Found Symp*. 1998;147:23–31.
37. Adkinson NF, Bochner BS, Busse WW, et al. *Middleton's Allergy, Principles and Practice*. 8th ed, Philadelphia, PA: Elsevier; 2014.
38. Yoshimoto T Okamura H, Tagawa YI, Iwakura Y, Nakanishi K. Interleukin 18 together with interleukin 12 inhibits IgE production by induction of interferon-gamma production from activated B cells. *Proc Natl Acad Sci USA*. 1997;94(8):3948–3953.
39. Suto A, Nakajima H, Hirose K, et al. Interleukin 21 prevents antigen-induced IgE production by inhibiting germ line C(epsilon) transcription of IL-4-stimulated B cells. *Blood*. 2002;100(13):4565–4573.
40. Melo RC, Spencer LA, Perez SA, Ghiran I, Dvorak AM, Weller PF. Human eosinophils secrete preformed, granule-stored interleukin-4 through distinct vesicular compartments. *Traffic*. 2005;6(11):1047–1057.
41. Schleimer RP, Sterbinsky SA, Kaiser J, et al. IL-4 induces adherence of human eosinophils and basophils but not neutrophils to endothelium. Association with expression of VCAM-1. *J Immunol*. 148(4):1086–1092.
42. Wise SK, Laury AM, Katz EH, Den Beste KA, Parkos CA, Nusrat. A Interleukin-4 and interleukin-13 compromise the sinonasal epithelial barrier and perturb intercellular junction protein expression. *Int Forum Allergy Rhinol*. 2014;4(5):361–370.
43. Ohashi Y, Nakai Y, Okamoto H, et al. Serum level of interleukin-4 in patients with perennial allergic rhinitis during allergen-specific immunotherapy. *Scand J Immunol*. 1996 Jun;43(6):680–686.
44. Kuperman DA, Huang X, Koth LL, et al. Direct effects of interleukin-13 on epithelial cells cause airway hyperreactivity and mucus overproduction in asthma. *Nat Med*. 2002;8(8):885–889.
45. Nabavi M, Arshi S, Bahrami A, et al. Increased level of interleukin-13, but not interleukin-4 and interferon-γ in chronic rhinosinusitis with nasal polyps. *Allergol Immunopathol (Madr)*. 2014;42(5):465–471.
46. Xu L, Rothman P. IFN-gamma represses epsilon germline transcription and subsequently down-regulates switch recombination to epsilon. *Int Immunol*. 1994;6(4): 515–521.
47. Ciprandi G, Fenoglio D, Di Gioacchino M, et al. Sublingual immunotherapy provides an early increase of interferon-gamma production. *J Biol Regul Homeost Agents*. 2008;22(3):169–173.
48. Akoum H, Tsicopoulos A, Vorng H, et al. Venom immunotherapy modulates interleukin-4 and interferon-gamma messenger RNA expression of peripheral T lymphocytes. *Immunology*. 1996;87(4):593–598.
49. Jacobsen L, Wahn U, Bilo MB. Allergen-specific immunotherapy provides immediate, long-term and preventive clinical effects in children and adults: the effects of immunotherapy can be categorised by level of benefit-the centenary of allergen specific subcutaneous immunotherapy. *Clin Transl Allergy*. 2012;2:8.

50. Kinet JP. The essential role of mast cells in orchestrating inflammation. *Immunol Rev.* 2007;217(1):5–7.
51. Galli SJ, Tsai M. IgE and mast cells in allergic disease. *Nature Med.* 2012;18:693–704.
52. Metcalfe DD, Baram D, Mekori YA. Mast cells. *Physiol Rev.* 1997;77(4):1033–1079.
53. Irani A, Schwartz LB. Mast cell heterogeneity. *Clin Exp Allergy.* 1989;19:143.
54. Bradding P, Okayama Y, Howarth PH, Church MK, Holgate ST. Heterogeneity of human mast cells based on cytokine content. *J Immunol.* 1995;155(1):297–307.
55. Yang TQ, Takeuchi K, Hayashi S, Majima Y. Effect of histamine on the permeability of the nasal mucosa in vivo. *Acta Otolaryngol.* 2003;123(3):401–405.
56. Simon FER, Simmons KJ. H_1 Antihistamines: current status and future directions. *World Allergy Organ J.* Sep 2008;1(9):145–155.
57. Holmberg K, Pipkorn U, Bake B, Blychert LO. Effects of topical treatment with H1 and H2 antagonists on clinical symptoms and nasal vascular reactions in patients with allergic rhinitis. *Allergy.* 1989;44:281–287.
58. McLeod RL, Mingo GG, Herczku C, et al. Combined histamine H1 and H3 receptor blockade produces nasal decongestion in an experimental model of nasal congestion. *Am J Rhinol.* 1999;13:391–399.
59. Nakaya M, Takeuchi N, Kondo K. Immunohistochemical localization of histamine receptor subtypes in human inferior turbinates. *Ann Otol Rhinol Laryngol.* 2004;113:552–557.
60. Miadonna A, Tedeschi A, Leggieri E, et al. Behavior and clinical relevance of histamine and leukotrienes C4 and B4 in grass pollen-induced rhinitis. *Am Rev Respir Dis.* 1987;136:357–362.
61. Okuda M, Watase T, Mezawa A, Liu CM. The role of leukotriene D4 in allergic rhinitis. *Ann Allergy.* 1988;60(6):537–540.
62. McMains KC, Kountakis SE. Medical and surgical considerations in patients with Samter's triad. *Am J Rhinol.* 2006;20:573–576.
63. Peters-Golden M, Henderson WR, Jr. The role of leukotrienes in allergic rhinitis. *Ann Allergy Asthma Immunol.* 2005;94(6):609–618.
64. Ishizaka T, De Bernardo R, Tomioka H, Lichtenstein LM, Ishizaka K. Identification of basophil granulocytes as a site of allergic histamine release. *J Immunol.* 1972;108(4):1000–1008.
65. Hogan SP, Rosenberg HF, Moqbel R, et al. Eosinophils: biological properties and role in health and disease. *Clin Exp Allergy.* 2008;38(5):709–750.
66. Hisamatsu K, Ganbo T, Nakazawa T, et al. Cytotoxicity of human eosinophil granule major basic protein to human nasal sinus mucosa in vitro. *J Allergy Clin Immunol.* 1990;86(1):52–63.
67. Lacy P, Abdel-Latif D, Steward M, Musat-Marcu S, Man SF, Moqbel R. Divergence of mechanisms regulating respiratory burst in blood and sputum eosinophils and neutrophils from atopic subjects. *J Immunol.* 2003;170(5):2670–2679.
68. Dor PJ, Ackerman SJ, Gleich GJ. Charcot-Leyden crystal protein and eosinophil granule major basic protein in sputum of patients with respiratory diseases. *Am Rev Respir Dis.* 1984 Dec;130(6):1072–1077.
69. Granville L, Chirala M, Cernoch P, Ostrowski M, Truong LD. Fungal sinusitis: histologic spectrum and correlation with culture. *Hum Pathol.* 2004;35(4):474–481.
70. Pantanowitz L, Balogh K. Charcot-Leyden crystals: pathology and diagnostic utility. *Ear Nose Throat J.* 2004;83(7):489–490.
71. Chapman MD, Pomés A, Breiteneder H, Ferreira F. Nomenclature and structural biology of allergens. *J Allergy Clin Immunol.* 2007 Feb;119(2):414–420.
72. Gendel SM, Jenkins JA. Allergen sequence databases. *Mol Nutr Food Res.* 2006 Jul;50(7):633–637.
73. King TP, Hoffman D, Lowenstein H, Marsh DG, Platts-Mills TA, Thomas W. Allergen nomenclature. WHO/IUIS Allergen Nomenclature Subcommittee. *Int Arch Allergy Immunol.* 1994 Nov;105(3):224–233.
74. Radauer C, Bublin M, Wagner S, Mari A, Breiteneder H. Allergens are distributed into few protein families and possess a restricted number of biochemical functions. *J Allergy Clin Immunol.* 2008 Apr;121(4):847–852.e7.
75. Weber RW. Guidelines for using pollen cross-reactivity in formulating allergen immunotherapy. *J Allergy Clin Immunol.* 2008 Jul;122(1):219–221.
76. Sporik R, Ingram JM, Price W, Sussman JH, Honsinger RW, Platts-Mills TA. Association of asthma with serum IgE and skin test reactivity to allergens among children living at high altitude. Tickling the dragon's breath. *Am J Respir Crit Care Med.* 1995 May;151(5):1388–1392.
77. Hilger C, Kuehn A, Hentges F. Animal lipocalin allergens. *Curr Allergy Asthma Rep.* 2012 Oct;12(5):438–447.
78. Bush RK, Wood RA, Eggleston PA. Laboratory animal allergy. *J Allergy Clin Immunol.* 1998 Jul;102(1):99–112.
79. Custovic A, Green R, Fletcher A, et al. Aerodynamic properties of the major dog allergen Can f 1: distribution in homes, concentration, and particle size of allergen in the air. *Am J Respir Crit Care Med.* 1997 Jan;155(1):94–98.
80. Perzanowski MS, Rönmark E, Platts-Mills TA, Lundbäck B. Effect of cat and dog ownership on sensitization and development of asthma among preteenage children. *Am J Respir Crit Care Med.* 2002 Sep 1;166(5):696–702.
81. Ownby DR, Johnson CC, Peterson EL. Exposure to dogs and cats in the first year of life and risk of allergic sensitization at 6 to 7 years of age. *JAMA.* 2002 Aug 28;288(8):963–972.
82. Patchett K, Lewis S, Crane J, Fitzharris P. Cat allergen (Fel d 1) levels on school children's clothing and in primary school classrooms in Wellington, New Zealand. *J Allergy Clin Immunol.* 1997 Dec;100(6, pt 1):755–759.
83. Almqvist C, Larsson PH, Egmar AC, Hedrén M, Malmberg P, Wickman M. School as a risk environment for children allergic to cats and a site for transfer of cat allergen to homes. *J Allergy Clin Immunol.* 1999 Jun;103(6):1012–1017.
84. Phipatanakul W, Matsui E, Portnoy J, et al. Environmental assessment and exposure reduction of rodents:

a practice parameter. *Ann Allergy Asthma Immunol*. 2012 Dec;109(6):375–387.

85. Matsui EC, Sampson HA, Bahnson HT, et al. Allergen-specific IgE as a biomarker of exposure plus sensitization in inner-city adolescents with asthma. *Allergy*. 2010 Nov;65(11):1414–1422.
86. Sporik R, Holgate ST, Platts-Mills TA, Cogswell JJ. Exposure to house-dust mite allergen (Der p I) and the development of asthma in childhood. A prospective study. *N Engl J Med*. 1990 Aug 23;323(8):502–507.
87. Rosenstreich DL, Eggleston P, Kattan M, et al. The role of cockroach allergy and exposure to cockroach allergen in causing morbidity among inner-city children with asthma. *N Engl J Med*. 1997 May 8;336(19):1356–1363.
88. Bloom KA, Huang FR, Bencharitiwong R, et al. Effect of heat treatment on milk and egg proteins allergenicity [published online December 18, 2014]. *Pediatr Allergy Immunol*. 2014 Dec;25(8):740–746. doi:10.1111/pai.12283.
89. Bellioni-Businco B, Paganelli R, Lucenti P, Giampietro PG, Perborn H, Businco L. Allergenicity of goat's milk in children with cow's milk allergy. *J Allergy Clin Immunol*. 1999 Jun;103(6):1191–1194.
90. Cooke SK, Sampson HA. Allergenic properties of ovomucoid in man. *J Immunol*. 1997 Aug 15;159(4):2026–2032.
91. Nicolaou N, Poorafshar M, Murray C, et al. Allergy or tolerance in children sensitized to peanut: prevalence and differentiation using component-resolved diagnostics. *J Allergy Clin Immunol*. 2010 Jan;125(1):191–197.e1–13.
92. Koppelman SJ, Wensing M, Ertmann M, Knulst AC, Knol EF. Relevance of Ara h1, Ara h2 and Ara h3 in peanut-allergic patients, as determined by immunoglobulin E Western blotting, basophil-histamine release and intracutaneous testing: Ara h2 is the most important peanut allergen. *Clin Exp Allergy*. 2004 Apr;34(4):583–590.
93. Shreffler WG, Castro RR, Kucuk ZY, et al. The major glycoprotein allergen from *Arachis hypogaea*, Ara h 1, is a ligand of dendritic cell-specific ICAM-grabbing non-integrin and acts as a Th2 adjuvant in vitro. *J Immunol*. 2006 Sep 15;177(6):3677–3685.
94. Sicherer SH, Muñoz-Furlong A, Godbold JH, Sampson HA. US prevalence of self-reported peanut, tree nut, and sesame allergy: 11-year follow-up. *J Allergy Clin Immunol*. 2010 Jun;125(6):1322–1326.
95. Matsuo H, Morita E, Tatham AS, et al. Identification of the IgE-binding epitope in omega-5 gliadin, a major allergen in wheat-dependent exercise-induced anaphylaxis. *J Biol Chem*. 2004 Mar 26;279(13):12135–12140.
96. Kuehn A, Swoboda I, Arumugam K, Hilger C, Hentges F. Fish allergens at a glance: variable allergenicity of parvalbumins, the major fish allergens. *Front Immunol*. 2014 Apr 22;5:179.
97. Nieuwenhuizen NE, Lopata AL. Allergic reactions to Anisakis found in fish. *Curr Allergy Asthma Rep*. 2014 Aug;14(8):455.
98. Muñoz-Furlong A, Sampson HA, Sicherer SH. Prevalence of self-reported seafood allergy in the US. *J Allergy Clin Immunol*. 2004;113(2):S100.
99. Reese G, Ayuso R, Lehrer SB. Tropomyosin: an invertebrate pan-allergen. *Int Arch Allergy Immunol*. 1999 Aug;119(4):247–258.
100. Pascal M, Grishina G, Yang AC, et al. Molecular diagnosis of shrimp allergy: efficiency of several allergens to predict clinical reactivity. *J Allergy Clin Immunol Pract*. 2015 Mar 11. doi:http://dx.doi.org/10.1016/j.jaip.2015.02.001.
101. Steinke JW, Platts-Mills TA, Commins SP. The alpha-gal story: lessons learned from connecting the dots. *J Allergy Clin Immunol*. 2015 Mar;135(3):589–596.
102. Capron M, Capron A. Immunoglobulin E and effector cells in schistosomiasis. *Science*. 1994;264(5167):1876–1877.
103. Gurish MF, Bryce PJ, Tao H, et al. IgE enhances parasite clearance and regulates mast cell responses in mice infected with *Trichinella spiralis*. *J Immunol*. 2004;172(2):1139–1145.
104. Bryce PJ, Oettgen HC. Antigen-independent effects of immunoglobulin E. *Curr Allergy Asthma Rep*. 2005;5(3):186–190.
105. Kalesnikoff J, Huber M, Lam V, Damen JE, Zhang J, Siraganian RP, Krystal G. Monomeric IgE stimulates signaling pathways in mast cells that lead to cytokine production and cell survival. *Immunity*. 2001 Jun;14(6):801–811.
106. Nagy E, Berczi I, Sehon AH. Growth inhibition of murine mammary carcinoma by monoclonal IgE antibodies specific for the mammary tumor virus. *Cancer Immunol. Immunother*. 1991;34:63–69.
107. Kershaw MH, Darcy PK,Trapani JA, MacGregor D, Smyth MJ. Tumor-specific IgE-mediated inhibition of human colorectal carcinoma xenograft growth. *Oncol Res*. 1998;10:133–142.
108. Gould HJ, Mackay GA, Karagiannis SN, et al. Comparison of IgE and IgG antibody-dependent cytotoxicity in vitro and in a SCID mouse xenograft model of ovarian carcinoma. *Eur J Immunol*. 1999;29:3527–3537.
109. Rondon C, Romero JJ, Lopez S, et al. Local IgE production and positive nasal provocation test in patients with persistent nonallergic rhinitis. *J Allergy Clin Immunol*. 2007;119:899–905.
110. Rondon C, Dona I, Lopez S, Campo P, Romero JJ, Torres MJ. Seasonal idiopathic rhinitis with local inflammatory response and specific IgE in absence of systemic response. *Allergy*. 2008;63:1352–1358.
111. *Guidelines for the Diagnosis and Management of Asthma (EPR-3)*. Bethesda, MD: National Heart Lung and Blood Institute; 2007.
112. Morgan WJ, Crain EF, Gruchalla, RS, et al. Results of a home-based environmental intervention for inner-city children with asthma. *N Engl J Med*. 2004;351:1068–1080.
113. Avner DB, Perzanowski MS, Platts-Mills TA, Woodfolk, JA. Evaluation of different techniques for washing cats: quantification of allergen removed from the cat and the effect on airborne Fel d 1. *J Allergy Clin Immunol*. 1997;100:307–312.

114. Lockey RF. The myth of hypoallergenic dogs (and cats). *J Allergy Clin Immunol*. 2012;130:910–911.
115. Smallwood J, Ownby D. Exposure to dog allergens and subsequent allergic sensitization: an updated review. *Curr Allergy Asthma Rep*. 2012;12:424–428.
116. Chen YC, Tsai CH, Lee YL. Early-life indoor environmental exposures increase the risk of childhood asthma. *Int J Hyg Environ Health*. 2011;215:19–25.
117. Koschel D, Wittstruck H, Renck T, Muller-Wening D, Hoffken G. Presenting features of feather duvet lung. *Int Arch Allergy Immunol*. 2010;152:264–270.
118. Korsgaard J. House dust mites and absolute indoor humidity. *Allergy*. 1983;38:85–92.
119. Vaughan JW, McLaughlin TE, Perzanowski, MS, Platts-Mills TA. Evaluation of materials used for bedding encasement: effect of pore size in blocking cat and dust mite allergen. *J Allergy Clin Immunol*. 1999;103:227–231.
120. McDonald LG, Tovey E. The role of water temperature and laundry procedures in reducing house dust mite populations and allergen content of bedding. *J Allergy Clin Immunol*. 1992;90:599–608.
121. Popplewell EJ, Innes VA, Lloyd-Hughes S, et al. The effect of high-efficiency and standard vacuum cleaners on mite, cat and dog allergen levels and clinical progress. *Pediatr Allergy Immunol*. 2000;11:142–148.
122. Sublett JL, Seltzer J, Burkhead R, et al. Air filters and air cleaners: rostrum by the American Academy of Allergy, Asthma and Immunology Indoor Allergen Committee. *J Allergy Clin Immunol*. 2010;125:32–38.
123. Burr ML, Matthews IP, Arthur RA, et al. Effects on patients with asthma of eradicating visible indoor mould: a randomized controlled trial. *Thorax*. 2007;62:767–772.
124. Kang B, Vellody D, Homburger H, Yunginger JW. Cockroach cause of allergic asthma. Its specificity and immunologic profile. *J Allergy Clin Immunol*. 1979;63:80–86.
125. Rosenstreich DL, Eggleston P, Kattan M, et al. The role of cockroach allergy and exposure to cockroach allergen in causing morbidity among inner-city children with asthma. *N Engl J Med*. 1997;336:1356–1363.
126. Portnoy J, Chew GL, Phipatanakul W, et al. Environmental assessment and exposure reduction of cockroaches: a practice parameter. *J Allergy Clin Immunol*. 2013;132:802–808.
127. Matsui EC, Simons E, Rand C, et al. Airborne mouse allergen in the homes of inner-city children with asthma. *J Allergy Clin Immunol*. 2005;115:358–363.
128. Sheehan WJ, Rangsithienchai PA, Wood RA, et al. Pest and allergen exposure and abatement in inner-city asthma: a work group report of the American Academy of Allergy, Asthma and Immunology Indoor Allergy/Air Pollution Committee. *J Allergy Clin Immunol*. 2010;125:575–581.
129. Nakazawa T, Satinover SM, Naccara L, et al. Asian ladybugs (*Harmonia axyridis*): a new seasonal indoor allergen. *J Allergy Clin Immunol*. 2007;119:421–427.
130. Mertz TL, Jacobs SB, Craig TJ, Ishmael FT. The brown marmorated stink bug as a new aeroallergen. *J Allergy Clin Immunol*. 2012;130:999–1001.
131. Leurs R, Church MK, Taglialatela M. H_1-antihistamines: inverse agonism, anti-inflammatory actions and cardiac effects. *Clin Exp Allergy*. 2002;32:489–498.
132. Carson S, Lee N, Thakurta S. *Drug Class Review: Newer Antihistamines: Final Report Update 2* [Internet]. May 2010.
133. Estelle F, Simons R. Advances in H_1-Antihistamines. *N Engl J Med*. 2004;351:2203–2217.
134. Bakker RA, Schoonus SB, Smit MJ, Timmerman H, Leurs R. Histamine H_1-receptor activation of nuclear factor-kappa B: roles for G beta gamma- and G alpha(q/11)-subunits in constitutive and agonist-mediated signaling. *Mol Pharmacol*. 2001;60:1133–1142.
135. Van Schoor J. Antihistamines: a brief review. *Prof Nurs Today*. 2012;16(5);16:21.
136. Van Cauwenberge P, Juniper EF. Comparison of the efficacy, safety and quality of life provided by fexofenadine hydrochloride 120 mg, loratadine 10 mg, and placebo administered once daily for the treatment of seasonal allergic rhinitis. *Clin Exp Allergy*. 2000;30:891–899.
137. Lieberman P. The basics of histamine biology. *Ann Allergy Asthma Immunol*. 2011;106(2, suppl):S2–S5.
138. van der Velden VH. Glucocorticoids: mechanisms of action and anti-inflammatory potential in asthma. *Mediators Inflamm*. 1998;7(4):229–237.
139. Townley RG, Suliaman F. The mechanism of corticosteroids in treating asthma. *Ann Allergy*. 1987;58(1):1–6.
140. Trangsrud AJ, Whitaker AL, Small RE. Intranasal corticosteroids for allergic rhinitis. *Pharmacotherapy*. 2002; 22(11):1458–1467.
141. Rodrigo GJ, Yañez A. The role of antileukotriene therapy in seasonal allergic rhinitis: a systematic review of randomized trials. *Ann Allergy Asthma Immunol*. 2006;96(6): 779–786.
142. Mastalerz L, Kumik J. Antileukotriene drugs in the treatment of asthma. *Pol Arch Med Wewn*. 2010;120(3):103–108.
143. Berges-Gimeno MP, Simon RA, Stevenson DD. The effect of leukotriene-modifier drugs on aspirin-induced asthma and rhinitis reactions. *Clin Exp Allergy*. 2002; 32(10):1491–1496.
144. Wentzel JL, Soler ZM, DeYoung K, Nguyen SA, Lohia S, Schlosser RJ. Leukotriene antagonists in nasal polyposis: a meta-analysis and systematic review. *Am J Rhinol Allergy*. 2013 Nov–Dec;27(6):482–489.
145. Lieberman P, Nicklas RA, Oppenheimer J, et al. The diagnosis and management of anaphylaxis practice parameter: 2010 update. *J Allergy Clin Immunol*. 2010 Sep;126(3):477–480.
146. Casale TB, Condemi J, LaForce C, et al. Effect of omalizumab on symptoms of seasonal allergic rhinitis: a randomized controlled trial. *JAMA*. 2001 Dec;286(23): 2956–2967.
147. Gevaert P, Calus L, Van Zele T, et al. Omalizumab is effective in allergic and nonallergic patients with nasal polyposis and asthma. *J Allergy Clin Immunol*. 2013; 131(1):110–116.
148. MacGlashan DW, Bochner BS, Adelman DC, et al. Down-regulation of Fc(epsilon)RI expression on human

basophils during in vivo treatment of atopic patients with anti-IgE antibody. *J Immunol*. 1997;158(3):1438–1445.
149. Shamji MH, Durham SR. Mechanisms of immunotherapy to aeroallergens. *Clin Exp Allergy*. 2011 Sep;41(9): 1235–1246.
150. Kepley CL. Antigen-induced reduction in mast cell and basophil functional responses due to reduced Syk protein levels. *Int Arch Allergy Immunol*. 2005;138:29.
151. Castells M. Rapid desensitization for hypersensitivity reactions to medications. *Immunol Allergy Clin North Am*. 2009;29:585.
152. Solensky R. Drug desensitization. *Immunol Allergy Clin North Am*. 2004;24:425.
153. Cernadas JR, Brockow K, Romano A, et al. General considerations on rapid desensitization for drug hypersensitivity—a consensus statement. *Allergy*. 2010;65:1357.
154. Gross WL, Trabandt A, Csernok E. Pathogenesis of Wegener's granulomatosis. *Ann Med Interne*. 1998 Sep; 149(5):280–286.
155. Joint Task Force on Practice Parameters; American Academy of Allergy, Asthma and Immunology; American College of Allergy, Asthma and Immunology; Joint Council of Allergy, Asthma and Immunology. Drug allergy: an updated practice parameter. *Ann Allergy Asthma Immunol*. 2010 Oct;105(4):259–273.
156. Warrington R, Watson W, Kim HL, Antonetti FR. An introduction to immunology and immunopathology. *Allergy Asthma Clin Immunol*. 2011;7(suppl 1):S1.
157. Theofilopoulos AN. Immune complexes in autoimmunity. In: Bona CA, Siminovitch KA, Zanetti M, Theofilopoulos AN, eds. *The Molecular Pathology of Autoimmune Diseases*. Chur, Switzerland: Harwood Academic Publishers, 1993:229–244.
158. Pitsios C, Stefanaki EC, Helbling A. Type IV delayed-type hypersensitivity of the respiratory tract due to budesonide use: report of two cases and a literature review. *Prim Care Respir J*. 2010 Jun;19(2):185–188.
159. Yawalkar N, Hari Y, Frutig K, et al. T cells isolated from positive epicutaneous test reactions to amoxicillin and ceftriaxone are drug specific and cytotoxic. *J Invest Dermatol*. 2000 Oct; 115(4):647–652.
160. Britschgi M, Steiner UC, Schmid S, et al. T-cell involvement in drug-induced acute generalized exanthematous pustulosis. *J Clin Invest*. 2001 Jun; 107(11):1433–1441.
161. Pecina JL, Cappel MA. Acute generalized exanthematous pustulosis. *Skinmed*. 2010;8(4):210–214.
162. Saissi EH, Beau-Salinas F, Jonville-Béra AP, Lorette G, Autret-Leca E. Drugs associated with acute generalized exanthematic pustulosis. *Ann Dermatol Venereol*. 2003 Jun–Jul;130(6–7):612–618.

3

Skin Testing and Laboratory Evaluation of Hypersensitivity

Gabriele S. de Vos and Joseph E. Jones

INTRODUCTION

The aim of skin and laboratory allergy testing is to detect allergic sensitization. Allergic sensitization refers to the presence of allergen specific immune receptors within the host that are able to specifically recognize and bind allergen. Allergic sensitization alone does not mean that allergen exposure will necessarily lead to clinical manifestation of allergy because many, mostly unknown factors are involved in regulating the inflammatory cascade between allergen recognition and a full inflammatory immune response. Nevertheless, allergic sensitization represents a risk for an allergic reaction. In most cases of allergic diseases relevant to the otolaryngologist, the relevant immune receptors consist of allergen specific IgE antibodies. Allergen-specific IgE is the hallmark of type I, or immediate-type allergic reactions, the predominant reaction type in allergic rhinitis, conjunctivitis, oral allergy syndrome, and allergic angioedema (see Chapter 2), and can be detected by prick or intradermal skin testing or by the serum-specific IgE laboratory tests that are the main subject of this chapter.

> A positive skin or serum-specific IgE test indicates that the patient has allergen-specific IgE to the test allergen. This does not necessarily mean that the patient also develops symptoms when exposed to this allergen.

SKIN TESTING

Skin testing was first described by Dr. Charles Blackley in 1865 and has since evolved into a cost-effective, low-risk method of detecting allergic sensitization.

Skin Prick Testing

In skin prick testing (also termed *skin puncture testing*) allergens are introduced into the epidermis using a sharp tool such as a lancet, the tip of an injection needle, or commercially available skin test applicators carrying one or more spikes at their head (Figure 3–1). Tests are typically performed at the volar site of the forearm or upper back. When using single prick devices (eg, lancet), a drop of allergen is first applied to the skin and the lancet is then passed through the drop, onto the skin, gently spiking into the upper layer of the epidermis, lifting the skin slightly, thereby introducing a small amount of antigen solution into the epidermis. In multitest devices, all heads of the device are typically loaded with allergen solution first. The device is then perpendicularly pressed onto the skin with sufficient pressure to allow the spikes to puncture the upper layer of the epidermis (Figure 3–2).

Epidermal mast cells that carry allergen-specific surface IgE degranulate and release large amounts of histamine into the surrounding tissue (see Chapter 2). Histamine binds to H1 (and fewer H2) receptors

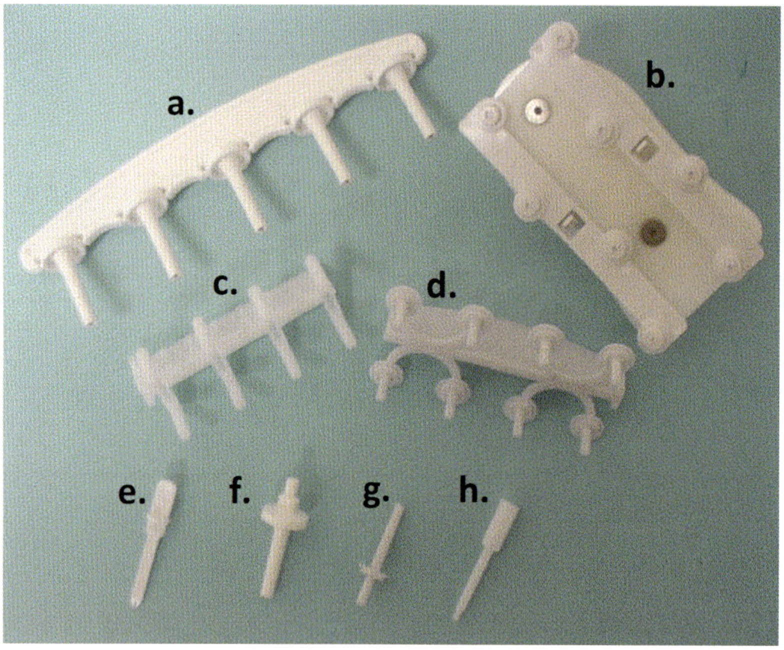

Figure 3–1. Examples of single-prick and multitest devices. **a.** Quintest, **b.** Greer Track, **c.** Multi-Test II, **d.** Quantitest, **e.** Accuset, **f.** Quintip, **g.** Sharptest, and **h.** Greer Pick. Adapted and reprinted with permission from from Carr WW, Martin B, Howard RS, et al. Comparison of test devices for skin prick testing. *J Allergy Clin Immunol.* Aug 2005;116(2):341–346.

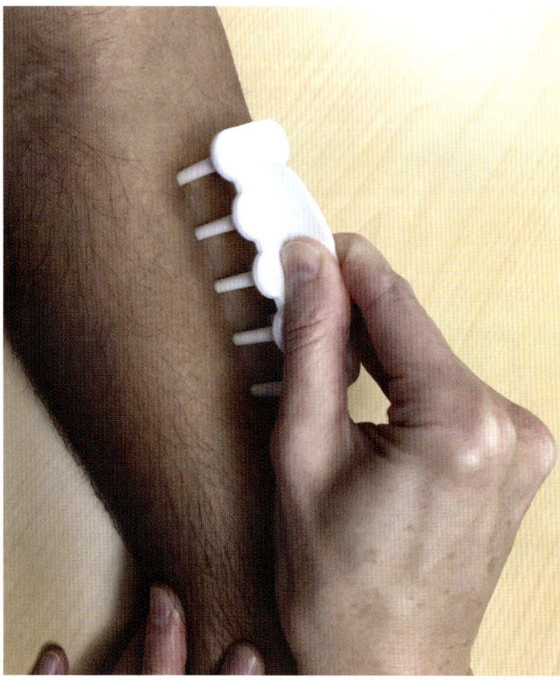

Figure 3–2. Application of the skin prick test using a multitest device (here ComforTen).

on endothelial cells and nerve endings, leading to an itchy "wheal and flare" reaction (Figure 3–3). Positive reactions become apparent within minutes and are typically fully developed after 15 to 20 minutes.

Defining a Positive Skin Prick Test

Conventionally, most researchers define a positive skin test as a wheal and flare reaction with a wheal diameter that is at least 3 mm larger than the wheal produced by a negative control solution (consisting of allergen-free diluent, eg, glycerin-saline). Occasionally, other cutoff levels may be used (eg, a 2-mm cutoff may be used to define a positive reaction if the skin test applicator produces small wheal sizes due to inherent mechanical characteristics or in younger patients).[1] In general, a wheal alone is not considered to represent a positive reaction. Instead, a flare surrounding the wheal indicates activation of endothelial and neuronal histamine receptors. However, in certain skin types (ie, very dark skin), a flare can be hard to distinguish, rendering the interpretation of a skin test difficult (see Figure 3–3). Typically, positive skin tests are accompanied by intense itching due to activation of nerve-ending histamine receptors. The presence of itching is not used for interpretation of skin test results but generally is supportive of a positive result.

> Conventional definition of a positive skin test is a wheal diameter 3 mm larger than the negative control. The presence of a flare supports a positive test.

Quantifying Positive Skin Prick Test Results

Skin test results are quantified by measuring the wheal diameter and flare diameter in millimeters. Some practitioners choose the largest diameter, and some others use the average between largest and orthogonal diameters. Both approaches are valid as long as they are used consistently. However, measuring the exact diameters can be time consuming and sometimes impractical (eg, when skin prick testing small children who may not stay still when trying to measure the results). Because of this, most practitioners use grading systems (example shown in Table 3–1). The major disadvantage of such grading systems is that they are not standardized (ie, every practitioner may use their own grading system), and thus do not allow accurate comparison of skin test results between different allergy practitioners. In addition, when using grading systems, the wheal diameters are typically visually estimated rather than exactly measured, allowing a certain degree of imprecision.

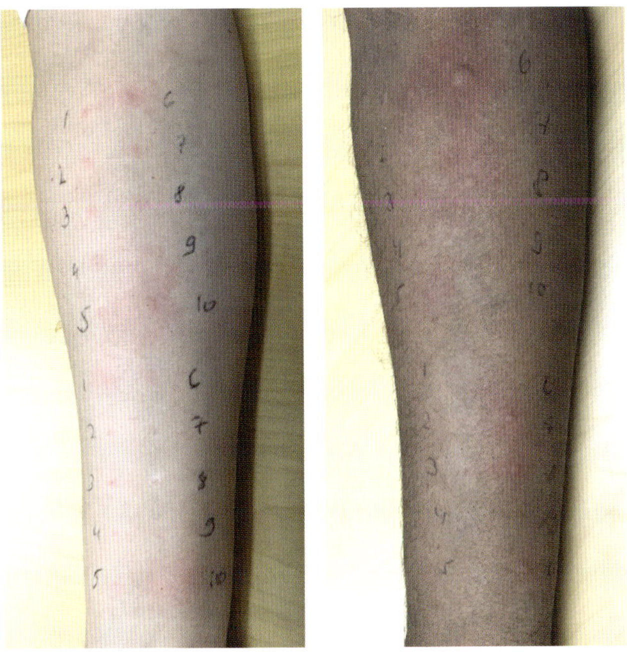

A B

Figure 3–3. Skin-prick test results in different skin types. **A.** Note that on very pale skin types, erythema may be seen due to mechanical irritation alone. **B.** In contrast, it can be difficult to distinguish flares on very dark skin.

Factors That Can Significantly Alter Skin Prick Test Results

To correctly interpret skin test results, it is important to be aware of factors that can significantly influence skin test results (ie, produce "false-positive" wheal and flares or suppress reactions) (summarized in Table 3–2).

Mechanical Trauma to the Skin. The mechanical trauma produced by the spikes of the skin test applicator alone can trigger histamine release from mast cells. This can result in a wheal and flare reaction (typically small) that does not involve IgE. This happens more commonly with skin test applicators that have multiple spikes (as opposed to one spike), and it is particularly prominent if the patient has also

Table 3–1. Example of Grading System for Skin Prick Test Reading

Grade	Wheal Size (Average of Largest and Orthogonal Diameter)
0	<3 mm than wheal size produced by diluent control
1	3–4 mm larger than wheal size produced by diluent control
2	5–7 mm wheal size produced by diluent control
3	8–10 mm
4	>10 mm

Note. "Grade 0" designates a negative skin test. "Grades 1–4" designate "positive" skin tests.

Table 3–2. Factors That Can Significantly Alter Skin Test Results

Factors leading to "false positive" or enhanced results
1. Nonspecific wheal and flare reactions due to mechanical irritation (dermographism)
Factors that can suppress skin test results
1. Medications that antagonize histamine receptors or suppress mast cell activity
2. Comorbidity: renal failure, recent venom anaphylaxis, peripheral nerve injury
Factors that can influence skin test in either way
1. Skin texture and skin diseases
2. Type of applicator and technique
3. Age (infants and elderly less reactive to allergens)
4. Location of skin test (upper back is slightly more reactive than the volar forearm)
5. Extract potency and composition

"dermographism" (ie, a general tendency to form local swelling and flaring with mechanical trauma). Therefore, a negative control skin test (with diluent, eg, glycerosaline) is necessary to compare the results produced by the mechanics of the skin test application alone.

Medications and Comorbidity. Many medications can suppress histamine-induced skin test reactions (Table 3–3).[2–12] The time and strength of suppression depends on the dose of the given medicine. For example, diphenhydramine 50 mg 4 times daily was shown to suppress skin testing for up to 5 days after discontinuation of this medicine. However, based on our own experience a single dose of diphenhydramine 25 mg may suppress skin testing for a substantially shorter time (12–24 hours).

In addition, certain medical conditions (eg, renal failure, anaphylactic shock after venom stings, strong vasovagal stimulation, or other conditions associated with peripheral hypoperfusion) can suppress histamine-induced skin reactions. Peripheral nerve injury may significantly suppress flare reactions. Normally, the histamine-induced signal received by peripheral nociceptive fibers is sent back to the skin through an axonal collateral in the peripheral ganglion. This "axonal reflex" causes vasodilation and contributes substantially to the flare reaction. If the peripheral fibers are disrupted, the flare reaction may be significantly inhibited. Therefore, a positive control using a histamine solution must accompany allergy skin testing. In most situations, a positive reaction to histamine solution (eg 2.5 mg/mL, for percutaneous testing) indicates that skin testing would have revealed any allergen-specific reactions if they were present.

Applicator and Technique. The size of wheal and flare reactions can vary widely depending on the skin test applicator used. For example, a recent study examined the responses to histamine alone ("positive control") of 2 multitest devices commonly used in the United States, the Multi-Test II (see Figure 3–1) which carries multiple spikes at each arm (Lincoln Diagnostics, Decatur, Illinois) and ComforTen (see Figure 3–2) which carries only one spike at each arm (Hollister-Stier Laboratories, Spokane, Washington). The Multi-Test II device produced significantly larger mean wheal sizes to histamine (7.5 mm, SD 1.7 mm) compared to the ComforTen device (3.9 mm, SD 1.6 mm). On the other hand, the Multi-Test II device also produced much larger wheal sizes to the negative control (glycerosaline) ranging from 0 to 4 mm compared to 0 to 1 mm with the ComforTen device.[13]

Similarly, single-prick devices can produce substantially different wheal sizes. A recent study of single prick devices commonly used in Europe showed that the median wheal diameters ranged from 1.4 mm (Stallerpoint device) to 5.4 mm (IV 23-gauge needle). In addition, the pressure and techniques with which the skin test is applied can substantially influence mechanically produced wheal-size diameters when using single or multiple test devices. Typically, when multitest devices are being used, the tester will not apply equal pressure to all sites of the applicator but often tilt it from site to site. This can result in larger wheal diameters at some positions (typically the corners) of the multitest applicator.[14] Similarly, when using single-prick devices, wheal diameters can largely differ depending on pressure and technique that is being applied.

It is important to take these differences in wheal sizes that are caused solely by the mechanical char-

Table 3-3. Examples of Medicines That Can Suppress Skin Test Results

Medication Name	Average Duration of Skin Test Suppression
H1-receptor antagonists, first generation	
Chlorpheniramine (4 mg 4×/day)	3 days (max. 6 days)
Cyproheptadine (8 mg/day)	9 days (max. 11 days)
Diphenhydramine (50 mg 4×/day)	2 days (max. 5 days)
Hydroxyzine (25 mg 4×/day)	5 days (max. 8 days)
Promethazine (25 mg 4×/day)	3 days (max. 5 days)
H1-receptor antagonists, second generation	
Azelastine nasal (1% 2×/day)	2 days
Cetirizine (10 mg/day)	3 days
Fexofenadine (60 mg 2×/day)	2 days
Loratadine (10 mg/day)	7 days
Tricyclic antidepressants	
Doxepin (25 mg, single dose)	6 days
Desipramine (25 mg, single dose)	2 days
Imipramines	>10 days
H2-receptor antagonists	
Ranitidine (150 mg, single dose)	12–24 hours
Leukotriene antagonists	
Montelukast (10 mg/day)	0
Zafirlukast (20 mg/day)	0
Glucocorticosteroids	
Systemic, short term (≤7 days)	0
Systemic, long term	Suppression of skin test likely
Inhaled, long term	0
Topical, clobetasol 0.05% (class 1, very potent) 2×/day × 7 days	Reduced allergen-induced wheal and flare response; no effect on histamine-induced wheal response, unclear duration
Topical anaesthetic	
EMLA (Prilocaine 2.5%, Lidocaine 2.5%) 1 hour prior to skin testing	0 reduction of wheal response, but 50%–100% reduction of flare response

acteristics of the testing tool and application into account when interpreting allergy test results.[15]

Another consideration when choosing a skin test applicator is the pain that the skin test produces. Multitest devices with only one spike at each arm produce generally less pain than multitest devices with multiple spikes, making them often the preferred tool in children.

Age. In general, infants exhibit less environmental sensitization and often have smaller wheal sizes compared to older children or adults.[16] On the other hand, responses to the histamine solution (positive control) are often large in infants, indicating that the small reaction sizes to allergens are truly due to lower amounts of IgE and/or fewer epidermal mast cells, and not merely due to lower skin reactivity to histamine. The prevalence of skin test positivity rises steadily through childhood, even though new sensitizations can occur at any point in life.[17,18] Skin test reactivity decreases again with older age, as do most allergic diseases (eg, allergic rhinitis) even though large reactions can still be found in adults over 65 years of age.[19]

Location. Regarding the location of testing, the upper back appears to show slightly larger wheal and flare reactivity compared to the inner forearms. We prefer testing on the forearms in adults and older children, because it allows the patient to visually appreciate the positive and negative results. In addition, the patient may wait for the evolution of the skin test in a more comfortable position than when the tests are placed on the back. In small children, however, testing on the upper back is necessary because the intense itching unavoidably makes them try to scratch the test site, thereby disturbing the results through mechanical irritation and cross contamination with the allergens of the other test sites.

Potency of Allergen Extracts. The potency of the allergen extract contributes to the skin test results. In general, high-potency (strongly concentrated and natural allergens) extracts are used for skin prick testing with environmental allergens. However, allergen potency can vary because of different factors such as the natural degradation of proteins.

Commercial allergen extract potency may decrease by up to 50% before their expiration date, due to natural decomposition and enzymatic degradation of proteins over time.[20] Preservatives and additives, such as human serum albumin and glycerin can help prevent the rapid decomposition of proteins and are typically included in allergen extracts (see Chapter 17).

Extract composition and individual sensitization profile also affect skin test reactions. A person allergic to a particular allergenic entity (eg, dust mite) is typically not only allergic to one dust mite protein but to multiple proteins. For most allergens, one or more so-called "major allergens" have been established (ie, allergens to which most people are sensitized, eg, Der p 1 in the dust mite *Dermatophagoides pteronyssinus*). However, currently there is no method that is able to clearly determine which is the most allergenic protein for a specific individual (ie, which one predominantly causes their allergy symptoms). That means that while in one dust mite allergic patient the allergen Der p 1 may trigger most of the patient's allergy symptoms, in another patient it may be Der p2, Der p4, etc. Not surprisingly, experiments in which patients were skin tested with single recombinant allergen proteins showed smaller skin test reactivity compared to natural extracts.[21] Therefore, skin test positivity will depend on how much of the relevant proteins are contained in the extract solution. For this reason, when the overall allergic potency of an extract is established, the "biologic potency" (based on patient's skin reactivity) of an extract is established by determining the overall allergenicity for most standardized extracts in the United States, instead of specific concentrations of allergen proteins. The concentrations of major allergens has been established as indicators of potency for only 2 aeroallergens, short ragweed and cat hair (see Chapter 2).

This complexity between the natural composition of the extract, the individual allergy profile to different proteins within an extract, and variable potency explains why many of the currently available extracts have yet not been standardized (ie, they contain a number of potentially allergenic proteins, each in unknown concentration). As a result, the concentration of these nonstandardized extracts is based on the total protein content (with units w:v or protein nitrogen units, PNU, per ml).

Clinically Irrelevant Skin Test Positivity Due to Cross-Reactive Antigens. Another consideration when interpreting skin (and serum) tests is the occurrence of positive results due to allergen cross-reactivity. Examples of cross-reactive allergens are tropomyosins in lobster, shrimp (Pen a 1), cockroach (Per a 7), and dust mite (Der p 10 and Der f 10).[22] Another example is positive skin test results to tree pollen in a subset of patients primarily sensitized to venom due to cross-reactive carbohydrate antigens.[23] To distinguish between irrelevant sensitizations and clinically relevant sensitizations, a careful history and sometimes, clinical challenge may be necessary, as described elsewhere.

Suppression of Skin Test Results After Anaphylaxis. In addition to the previously mentioned factors that can alter skin reactivity, there are reports that venom skin and serum IgE testing is suppressed for up to 6 weeks after venom (eg, bee sting) induced anaphylaxis. Similar findings have not been reported with environmental, food, or drug skin testing but should be considered when testing for any allergens following an episode of anaphylaxis.[24]

Skin Prick Test Results and the Correlation with Clinical Allergy

Allergic sensitization detected by skin prick, intradermal or serum specific IgE testing does not necessarily translate into the presence of clinical allergic symptoms. Approximately 10% to 20% of individuals without allergy symptoms may have positive skin prick test reactions to environmental allergens.[25] Even though such sensitizations predict an increased risk of developing allergic symptoms in the future, only 15% to 60% of such individuals may develop disease.[26] Therefore, the "proof" of which allergen is the true culprit of the patient's allergic symptoms can only be provided by allergen challenge or a strongly supportive history.

> Positive skin prick tests or serum-specific IgE tests indicate the presence of IgE, *not* clinical reactivity.

Allergen challenges are primarily performed in experimental settings by intranasal application of allergen extract, by controlled natural exposure, or by bronchial provocation (inhaling allergen in a nebulized suspension). These challenges can be time consuming and require close supervision because of potential asthma exacerbations or systemic reactions, and are therefore rarely done in daily practice. Instead, most practitioners rely on a careful history. While the history may be quite conclusive if sporadic exposures trigger symptoms (eg, sneezing and runny nose during pollen season or when exposed to specific pets), the relation between allergic sensitization and exposure is much more difficult to establish if the patient complains about perennial symptoms. Such patients may be exposed almost continuously to potential triggers such as dust mite, roach, mouse, or mold antigens. If allergic sensitization to these antigens is detected by skin testing, it is typically assumed that this may be the symptom trigger. However, nasal challenge studies have demonstrated that positive dust mite and mouse skin prick testing results predict nasal symptoms in only 40% to 80% of patients when using the conventional skin prick test cutoff point of a 3 mm wheal diameter larger than the negative control.[27] In one recent study, a positive cat skin prick test predicted the development of allergic symptoms during a cat bronchial provocation challenge in only 44% of patients. However, patients with a large wheal reaction (≥8 mm) to cat allergen had a 71% chance of also reacting to a cat bronchial challenge. It is noteworthy that in the same study 78% of patients with a positive bronchial challenge did not think that cats were a trigger of their allergy symptoms.[28]

In summary, allergen skin prick testing is predictive of a positive challenge about 70% of the time (range 45% to 95%, depending on the type and potency of the allergen extract, the type of challenge, and the study population). In general, the larger the skin prick test results, the higher the probability of being clinically allergic.[28–32] Skin testing can further classify the potentially offending allergen. For example, if a patient complains about seasonal allergic rhinitis, the skin test may not only confirm pollen sensitivity (presence of pollen specific IgE) but also help distinguish the exact pollen to which the patient may be allergic (eg, the exact tree, grass or weed pollen).

> Approximately 10% to 20% of asymptomatic individuals may have positive test results. Skin prick test and serum-specific IgE tests are about 70% predictive of specific clinical allergy confirmed by challenges.

Choice of Allergen Extracts for Skin Testing

Our environment contains thousands of substances to which we could potentially be allergic, but not all of these tend to elicit allergic responses. In general, the more intense the exposure to a particular antigen, the more likely it will become allergenic to a predisposed individual. For example, mouse or cockroach allergy is rarely found in individuals living in clean, noninfested environments, but is common in inner-city children living in sometimes highly mouse- or roach-infested neighborhoods.[33–35] On the other hand, horse allergy may be rare in inner-city populations but may occur more commonly in rural populations or those engaging in equestrian sports. Similarly, certain pollen are only present in certain areas, such as southern grasses that don't naturally grow in temperate northern climates. Therefore, the choice of allergen extracts for routine skin testing should be based on the common exposures in a given geographical area. The routine panel of test allergens may have to be expanded for patients with specific exposures (eg, testing for rabbit antigen if a patient reports symptoms at home where he or she keeps a pet rabbit).

> General principles in choosing allergen extracts for testing include the following: test allergens are relevant to the area and population; avoid unnecessary testing with multiple highly cross-reactive allergens; and consider testing with fresh material if skin and serum-specific IgE tests are negative but there is a high clinical suspicion of clinical allergy.

Cross-reactivity between allergens needs to be considered to avoid unnecessary testing. For example, northern grasses are highly cross-reactive, so it is sufficient to only test for one common northern grass or a northern grass mixture instead of individual northern grasses. Similarly, the most common dust mites found in homes are *Dermatophagoides pteronyssinus* and *D farinae*. Because of their high cross-reactivity, testing to a dust mite mixture instead of the individual dust mite species is sufficient. The same is true for the most common cockroach species found in homes: *Blatella germanica*, (German cockroach), and *Blatella americana* (and *Blatella orientalis* in southern regions). Table 3–4 shows an example of a routine panel of allergen extracts used in an inner-city practice in northeastern United States.

Beyond those considerations, the choice of allergy extracts for skin testing is limited by the commercial availability of extracts. Even commonly present environmental allergens may not be commercially available. For example, in addition to the house dust mites (*Dermatophagoides pteronyssinus* and *D farina*) that are found in 95% of house dust samples and are included in routine allergy skin testing panels worldwide, storage mites (eg, *Glycyphagus domesticus*) are also commonly found in house dust. Patients are commonly sensitized to these storage mites, and they have only limited cross-reactivity with other dust mites. However, extracts for those storage mites are currently not commercially available in every country.[36] In some instances, if testing to routine allergens and commercially available specific extracts do not reveal the suspected allergen, it is possible to produce a testing extract from material that the patient brings in (eg, dust samples, insects). While this approach may in some instances help to identify additional allergy triggers, this method is obviously nonstandardized and subject to variability in potency, purity, and interpretation.

Role of Food Allergy Testing in Evaluation of Allergic Otorhinolaryngologic Disorders

With the exception of food-induced angioedema or in rare instances allergic mucositis affecting the nasolaryngeal tract (see Chapter 11), food allergy testing is not usually required for common otorhinologic disorders (ie, rhinitis, rhinosinusitis, conjunctivitis, or otitis externa). Primary food allergies typically induce skin (urticaria, eczema, angioedema) and/or gastrointestinal (GI) symptoms (vomiting, diarrhea, particularly in infants). Common food allergies may involve the respiratory tract in some instances (eg, a highly fish allergic patients may experience rhinitis symptoms and/or an asthma attack when inhaling aerolized proteins from fish cooking), but are practically never the cause of isolated ear, nose, or throat symptoms. Therefore, food allergy testing (eg, to a panel of common food allergens) is usually not necessary in routine ear, nose, and throat (ENT) practice.

However, there is one important exception where food antigens may play a role in eliciting isolated mouth, laryngeal, or nasal symptoms. Those are food antigens that cross-react with environmental allergens. Most commonly, these are fruit

Table 3-4. Example of 40 Environmental Skin Testing Extracts for Use in an Inner-City Allergy Clinic in the Northeastern United States

Panel A	Panel B	Panel C	Panel D
Dermatophagoides mix (pteronyssinus/farina)	*Cladosporium sphaerospermum*	Ash, Red/Green	Cedar
Feathers	*Penicillium chrysogenum* (notatum)	Beech, American	Ragweed (giant, short)
Cat hair	*Aspergillus fumigatus*	Cottonwood, Eastern	Lamb's Quarter
Dog	*Aureobasidium pullulans*	Elm, American	Dock, sorrel
Cockroach mix (American/German)	*Fusarium moniliforme*	Hickory, Shagbark	English Plantain
Mouse epithelium	*Mucor plumbeus*	Maple, Red	Mugwort
Rat epithelium	Birch	Oak, White	Cocklebur
Alternaria alternata	Northern grass-mix[1]	Sycamore, American/ Eastern	Goldenrod
Aspergillus niger	Negative control (glycerin 50%)	Poplar, White	Marsh Elder
Bipolaris sorokiniana	Histamine (2.75 mg/mL)	Sweet Gum	Russian Thistle

[1]Kentucky Blue/June, Orchard, Redtop, Timothy, Sweet Vernal.

Note. "Panel" refers here to the allergens tested by one skin test applicator, in this case a 10-headed multitest device; of note, allergens that are known to induce large skin reactions in sensitized individuals should not be placed next to each other to facilitate interpretation. In this example, the patient would be tested with 4 multitest applicators. White = indoor allergens other than molds, Gray = mold, green = tree pollen, orange = weed pollen, red = grass pollen, yellow = negative and positive control.

or vegetable proteins that are similar in their conformational structure to pollen allergens. A common example is the "oral allergy syndrome," the most common presentation of "pollen associated food allergy." Through ingestion of certain antigens present in fruit or vegetables that have high structural similarities with pollen allergens, pollen-sensitized patients may experience mouth, tongue, or throat itching; oral burning; and even swelling when ingesting such food (see Chapter 11). One of the most common examples is birch-pollen allergy, which is widely prevalent in Northern Europe and the United States. Patients may experience oral itching when ingesting fresh apples, peaches, plums, cherries, or other related fruit. Less commonly, pollen allergic patients may experience isolated rhinitis symptoms when ingesting cross-reactive antigens (eg, a ragweed or mugwort pollen sensitized patient may experience rhinitis symptoms when ingesting chamomile or other herbal teas). Cases where pollen cross-reactive food allergens trigger isolated rhinitis symptoms are rare but should be considered in pollen-sensitized patients, because removing such cross-reactive food (eg, tea) from the diet may be clinically beneficial.

> Occasionally, IgE-mediated food allergy testing may play a role in ENT allergies. Conditions include pollen-associated "oral allergy syndrome" (pollen cross-reactive fruit, vegetables, or herbs), pollen-associated food-induced allergic rhinitis without skin symptoms (rare) and food-induced angioedema of ENT organs.

Testing to such pollen-associated food antigens is typically not necessary because the history alone together with pollen sensitization on environmental skin testing establishes the diagnosis in most patients. Skin or serum-specific IgE testing to commercial extracts of fruit and vegetables may not always reveal allergic sensitization, in part because of instability (mostly heat lability) of these allergens. A reasonable alternative is to perform "prick to prick" testing using fresh fruit: the practitioner pricks the fruit first (eg, apple, near the stalk where most of the relevant allergens are found), so that some of the fruit material is collected on the tip of the testing device, and then pricks the patient's skin, thereby introducing the fresh fruit material into the epidermis.[37] On the other hand, skin tests with herbs or seasoning are often negative, even if patient are truly sensitized to these materials.[38]

Safety of Skin Prick Testing

Skin prick testing with environmental allergen extracts is very safe. Systemic allergic reactions are extremely rare (and if they occur, are mild, such as hives or mild rhinitis symptoms). However, because of the theoretical risk of worsening asthma symptoms in patients with uncontrolled or acute asthma symptoms (ie, wheezing, shortness of breath) it is generally recommended to avoid doing skin testing on such patients. In these situations, serum-specific IgE testing is preferred. Similarly, infections due to skin prick testing have not been described. This may be due to the fact that most commercial allergen extracts contain phenol or other disinfectant preservatives. Nevertheless, skin hygiene should be performed similar to what is done with needle injections.

Skin prick testing to environmental allergens is extremely unlikely to cause anaphylaxis. However, food allergy skin testing has been reported to cause anaphylaxis, with even one reported fatal case in a highly sensitized child. Therefore, food allergy skin testing should be only done in absence of risk factors for severe anaphylaxis (eg, history of severe anaphylaxis upon exposure, uncontrolled asthma, etc; see also Chapter 9). Laboratory serum-specific IgE testing may therefore be preferable in such patients.

The most common (although still very rare) systemic reaction to skin prick testing is vasovagal syncope. Patients with fear of needles or history of "fainting with needle sticks" may be prone to such reactions. For a detailed description of how to distinguish a vasovagal syncope from anaphylaxis and how to treat it see Chapter 9 (Differential Diagnosis of Anaphylaxis).

> Skin prick testing with environmental allergens has a negligible risk of anaphylaxis. Intradermal testing with environmental allergens carries a very low risk of anaphylaxis if preceded by negative skin prick or very low dose intradermal testing (intradermal dilutional testing). Therefore, avoid skin testing in patients with unstable asthma or asthma exacerbations.

Intradermal (Intracutaneous) Testing

There are 2 different approaches to intradermal allergy testing: the first uses fixed, relatively strong concentrations of allergen extracts for which the patient tested negative on skin prick testing. The second approach forgoes skin prick testing and uses instead highly diluted extracts for initial intradermal testing. If negative, a sequence of higher concentrations will be tested until 2 sequential positive responses occur (intradermal dilutional testing, IDT).

Generally, intradermal testing may pick up 20% to 30% of sensitizations that would have otherwise been missed if skin prick testing alone had been performed.[39] However, intradermal testing is also less specific in predicting the presence of clinical allergy.

Intradermal Testing Techniques

Intradermal Testing Using Fixed Allergen Concentrations. Intradermal testing with fixed, high extract concentrations to environmental allergens is performed when skin prick tests are negative to specific allergens, yet the history suggests allergy. Intradermal tests are more sensitive in revealing allergic sensitization than skin prick testing. However, intradermal tests are also less specific in terms of predicting clinical allergy symptoms and are more likely to produce systemic allergic reactions than skin prick tests. That is why intradermal testing at fixed concentrations should never be performed without preceding skin prick testing. Because skin prick testing with subsequent intradermal testing at fixed concentrations is time and cost efficient, it is the most common approach practiced by allergists in the United States.

In general, intradermal testing carries a small risk of systemic allergic reactions. The higher the amount of allergen injected, the higher the risk of allergic reaction. The optimal testing concentration (ie, the concentration that carries the lowest risk of systemic allergic reactions) depends on the allergenic potency of the individual extract. Hence, one way to determine a suitable extract concentration for intradermal testing is to chose a testing concentration between 1:10 to 1:100 vol/vol dilution of recommended immunotherapy maintenance concentrations (Chapter 17) or a 1:100 to 1:1000 dilution of skin prick test concentrations, which, after negative skin prick tests, can be considered safe in clinical practice.[16] Typically, concentrations between 1:40 to 1:1000 vol/vol dilutions from the manufacturer's stock solutions are used.

A small volume (~0.02 mL) of the test concentrate is injected into the patient's arm (forearm or upper arm), using a 27- to 30-gauge syringe, producing a small (3 mm) visible bump (Figure 3–4). Initial skin irritation can produce a temporary flare reaction, which should not be confused with a "positive" allergic skin test response that develops within the next 15 to 20 minutes. By that time, nonspecific flare responses due to irritation have usually completely resolved (Figure 3–5). Positive reactions are quantified the same way as skin prick tests (wheal and flare diameters in millimeters).

Quantitative Intradermal Testing Methods. Intradermal dilutional testing (IDT) refers to the second approach to intradermal testing and consists of sequential intradermal testing starting with highly diluted extracts and stepwise increase of intradermal doses (Figure 3–6). Typically, IDT is performed without having done previous skin prick testing. The IDT extract concentrations that achieve similar results as skin prick testing (and are probably as

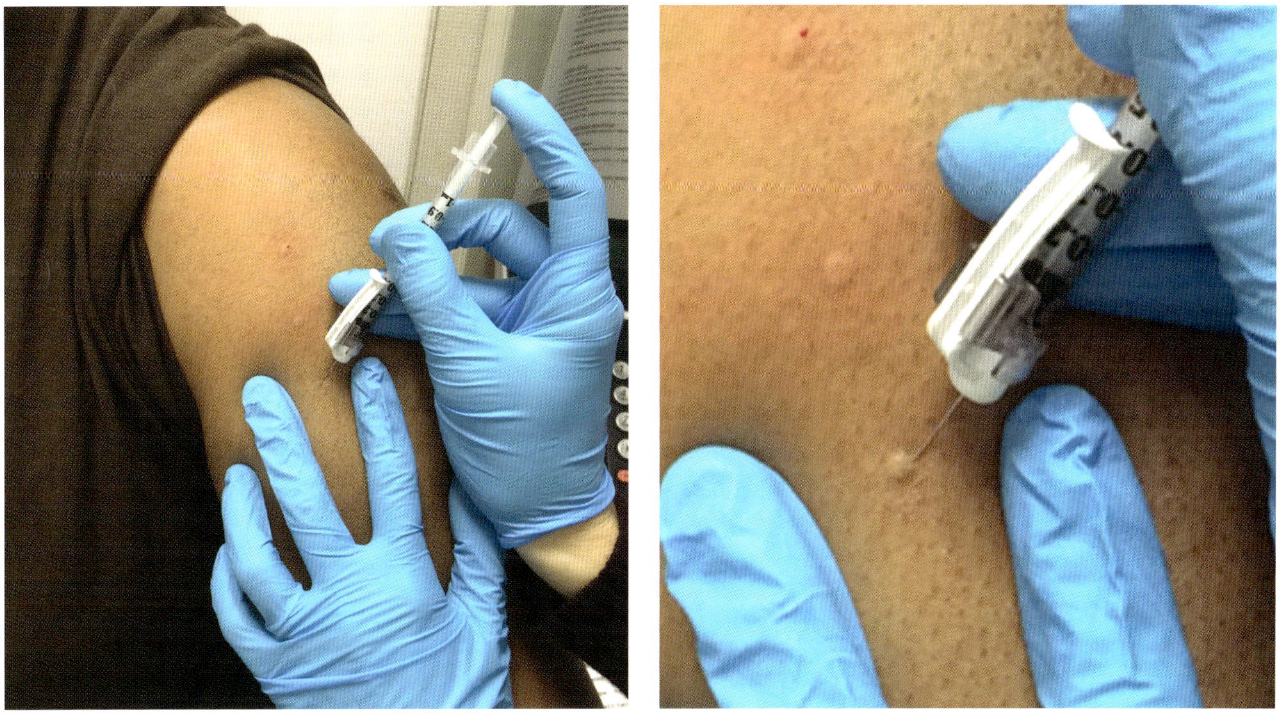

Figure 3–4. Intradermal testing. A small amount of diluted allergen extract is injected into the epidermis, producing a small wheal and irritative flare. These traumatic skin responses are not to be confused with allergic skin reactions that develop within the next 15 to 20 minutes (see Figure 3–5).

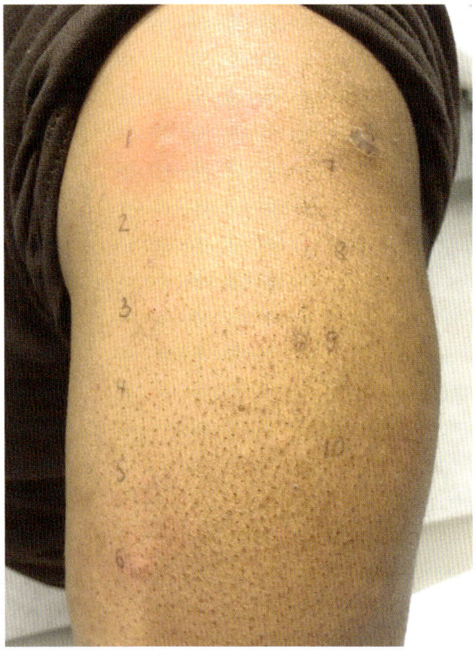

Figure 3–5. Intradermal skin test results 15 to 20 minutes after placement in the patient from Figure 3–4. Note the disappearance of the initial traumatic wheal and flare reactions and appearance of true allergic skin reactions on positions 1 and 6.

safe as SPT) range from 1:12 500 wt:vol to 1:312 000 wt:vol.[16] Note that these initial concentrations in IDT are about 10 to 100 times lower compared to extract concentrations used for fixed-concentration intradermal testing after negative skin tests. The IDT results are read after 10 to 15 minutes. After intradermal testing with the initial, most diluted extract, a second, 5-fold more concentrated, dilution is used to repeat the intradermal test. This is repeated until a wheal is observed that is at least 2 mm larger than the preceding skin reaction; an additional intradermal test is then performed with the next 5-fold higher concentration; if this again produces a wheal 2 mm larger than the preceding result, the skin test is confirmed to be positive (see Figure 3–6).[40] If the intradermal test result in IDT is negative, the intradermal test is repeated using the same allergen at a higher concentration and so forth until 2 sequential positive responses are found. If after a negative intradermal test dose, the next higher concentration elicits a very large skin reaction ("flash response"), no further testing is done. Occasionally, a response that is positive at one concentration is not larger at the next higher concentration but instead remains

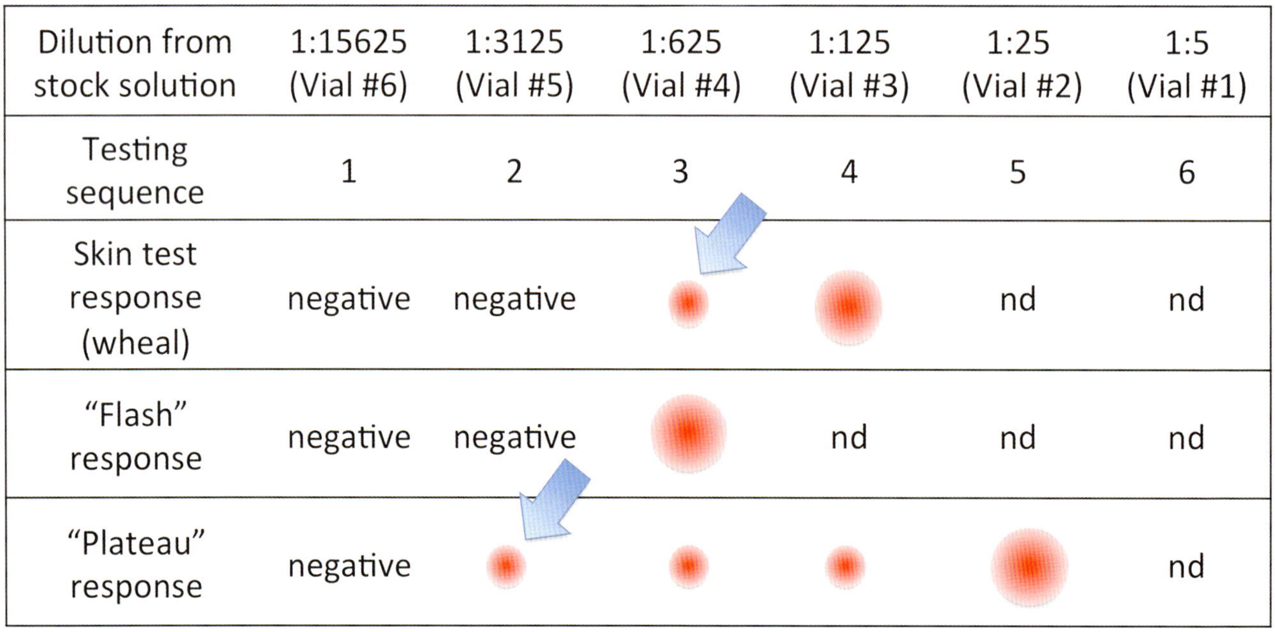

Dilution from stock solution	1:15625 (Vial #6)	1:3125 (Vial #5)	1:625 (Vial #4)	1:125 (Vial #3)	1:25 (Vial #2)	1:5 (Vial #1)
Testing sequence	1	2	3	4	5	6
Skin test response (wheal)	negative	negative			nd	nd
"Flash" response	negative	negative		nd	nd	nd
"Plateau" response	negative					nd

Figure 3–6. Intradermal dilutional testing (IDT). The manufacturer's stock solution is diluted in 5-fold steps. The strongest concentration (1:5) is named "vial #1." Intradermal testing starts with the weakest concentration (vial #6) and results are read after 10 to 15 minutes. before the next higher concentration is being tested. *Nd* = not done; blue arrows indicate the "endpoint" (ie, the concentration at which subcutaneous immunotherapy can be started safely). If a "flash response" occurs, repeat testing is recommended at another time point.

at the same size ("plateau response"). In this case, subsequent higher concentrations are used for testing until a larger reaction confirms the previous skin test. The principal aim of this method is not only to detect allergic sensitizations but also to establish a safe dose starting point for subcutaneous allergy immunotherapy ("endpoint"). Typically, the concentration of the extract vial that produced the first positive reaction is considered to be the "endpoint" concentration (see Figure 3–6). However, to date, no advantage regarding safety or efficacy of immunotherapy based on IDT has been demonstrated compared to immunotherapy based on skin prick testing.[40]

Because IDT is less time and cost efficient compared to skin prick testing, a newer, modified skin testing approach combining skin prick testing with IDT has been proposed, the modified quantitative test (MQT).[41] In MQT, skin prick testing is performed first. Depending on the result, intradermal testing at specific concentrations will be performed, following a specific algorithm (Figure 3–7). MQT has been shown to predict endpoints (ie, immunotherapy starting doses) more conservatively than IDT.[39] The clinical advantages of this testing method have yet to be established.

The reproducibility of intradermal tests is largely subject to the same factors as described above for skin prick testing, including suppression by certain medications, age, and allergen potency. Intradermal testing almost never causes a dermographic response so a negative control (intradermal injection of extract diluent) is usually not necessary, particularly if a preceding skin prick test did not show any dermographism. Similarly, if the histamine control in the preceding skin prick test showed a good positive response, it may not be necessary to include a histamine control for intradermal testing unless the patient has been exposed to factors that may influence histamine reactivity (eg, antihistamines). Nevertheless, including a negative and a positive control (histamine at 0.1 mg/mL of histamine base for intradermal testing) represents the most conservative and accurate approach. Intradermal tests are read after 15 to 20 minutes, and wheal and flare reactions are quantified in the same manner as skin prick testing.

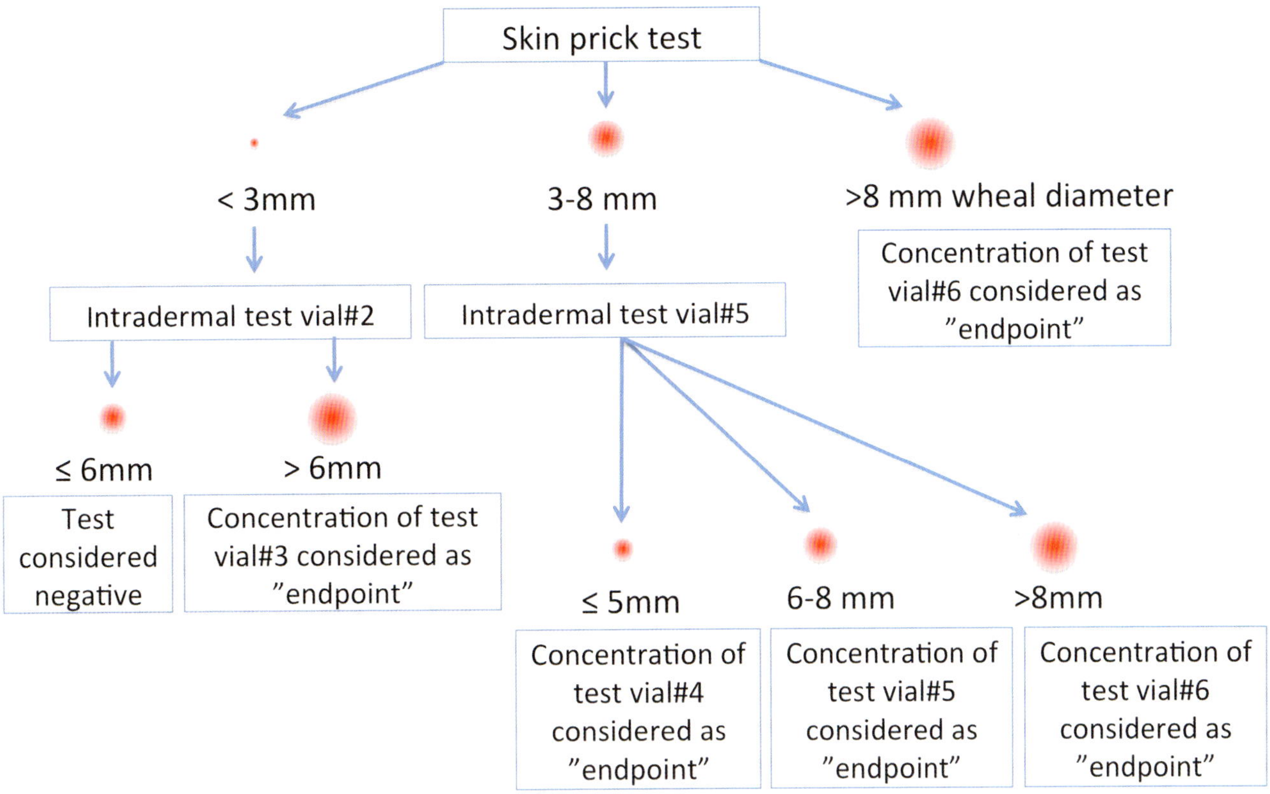

Figure 3–7. Algorithm of the modified quantitative testing method (MQT).

Correlation of Intradermal Test Results and Clinical Allergies

In comparison to skin prick and serum-specific IgE testing (see below), intradermal testing at high concentrations (when SPT or serum IgE testing was negative) predicts immediate clinical allergy relatively poorly. Researchers using cutoff points of 5-mm wheal size larger than the negative control found that such positive results predicted positive acute allergen challenges only about 40% of the time (12% to 68%, depending on allergen and extract concentrations).[27] However, large positive results (wheal size >12 mm) correlate with clinical allergy symptoms nearly 100% of the time. A number of studies showed that a negative intradermal test predicts a negative challenge in 53% to 100% (lowest for mouse, highest for dust mite).

In summary, intradermal testing at relatively high concentrations as customarily done by most allergy practitioners poorly predicts outcomes of acute clinical challenges. The use of intradermal testing at high concentrations (ie, as used in fixed concentration intradermal testing or concentrated vials in intradermal testing) should therefore be reserved for situations where the history strongly suggests a particular allergy but skin prick test results are negative. Intradermal testing may also be helpful when a positive intradermal test result will influence treatment (eg, removal of certain allergen sources or choice of allergens for allergy immunotherapy). However, to date it is unknown if inclusion of allergens into allergy immunotherapy regimens, for which the patient tested positive on intradermal but not skin prick testing and for which challenge results are unknown, provides any clinical benefits.

> After negative skin prick testing, intradermal testing with highly concentrated extracts poorly predicts acute specific clinical allergy. However, intradermal testing may be helpful in cases where clinical suspicion remains high despite negative skin prick or serum-specific IgE testing.

Intradermal dilutional testing (IDT) predicts clinical allergies in about 75%, similar to skin prick testing. Negative IDT excluded clinical allergy in about 73% of patients.[16] More trials directly comparing skin prick testing with IDT would be necessary to better gauge and compare their values in predicting clinical allergy for specific allergens.

Safety of Intradermal Testing

When testing with environmental allergens, systemic allergic reactions are rare, provided that low threshold reactions have been excluded by preceding skin prick test or low-concentration IDT. If systemic allergic reactions still occur, they are typically mild (ie, limited to the skin with local and few spreading hives without other symptoms) and readily treated with antihistamines. If anaphylaxis is suspected, treatment should be initiated accordingly (see Chapter 9).

Late-Phase Cutaneous Reactions to Skin Testing

Late-phase reactions to skin prick or intradermal testing can occur hours after the initial skin test, regardless of whether the immediate results were positive. Late-phase reactions are not necessarily allergen specific as they can also occur as a consequence of nonspecific experimental mast cell activation (eg, by substance 48/80 or kallikrein).[42] These reactions consist of wheal (and sometimes flare) reactions and typically evolve to full size within 6 to 12 hours after skin testing, plateau at 24 hours, and resolve after 2 to 7 days. In some cases, a hyperpigmented mark may remain for weeks but will eventually completely resolve. Although these reactions may occur as a consequence of an allergen specific, non-IgE-mediated mechanisms (ie, allergen-specific T-cell response), to date it is uncertain if these tests truly predict clinical allergy. Therefore, isolated late-phase reactions are typically not used as base for allergen-specific treatment (ie, allergy immunotherapy), even though reduction of late-phase reactions may correlate with clinical improvement in response to allergy immunotherapy.[43]

Other types of skin testing (ie, allergen patch testing) are covered in Chapter 10, since they are being used in the diagnosis of contact dermatitis. Patch testing has no role in the workup of allergic rhinitis, conjunctivitis, or asthma.

LABORATORY EVALUATION OF ALLERGIC SENSITIZATION

Allergic sensitization can also be assessed by in vitro assays. The primary method to detect specific immediate-type hypersensitivity is the quantification of allergen-specific IgE in the patient's serum. Other in vitro tests, such as basophil activation, are used experimentally to measure specific and nonspecific hypersensitivity. In addition, in vitro lymphocyte stimulation tests have been used experimentally to assess cell-mediated hypersensitivity; however, their role has not yet been established in the clinical evaluation of allergic disorders.

Allergen-Specific Serum IgE

Like skin testing, serum testing aims to detect allergen-specific IgE. While skin testing was long considered to be superior to serum testing, this no longer appears to be true since the development of more sensitive, commercially available, standard laboratory methods. Instead, each method carries its own advantages and rather than considering them interchangeable, skin and serum testing may actually complement each other (discussed later in this chapter) (Table 3–5).

Detection of allergen-specific IgE in serum (serum-specific IgE) was first developed in the late 1960s. The initial testing laboratory methods used radioactive labels and were termed *radioallergosorbent tests* (RAST). Today, most manufacturers have replaced radioactive signals with other detection methods (eg, chemiluminescence) and have added other improvements that allow for more accurate quantification of allergen-specific serum IgE (Figure 3–8). Moreover, commercial assays are calibrated using interpolation against a standardized human serum IgE (WHO 75/502) so that a uniform system of reporting is possible (1 unit of serum IgE = 1 IU/mL = 1 kU/L). Table 3–6 lists commonly used commercial assays quantifying serum-specific IgE.

Nevertheless, different commercial assays may still show significant differences in specific IgE levels in comparison studies.[44,45] These differences need to be considered when interpreting serum-specific IgE levels. For example, certain food-specific IgE levels measured by the ImmunoCAP method have been associated with predictive values of clinical reactivity (eg, having an allergic reaction when ingesting that food; see Chapter 11). These levels cannot be directly compared to specific IgE levels measured by other commercial methods, as other assays may result in higher or lower specific IgE levels. Similarly, different laboratory methods have been used to predict clinical respiratory allergies (ie, rhinitis or asthma) based on specific aeroallergen-specific IgE levels. Comparison studies between laboratory methods are needed to extrapolate these results to serum-specific IgE levels.

Very high total serum IgE levels may result in nonspecific IgE binding. This should be suspected if

Table 3–5. Advantages of Skin Testing Compared to Serum Testing for IgE-Mediated Hypersensitivity

Skin Prick Testing	Serum-Specific IgE Testing
Less expensive	Does not require knowledge of skin testing technique
Fast results (20 minutes)	Results not influenced by technique, tools, antihistamines/antidepressants, skin conditions
Equally sensitive as in vitro test; however, some sensitizations may be missed if skin prick testing alone is done.	Does not require availability and handling of allergen extracts
Results are visible to the patient. This may encourage compliance with environmental remediation measures or allergy immunotherapy.	Disadvantage: Some sensitizations may be missed if serum-specific IgE testing alone is done

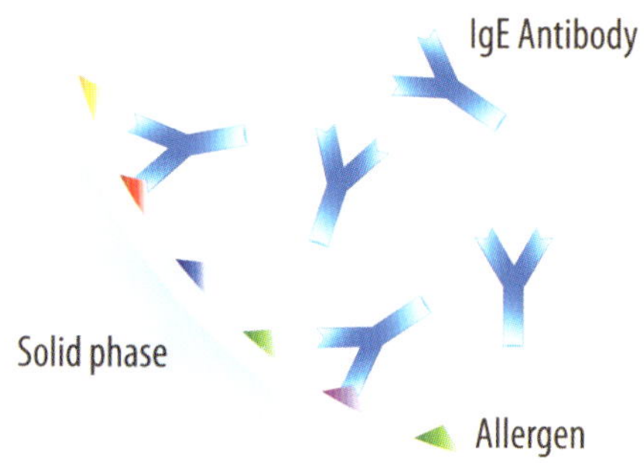

A

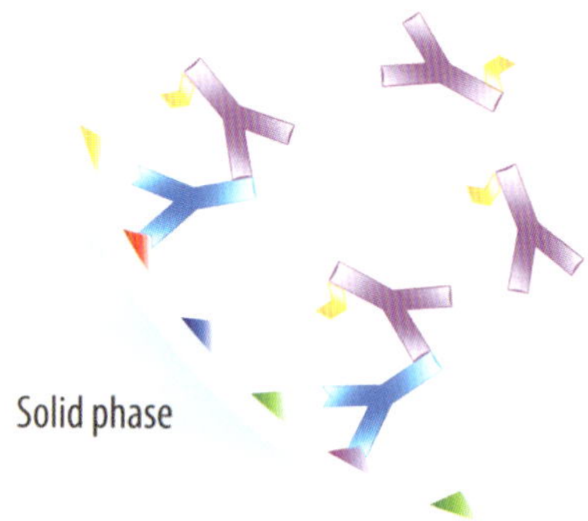

B

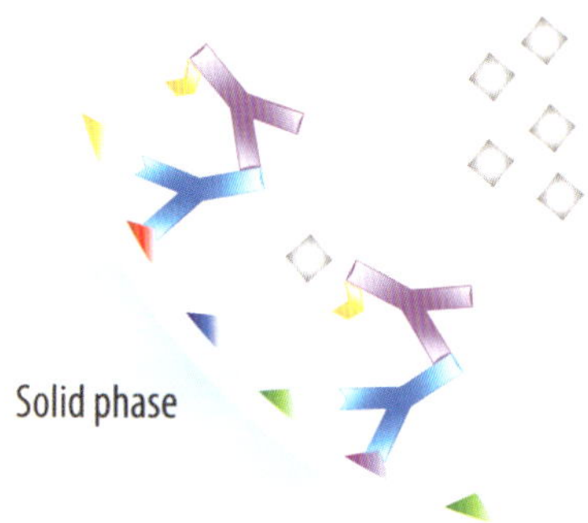

C

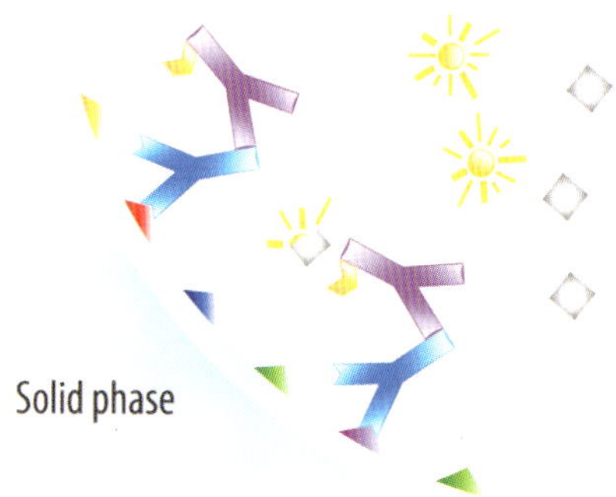

D

Figure 3-8. Principle of serum specific IgE detection (ImmunoCAP). **A.** The CAP contains a solid phase (cellulose polymer) coated with allergen extract (eg, dust mite (*triangle shapes*)). Note that the allergen extract consists of different proteins (eg, Der p1, Der p2, Der p5, etc, *depicted as triangle shapes in different colors*). The patient's serum is added to the solid phase. Specific IgE of the patient (*blue IgE antibodies*) bind to allergens. **B.** An Anti-IgE antibody is added (*purple*), flagged with an enzyme (*yellow*). **C.** A substrate is added (*gray squares*). **D.** Luminescent signals are created by enzymatic processing of the substrate. These signals can now be quantified. Reprinted with permission from Thermo Fisher Scientific. © Phadia US Inc. Phadia®, EliA™ and ImmunoCAP® are registered US trademarks of Phadia US Inc, or its affiliated entities, and are used herein pursuant to a limited license with Phadia US Inc.

Table 3–6. Examples of Commercial Technologies Used to Measure Serum-Specific IgE

Method
ImmunoCAP systems (Thermo Fisher Scientific/Phadia, FEIA, automatic)
Immulite 2000 (Siemens, chemiluminescence, automatic)
Hytec 288 Plus (Hycor Biomedical, EIA, automatic)

low-level serum-specific IgE levels to many allergens without clinical correlation are observed. Another explanation for high total IgE levels but low specific IgE levels is that total IgE is composed largely of low-affinity IgE which does not bind strong enough to allergen for detection on laboratory or skin tests. The clinical relevance of such low-affinity IgE antibodies is not clear. The different manufacturers may guide the user at what total IgE levels nonspecific IgE binding may occur.

In some cases, low specific IgE results may be explained by the allergen composition present in the assay. For example, similar to the situation in skin testing, when a patient is allergic to a particular protein that is either labile or only represented in small amounts in the entire allergen preparation, serum-specific IgE levels may be low or undetectable. In addition, if a person has high IgG levels against a particular allergen, which may occur as a result of natural allergen exposure in some patients or in patients receiving allergy immunotherapy, those IgG molecules may bind to the allergen instead of IgE, thereby "blocking" the binding of IgE, resulting in low specific IgE levels. Other factors related to the allergen that were described under allergen skin testing, and that may also influence the interpretation of serum-specific IgE levels (ie, cross-reactivity of allergens) apply to the interpretation of serum tests.

Allergen Component Testing

As was reviewed earlier, in vivo and in vitro allergen extract tests detect allergen-specific antibodies (sensitization), which may or may not be clinically relevant. Making a diagnosis can be difficult when the history is not clear, such as in perennial allergic rhinitis or in some cases of food allergies. Generally, as was shown above, traditional extract IgE tests offer high sensitivity and low specificity for the diagnosis of allergic disease. Component testing may improve diagnostic accuracy in the allergy workup (Figure 3–9).

The principle of component testing is to detect specific serum IgE to not only the entire allergen extract (eg, birch pollen) but also to different relevant proteins within the extract (eg, birch pollen proteins) (see Figure 3–9). Allergen component testing or component-resolved diagnostics (ie, testing for specific protein components within an allergen source) has recently gained an important role in the diagnosis and prognosis of certain food allergies (eg, peanut, egg, and milk, see also Chapter 11). Component testing has recently become an important tool in daily allergy practice for distinguishing true food allergy from tolerance in patients without clear histories.[46–49] Research into its role in environmental testing and prediction of rhinitis and asthma as well as predicting treatment outcomes to allergy immunotherapy is ongoing. These assays may pave the way to more specific, efficient, and precise diagnosis of IgE-mediated allergies in the future.

Recently, a highly efficient method has been developed using biochip technology ("multiplex assay"). In this method, allergens and allergen components are immobilized in a microarray. Only a minimal volume of serum (~30 uL) is needed to detect IgE against more than 100 components of more than 50 allergens (Figure 3–10). However, this method has not yet been approved for commercial use in the United States.

Comparison Between Allergen Skin Testing and Specific Serum IgE Testing

Until recently, it was thought that skin prick testing was superior to specific serum IgE testing for detecting allergic sensitization and predicting clinical allergy. However, with modern advancements in automation, reagent preparation, and refined methods of in vitro methods of measuring specific IgE in serum, this appears no longer to be true.[16,50,51] A number of studies comparing modern methods of serum-specific IgE testing and skin prick testing showed substantial discordance between skin and serum test results.[1,27,52] On average, about 25% of sensitizations (presuming a patient is truly sensitized) may be missed if only one of the 2 testing methods is performed (serum-specific IgE or skin

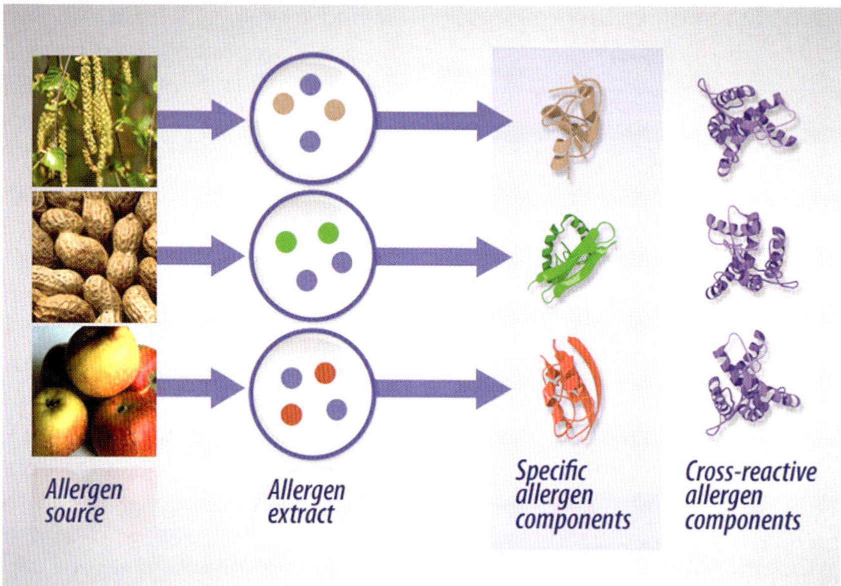

Figure 3–9. Component resolved testing. Allergen extracts consist of many different proteins. Some proteins are unique to that substance (*brown, green, or red dots*) and some proteins are common to different substances (ie, panallergen, *purple dots*). Each patient may be sensitized to different proteins within the same extract. Depending on the specific proteins the patient is sensitized to, allergies may be less or more severe. If a patient is allergic to a panallergen, the patient may experience allergic reactions when exposed to any substance that contains that panallergen. Reprinted with permission from Thermo Fisher Scientific. © Phadia US Inc. Phadia®, EliA™ and ImmunoCAP® are registered US trademarks of Phadia US Inc, or its affiliated entities, and are used herein pursuant to a limited license with Phadia US Inc.

prick testing). Relatively few studies have been done comparing modern methods of serum allergen–specific IgE with skin prick testing to predict clinical allergy. Great variation was found between allergens tested and study populations. For example, serum-specific IgE testing was found superior compared to skin prick testing for predicting clinical dust mite allergy in adults <60 years of age.[30] Whereas, sensitivity to the mold *Alternaria* detected by skin prick testing predicted a positive challenge outcome better than serum-specific IgE testing.[29]

> About 25% of sensitizations (presuming a patient is truly sensitized) may be missed if only one of the two testing methods (serum specific IgE or skin prick testing) is performed.

Even though the role of intradermal testing in comparison with modern methods of serum-specific IgE testing has not been well studied, we found in a preliminary analysis that intradermal testing will almost always reveal sensitizations that were not revealed by skin prick testing and/or specific sIgE testing.[53] In other words, intradermal testing appears to be most sensitive in detecting allergen sensitization when compared to skin prick and/or specific sIgE testing. However, clinical correlation is strongly advised because intradermal testing is also likely to reveal low-level sensitizations that may not be clinically relevant.

In conclusion, modern methods of detecting allergen-specific IgE in the patient's serum may be comparable with skin prick testing in terms of its power to predict clinical allergy symptoms. However, if clinical suspicion is high for the presence of

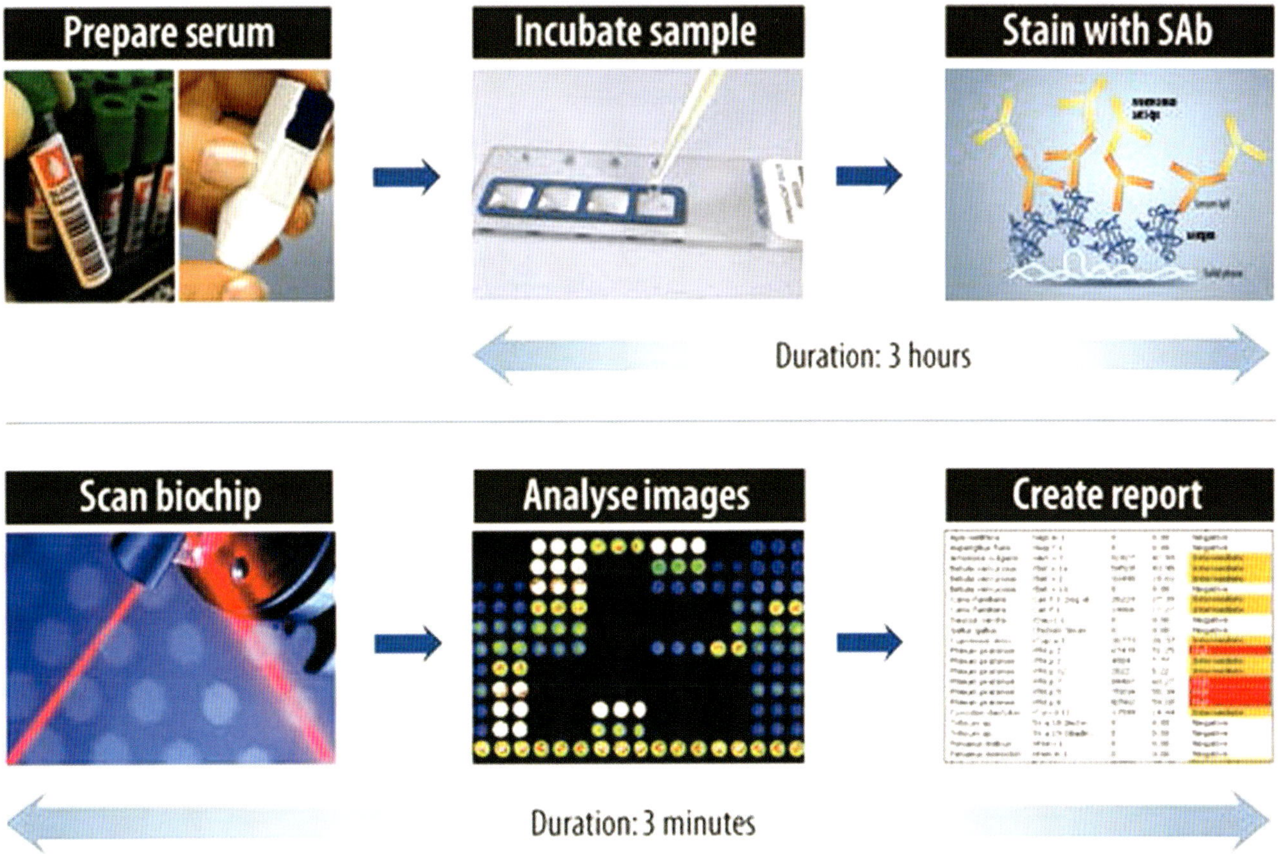

Figure 3–10. Microchip technology for measurement of allergen and allergen-component specific IgE. Purified allergen components are immobilized on the biochip. In a 2-step assay, antibodies from the patient's serum bind to the immobilized allergen components. After a short washing step, allergen bound antibodies are detected by a fluorescence-labeled antibody. Test results are measured with a biochip scanner and evaluated using the Phadia MIA software. Reprinted with permission from Thermo Fisher Scientific. © Phadia US Inc. Phadia®, EliA™ and ImmunoCAP® are registered US trademarks of Phadia US Inc, or its affiliated entities, and are used herein pursuant to a limited license with Phadia US Inc.

a specific allergy, but the initial test (skin prick or serum-specific IgE) is negative, there is a 25% chance of detecting the allergy with a second method (serum-specific IgE or skin prick test). Hence, at present, if a patient with high clinical suspicion has negative skin prick test results, it is reasonable to perform additional serum-specific IgE and/or intradermal testing in order to establish the diagnosis of specific hypersensitivity (Figure 3–11).

Total Serum IgE

Measuring the total IgE antibody level in peripheral blood has by itself only modest value in predicting allergic disease. Elevated IgE levels can be caused by conditions other than allergy, such as parasitic disease, malignancy, immune deficiency disorders, or certain chronic infections (Table 3–7). Total IgE levels can therefore only be interpreted in the context of clinical history and other diagnostic criteria. Nevertheless, elevated total IgE has been associated with asthma, allergic rhinitis, atopic dermatitis, allergic bronchopulmonary aspergillosis (ABPA, IgE often 1000 to 4000 IU/l) and allergic fungal rhinosinusitis (AFRS, IgE often 500 to 1000 IU/l). In ABPA and AFRS, IgE levels typically correspond with disease activity and may be suppressed during immune suppression with systemic glucocorticosteroids.[54] Total

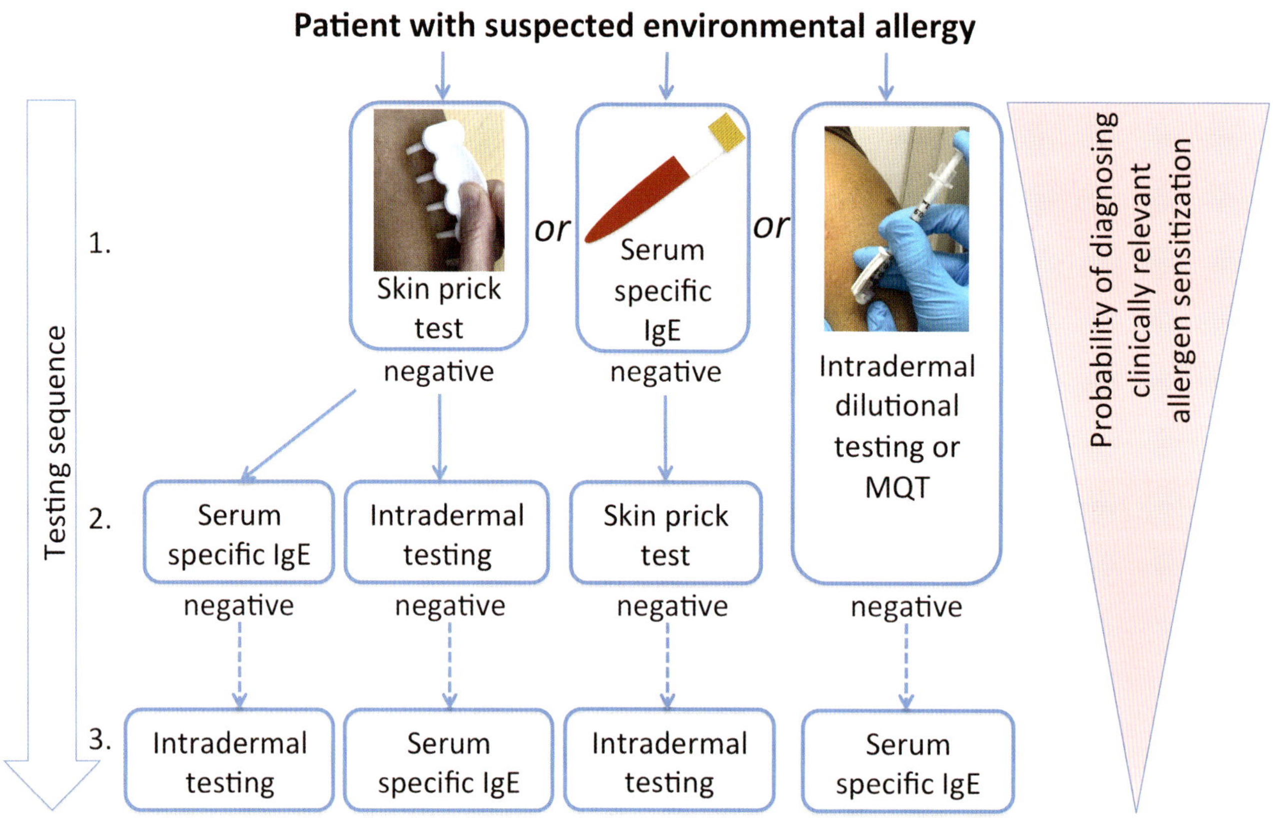

Figure 3–11. Diagnostic approach to a patient with high suspicion of type-1 allergic disease (eg allergic rhinitis, rhinoconjunctivitis). Based on current evidence it is most likely that clinically relevant sensitizations will be found with one testing method at the first level of testing (skin prick or serum-specific IgE testing or intradermal dilutional testing at low concentrations). If the first level of testing is negative but the suspicion for specific allergy high, it is reasonable to proceed with a second level of testing. To date it is not clear if adding a third level of testing adds meaningful information (*dashed arrows*). If all levels fail to diagnose the specific allergy but clinical suspicion remains high, skin prick testing with fresh material may be considered. *MQT,* modified quantitative testing.

Table 3–7. Causes for Elevated Total Serum IgE

1. Allergies
2. Parasitic disease
3. Certain bacterial and viral infections (eg, HIV, *Mycobacterium tuberculosis*, cytomegalovirus, Epstein-Barr virus, candidiasis)
4. Immunodeficiencies (rare): Hyper-IgE syndrome, Wiskott-Aldrich syndrome, Netherton disease, IPEX, Omenn syndrome, atypical DiGeorge syndrome
5. Certain neoplasms (eg, Hodgkin lymphoma, IgE myeloma)
6. Other: Tobacco smoker, cystic fibrosis, nephrotic syndrome, bone marrow transplantation, bullous pemphigoid

serum IgE levels are also used to establish the indication for omalizumab (Xolair, anti-IgE antibody) for allergic asthma and may be used in a similar way in the treatment of ABPA.[55]

Other Laboratory Tests Assessing Hypersensitivity

Allergen-Specific IgG

Allergen-specific IgG levels have limited clinical utility for the diagnosis of allergic diseases that are relevant to the otolaryngologist. Fungal-specific IgG antibodies and precipitins can be found in many patients with AFRS, but a negative result does not necessarily exclude the diagnosis of AFRS.[54] Nevertheless, positive results may support the diagnosis if the history and clinical findings are consistent. Pulmonary diseases in which the role of allergen-specific IgG testing has been scientifically well established are ABPA and hypersensitivity pneumonitis. Hypersensitivity pneumonitis is a non-IgE–mediated interstitial inflammation of the lungs in response to specific allergens in the environment that can progress to interstitial fibrosis and respiratory failure. The IgG testing panels against relatively common allergens that have been associated with this disease are commercially available (ie, specific fungi, bacteria, and feather/bird allergens) but do not exclude the disease if negative because other allergens that are not included in these panels may be causative.

Furthermore, most immunotherapy studies have shown that allergy immunotherapy produces an increase in allergen-specific serum IgG4 levels. However, correlation with clinical response to allergy immunotherapy has been inconsistent.

Local Specific IgE Measurement

Research is ongoing into diagnostic tests that detect and measure IgE locally at the site of inflammation rather than in serum. This may have an important role in a subset of patients diagnosed with nonallergic rhinitis. Novel methods of harvesting local IgE from nasal mucosa are being developed. Preliminary studies have found that a substantial proportion of patients previously labeled as "nonallergic" may have local allergic rhinitis with production of allergen-specific IgE in their nasal mucosa.[56–58]

Allergen-Triggered Basophil Activation Tests

After incubation with relevant allergens, histamine and leukotriene C4 release from peripheral basophils can be measured in blood samples of atopic patients. Alternatively, basophil activation can be determined by flow cytometry, by measuring the CD63 or CD203C markers that are expressed on the surface of activated basophils. Even though relatively good correlation with skin and IgE testing has been demonstrated, these allergen-specific basophil tests are presently being used for research purposes only.[59]

> There are a number of nonstandardized laboratory methods for investigating specific hypersensitivity that are not recommended for routine evaluation of hypersensitivity. These include basophil activation tests, lymphocyte stimulation tests, markers of eosinophil activation, allergen-specific IgG/IgG4, and cytotoxicity assays.

Chronic Urticaria Index

Non-allergen–specific basophil activation is often measured in patients with chronic urticaria. Patients with chronic urticaria (CU) suffer from recurrent hives with or without angioedema that may occasionally involve the lips or face. Many patients with chronic urticaria respond to the treatment with antihistamines, indicating that histamine release from mast cells and basophils plays a pathogenic role. Nevertheless, neither food nor environmental allergies seem to play a significant role in many patients with this disease suggesting that mast cells and basophils are activated by other mechanisms than allergen stimulation. It was shown that a subset of patients produce autoantibodies against the IgE receptor on mast cells and basophils that may explain the disease. For the CU index, the patient's serum (which may contain these autoantibodies) is incubated in vitro together with basophils (from healthy donors). Basophil activation can then be determined by histamine release into the supernatant or flow cytometric measurement of activation markers (eg, CD63 and CD203c). The anti-IgE or anti-IgE-receptor autoantibodies in the serum of the patient with chronic urticaria will activate the basophils, resulting in a high CU index. However, it should be noted that basophils and mast cells may release histamine through non-IgE/IgE receptor mechanisms as well.[60] Therefore, an elevated CU index may not always reflect the presence of autoantibodies.

Markers of Anaphylaxis and Mast Cell Disorders

Several markers can be measured in plasma or urine to confirm the diagnosis of anaphylaxis (ie, tryptase, histamine, and urine *N*-methyl histamine). If elevated in absence of anaphylaxis they may give rise to suspicion of mast cell disorders. These laboratory markers are discussed in detail in Chapter 9 (Anaphylaxis and Mast Cell Disorders; Laboratory Tests).

Eosinophil Activation

Eosinophils are key cells in allergic inflammation. Eosinophils in the nasal smear correlate well with active allergen exposure symptoms, positive skin prick test or serum-specific IgE, release of inflammatory cytokines, and spirometry/methacholine challenges. Eosinophils are attracted to the site of allergic reaction within hours. Eosinophilic cationic protein (ECP, a measurable marker of eosinophil activation) in serum, sputum, and nasal secretions, can be detected in patients experiencing late-phase allergic reactions. However, ECP has not shown to be clinically useful in the diagnosis or in monitoring of allergic disease.

In Vitro Cell-Mediated Hypersensitivity Tests

Predominantly used in research settings, patient lymphocytes can be incubated with allergens and subsequent lymphocyte proliferation /transformation, and cytokine or chemokine production, can be measured. Allergen-induced lymphocyte proliferation as well as production of certain chemokines (eg, macrophage migration inhibitory factor, MIF) correlates with specific delayed hypersensitivity reactions on skin testing. Allergen-specific lymphocyte stimulation and eosinophil activation tests are primarily used in research settings.[16]

REFERENCES

1. de Vos G, Nazari R, Ferastraoaru D, et al. Discordance between aeroallergen specific serum IgE and skin testing in children younger than 4 years. *Ann Allergy Asthma Immunol.* Jun 2013;110(6):438–443.
2. Cook TJ, MacQueen DM, Wittig HJ, Thornby JI, Lantos RL, Virtue CM. Degree and duration of skin test suppression and side effects with antihistamines. A double blind controlled study with five antihistamines. *J Allergy Clin Immunol.* Feb 1973;51(2):71–77.
3. Almind M, Dirksen A, Nielsen NH, Svendsen UG. Duration of the inhibitory activity on histamine-induced skin weals of sedative and non-sedative antihistamines. *Allergy.* Nov 1988;43(8):593–596.
4. Pearlman DS, Grossman J, Meltzer EO. Histamine skin test reactivity following single and multiple doses of azelastine nasal spray in patients with seasonal allergic rhinitis. *Ann Allergy Asthma Immunol.* Sep 2003;91(3):258–262.
5. Sicherer SH, Eggleston PA. EMLA cream for pain reduction in diagnostic allergy skin testing: effects on wheal and flare responses. *Ann Allergy Asthma Immunol.* Jan 1997;78(1):64–68.
6. Simons FE, Simons KJ. Clinical pharmacology of new histamine H1 receptor antagonists. *Clin Pharmacokinet.* May 1999;36(5):329–352.
7. Rao KS, Menon PK, Hilman BC, Sebastian CS, Bairnsfather L. Duration of the suppressive effect of tricyclic antidepressants on histamine-induced wheal-and-flare reactions in human skin. *J Allergy Clin Immunol.* Nov 1988;82(5, pt 1):752–757.
8. Wolfe HI, Fontana VJ. The effect of tranquilizers on the immediate skin wheal reaction. A preliminary report. *J. Allergy.* May–Jun 1964;35:271–273.
9. Simons FE, Johnston L, Gu X, Simons KJ. Suppression of the early and late cutaneous allergic responses using fexofenadine and montelukast. *Ann Allergy Asthma Immunol.* Jan 2001;86(1):44–50.
10. Saarinen JV, Harvima RJ, Horsmanheimo M, Harvima IT. Modulation of the immediate allergic wheal reaction in the skin by drugs inhibiting the effects of leukotriene C4 and prostaglandin D2. *Eur J Clin Pharmacol.* Apr 2001; 57(1):1–4.
11. Andersson M, Pipkorn U. Inhibition of the dermal immediate allergic reaction through prolonged treatment with topical glucocorticosteroids. *J Allergy Clin Immunol.* Feb 1987;79(2):345–349.
12. Bousquet J, Heinzerling L, Bachert C, et al. Practical guide to skin prick tests in allergy to aeroallergens. *Allergy.* Jan 2012;67(1):18–24.
13. Dykewicz MS, Dooms KT, Chassaing DL. Comparison of the Multi-Test II and ComforTen allergy skin test devices. *Allergy Asthma Proc.* May–Jun 2011;32(3):198–202.
14. Dykewicz MS, Lemmon JK, Keaney DL. Comparison of the Multi-Test II and Skintestor Omni allergy skin test devices. *Ann Allergy Asthma Immunol.* Jun 2007;98(6):559–562.
15. Nelson HS. Variables in allergy skin testing. *Allergy Proc.* Nov–Dec 1994;15(6):265–268.
16. Bernstein IL, Li JT, Bernstein DI, et al. Allergy diagnostic testing: an updated practice parameter. *Ann Allergy Asthma Immunol.* Mar 2008;100(3, suppl 3):S1–148.
17. Havstad S, Wegienka G, Zoratti EM, et al. Effect of prenatal indoor pet exposure on the trajectory of total IgE levels in early childhood. *J Allergy Clin Immunol.* Oct 2011;128(4):880–885.e884.
18. Lau S, Illi S, Sommerfeld C, et al. Early exposure to house-dust mite and cat allergens and development of childhood asthma: a cohort study. Multicentre Allergy Study Group. *Lancet.* Oct 21 2000;356(9239):1392–1397.
19. Di Lorenzo G, Leto-Barone MS, La Piana S, Ditta V, Di Fede G, Rini GB. Clinical course of rhinitis and changes

in vivo and in vitro of allergic parameters in elderly patients: a long-term follow-up study. *Clin Exp Med.* Feb 2013;13(1):67–73.
20. Morrow KS, Slater JE. Regulatory aspects of allergen vaccines in the US. *Clin Rev Allergy Immunol.* Oct 2001; 21(2–3):141–152.
21. Schmid-Grendelmeier P, Crameri R. Recombinant allergens for skin testing. *Int Arch Allergy Immunol.* Jun 2001;125(2):96–111.
22. Ayuso R, Reese G, Leong-Kee S, Plante M, Lehrer SB. Molecular basis of arthropod cross-reactivity: IgE-binding cross-reactive epitopes of shrimp, house dust mite and cockroach tropomyosins. *Int Arch Allergy Immunol.* Sep 2002;129(1):38–48.
23. Kochuyt AM, Van Hoeyveld EM, Stevens EA. Prevalence and clinical relevance of specific immunoglobulin E to pollen caused by sting- induced specific immunoglobulin E to cross-reacting carbohydrate determinants in Hymenoptera venoms. *Clin Exp Allergy.* Apr 2005;35(4):441–447.
24. Goldberg A, Confino-Cohen R. Timing of venom skin tests and IgE determinations after insect sting anaphylaxis. *J Allergy Clin Immunol.* Aug 1997;100(2):182–184.
25. Salo PM, Calatroni A, Gergen PJ, et al. Allergy-related outcomes in relation to serum IgE: results from the National Health and Nutrition Examination Survey 2005–2006. *J Allergy Clin Immunol.* May 2011;127(5):1226–1235, e1227.
26. Bodtger U, Poulsen LK, Malling HJ. Asymptomatic skin sensitization to birch predicts later development of birch pollen allergy in adults: a 3-year follow-up study. *J Allergy Clin Immunol.* Jan 2003;111(1):149–154.
27. de Vos G. Skin testing versus serum-specific IgE testing: which is better for diagnosing aeroallergen sensitization and predicting clinical allergy? *Curr Allergy Asthma Rep.* May 2014;14(5):430.
28. Fernandez C, Cardenas R, Martin D, et al. Analysis of skin testing and serum specific immunoglobulin E to predict airway reactivity to cat allergens. *Clin Exp Allergy.* Mar 2007;37(3):391–399.
29. Fernandez C, Bevilacqua E, Fernandez N, et al. Asthma related to Alternaria sensitization: an analysis of skin-test and serum-specific IgE efficiency based on the bronchial provocation test. *Clin Exp Allergy.* May 2011;41(5): 649–656.
30. King MJ, Tamulis T, Lockey RF. Prick puncture skin tests and serum specific IgE as predictors of nasal challenge response to dermatophagoides pteronyssinus in older adults. *Ann Allergy Asthma Immunol.* Jul 2008;101(1):12–17.
31. Sharma HP, Wood RA, Bravo AR, Matsui EC. A comparison of skin prick tests, intradermal skin tests, and specific IgE in the diagnosis of mouse allergy. *J Allergy Clin Immunol.* Apr 2008;121(4):933–939.
32. Wood RA, Phipatanakul W, Hamilton RG, Eggleston PA. A comparison of skin prick tests, intradermal skin tests, and RASTs in the diagnosis of cat allergy. *J Allergy Clin Immunol.* May 1999;103(5, pt 1):773–779.
33. Phipatanakul W, Eggleston PA, Wright EC, Wood RA, National Coooperative Inner-City Asthma S. Mouse allergen. II. The relationship of mouse allergen exposure to mouse sensitization and asthma morbidity in inner-city children with asthma. *J Allergy Clin Immunol.* Dec 2000;106(6):1075–1080.
34. Matsui EC, Eggleston PA, Buckley TJ, et al. Household mouse allergen exposure and asthma morbidity in inner-city preschool children. *Ann Allergy Asthma Immunol.* Oct 2006;97(4):514–520.
35. Rosenstreich DL, Eggleston P, Kattan M, et al. The role of cockroach allergy and exposure to cockroach allergen in causing morbidity among inner-city children with asthma. *N Engl J Med.* May 8 1997;336(19):1356–1363.
36. Arias-Irigoyen J, Lombardero M, Arteaga C, Carpizo JA, Barber D. Limited IgE cross-reactivity between *Dermatophagoides pteronyssinus* and *Glycyphagus domesticus* in patients naturally exposed to both mite species. *J Allergy Clin Immunol.* Jul 2007;120(1):98–104.
37. Vlieg-Boerstra BJ, van de Weg WE, van der Heide S, Dubois AE. Where to prick the apple for skin testing? *Allergy.* Sep 2013;68(9):1196–1198.
38. Chen JL, Bahna SL. Spice allergy. *Ann Allergy Asthma Immunol.* Sep 2011;107(3):191–199; quiz 199, 265.
39. Peltier J, Ryan MW. Comparison of intradermal dilutional testing, skin prick testing, and modified quantitative testing for common allergens. *Otolaryngol Head Neck Surg.* Aug 2007;137(2):246–249.
40. Fornadley JA. Skin testing for inhalant allergy. *Int Forum Allergy Rhinol.* Sep 2014;(4, suppl 2):S41–45.
41. Krouse JH, Krouse HJ. Modulation of immune mediators with MQT-based immunotherapy. *Otolaryngol Head Neck Surg.* May 2006;134(5):746–750.
42. Lemanske RF, Jr., Kaliner MA. Late phase allergic reactions. *Int J Dermatol.* Sep 1983;22(7):401–409.
43. Parker WA, Jr., Whisman BA, Apaliski SJ, Reid MJ. The relationships between late cutaneous responses and specific antibody responses with outcome of immunotherapy for seasonal allergic rhinitis. *J Allergy Clin Immunol.* Nov 1989;84(5, pt 1):667–677.
44. Kontis KJ, Valcour A, Patel A, et al. Correlation of the turbo-MP RIA with ImmunoCAP FEIA for determination of food allergen-specific immunoglobulin E. *Ann Clin Lab Sci.* Winter 2006;36(1):79–87.
45. Hamilton RG, Mudd K, White MA, Wood RA. Extension of food allergen specific IgE ranges from the ImmunoCAP to the IMMULITE systems. *Ann Allergy Asthma Immunol.* Aug 2011;107(2):139–144.
46. Dang TD, Tang M, Choo S, et al. Increasing the accuracy of peanut allergy diagnosis by using Ara h 2. *J Allergy Clin Immunol.* Apr 2012;129(4):1056–1063.
47. Nicolaou N, Murray C, Belgrave D, Poorafshar M, Simpson A, Custovic A. Quantification of specific IgE to whole peanut extract and peanut components in prediction of peanut allergy. *J Allergy Clin Immunol.* Mar 2011;127(3): 684–685.
48. Masthoff LJ, Mattsson L, Zuidmeer-Jongejan L, et al. Sensitization to Cor a 9 and Cor a 14 is highly specific for a hazelnut allergy with objective symptoms in Dutch children and adults. *J Allergy Clin Immunol.* Aug 2013;132(2): 393–399.

49. Kattan JD, Sicherer SH, Sampson HA. Clinical reactivity to hazelnut may be better identified by component testing than traditional testing methods. *J Allergy Clin Immunol.* Sep–Oct 2014;2(5):633–634, e631.
50. National Asthma E, Prevention P. Expert Panel Report 3 (EPR-3): Guidelines for the Diagnosis and Management of Asthma-Summary Report 2007. *J Allergy Clin Immunol.* Nov 2007;120(5, suppl):S94–138.
51. Burks AW, Jones SM, Boyce JA, et al. NIAID-sponsored 2010 guidelines for managing food allergy: applications in the pediatric population. *Pediatrics.* Nov 2011;128(5):955–965.
52. Schoos AM, Chawes BL, Folsgaard NV, Samandari N, Bonnelykke K, Bisgaard H. Disagreement between skin prick test and specific IgE in young children. *Allergy.* Jan 2015;70(1):41–48.
53. Ferastraoaru D, Shtessel M, Hudes G, de Vos G. *Comparison between intradermal skin testing and serum specific immunoglobulin E in detecting allergic sensitization in patients with negative skin prick tests.* Abstract presented at: Meeting of the American Academy of Allergy, Asthma and Immunology; February 2015; Houston, TX.
54. Callejas CA, Douglas RG. Fungal rhinosinusitis: what every allergist should know. *Clin Exp Allergy.* Aug 2013;43(8):835–849.
55. Collins J, Devos G, Hudes G, Rosenstreich D. Allergic bronchopulmonary aspergillosis treated successfully for one year with omalizumab. *J Asthma Allergy.* 2012;5:65–70.
56. Reisacher WR. Mucosal brush biopsy testing of the inferior turbinate to detect local, antigen-specific immunoglobulin E. *Int Forum Allergy Rhinol.* Jan–Feb 2012;2(1):69–74.
57. Reisacher WR. Detecting local immunoglobulin E from mucosal brush biopsy of the inferior turbinates using microarray analysis. *Int Forum Allergy Rhinol.* May 2013;3(5):399–403.
58. Reisacher WR, Bremberg MG. Prevalence of antigen-specific immunoglobulin E on mucosal brush biopsy of the inferior turbinates in patients with nonallergic rhinitis. *Int Forum Allergy Rhinol.* Apr 2014;4(4):292–297.
59. Moneret-Vautrin DA, Sainte-Laudy J, Kanny G, Fremont S. Human basophil activation measured by CD63 expression and LTC4 release in IgE-mediated food allergy. *Ann Allergy Asthma Immunol.* Jan 1999;82(1):33–40.
60. Bossi F, Frossi B, Radillo O, et al. Mast cells are critically involved in serum-mediated vascular leakage in chronic urticaria beyond high-affinity IgE receptor stimulation. *Allergy.* Dec 2011;66(12):1538–1545.

4

Genetics of Allergic Disorders

C. Doriene van Ginkel, Anthony E.J. Dubois, and Gerard H. Koppelman

INTRODUCTION TO THE HERITABILITY OF ALLERGIC DISEASES

Multifactorial Etiology

With an estimated prevalence ranging between 16% and 57% in the United States, Europe, Australia, New Zealand, and Taiwan, atopy is the most common disorder of the immune system[1] and is defined as sensitization to atopic allergens. Sensitization is defined as the production of specific immunoglobulin E (sIgE), and atopic allergens are defined as allergens that may show epidemiologically significant cosensitization with known "reference" atopic allergens such as house dust mite.[2] Despite the high prevalence of atopic allergic diseases such as asthma, rhinitis, food allergy, and atopic dermatitis, the pathogenesis of these disorders remains poorly understood.

Atopic diseases have a multifactorial etiology, with a complex interaction of genetic risk factors and environmental triggers. A well-known purported environmental influence is described in the hygiene hypothesis, which states that exposure to microbes and microbial products early in life is associated with a decrease in risk of developing allergic disease. This is supported by multiple epidemiological studies which have shown that there is an inverse relationship between markers of early life exposure to microbes and microbial products (such as number of siblings, day care attendance or growing up on a farm) and allergic disease.[1]

Heritability

The genetic basis of atopy is widely established, and in the past, atopy was even defined as "a personal or familial tendency to produce IgE antibodies in response to low doses of allergens."[3] Atopic diseases coexist in individuals and are clustered in families and populations. As early as in 1916, positive family histories were reported in half of asthmatic patients.[4] Since then, numerous epidemiologic studies have reported familial clustering of atopic diseases as well as higher concordance rates among monozygotic twins than dizygotic twins. For example, one study reported a 5-fold increase for the risk of peanut allergy for a child with a peanut allergic sibling or parents.[5] For atopy in general, current heritability estimations vary between 34% and 84%,[1] which means that this proportion of variance is due to heritable factors. Heritability estimates of allergic diseases vary between 35% and 95% for asthma, 33% and 91% for allergic rhinitis, and 71% and 84% for atopic dermatitis.[1]

Furthermore, many patients suffer from multiple atopic diseases. For example, 90% of all children referred to a tertiary clinic for food allergy have been diagnosed with atopic diseases other than food allergy, most commonly atopic dermatitis.[6] Is the co-occurrence of atopic diseases due to a shared etiology, or they can be regarded as different clinical manifestations of atopy? The answer to this question is as yet unknown although a recent report on 12 European birth cohorts with over 27 000 children showed that the population attributable risk of IgE sensitization was only 38% for having an atopic comorbidity (asthma, atopic dermatitis, and rhinitis).[7] This suggests that IgE sensitization can no longer be considered the only causal mechanism for comorbidity in allergic diseases.

In this chapter, we will provide an overview of the genetics of allergic disease, and start with an introduction into genetic and epigenetic research that has revolutionized our knowledge about atopy and atopic diseases over the past 2 decades. In addition, we will explain the pathway leading to IgE sensitization and genetic markers associated with the different atopic diseases. Emphasis will be on the causal mechanism behind the genetic markers, and different causal theories will be discussed.

> Atopic diseases have a multifactorial etiology, with a complex interaction of genetic risk factors and environmental triggers. For atopy in general, current heritability estimations vary between 34% and 84%.[1] Genetic studies may provide an answer to the question whether the co-occurrence of atopic diseases is due to a shared etiology or if they can be regarded as different clinical manifestations of atopy.

RESEARCH ON THE GENETICS OF ATOPY AND ALLERGY

In the last 2 decades, approaches to studying the genetics of allergy have evolved enormously. Since the first study reporting an association between a genetic locus and atopic disease in 1989,[8] over 1000 candidate gene studies have been published. These candidate gene studies are hypothesis driven and therefore focus on preidentified genetic variations, which have been selected based on their function in known pathways leading to allergy. The genetic markers used are single nucleotide polymorphisms (SNPs), which are changes of one base pair in the genome that account for over 90% of all genetic variation. Alternatively, other sources of genetic variation, such as insertions, deletions, or copy number variants can be studied. The study design is usually a comparison of the frequency of a gene variant in a population of cases versus a population of healthy controls. Replicating findings from these candidate gene studies has proved to be challenging due to a variety of reasons, such as lack of standardized phenotyping and lack of power.[1] An important aspect of genetic studies is that the identified genetic variants can have a direct, functional effect in a gene, and thereby increase disease risk. Alternatively, a SNP can be only indirectly involved by being in linkage disequilibrium (LD) with the pathogenic variant. The LD is the association of 2 genetic variants, in which both are inherited together, mostly because they are close to each other on the genome.

To generate information on new, as yet undiscovered pathways, genome-wide approaches were then developed which analyze all regions of the genome and are therefore hypothesis free. The first approach that was used is called *positional cloning*, which combines linkage studies in families with subsequent fine mapping studies using a case-control approach. In linkage studies, genetic markers evenly spaced across the genome are studied for cosegregation in affected relatives. This method is based on the hypothesis that the "disease variant" is inherited and therefore similar in affected relatives. Combining data in different families provides information on large chromosomal regions associated with allergy of several millions of base pairs, which generally contain dozens to hundreds of genes. Therefore, with linkage studies it is difficult to pinpoint one or more genes, and this method is then followed up by positional candidate gene studies, where genes in the linked regions are investigated for association with the disease using a case-control design.

Although several interesting genes have been identified with this method, the current method of choice is called the Genome Wide Association study (GWAS). In a GWAS, between three hundred thousand and one million SNPs are analyzed using DNA chips. The number of SNPs tested requires statistical correction for multiple testing errors and therefore requires large sample sizes. The GWAS select for prevalent genetic variations (ie, present in >5% in the general population). A recent development is the use of resequencing studies. Because GWAS are only sensitive to common variants, this method aims for rare variants that may have a relatively strong effect on the risk of developing the disease. These rare variants are studied for enrichment in cases compared to controls.

All approaches have advantages and disadvantages (Table 4–1) and provide relevant information on the genetic origins of atopy. Study outcomes are discussed below.

In the last 2 decades, approaches to studying the genetics of allergy have evolved from the hypothesis-driven candidate gene studies toward hypothesis-free genome-wide association studies. Identified genetic variants can have a direct, functional effect in a gene, and thereby increase disease risk, or can be only indirectly involved by being associated with the pathogenic variant.

Gene-Environment Interactions and Epigenetics

Although results from candidate gene and genome-wide analyses are promising, the SNPs currently identified can only explain a few percent of the total estimated heritability of atopy. Therefore, current research is directed at the cause of this "missing heritability." This can be due to as yet unidentified prevalent variants with very modest effects, rare variants with strong effects, or other sources of genetic variation such as copy number variation. Furthermore, interactions between genes and environment and gene-gene interactions have been proposed.

Table 4-1. Approaches for Gene Discovery

Approach	Advantages	Disadvantages
Candidate gene association studies (1979s–present)	Hypothesis driven Results easy to interpret Detects genes with modest effect sizes	Limited to what we know Cannot discover novel genes or pathways Requires LD between markers and causal variants
Genome-wide linkage studies (1980–1990s) (positional cloning)	Genome wide Can discover novel genes and pathways Requires relatively few genetic markers Does not rely on LD between markers and causal variants Can detect genes harboring rare risk variants	Requires families Poor resolution Low power to detect genes with modest effects
Genome-wide association studies (2007–present)	Genome wide Can discover novel genes and pathways Excellent resolution Can detect loci with modest effect sizes	Requires dense marker typing and very large sample sizes Requires LD between markers and causal variants Limited to common variants
Resequencing studies in genes, exomes, or whole genomes (ongoing)	Reveals all variation (rare and common)	Costly Requires large sample sizes Computationally and analytically challenging Difficult to interpret

Source: Reprinted with permission from John Wiley and Sons. Ober C, Yao T-C. The genetics of asthma and allergic disease: a 21st century perspective. *Immunol Rev.* 2011;242:10–30.

Currently, epigenetics as a cause of missing heritability is an emerging field of research. Epigenetics refers to the regulation of DNA expression by methylation, chromatin modifications, or regulatory RNA molecules, which do not affect the DNA sequence itself, yet are heritable. It has been shown that environmental factors can influence epigenetic mechanisms, such as the expression of DNA by influencing the degree of DNA compaction and accessibility for gene transcription, regulating gene expression in a temporal and tissue-specific manner. The epigenetic regulation of DNA may be transmitted through multiple generations. Technology to study epigenetic regulation on a genome-wide scale has recently emerged. The best described epigenetic mechanisms are microRNAs, DNA methylation, and histone modifications, which are explained briefly below.

DNA is transcribed into messenger RNA (mRNA) and undergoes splicing, a RNA processing event in which the introns are removed and exons joined together. After splicing, mRNA is transcribed into proteins. Specific parts of DNA can also be transcribed into regulatory RNAs, which include long noncoding RNAs and microRNAs (miRNA). The latter are small RNAs that do not code for a protein but can bind to mRNA and thereby degrade or modify the mRNA and inhibit the protein transcription. One miRNA can modify multiple mRNAs, and one mRNA can be modified by multiple miRNAs, which indicates the complexity of this regulation.[9]

DNA methylation is the best studied epigenetic modification of DNA, and it occurs predominantly on CpG dinucleotides. Methylation describes the addition of a methyl group to a cytosine to form a 5′-methylcytosine. Approximately 75% of all CpG dinucleotides in the genome are methylated, and methylation is more prevalent in gene bodies and exons. CpG islands are generally less methylated regions where CpG dinucleotides cluster, and these are frequently located in regulatory regions such as promotor regions which are the starting point of DNA transcription. When methylated, the CpG islands in promotor regions inhibit DNA transcription by blocking the binding of transcription factors.[10] Methylation in gene bodies might stimulate transcription or influence splicing or chromosomal stability.[11]

DNA is wrapped around histones, which are proteins that interact with the long DNA chain to organize it into tightly wound nucleosomes. The amino acid tails of histones can be methylated, acetylated, phosphorylated, or otherwise modified causing changes in the structure of the DNA wrapping. These changes influence the accessibility of DNA for gene transcription. Histone acetylation has been most extensively studied and is associated with transcriptional activation. Histone acetyltransferase promotes transcription by attaching an acetyl group to lysine residues, which indirectly recruits activator proteins to the DNA. The acetyl group can be removed from histones by histone deacetylase enzyme, which leads to decreased gene expression.[10] Levels of histone acetyltransferase and histone deacetylase enzyme are therefore indicators for gene expression, and their role in atopy and atopic diseases is currently under investigation.

> Genetic studies conducted so far are not able to account for all the estimated heritability. Epigenetic influences and gene-environment interaction are therefore proposed to partly explain this "missing heritability." Epigenetics refers to the regulation of DNA expression by methylation, chromatin modifications, or regulatory RNA molecules, which do not affect the DNA sequence itself, yet are heritable.

Difference Between Sensitization and Clinical Disease

Defining Sensitization

Atopic individuals produce specific immunoglobulin E (sIgE) after exposure to atopic allergens, which is termed *sensitization*. The sIgE may then bind to mast cells and/or basophils which may then, in turn, initiate an allergic reaction after re-encountering the allergen.

The prevalence of IgE sensitization differs between populations, with reported prevalences varying between 16% and 57% in the United States, Europe, Australia, New Zealand, and Taiwan.[1] Sensitization is a strong risk factor for allergic disease although it is well established that sensitization does not always lead to symptoms, or clinical disease. The exact prevalence of asymptomatic sensitization is not really known. However, in the case of food allergy, only approximately 50% of children highly suspected of being food allergic and commonly sensitized to that suspect food are found to be clinically reactive to that food, as ascertained by a positive reaction to a double-blind placebo-controlled food challenge.[6] The prevalence of sensitization among asthma patients is about 60% to 80%,[1] and the ratio of rhinitis associated with and without sensitization is 3:1.[12] Approximately 20% of patients with atopic dermatitis are not sensitized to any allergen.[13] These data indicate that not all patients with atopic diseases are sensitized.

The mechanisms that result in atopy and the pathway driving sensitized individuals to become clinically allergic remain unknown. Since the genetic makeup of a child influences these differences it is likely that the genetic studies on these phenotypes may lead to knowledge on the pathogenetic mechanisms of allergy.

Importance of Disease Definition

The definition of the phenotype used is of great importance when interpreting data on genetics of atopy and allergic diseases. Moreover, there is an important difference between atopic sensitization and atopic disease. Sensitization is usually defined as either a specific IgE level above 0.35 kU/l, a positive allergen skin prick test, a high total serum IgE, or a combination of these tests. High total serum IgE is not always associated with atopy, since it can also be associated with helminthic infections or dermatitis without evidence of atopy. Moreover, no proper cutoff for total serum IgE has been defined above which the diagnosis of atopy may be reliably made and the upper limit of "normal" is unknown.

There are several diagnostic methods used to diagnose each atopic disease. When comparing studies, different definitions have been used, which complicates the replication of genetic findings. Asthma is difficult to define, especially in young children with symptoms of wheeze that may also be due to viral respiratory infections. Furthermore, there are several subgroups, including allergic asthma, exercise-induced asthma, and occupational asthma. These diseases are highly likely to have different pathophysiologies, which may be difficult to distinguish in genetic studies where the phenotypes have not been specifically defined. Allergic rhinitis is diagnosed based on symptoms, temporal pattern (seasonal or chronic), skin prick tests and response to medications. There are nonallergic rhinitis syndromes such as idiopathic rhinitis, infectious rhinitis and hormonal, alcohol, food or drug-induced rhinitis which are sometimes difficult to differentiate from allergic rhinitis.[12] For food allergy, one can use open food challenges or the double-blind placebo controlled food challenge, the latter being the gold standard. Open food challenges have a higher false-positive rate than double-blind placebo controlled challenges,[14,15] and studies using the former for case definition of food allergy may therefore fail to differentiate between asymptomatic sensitization and clinical reactivity to foods. This difference is clinically relevant since asymptomatic sensitization does not require therapy. The diagnosis of atopic dermatitis is not based on a specific test but is instead based on physical examination, history, and reported symptoms. The prevalence based on skin examination is approximately two-thirds of the prevalence of self-reported or questionnaire-based atopic dermatitis.[16]

To differentiate between the specific atopic diseases, the control group selected is also important. Are patients with one atopic disease compared to nonatopic healthy controls or are different groups of patients with a specific atopic disease compared? To differentiate between sensitization and atopic disease, a sufficient number of asymptomatically sensitized patients should be included in the study. For example, when comparing food allergic patients to the general population, genetic markers thought to be associated with food allergy may in reality be associated with sensitization to foods since both of these traits are often seen together in the cases but are generally both lacking in (nonatopic) controls.

> Sensitization does not always lead to symptoms or atopic disease. It is therefore highly important to distinguish these phenotypes from one another. Genetic studies may give insight in the pathway(s) driving sensitized individuals to become clinically allergic.

Genes Important in the Pathway Leading to Atopy and Allergy

In this section, we briefly describe the pathway leading to sensitization. We then describe current knowledge on the mechanisms of atopy, and how genetic and epigenetic (candidate) gene studies have provided a model to understand the relationship between (epi)genetic variation and disease development. We cannot provide a complete overview of all candidate gene studies, but have selected well-replicated genes to illustrate novel insights that such studies have provided.

Pathway Leading to Sensitization. Individuals may become sensitized by skin contact, inhalation, or ingestion of (glyco-)proteins. Dendritic cells are specialized in antigen presentation and capture these proteins in the gut or other sites of entry, after which they home to secondary lymphoid organs such as lymph nodes. The dendritic cell processes the protein and presents an allergen peptide on a major histocompatibility complex (MHC) class II molecule to naïve $CD4^+$ T lymphocytes. In immune responses to atopic allergens, dendritic cells concurrently secrete the cytokine interleukin-4 (IL-4). Both the peptide containing MHC receptor and IL-4 bind to $CD4^+$ T cells, which induces expression of signal transducer and activator of transcription 6 molecule (STAT6). This in turn stimulates the $CD4^+$ T cells to differentiate into T helper 2 cells (Th2).[17] The Th2 cells then activate B cells by producing CD40 ligand, IL-4, IL-5, and IL-13. Naïve mature B cells also present antigens in the lymph nodes and are activated by Th2 cells to undergo IL-4 and IL-13 induced immunoglobulin class-switching. This results in the production of allergen-specific IgE antibodies by the activated B cells. The allergen-specific IgE (sIgE) antibodies may then bind to resident tissue mast cells as can be demonstrated by immediate skin testing, or the sIgE may also be measured directly in many body fluids including blood.

Epithelial Barrier. The epithelia of the skin, lung, and gastrointestinal tract are the first sites to encounter allergens. An impaired barrier function may therefore permit intact proteins to pass the barrier and to elicit an immune response. The filaggrin (*FLG*) gene on chromosome 1q21 lies within the epidermal differentiation complex. These genes play an important role in skin barrier function since the filaggrin protein helps aggregate the epidermal cytoskeleton to form a protein-lipid barrier. Loss of function (LOF) variants of the *FLG* gene result in a defective form of the filaggrin protein and have a prevalence of about 10% in Western populations.[18] *FLG* LOF variants are associated with ichthyosis vulgaris, characterized by palmar hyperlinearity, keratosis pilaris, and a fine white scale on the extremities. Ichthyosis vulgaris is strongly associated with atopy; 37% to 50% of people with ichthyosis vulgaris have atopic diseases and about 8% of atopic dermatitis patients have ichthyosis vulgaris.[19] Furthermore, the *FLG* LOF variants are strong risk factors for atopic dermatitis[20] and are associated with allergic rhinitis and sensitization.[21] In children with atopic dermatitis, they are also associated with asthma.[22] Other studies suggest a role of *FLG* in sensitization to foods and clinical food allergy.[23] The genetic findings of *FLG* being an important gene for food allergy have led to the dual-allergen exposure hypothesis for the pathogenesis of food allergy. This proposes that low-dose cutaneous exposure to food allergens triggers Th2 responses and IgE production by B cells while early oral exposure induces tolerance by stimulating regulatory T cells and Th1 cells.[24] This hypothesis is supported by a study showing that epicutaneous exposure to peanut protein causes Th2-type immunity with high levels of peanut-specific IgE and prevents the development of oral tolerance to peanut.[25] A recent study showed that early life environmental exposure to peanuts, as measured by peanut in household dust, is indeed associated with peanut sensitization and allergy as confirmed by open food challenges, but only in children carrying *FLG* mutations.[26] This percutaneous priming is also proposed for the role of *FLG* in asthma and rhinitis.[21] However, future studies are needed to define the effect of *FLG* loss of function variants on sensitization and atopic diseases since it is yet unclear whether *FLG* is important only in the pathway leading to sensitization or also in the pathway leading from sensitization to specific allergic diseases. The GWAS on asthma have identified other SNPs important in the epithelial barrier (see below under Asthma).

> Recent studies have identified genetic markers important in epithelial barrier function, such as the filaggrin gene, to be associated with atopic diseases. It is therefore hypothesized that cutaneous exposure to allergens in individuals with an impaired barrier function may trigger Th2 responses and allergy.

T and B Cell Differentiation. Genes encoding STAT6, IL-4, IL-13, and the IL-4 receptor alpha chain are among the best-replicated candidate genes in allergic disease. As discussed above, the IL-4 cytokine stimulates T cells to differentiate into Th2 cells, and IL-4 and IL-13 stimulate B cells to produce IgE. Several chromosome 5q SNPs located in the gene coding for IL-4, IL-13, and another chromosome 16 (IL-4RA) gene that codes for their receptor have been reproducibly associated with sensitization and asthma.[9,27–29] Variants in the *IL-13* gene have been associated with sensitization to both allergenic foods[30] and inhalants.[31] Interestingly, epigenetic mechanisms may also be important, since recent data have shown that early farm exposure is associated with hypomethylation of the *IL-13* gene.[32] Studies have also shown that Th2 polarization occurs through epigenetic regulation of the *IL-4* gene by demethylation and active histone modifications, leading to greater IL-4 expression.[10] The *RHS7* gene, one of the 4 RAD50 DNase I hypersensitivity sites (RHS4-7) is located closely to Th2 associated cytokines. It was reported to affect methylation of the *IL-13* promotor and expression of IL-4. Variants of the *RHS7* gene were also associated with total serum IgE levels. Because of these findings, DNA methylation of the *IL-13* promotor has been suggested to mediate this genetic effect on IgE levels.[33]

Variants in the *STAT6* gene located on chromosome 12q are associated with total serum IgE levels,[34] allergic sensitization,[35] as well as a tree nut allergy.[36] In another study, early exposure to a farm environment was associated with hypomethylation of this gene.[32]

The *CD14* gene encodes a lipopolysaccharide receptor. Lipopolysaccharides are the main component of endotoxin, which is present in house dust. *CD14* gene variants are reported to be associated with atopy, and thought to influence the balance between Th1 and Th2 responses to antigens. The -159T promoter variant of the *CD14* gene is associated with asthma in patients highly exposed to microbes and endotoxin and the -159C variant is associated with this phenotype among patients with low exposure.[9,37] Thus, gene variants in this gene may interact with the environment, in particular microbial exposures.[38] Figure 4–1 illustrates the association between the -159C/T genotype and IgE sensitization among exposed and nonexposed patients in the Manchester Asthma and Allergy study.[39]

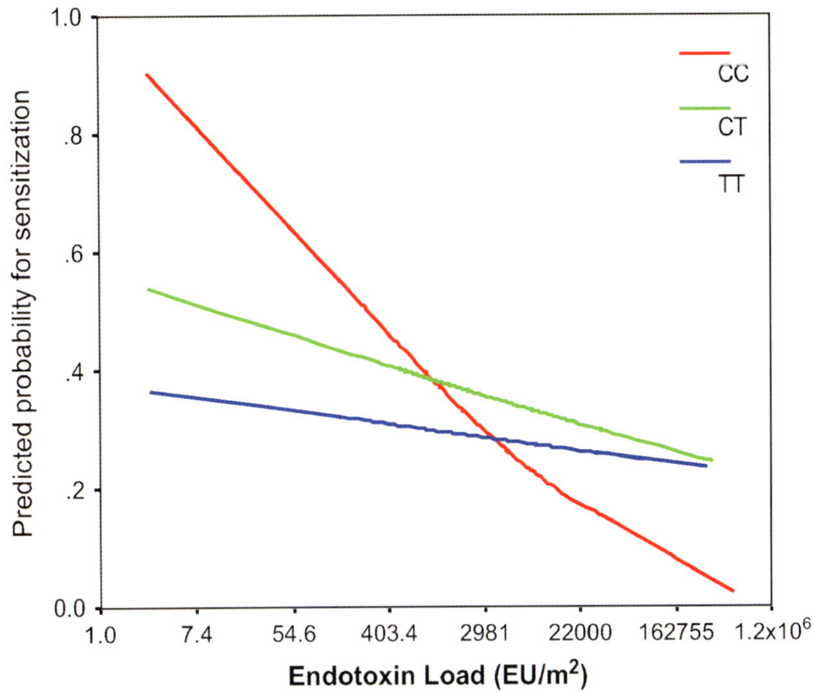

Figure 4–1. Fitted predicted probability curves for allergic sensitization at 5 years of age in relation to environmental endotoxin load in children with CC, CT, and TT genotypes in the promoter region of the *CD14* gene (CD14/-159 C to T) derived from the logistic regression analysis. Reprinted with permission from the American Thoracic Society. Copyright © 2014 American Thoracic Society. Simpson A, et al. Endotoxin exposure, CD14, and allergic disease: an interaction between genes and the environment. *Am J Respir Crit Care Med.* 2006;174:386–392. Official Journal of the American Thoracic Society.

> Genetic variation in genes coding for cytokines such as IL-4 and IL-13, important in B and T cell differentiation, is associated with sensitization. An individual's response to environmental factors such as house dust may be influenced by their genetic makeup, such as shown for the *CD14* gene.

Antigen Presentation. Major histocompatibility class II (MHC II) antigens are cell surface proteins expressed on antigen-presenting cells such as dendritic cells. In humans, these are termed human leukocyte antigens (HLA). As explained above, antigens captured by antigen-presenting cells are degraded to peptides and the resulting peptide fragments are inserted into the cleft of an appropriate MHC class II molecule (Figure 4–2). The resulting complex is transported to the surface of the antigen-presenting cell where it is presented to naïve $CD4^+$ T cells with receptors recognizing the peptide MHC II complex. In the case of responses to allergens, these $CD4^+$ cells are activated and then differentiate into Th2 cells. Genetic variation in the HLA region (*HLA-DQ* and *HLA-DR*) is strongly associated with (adult) onset asthma and IgE levels, respectively.[40,41]

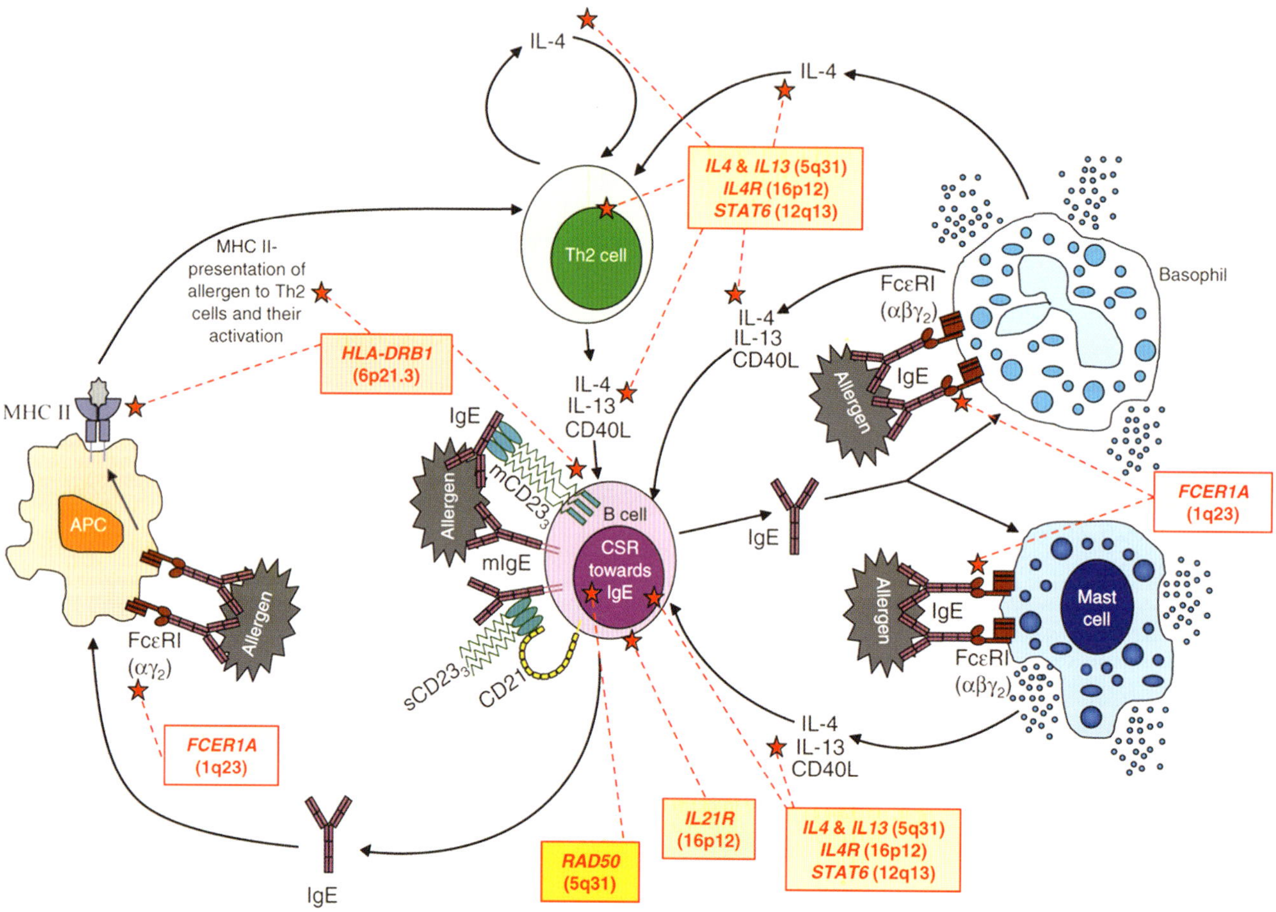

Figure 4–2. Basic molecules and cells contributing to the IgE network, IgE function, and IgE regulation. Gene products identified by GWA studies on total serum IgE are depicted in red (with chromosomal loci provided). IL-4 denotes interleukin-4; MHC II, major histocompatibility complex, class II; APC, antigen-presenting cell; IL-13, interleukin-13; CD40L, CD40 ligand; mIgE, membrane IgE; FceRI, the high-affinity IgE receptor; CSR, class-switch recombination; (m/s) CD233, (membrane/soluble) low-affinity IgE receptor, trimeric form. Reprinted with permission from John Wiley and Sons. Potaczek DP, Kabesch M. Current concepts of IgE regulation and impact of genetic determinants. *Clin Exp Allergy*. 2012;42:852–871.

Since the structure of the MHC II molecule determines which antigen peptides are presented to $CD4^+$ cells and which are not, they may be important in explaining why certain antigenic proteins have a tendency to elicit production of IgE antibodies (ie, allergens) and others do not (ie, nonallergens). One hypothesis is that allergens are distinguished from other antigens by the fact that they do not trigger danger signals that result in Th1 or Th17 cytokine production. However, studies showing associations between MHC II and sensitization suggest that multiple disease mechanisms may be important. Furthermore, due to the strong linkage disequilibrium on chromosome 6 (the HLA gene repertoire) it has been difficult to pinpoint which genes are important.

FcεRI Receptor. Activated B cells produce antigen-specific IgE antibodies which bind to the high-affinity FcεRI receptor on mast cells, basophils, and eosinophils. When IgE binds to the high-affinity FcεRI receptor and subsequently binds the allergen, these resulting complexes cross-link and activate the mast cell or basophil, which will then release pro-inflammatory substances such as

- Biogenic amines such as histamine which increase vascular permeability, vascular smooth muscle cell relaxation, bronchial smooth muscle contraction, and peristalsis
- Granule enzymes and proteoglycans such as tryptase and chymase which induce tissue damage and mucus secretion
- Lipid mediators such as prostaglandin D2 which act as a vasodilator and bronchoconstrictor and promote neutrophil accumulation at inflammatory sites
- Cytokines such as IL-4, IL-5 (the latter induces eosinophil activation), IL-6, IL-13 (the latter induces mucus production) which all induce inflammation. TNF-α enhances the expression of adhesion molecules on endothelial cells, allowing influx of inflammatory cells at sites of inflammation.

Candidate gene studies of the beta chain of the FcεRI (published in 1993) that showed an association with asthma, were among the first genetic studies in asthma.[42] However, subsequent replication studies have produced inconsistent results, with some reports confirming, and other refuting this association.

Regulatory T Cells. Allergy can also be defined as the failure to tolerate allergens and regulatory T cells are important in the induction of tolerance. There are several types of regulatory T cells, including $CD4^+CD25$ regulatory T cells, which express the transcription factor, forkhead/winged helix transcription factor box protein 3 (FOXP3). The levels of *FOXP3* gene expression are considered the most reliable marker for the functionality of regulatory T cells and correlate with their suppressive activity. SNPs in the X chromosomal *FOXP3* gene were reported to have opposite effects among different sexes since they were associated with sensitization to egg and inhalant allergens in girls, and remission of sensitization in boys.[43]

Secondhand smoking and air pollution exposure in children are reported to be associated with increased methylation levels of the promotor of the *FOXP3* gene.[44,45] This increased methylation is associated with a decreased expression of FOXP3 and has been reported to be associated with a higher risk of asthma and/or persistent wheezing.[44] Furthermore, *FOXP3* methylation was significantly decreased in peanut-allergic patients undergoing peanut oral immunotherapy compared to patients undergoing regular care. Interestingly, in patients who remained tolerant to peanut 6 months after oral immunotherapy (as shown by open food challenges), the *FOXP3* DNA methylation level was lower compared to those patients who lost their peanut tolerance.[46] A similar phenomenon occurs in allergic rhinitis patients receiving sublingual immunotherapy for grass and dust mites who also show decreased methylation of *FOXP3* in regulatory T cells compared to those on placebo.[47] These findings suggest that *FOXP3* methylation is influenced by environmental factors and may be associated with the development of clinical tolerance to allergens.

> Failure to tolerate allergens can be due to an impaired function of regulatory T cells. *FOXP3* expression is associated with regulatory T cell function and genetic variation in the gene encoding *FOXP3* is associated with asthma. There is substantial evidence that *FOXP3* is important in acquiring tolerance, as is the goal of immunotherapy.

Specific Atopic Disease Genes Identified by GWAS

Aside from genes that have been associated with atopic sensitization and genes that are shared between atopic diseases, there are also disease-specific genes (as discussed above and in Figure 4–3 and Table 4–2). GWA studies that systematically compare sensitization, asthma, allergic rhinitis, and atopic dermatitis have provided more insight into the genetic overlap of these diseases (shown in Figure 4–3). Importantly, some of the genetic markers found to be associated with a specific atopic disease are not associated with specific or total serum IgE levels, indicating that mechanisms unrelated to IgE may also be important in asthma and atopic dermatitis.

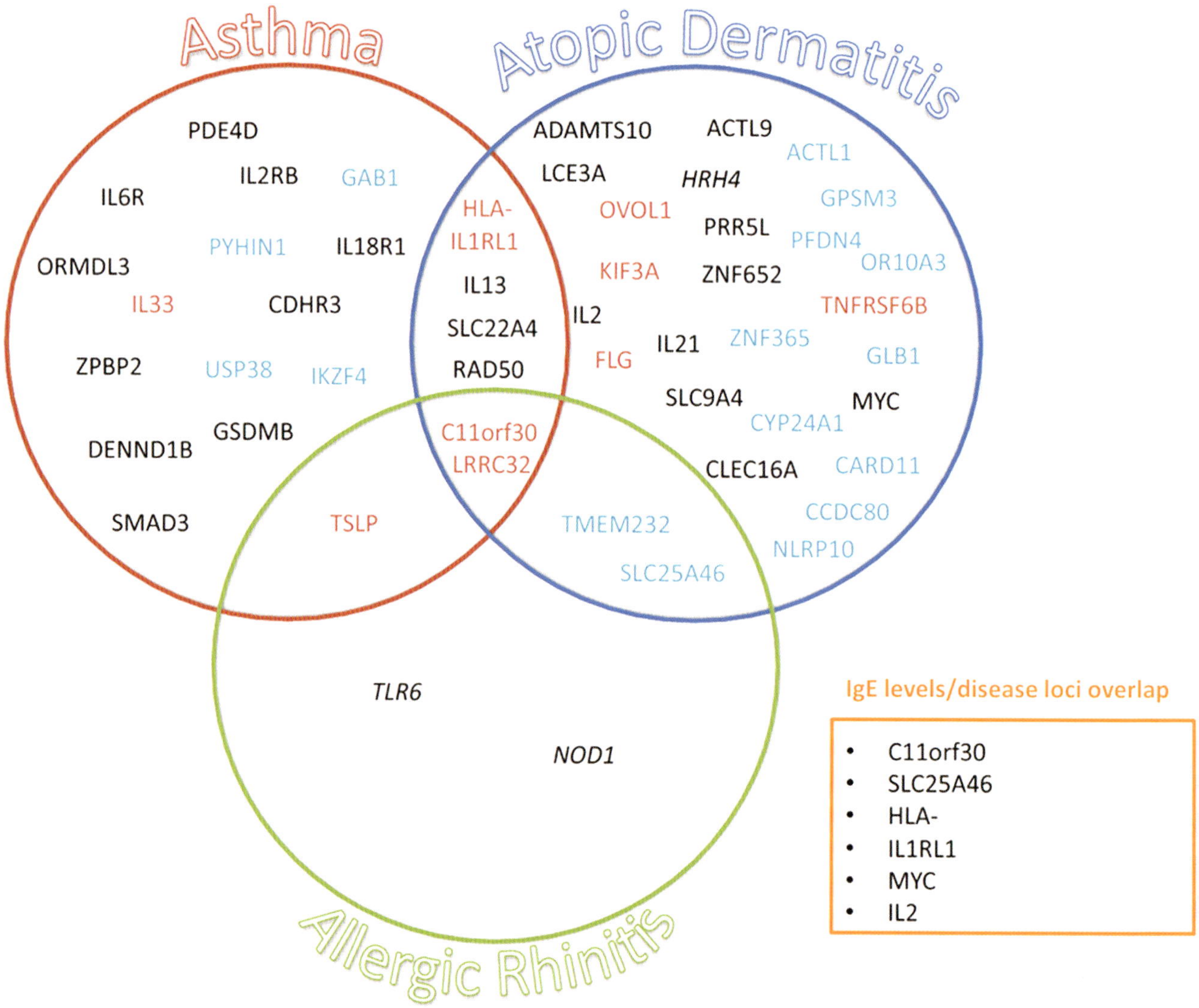

Figure 4–3. Venn diagram illustrating genes identified through genome-wide association studies as associated with the allergic diseases asthma, atopic dermatitis, and allergic rhinitis. Genes highlighted in black identify those discovered in Caucasian populations, with italics defining promising genes that did not quite achieve genome-wide significance. Genes highlighted in blue identify those genes discovered in non-Caucasian populations, while those in red identify those genes discovered in both Caucasian and other ancestry populations. Reprinted with permission from John Wiley and Sons. Portelli MA, Hodge E, Sayers I. Genetic risk factors for the development of allergic disease identified by genome wide association. *Clin Exp Allergy*. 2014;44.

Table 4-2. Susceptibility Genes for Asthma, Allergic Rhinitis, and Atopic Dermatitis Recently Identified by GWAS

Gene(s)	Chrs	Association	Potential Function	GWAS
IL6R	1q21	Asthma	Regulatory T cell function, T cell differentiation	[58]
DENND1B	1q31		Memory T cell functions.	[59]B
IL1RL1	2q11		IL-33 receptor-recruitment of inflammatory cells	[41], [60], [61]A, [62]B, [63]
PDE4D	5q12		Cell signaling, inflammation, ASM function	64
TSLP	5q22		Activates dendritic cells, Th2 immune responses	41
SLC22A4/RAD50/IL13	5q31		Organic cationic transporter/DNA repair/ Th2 cytokine	[62]B, [65]A, [41], [63]
HLA-DRA/DRQ	6p21*		T cell responses/many additional genes in region	[62]B
CDHR3	7q22		Epithelial polarity, cell-cell contact and differentiation	[41], [60], [62]B
IL33	9p24		Recruitment/activation of inflammatory cells	58
C11orf30/LRRC32	11q13		Regulates gene expression, epithelial barrier/regulatory T cell function	41
SMAD3	15q22		TGF-β signaling intermediate, fibrosis	[41], [61]A, [62]B
ORMDL3/GSDMB	17q21		Sphingolipid synthesis/cell apoptosis	[52]C
IL2RB	22q12		Binds IL-2/IL-15, lymphoid cell differentiation	[59], [41]
C11orf30/LRRC32	11q13	Allergic rhinitis	Regulates gene expression, epithelial barrier/regulatory T cell function	66
FLG, LCE3A	1q21*	Atopic dermatitis	Epidermal differentiation and structure	[67], [68], [69]Λ, [70]
IL1RL1, SLC9A4	2q12*		IL-33 receptor/sodium-hydrogen exchanger	[69]Λ
IL2-IL21	4q27		T cell survival/B cell proliferation and IgE production	[69]Λ
SLC22A4/RAD50/ IL13/KIF3A	5q31		Organic cationic transporter/DNA repair/ Th2 cytokine/cilia protein	[68], [69], [70]
HLA-B (BAT1/TNXB/CREBL1)	6p21		T cell responses/many additional genes in region	[70]
PRR5L	11p13		Cellular apoptosis	[69]Λ
OVOL1	11q13*		Development and differentiation of epidermal/epithelial tissues	[68]
C11orf30/LRRC32	11q13*		Regulates gene expression, epithelial barrier/regulatory T cell function	[67], [69]Λ, [70]

continues

Table 4–2. *continued*

Gene(s)	Chrs	Association	Potential Function	GWAS
CLEC16A	16p13	Atopic dermatitis *continued*	Inflammatory cell function (ITAM receptor)	69^
ZNF652	17q21		Transcriptional repressor in epithelial cancers	69^
ADAMTS10/ACTL9	19p13*		Extracellular matrix cleavage/epithelial morphology	68
TNFRSF6B	20q13*		Decoy receptor, immunomodulation of T cells	68, 69^

Source: Reprinted with permission from John Wiley and Sons. Portelli MA, Hodge E, Sayers I. Genetic risk factors for the development of allergic disease identified by genome wide association. *Clin Exp Allergy.* 2014;44.

Note. Genes focused to those meeting conventional genome-wide significance ($P<5 \times 10^{-8}$) and/or independent replication in Caucasian studies only. [A]Severe Asthma, [B]Childhood severe asthma with exacerbation, and [C]Childhood onset asthma. Data taken from Asthma: 1. (1), 2. (2), 3. (3), 4. (4), 5. (5)[A], 6. (6)[B], 7. (7), 8. (8), 9. (9), 10. (10), 11. (11). Allergic Rhinitis: 12. (12). Atopic Dermatitis: 13. (13), 14. (14), 15. (15) ^using Immunochip array, 16. (16). *Association also observed in the Asian population GWAS.

IL, interleukin; *IL6R*, IL-6 receptor; *DENND1B*, Denn/madd domain-containing 1b; *IL1RL1*, IL-1 receptor like 1; *PDE4D*, phosphodiesterase 4d, cAMP specific; ASM, airway smooth muscle; *TSLP*, thymic stromal lymphopoietin; Th2, T helper 2; *SLC22A4*, solute carrier family 22 (organic cation/zwitterion transporter), member 4; *RAD50, S. cerevisiae, homolog of (DNA repair)*; IL13. IL-13; *HLA-*, major histocompatibility complex, class II; *CDHR3*, cadherin-related family member 3; *IL33*, IL-33; *C11orf30*, chromosome 11 open reading frame 30; *LRRC32*, leucine-rich repeat containing 32; *SMAD3*, mothers against decapentaplegic drosophila homolog3; TGF-β, transforming growth factor beta; *ORMDL3*, orm1-like protein 3; *GSDMB*, gasdermin b; *IL2RB*, IL-2 receptor beta; Ig, immunoglobulin; *FLG*, filaggrin; *LCE3A*, late cornified envelope 3A; *IL1RL1*, interleukin receptor-like 1; *SLC9A4*, solute carrier family 9, subfamily A (NHE4, cation proton antiporter 4), member 4; *IL2-IL21*, interleukin 2/21; *KIF3A*, kinesin family member 3A; *PRR5L*, proline rich 5-like; *OVOL1*, ovo-like 1(Drosophila); *CLEC16A*, C-type lectin domain family 16, member A; *ZNF652*, zinc finger protein 652; *ADAMTS10*, ADAM metallopeptidase with thrombospondin type 1 motif, 10; *ACTL9*, actin-like 9; *TNFRSF6B*, tumor necrosis factor receptor superfamily, member 6b, decoy.

The specific symptoms that occur following a particular allergen encounter are determined by several factors that currently remain largely unknown. Tissue-specific expression of atopy may relate to the route of allergen exposure or the local presence and activation of inflammatory cells, including mast cells, or relate to the homing of active T cells to the target tissue. Genetic factors related to the microstructure of the target tissues may thus be important in determining the organ specificity of allergic disease. In addition to factors that relate to increased risk, it is tempting to speculate that local protective factors exist, that may be either genetic or epigenetic. The next section provides an overview how genetic studies have increased our understanding of the unique and shared origin of these diseases.

Asthma. Asthma is a chronic inflammation of the airways with a prevalence of 8% in the US population that is characterized by reversible bronchial airway obstruction, chronic bronchial inflammation, and associated airway remodelling. The airway obstruction is partly caused by bronchial smooth muscle cell contraction and hypertrophy, mucosal edema, and by the production of mucus. The inflammation is characterized by mast cell, basophil, and eosinophil activation. These produce mediators of inflammation and airway remodelling.[40,48–50]

Family-based linkage studies were the first approach that could be used to identify novel genes that were previously not implicated in asthma. The first gene discovered by this approach was *ADAM33* (a disintegrin and matrix metalloproteinase 33).[51] *ADAM33* was associated with asthma and bronchial hyperresponsiveness, but not sensitization, and subsequent functional studies showed a role in smooth muscle and vascular remodeling.[1] Several other asthma genes found by positional cloning were mainly expressed in structural cells of the airways. This suggests that these cells, in particular the airway epithelial cells, are important in asthma susceptibility.[50]

The GWA studies have now provided a replicable set of genes that are associated with asthma (see Table 4–2). The first GWA study in asthma in 2007 revealed that SNPs on chromosome 17q12-21 were associated with childhood onset asthma.[52] These SNPs regulate *ORMDL3* and *GSDMB* expression, genes of unknown function but potentially of importance to eosinophil trafficking, endoplasmic reticulum stress, and epithelial cell remodelling.[1,48] The 17q12-21 locus is strongly associated with childhood-onset asthma, and to a lesser extent with allergic rhinitis, but not with atopic dermatitis or sensitization.[1]

The GWA studies of asthma have revealed three genes that are in one single functional pathway: The *IL33* gene encodes the IL-33 cytokine released by damaged cells, whereas *IL1RL1* encodes the IL-33 receptor complex.[48] Studies indicate that IL-33 acts on cells of both the adaptive and innate immune systems. The *IL33* and *IL1RL1* genes may exert their function in a recently discovered population of *IL-33*-responsive innate immune cells, the type 2 innate lymphoid cells, that are important sources of hallmark Th2 cytokines, such as IL-5 and IL-13.[48] Other asthma-associated genes discovered by GWA analysis include *SMAD3*, which is a signaling intermediate of TGF beta, a cytokine important in airway wall remodeling.[48] The relevance of epithelial cytokines in asthma was underscored by the finding that TSLP, an epithelial cytokine, is also associated with asthma.[48]

The first resequencing study on asthma was published in 2012, hypothesizing that rare variants with a low frequency (<5%) have a large effect on disease susceptibility. This first study focused on 9 candidate genes and showed that indeed 4 of these rare variants contribute to asthma susceptibility.[53] However, large resequencing projects are needed to define if and how often, these rare genetic variants contribute to diseases such as asthma.

Rhinitis. Allergic rhinitis, or "hay fever," is often accompanied by allergic conjunctivitis. Common allergens are house dust mite, animal danders, and plant pollens. Patients suffer from mucosal edema, sneezing, mucus secretion, and itchy eyes. There is a strong and almost complete overlap between genes that associate with IgE sensitization and allergic rhinitis.[35,54] A recent meta-analysis of GWA studies on both asthma and allergic rhinitis identified 11 independent SNPs associated with the combined phenotype of asthma and allergic rhinitis. Two GWA studies on allergic rhinitis identified the *LRRC32* gene variant, that was associated with the phenotype of allergic rhinitis without asthma.[55] The *LRRC32* gene variant is reported to encode a cell surface molecule expressed on regulatory T cells which induces *FOXP3* expression.[56]

Food Allergy. Food allergies are most commonly IgE-mediated immediate-type reactions that occur after ingestion of allergenic foods such as peanut, apple, or cow's milk. Gastrointestinal symptoms such as vomiting and diarrhea are the most common, although respiratory symptoms, urticaria, and atopic dermatitis are often seen as well. Food allergy is potentially lethal since it can lead to anaphylaxis. This is a systemic allergic reaction characterized by vasodilatation, edema in several tissues, and bronchial obstruction, which can result in redistributive shock and respiratory impairment. Patients suffering from both asthma and food allergy are at high risk for anaphylaxis. Although this is an important clinical problem, compared to other atopic diseases, food allergy has been studied to a lesser extent, and no genome-wide associated studies are available.

> The GWA studies have now provided a replicable set of genes that are associated with asthma and atopic dermatitis. There is a strong and almost complete overlap in genes associated with sensitization and allergic rhinitis, and some genes overlap with asthma and rhinitis. No genome-wide associated studies are yet available for food allergy.

Atopic Dermatitis. Atopic dermatitis or eczema is characterized by dry skin, intense pruritus, and a characteristic age-related distribution of inflammatory lesions. The pathophysiology is thought to be based on an impaired skin barrier, abnormal immune reactivity, and environmental factors such as allergens and microbes.[57] However, the initial events in AD remain unclear. More progress has been made in identifying the effector pathway since it is now known that among other cytokines, IL-4 and IL-13 act on endothelial cells to promote cutaneous inflammation.[57]

The genes identified in atopic dermatitis GWA studies show little overlap with genes for IgE[71] sensitization, asthma, or rhinitis. As described above, an impaired epithelial barrier may be important in the development of atopic dermatitis. The strongest evidence comes from the *FLG* gene but also other genes from the epidermal differentiation complex may be important. Furthermore a defective antimicrobial immune response predispose patients with atopic dermatitis to infections.[57]

SUMMARY AND CLINICAL IMPLICATIONS

Atopy and atopic diseases have a multifactorial etiology with influences from both environmental and (epi)genetic factors. In the last century, research has identified many genes and several pathways associated with IgE levels and each specific allergic disease. There is an overlap in genes associated with the different allergic diseases, although there are genes reported which are disease specific as well. Genetic studies have thus provided more insight into the basic mechanisms leading to different allergic diseases. However, future studies are indicated to identify genetic markers associated with food allergy and to further explore the mechanism leading from sensitization to atopic diseases. Promising fields are the role of regulatory T cells and epithelial integrity in the pathophysiology of sensitization, asthma, rhinitis, food allergy, and atopic dermatitis.

Gene-environment interactions and epigenetic influences add another layer of complexity to this pathogenesis. Understanding the genetic and epigenetic basis and thereby the pathophysiology of allergy may improve diagnosis and treatment by predicting disease onset and providing targets for personalized treatment of patients. Specifically, genetic variation may affect treatment response and should therefore be taken into account. Identification of environmental factors influencing epigenetic regulation of genes can provide evidence for how exposure may regulate genes in atopy, which may in turn lead to better forms of prevention.

REFERENCES

1. Ober C, Yao T-C. The genetics of asthma and allergic disease: a 21st century perspective. *Immunol Rev*. 2011;242:10–30.
2. Dubois AEJ, de Monchy SJGR, Schouten JP, et al. Basic concepts relating to the field of allergology. *Allergy*. 1999;54:760–762.
3. Muraro A, Dreborg S, Halken S, et al. Dietary prevention of allergic diseases in infants and small children. Part III: critical review of published peer- reviewed observational and interventional studies and final recommendations. *Pediatr Allergy Immunol*. 2004;15:291–307.
4. Cooke RA, Veer, AV. Human sensitization. *J Immunol*. 1916;1:201–305.
5. Hourihane JO, Dean TP, Warner JO. Peanut allergy in relation to heredity, maternal diet, and other atopic diseases: results of a questionnaire survey, skin prick testing, and food challenges. *BMJ*. 1996;313:518–521.
6. Van den Berg ME, Flokstra-de Blok BMJ, Vlieg-Boerstra BJ, et al. Parental eczema increases the risk of double-blind, placebo-controlled reactions to milk but not to egg, peanut or hazelnut. *Int Arch Allergy Immunol*. 2012;158:77–83.
7. Pinart M, Benet M, Maesano I, et al. Comorbidity of eczema, rhinitis, and asthma in IgE-sensitised and non-IgE-sensitised children: an international population-based cohort study. *Lancet*. 2013;2600:1–10.
8. Cookson WOCM, Faux JA, Sharp PA, Hopkin JM. Linkage between immunoglobulin E responses underlying asthma and rhinitis and chromosome 11q. *Lancet*. 1989;June:1292–1295.
9. Munthe-Kaas MC, Willemse BWM, Koppelman GH. Genetics and epigenetics of childhood asthma. *Eur Respir Monogr*. 2012;56:97–114.
10. North ML, Ellis AK. The role of epigenetics in the developmental origins of allergic disease. *Ann Allergy Asthma Immunol*. 2011;106:355–361; quiz 362.
11. Hong X, Wang X. Epigenetics and development of food allergy (FA) in early childhood. *Curr Allergy Asthma Rep*. 2014;14:460.
12. Wallace DV, Dykewicz M, Bernstein D, et al. The diagnosis and management of rhinitis: an updated practice parameter. *J Allergy Clin Immunol*. 2008;122:S1–84.
13. Eichenfield LF, Tom W, Chamlin S, et al. Guidelines of care for the management of atopic dermatitis: section 1. Diagnosis and assessment of atopic dermatitis. *J Am Acad Dermatol*. 2014;70:338–351.
14. Muraro A, Halken S, Arshad SH, et al. EAACI Food Allergy and Anaphylaxis Guidelines. Primary prevention of food allergy. *Allergy*. 2014;69:590–601.
15. Brouwer ML, Wolt-Plompen S, Dubois AEJ, et al. No effects of probiotics on atopic dermatitis in infancy: a randomized clinical and experimental allergy. *Clin Exp Allergy*. 2006;36:899–906.
16. Caroll CL, Balkrishnan R, Feldman SR, Fleischer AB, Manuel JC. The burden of atopic dermatitis: impact on

the patient, family, and society. *Pediatr Dermatol*. 2005;22: 192–199.
17. Potaczek DP, Kabesch M. Current concepts of IgE regulation and impact of genetic determinants. *Clin Exp Allergy*. 2012;42:852–871.
18. Van den Oord RA, Sheikh A. Filaggrin gene defects and risk of developing allergic sensitisation and allergic disorders: systematic review and meta-analysis. *BMJ*, 2009; 339:b2433.
19. Smith FJD, Irvine A, Terron-Kwiatkowski A, et al. Loss-of-function mutations in the gene encoding filaggrin cause ichthyosis vulgaris. *Nat Genet*. 2006;38:337–342.
20. Sandilands A, Terron-Kwiatkowski A, Hull P, et al. Comprehensive analysis of the gene encoding filaggrin uncovers prevalent and rare mutations in ichthyosis vulgaris and atopic eczema. *Nat Genet*. 2007;39:650–654.
21. Weidinger S, O'Sullivan M, Illig T, et al. Filaggrin mutations, atopic eczema, hay fever, and asthma in children. *J Allergy Clin Immunol*. 2008;121:1203–1209.e1.
22. Rodríguez E,Baurecht H, Herberich E, et al. Meta-analysis of filaggrin polymorphisms in eczema and asthma: robust risk factors in atopic disease. *J Allergy Clin Immunol*. 2009;123:1361–1370.e7.
23. Brown SJ, Asai H, Cordell H, et al. Loss-of-function variants in the filaggrin gene are a significant risk factor for peanut allergy. *J Allergy Clin Immunol*. 2011;127:661–667.
24. Lack G. Update on risk factors for food allergy. *J Allergy Clin Immunol*. 2012;129:1187–1197.
25. Strid J, Hourihane J, Kimber I, Callard R, Strobel S. Epicutaneous exposure to peanut protein prevents oral tolerance and enhances allergic sensitization. *Clin Exp Allergy*, 2005;35:757–766.
26. Brough H, Simpson A, Makinson K, et al. Peanut allergy: effect of environmental peanut exposure in children with filaggrin loss-of-function mutations. *J Allergy Clin Immunol*. 2014;134:867 875.e1.
27. Ober C, Leavitt S, Tsalenko A, et al. Variation in the interleukin 4-receptor alpha gene confers susceptibility to asthma and atopy in ethnically diverse populations. *Am J Hum Genet*. 2000;606:517–526.
28. Khurana hershey GK, Friedrich MF, Esswein LA, Thomas ML, Chatila TA. The association of atopy with a gain-of-function mutation in the a subunit of the interleukin-4 receptor. *N Engl J Med*. 1997;337:1720–1725.
29. Heinzmann A, Mao S, Akaiwa M, et al. Genetic variants of IL-13 signalling and human asthma and atopy. *Hum Mol Genet*. 2000;9:549–559.
30. Zitnik SE, Ruschendorf F, Muller S, et al. IL13 variants are associated with total serum IgE and early sensitization to food allergens in children with atopic dermatitis. *Pediatr Allergy Immunol*. 2009;20:551–555.
31. Liu, X, Beaty T, Deindl P, et al. Associations between specific serum IgE response and 6 variants within the genes IL4, IL13, and IL4RA in German children: the German Multicenter Atopy Study. *J Allergy Clin Immunol*. 2004; 113:489–495.
32. Michel S, Busato F, Genuneit J, et al. Farm exposure and time trends in early childhood may influence DNA methylation in genes related to asthma and allergy. *Allergy*. 2013;68:355–364.
33. Schieck M, Sharma V, Michel S, et al. A polymorphism in the TH 2 locus control region is associated with changes in DNA methylation and gene expression. *Allergy*. 2014; 69:1171–1180.
34. Weidinger S, Gieger C, Rodriguez E, et al. Genome-wide scan on total serum IgE levels identifies FCER1A as novel susceptibility locus. *PLoS Genet*. 2008;4(8):e1000166.
35. Bønnelykke K, Matheson M, Pers T, et al. Meta-analysis of genome-wide association studies identifies ten loci influencing allergic sensitization. *Nat Genet*. 2013;45:902–906.
36. Amoli MM, Hand S, Majeer A, et al. Polymorphism in the STAT6 gene encodes risk for nut allergy. *Genes Immun*. 2002;3:220–224.
37. Ober C, Vercelli D. Gene-environment interactions in human disease: nuisance or opportunity? *Trends Genet*. 2011;27:107–115.
38. Lau MYZ, Dharmage S, Burgess J, et al. CD14 polymorphisms, microbial exposure and allergic diseases: a systematic review of gene–environment interactions. *Allergy*. 2014;69:1440–1453.
39. Simpson A, John S, Jury F, et al. Endotoxin exposure, CD14, and allergic disease: an interaction between genes and the environment. *Am J Respir Crit Care Med*. 2006;174: 386–392.
40. Abbas AK, Lichtman AH, Pillai S. *Cellular and Molecular Immunology*. Philadelphia, PA: Elsevier, Saunders; 2012.
41. Moffatt MF, Phil D, Gut I, et al. A large-scale, consortium-based genomewide association study of asthma. *N Engl J Med*. 2010;363:1211–1221.
42. Stanford AJ, Shirakawa T, Mofatt M, et al. Localisation of atopy and β subunit of high-affinity IgE receptor (FcERI) on chromosome 11q. *Lancet*. 1993;341:332–334.
43. Bottema RWB, Kerkhof M, Reijmerink N, et al. X-chromosome Forkhead Box P3 polymorphisms associate with atopy in girls in three Dutch birth cohorts. *Allergy*. 2010; 65:865–874.
44. Brunst KJ, Leung Y, Ryan P, et al. Forkhead box protein 3 (FOXP3) hypermethylation is associated with diesel exhaust exposure and risk for childhood asthma. *J Allergy Clin Immunol*. 2013;131:592–594.e1–3.
45. Kohli A, Garcia M, Miller R, et al. Secondhand smoke in combination with ambient air pollution exposure is associated with increasedx CpG methylation and decreased expression of IFN-γ in T effector cells and Foxp3 in T regulatory cells in children. *Clin Epigenetics*. 2012;4:17.
46. Syed A, Garcia M, Lyu S, et al. Peanut oral immunotherapy results in increased antigen-induced regulatory T-cell function and hypomethylation of forkhead box protein 3 (FOXP3). *J Allergy Clin Immunol*. 2014;133:500–510.
47. Swamy RS, Reshamwala N, Hunter T, et al. Epigenetic modifications and improved regulatory T-cell function in subjects undergoing dual sublingual immunotherapy. *J Allergy Clin Immunol*. 2012;130:215–224.e7.
48. Portelli MA, Hodge E, Sayers I. Genetic risk factors for the development of allergic disease identified by genome wide association. *Clin Exp Allergy*. 2014;45:21–31.

49. Yang IV, Schwartz D. Epigenetic mechanisms and the development of asthma. *J Allergy Clin Immunol*. 2012;130: 1243–1255.
50. Holgate ST, Yang Y, Haitchi H, et al. The genetics of asthma: ADAM33 as an example of a susceptibility gene. *Proc Am Thorac Soc*. 2006;3:440–443.
51. Eerdewegh P, Little R, Mastro R, et al. Association of the ADAM33 gene with asthma and bronchial hyperresponsiveness. *Nature*. 2002;418; 426–430.
52. Moffatt MF, Kabesch M, Liang L, et al. Genetic variants regulating ORMDL3 expression contribute to the risk of childhood asthma. *Nature*. 2007;448:470–473.
53. Torgerson DG, Capurso D, Mathias R, et al. Resequencing candidate genes implicates rare variants in asthma susceptibility. *Am J Hum Genet*. 2012;90:273–281.
54. Hinds D, McMahon G, Kiefer A, et al. A genome-wide association meta-analysis of self-reported allergy identifies shared and allergy-specific susceptibility loci. *Nat Genet*. 2013;45:907–911.
55. Ferreira MAR, Matheson M, Tang C, et al. Genome-wide association analysis identifies 11 risk variants associated with the asthma with hay fever phenotype. *J Allergy Clin Immunol*. 2014;133:1564–1571.
56. Wang R, Wan Q, Kozhaya L, Fujii H, Unutmaz D. Identification of a regulatory T cell specific cell surface molecule that mediates suppressive signals and induces Foxp3 expression. *PLoS One*. 2008;3:e2705.
57. Dubrac S, Schmuth M, Ebner S. Atopic dermatitis: the role of Langerhans cells in disease pathogenesis. *Immunol Cell Biol*. 2010;88:400–409.
58. Ferreira MAR, Matheson M, Duff D, et al. Identification of IL6R and chromosome 11q13.5 as risk loci for asthma. *Lancet*. 2011;378:1006–1114.
59. Sleiman P, Flory J, Imielinksi M, et al. Variants of DENND1B associated with asthma in children. *N Engl J Med*. 2010;362:36–44.
60. Gudbjartsson DF, Bjornsdottir US, Halapi E, et al. Sequence variants affecting eosinophil numbers associate with asthma and myocardial infarction. *Nature Genetics*. 2009;41:342–347.
61. Wan YI, Shrine N, Artigas M, et al. Genome-wide association study to identify genetic determinants of severe asthma. *Thorax*. 2012. doi:10.1136/thoraxjnl-2011-201262
62. Bønnelykke K, Sleiman P, Nielsen K, et al. A genome-wide association study identifies CDHR3 as a susceptibility locus for early childhood asthma with severe exacerbations. *Nat Genet*. 2014;46:51–55.
63. Ramasamy A, Kuokkanen M, Vedantam S, et al. Genome-wide association studies of asthma in population-based cohorts confirm known and suggested loci and identify an additional association near HLA. *PLoS One*. 2012;7: e44008.
64. Himes BE, Hunninghake G, Baurley J, et al. Genome-wide association analysis identifies PDE4D as an asthma-susceptibility gene. *Am J Hum Genet*. 2009;84:581–593.
65. Li X, Howard T, Zheng S, et al. Genome-wide association study of asthma identifies RAD50-IL13 and HLA-DR/DQ regions. *J Allergy Clin Immunol*. 2010;125:328–335.e11.
66. Ramasamy A, Curjuric I, Coin L, et al. A genome-wide meta-analysis of genetic variants associated with allergic rhinitis and grass sensitization and their interaction with birth order. *J Allergy Clin Immunol*. 2011;128:996–1005.
67. Esparza-Gordillo J, Weidinger S, Folster-Holst R, et al. A common variant on chromosome 11q13 is associated with atopic dermatitis. *Nat Genet*. 2009;41:596–601.
68. Paternoster L,Standl M, Chen C, et al. Meta-analysis of genome-wide association studies identifies three new risk loci for atopic dermatitis. *Nat Genet*. 2011;44:187–192.
69. Ellinghaus D, Baurecht H, Esparza-Gordillo J, et al. High-density genotyping study identifies four new susceptibility loci for atopic dermatitis. *Nat Genet*. 2013;45:808–812.
70. Weidinger S, Willis-Owen S, Kamatani Y, et al. A genome-wide association study of atopic dermatitis identifies loci with overlapping effects on asthma and psoriasis. *Hum Mol Genet*. 2013;22:4841–4856.
71. Granada M, Wilk J, Tuzova M, et al. A genome-wide association study of plasma total IgE concentrations in the Framingham Heart Study. *J Allergy Clin Immunol*. 2012; 129:840–845.e21.

5

Rhinitis and Rhinosinusitis

Judd H. Fastenberg and Alexis H. Jackman

INTRODUCTION

Rhinitis and rhinosinusitis are among the most common medical problems in the United States and refer to inflammation of the nose and paranasal sinuses, respectively. Both may result from several different pathologic processes, one of the most significant of which is allergy. Although an allergic connection to both conditions has long been recognized, our scientific understanding of allergy's contribution is incompletely understood and continues to evolve.

RHINITIS

Rhinitis is divided into allergic and nonallergic subtypes. According to the 2008 Allergic Rhinitis and its Impact on Asthma (ARIA) Guidelines, allergic rhinitis is defined as a "symptomatic disorder of the nose induced after allergen exposure by an IgE-mediated inflammation."[1] Nonallergic rhinitis (NAR) generally refers to syndromes with nasal inflammation with no allergic or infectious trigger.

Allergic Rhinitis

Epidemiology

Allergic rhinitis is the second leading cause of chronic disease in the United States, affecting up to 60 million Americans.[2] Its prevalence is difficult to precisely estimate due to the variability of how the condition is diagnosed, as well as its significant geographic variations. The 2009 National Health Interview Survey conducted by the Centers for Disease Control and Prevention (CDC) reported that approximately 8% of those surveyed, or roughly 17.7 million adults, had been diagnosed with "hay fever" in the preceding 12 months.[3] Over 7 million children were similarly reported to have "hay fever," and an addition 8.2 million were reported to have "respiratory allergy" during that same time period.[4] Other studies have quoted rates as high as 10% to 30% among adults and up to 40% in children.[5] The financial burden of allergic rhinitis on the American health care system is immense. Most of the direct cost is attributable to physician charges and medication/pharmaceutical costs. In 2011, this was estimated to be approximately $3.4 billion in the United States alone.[6] Indirect costs are more difficult to estimate but one 2004 study estimated that the total yearly cost attributable to allergic rhinitis exceeded $11 billion.[7]

Several controversial theories exist to explain the rising prevalence of allergic rhinitis. Allergic rhinitis is part of the "atopic march," which refers to observation that young children with atopic dermatitis and food allergies are at a great risk later in life to develop asthma and allergic rhinitis.[8] One of the most studied explanations for this effect is the "hygiene hypothesis," which postulates that a lack of early exposure to infections increases the chance of developing atopy later in life.[9] One pathophysiologic explanation for this is that early infections shift the bias of T cells from allergic inflammation (TH2) at birth to a nonallergic (TH1) bias.[10]

Pathophysiology

The pathophysiology of allergic rhinitis initially involves patient sensitization to allergens. Antigen-presenting cells (APCs) located in the mucosa process antigens and present the generated allergenic peptides bound to major histocompatibility complex (MHC) class II molecules. MHC Class II molecules and antigen complex then bind to the T-cell receptors of $CD4^+$ T cells that stimulates their differentiation into allergen-specific TH2 cells. These allergen-specific T cells then secrete cytokines, which induce isotype switching of B cells to produce IgE, and the migration and activation of eosinophils, mast cells, and neutrophils. The antigen-specific IgE then bind to receptors on mast cells and basophils.

Allergic reactions in allergic rhinitis patients can be early or late. The early reaction is a type I hypersensitivity reaction mediated by histamine, prostaglandins, and leukotrienes released by mast cells in response to allergens. It typically occurs within 30 minutes of allergen exposure, includes symptoms such as sneezing and rhinorrhea, and is generally short lived. The late reaction is caused by eosinophil chemotaxis mediated by the same chemical mediators as the early reaction. Inflammatory cells, eosinophils, and mast cells migrate into the nasal mucosa as a result, and remodel the normal tissue. This eventually leads to symptoms of nasal obstruction. The late reaction typically occurs 6 hours after exposure and slowly improves over time.

Nonspecific hyper-responsiveness is one of the major clinical characteristics of allergic inflammation. Due to eosinophilic inflammation and damage of the nasal mucosa, exposed nerve fibers within the mucosa become hyperactive to normal stimuli. This process of neurogenic inflammation leads to the increased secretion of neuropeptides such as substance P and neurokinin A, which induces contraction of smooth muscle, mucous secretions of goblet cells, and plasma exudation from capillaries, further potentiating symptoms.

Classification of Rhinitis

Classification of allergic rhinitis, as defined by the 2008 ARIA guidelines, is based on the severity of symptoms and whether they are intermittent or persistent in nature. This represents a shift away from an earlier classification system that relied upon seasonal versus perennial nature of symptoms and which was felt to poorly describe certain disease subtypes. Persistent allergic rhinitis (PAR) is a condition where symptoms are present for more than 4 consecutive days per week or for more than 4 consecutive weeks. Intermittent allergic rhinitis (IAR) is defined by symptoms that occur over shorter time periods. Persistent patients typically tend to complain primarily of nasal obstruction symptoms, while those with intermittent disease tend to have more sneezing, itching, and rhinorrhea.[11] Symptoms may be classified as moderate/severe if they include one or more of the following: sleep disturbance, impairment of daily activities, impairment of school/work, or other troublesome symptoms.

Diagnosis

The diagnosis of allergic rhinitis relies significantly on history, as well as physical examination and objective testing. History is the most important source of information and relies on 3 essential components: symptoms, timing, and location. The 3 primary symptoms of allergic rhinitis are rhinorrhea, sneezing, and nasal congestion. More general allergic symptoms such as eye itching, watering, redness and swelling, increased mucus, muffled hearing, aural fullness, and hoarseness may also be present. Some of these symptoms may include other disease processes such as asthma, chronic rhinosinusitis, eustachian tube dysfunction, and otitis media, all of which may be worsened by allergies. Timing and location/environment are significant in terms of establishing potential allergic exposures and triggers. Timing of symptoms includes onset (age and duration), fluctuation, and seasonality. Location and environment of symptoms focuses on geography where certain pollens and outdoor allergens are common, as well as more local exposures such as indoor/outdoor, the presence of pets or other animals, tobacco use, carpeting, type of heating or air conditioning, and mold. Past medical history may elicit the presence of other allergic disorders, such as childhood food allergy, asthma, and atopic dermatitis. Asthma should be a specific concern since studies have demonstrated that a significant number of patients will be affected by both conditions. Of note, the use of validated scoring systems, such as the 8-parameter symptom questionnaire described by Ologe et al, may function as a simple, valid diagnostic tool.[12]

Physical examination should focus on comorbid conditions such as otitis, eustachian tube dysfunction, sinusitis, allergic conjunctivitis, and asthma. Affected children may have the typical "adenoid or allergic facies," including high-arched palate, dental malocclusion, and upper lip elevation.[13] Nasal examination including anterior rhinoscopy may demonstrate increased mucus and/or pale and "boggy" turbinates (Figure 5–1). Of note, although nasal polyps may be present in patients with chronic nasal inflammation, they are not seen more frequently in allergic rhinitis patients.[14] Ocular findings may include swelling and vascularity of the lower eyelids, commonly referred to as "allergic shiners," thickening of the scleral surfaces, as well as prominent conjunctival vessels. There also may be erythema of the posterior pharyngeal wall with or without the characteristic cobblestoned appearance. Several findings consistent with more general allergic disease may also be present.

> The 3 primary symptoms of allergic rhinitis are rhinorrhea, sneezing, and nasal congestion.

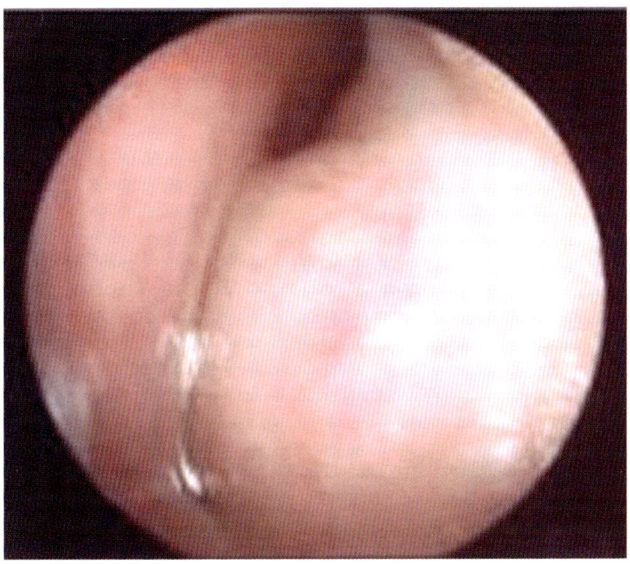

Figure 5–1. Swollen nasal turbinates in allergic rhinitis.

Treatment

Several treatment options are available to the otolaryngologist treating allergic rhinitis. Environment control and pharmacotherapy are the cornerstones of treatment with immunotherapy and surgery also playing a role in appropriate patients. A stepwise and tailored treatment approach should be based on each patient's disease and should rely on patient education and both physician and patient assessment of outcome.

Environmental control is predicated on patients understanding the causes and triggers of their allergic disease and refers to using strategies to avoid, reduce, or eliminate allergen exposure (reviewed in Chapter 2). Although the avoidance of inciting allergens is a logical key to treatment, studies have not consistently demonstrated a correlation between decreased allergen levels and decreased symptoms. Multiple forms of environmental controls exist and have varying degrees of effectiveness, including interventions such as high-efficiency particulate absorption (HEPA) filters, hard surface flooring, and barrier protection on pillows and mattresses.[15,16]

Pharmacological treatment, which is a billion-dollar industry in the United States, is geared toward symptom control and a stepwise approach is generally recommended. For example, patients may be asked to try one drug at a time and then can progressively add or replace medications based on their symptom response.

Combination therapy is very common. Intranasal corticosteroids help alleviate most primary symptoms and are generally considered to be the most effective class of medications. Studies have demonstrated that they are relatively safe to use in both adults and in children (starting at age 2). The side effect profile is relatively minor, primarily including epistaxis, headache, and nasal irritation, but they only rarely cause any of the serious systemic side effects of oral or parenteral corticosteroids. Because they have a slow onset of action, patients are required to use intranasal steroids daily and maximal benefit is not seen until 7 to 10 days of continuous use.[17] Oral corticosteroids are more potent, but their use is limited due to their side effect profile.

Antihistamines were first introduced in the 1940s and have long been a mainstay of treatment.[18] Oral antihistamines are generally effective against sneezing, rhinorrhea, nasal itching, and eye symptoms, but may be less effective for treating nasal congestion.[19] Topical intranasal antihistamine sprays such as azelastine and olopatadine were more recently introduced and are effective first-line agents.[20] They allow for the delivery of higher concentrations of the medication to the target area with less systemic absorption and resulting side effects, offer improved efficacy for nasal symptoms, and have a quicker onset of action than oral antihistamines.[21] Dual therapy with intranasal steroids and intranasal antihistamine has an additive effect and is effective in treating moderate-to-severe disease.[22,23] These can be delivered as individual sprays or by the use of a combined spray (Dymista).

Intranasal decongestants may offer short-term control of symptoms. Generally only 3 to 5 days of use are recommended given that long-term use has the potential for abuse, rebound nasal congestion, and the development of chronic nasal inflammation (rhinitis medicamentosa). Combining intranasal steroids with intranasal decongestants such as oxymetazoline has been demonstrated to enhance symptom control.[24] Nasal saline may provide symptomatic relief by thinning and clearing mucus and allergy particles from the nasal mucosa. Given that it has relatively few significant side effects, it is routinely added to nearly all treatment regimens.[25] Leukotriene modifiers are a good pharmacologic option for those patients affected by both allergic rhinitis and asthma, and have been shown to have an added effect when combined with intranasal antihistamines, similar to that of intranasal steroids.[26] Anticholinergics such as ipratropium nasal spray may be a good choice for patients whose primary symptom is clear rhinorrhea since its primary effect is to decrease nasal secretions.[27] Several other emerging therapies such as omalizumab (a monoclonal anti-IgE antibody),[28,29] anti-interleukin 5 (IL-5),[30] and botulism neurotoxin[31] are actively being investigated.

Immunotherapy, or allergy desensitization, is the only therapy that can permanently decrease or even eliminate allergic rhinitis symptoms. It modulates the body's immune system and enables it to tolerate exposure to known allergens.[32] It can be administered in a number of different forms, the most common of which are subcutaneous and sublingual administration (reviewed in Chapter 17). Both routes have been shown to be effective, however comparative effectiveness is still under investigation. Currently, there are no explicit practice guidelines for choosing between these 2 therapies.[33,34] Subcutaneous administration is considered the gold standard for the treatment of pharmacologically resistant allergic rhinitis. It is generally well tolerated; however, it causes a high frequency of mild adverse events (up to 71% of patients), although the rate of serious or fatal side effects related to anaphylaxis is rare (death in 1/2.5 million injections). Treatment is typically administered once weekly, but can be given more frequently if necessary, and must be done in a clinical setting. Given this constraint, many physicians reserve such treatment for patients with moderate-to-severe disease. Sublingual therapy (SLIT) was introduced more recently and has the benefit of being able to be self-administered at home and is typically taken daily. It has an improved safety profile although anaphylactic reactions have been reported.[35,36] Currently in the United States, SLIT is only US Food and Drug Administration (FDA)-approved for grass and ragweed pollen allergy. Alternative administration techniques such as intralymphatic immunotherapy are actively being investigated and may represent a more cost-effective and less time-consuming treatment option.[37]

> Immunotherapy has the potential to permanently decrease or eliminate allergic rhinitis symptoms by modulating the body's immune system.

The fourth treatment option, surgery, can be beneficial in the treatment of allergic rhinitis in select patients, including those with specific anatomic abnormalities and those with disease refractory to medical treatment. The inferior turbinate is the most important contributor to nasal obstruction and may become enlarged due to allergic inflammation. Several techniques for reduction of the inferior turbinate exist, including lateral outfracture, submucosal resection, laser vaporization, radiofrequency ablation, and coblation.[38] Radiofrequency turbinoplasty has been shown to safely and effectively decrease nasal resistance and improve congestion with good long-term outcomes.[39–41] Furthermore, it may lead to a quality of life benefit at 5 years.[42] Septoplasty has also been demonstrated to improve quality of life in allergic rhinitis patients with septal deviation.[43] Surgically addressing other anatomic abnormalities such as adenoid hypertrophy, nasal polyps, nasal valve collapse, concha bullosa, and sinus disease may also lead to a benefit in nasal obstruction symptoms.

> The inferior turbinate may be enlarged due to allergic inflammation and is a common target of surgical treatment.

Nonallergic Rhinitis

Nonallergic rhinitis (NAR) generally refers to nasal inflammatory syndromes with no allergic or infectious triggers, but increased symptoms from other triggers such as changes in weather or barometric pressure, or exposure to irritants such as fumes, caustic odors, or cigarette smoke. Our understanding of the underlying pathophysiology of nonallergic rhinitis is incomplete. As a result, the current classification system based largely on etiology is limited. It is further constrained by the fact that rhinitis symptoms are often multifactorial and that allergic and nonallergic etiologies often overlap. Concerted efforts are now being made to develop an improved classification system for NAR that is based on consensus definitions. In December 2008, the Nonallergic Rhinitis Consensus Panel Proceedings established 8 subtypes that fill the criteria for nonallergic rhinitis (Table 5–1).

While varied in etiology and underlying pathophysiology, there are several common clinical presentations of NAR. It is more prevalent after 20 years of age and is female predominant.[44–46] Individuals with nonallergic rhinitis have been shown to be increasingly sensitive to irritants. In addition, nasal eosinophilia can be demonstrated in approximately 33% of nonallergic rhinitis patients.[44]

Table 5–1. Nonallergic Rhinitis Subtypes

Subtypes	Clinical Presentation
Nonallergic rhinopathy (previously known as vasomotor rhinitis or idiopathic nonallergic rhinitis)	Chronic nasal symptoms without immunologic or infectious etiology or nasal eosinophilia
Nonallergic rhinitis with eosinophilia (NARES)	Typically year-round symptoms with nasal eosinophilia but negative skin tests/IgE antibodies
Atrophic rhinitis	Chronic, progressive atrophy of nasal mucosa with crusting and dryness
Senile rhinitis	Typically presents with watery rhinorrhea, may worsen after certain food/environmental triggers
Gustatory rhinitis	Occurs after eating, especially hot/spicy foods (due to cholinergic effect)
Drug-induced rhinitis (including rhinitis medicamentosa)	Typically occurs after repeated use of topic nasal decongestants (ie, oxymetazoline, phenylephrine)
Hormonal-induced rhinitis	Occurs in response to endogenous female hormones, such as with pregnancy
Cerebral spinal fluid leak	Should be considered with persistent clear rhinorrhea, especially if unilateral or in setting of recent craniofacial trauma

Source: Adapted from Tran NP, Vickery J, Blaiss MS. Management of rhinitis: allergic and nonallergic. *Allergy Asthma Immunol Res.* 2011;3:146–156.

The prevalence of NAR is even more difficult to estimate than that of allergic rhinitis, most likely because rhinitis symptoms are frequently underreported and because the disease is poorly classified. There is also frequently an overlap between nonallergic and allergic rhinitis, and many patients who are classified as having allergic rhinitis because of positive allergy testing or response to empiric pharmacologic therapy actually have multifactorial disease. Despite these limitations, it is extrapolated from population data that almost 20 million Americans suffer from nonallergic rhinitis. European studies demonstrate that nearly 50 million Europeans have nonallergic rhinitis and that worldwide the number of affected patients is close to 200 million.[47]

Much like with allergic disease, the economic burden of NAR is substantial. Schatz et al. reviewed the records of 1 million Kaiser Permanente Southern

California patients and found that 15% had at least 1 medical encounter because of rhinitis symptoms over a 3-year period, and that another 14% received rhinitis medications with no medical encounter at all. In addition, they found that the same patients tended to have significantly more health care visits and a higher prevalence of comorbid conditions such as acute and chronic sinusitis, asthma, sleep apnea, and fatigue.[48] Patients with rhinitis symptoms also report that their symptoms adversely impact their quality of daily living, sleep, and productivity.[49] In addition, there is significant cost associated with both inadequately diagnosed and incompletely treated NAR.[50]

Diagnosis is largely predicated on ruling out allergy, mechanical obstruction, and infection as a cause. The absence of allergic disease is typically determined by a negative skin prick test for relevant allergens and/or negative allergic-specific antibody tests. History is especially significant in differentiating allergic from nonallergic disease. This includes thoroughly reviewing alleviating and exacerbating factors, medication lists, irritation exposure, and other related medical problems. Anterior rhinoscopy and nasal endoscopy should rule out structural contributions. At this time, there is no definitive objective testing that differentiates between patients with different subtypes of disease.

Treatment has several different components. It is recommended that patients avoid environmental triggers such as strong odors and air pollutants that may be respiratory irritants. There are several pharmacologic therapies for symptom-directed treatment of idiopathic rhinitis. Intranasal antihistamines are generally considered to be first-line therapy. Several randomized control trials have demonstrated that azelastine, which is FDA approved for the treatment of nonallergic rhinitis, contributes to the symptomatic relief of nasal congestion, rhinorrhea, postnasal drip, and associated-sneezing.[51–53] The mechanism for this beneficial effect is unclear and may be related to the dual anti-inflammatory and anti-allergic activities of azelastine. Intranasal corticosteroids have also been found to be effective, specifically for nonallergic rhinopathy and nonallergic rhinitis with eosinophilia (NARES), although there is a subgroup of patients that fail to respond to this therapy, as demonstrated in a randomized control trial.[54] This class of drugs includes fluticasone propionate, triamcinolone acetonide, mometasone furoate, and beclomethasone dipropionate, all of which are FDA approved for treatment of NAR. Decongestants are generally considered to be an adjunctive therapy that can be used on an as-needed basis for refractory nasal congestion.[55] Nasal saline is generally accepted as another well-tolerated, low-risk, adjunct treatment for chronic rhinosinusitis symptoms. It is best performed immediately before the use of intranasal antihistamines or corticosteroids and can be especially helpful in reducing postnasal drip, sneezing, and congestion. Several other therapies have been investigated for a possible beneficial effect in NAR, including capsaicin, silver nitrate, and acupuncture.[56–58] After 6 to 12 months of failed medical therapy, surgical options may be considered and should focus on existing structural abnormalities that may contribute to disease.

> The diagnosis of nonallergic rhinitis is largely predicated on ruling out other causes, such as allergy, mechanical obstruction, and infection.

Rhinosinusitis

Rhinosinusitis is an umbrella term that refers to a continuum of inflammatory changes in the nose and sinuses that may result from several different pathological processes. In 1996, a multidisciplinary Rhinosinusitis Task Force (RSTF) defined 5 separate categories of disease: acute, subacute, chronic, recurrent acute, and acute exacerbation of chronic rhinosinusitis. These categories were defined according to specific major and minor signs, symptoms, and the time course over which they occurred, without regard to their specific pathogenesis. They have since been refined and updated by Task Forces reconvened in 2003 and 2007. Recently, consensus guidelines have been published jointly by multiple national societies.

Acute rhinosinusitis (ARS) is defined by the presence of specific signs and symptoms for duration of up to 4 weeks, subacute rhinosinusitis is defined as lasting between 4 and 12 weeks, and recurrent acute rhinosinusitis is defined by 4 or more episodes of acute sinusitis with complete symptom remission between episodes. Chronic rhinosinusitis (CRS) is defined by a presence of several clinical symptoms for duration of at least 12 weeks, while patients with sudden worsening of persistent symptoms were classified as having an acute exacerbation of chronic rhinosinusitis.[59]

Epidemiology

Rhinosinusitis is one of the most common diseases in the United States. Approximately 20 million cases of acute bacterial rhinosinusitis are diagnosed annually with another 30 million Americans suffering from chronic rhinosinusitis.[60] According to the 2007 National Health Interview Surveys, rhinosinusitis is one of the top 10 leading office visit diagnoses in the United States.[61] The resulting economic burden of disease on the US health care system is consequently immense. Direct health care expenditures associated with acute rhinosinusitis are estimated to be $3.5 billion and with chronic rhinosinusitis $4.3 billion.[62] This includes hospital and physician visits, the majority of which comes from the emergency and ambulatory settings with the most of the outpatient care provided by primary care physicians.[63] It also includes significant medication costs, including over $200 million for prescription medications and billions for over-the-counter medications.[64] This does not take into account indirect costs, including lost or restricted workdays and lost productivity. In 2007, the estimated opportunity cost attributed to acute rhinosinusitis alone was $18.3 billion.[65] For an individual CRS patient, the yearly indirect cost is estimated to be $1539.[66]

Acute Rhinosinusitis

Etiology. Acute rhinosinusitis (ARS) is most commonly associated with an infectious etiology in both adults and children. Viral agents tend to predominate, the most common of which is rhinovirus, followed in prevalence by influenza virus, parainfluenza virus, and adenovirus.[67] The viral mechanism of spread includes viral entry into the nose, incorporation into the mucus stream, activation of receptors on specialized lymphoepithelial cells, and a resulting inflammatory reaction.[68] This process leads to the sore throat, nasal obstruction, and rhinorrhea that are hallmarks of acute viral rhinosinusitis (AVRS) symptoms.

Acute bacterial rhinosinusitis (ABRS) classically presents as a superimposed infection in a patient with previous AVRS. Viral disease promotes bacterial infection by several mechanisms including impaired sinus ostia and mucus drainage secondary to inflamed and edematous mucosa, as well as inflammatory-mediated mucociliary dysfunction and mucus stasis. It is estimated that only 0.5% to 2% of AVRS are complicated by bacterial infections; however, given the significant number of patients affected by viral disease, this accounts for about 20 million cases of ABRS per year.[60,65]

The majority of ABRS infections are due to a single bacterial isolate; however, approximately 25% of cases are polymicrobial in nature.[69] The most common pathogens isolated from the maxillary sinuses of affected patients with uncomplicated disease in decreasing prevalence are *Streptococcus pneumoniae*, *Haemophilus influenzae*, and *Moraxella catarrhalis*.[70,71] Antibiotic resistance continues to be a key concern, including macrolide-resistant *S. pneumoniae*, which may contribute to treatment failure.[72,73] Concerns about beta-lactamase-producing *H. influenzae* have been mitigated by a decrease in the prevalence of resistant isolates. Anaerobic bacteria only account for 2% to 6% of ABRS and may arise from primary dental pathology. *Staphylococcus aureus* and *S. pyogenes* account for less than 5% of disease although they are generally overestimated based on nasal swab cultures and may have a high propensity to cause acute complications such as orbital extension of disease and intracranial abscesses. Nosocomial infections tend to have a higher prevalence of Gram-negative organisms such as *Pseudomonas aeruginosa*, *Klebsiella pneumoniae*, and *Enterobacter* species. Patients at high risk for nosocomial infection include those who require long periods of intensive care with prolonged endotracheal intubation or nasogastric tubing.[74]

> The most common bacterial pathogens in ABRS are *Streptococcus pneumoniae*, *Haemophilus influenzae*, and *Moraxella catarrhalis*.

Pathophysiology. The pathophysiologic reaction to infectious agents in ARS is the initiation of an inflammatory response, the purpose of which is to promote eradication of the pathogen. Ultimately this inflammatory cascade subsides and normal sinus function is restored. Pathologic changes include loss of cilia and respiratory epithelium with mucosal infiltrates of lymphocytes and plasma cells. Luminal exudates consist primarily of neutrophils with limited amounts of eosinophils.[75] Increased levels of several inflammatory cytokines have been demonstrated in conjunction with these histopathologic changes. Cytokines such as IL-1B, IL-6, and TNF-α are important in inducing expression of adhesion molecules and activating endothelial cells and T lymphocytes. Subsequently, these activated T lymphocytes release IL-8, a neutrophil chemotaxic factor, which further potentiates the inflammatory response and eventually leads to elimination of the initiating organism.[76–78] As the infection resolves, the inflammatory reaction subsides, and the physiologic state is restored.

Symptoms. ARS may present with a range of symptoms including nasal obstruction, nasal discharge, nasal purulence, postnasal drip, facial pressure and/or pain, alteration in the sense of smell, cough, fever, halitosis, dental pain, fatigue, ear pain, and headache. Clinical evaluation may focus specifically on differentiating between ABRS and AVRS, which may be very difficult in the first 3 to 4 days after disease onset. Recent efforts have been made to develop a model to help practitioners differentiate between the 2 entities to help facilitate treatment. This includes the replacement of major and minor symptoms of ABRS, as detailed by the RTSF, with a new concept that highlights 3 cardinal symptoms, which include (1) purulent nasal discharge; (2) nasal obstruction; (3) and facial pain, pressure, or fullness. These symptoms have been found to be highly sensitive and specific indicators of disease and correlate with radiologic and other objective testing measures.[79,80] Fever is not included as a cardinal symptom as it only has a specificity of approximately 50% for the diagnosis of ABRS. According to 2007 guidelines, ABRS is diagnosed when the aforementioned 3 cardinal symptoms are present for 10 days or longer beyond the onset of upper respiratory symptoms, or when the symptoms or signs of ABRS worsen within 10 days after a period of initial improvement (referred to as "double-worsening").[59] The presence of purulent nasal discharge is not an effective way to differentiate between bacterial and viral infection since it is indicative of the presence of neutrophils and general inflammation, and is not specific for bacteria. Symptoms related to inflammation and edema from AVRS should be improving within 10 days of onset of disease, otherwise ABRS should be considered.[59]

> The 3 cardinal symptoms of ABRS are purulent nasal discharge, nasal pain, and facial pain, pressure, or fullness.

Physical Examination and Imaging. Physical examination should include inspection of the face for signs of extension of disease into soft tissues with a focus on the cheeks and periorbital region. Nasal examination should be performed before and after topical decongestion, including anterior rhinoscopy inspecting for crusting, edema, pus in area of the middle meatus, and enlarged turbinates. However, the view may be limited by the presence of nasal polyps, other nasal masses, and/or septal deviation. Although directed cultures are not necessary for the diagnosis or treatment of ABRS, endoscopic-directed middle meatus cultures correlate well with cultures that have been obtained by direct maxillary sinus aspiration.[81] Nasopharyngeal or nasal cavity cultures are generally not reliable and may be contaminated by normal colonizing bacteria.[82]

Imaging for sinusitis usually begins with computed tomography (CT), which can provide information about the complex structure of the paranasal sinuses and bony structures. Findings including opacification of the sinus cavities, air-fluid levels, and moderate-to-severe mucosal thickening tend to correlate with ABRS.[83] The Lund-Mackay classification system, which quantitates sinus disease by the number of sinuses with any degree of opacification (with consideration of anatomic variants), is a well-accepted objective staging system.[84] While the presence of several of the previously mentioned findings on CT has a high positive predictive value (PPV), the use of CT in uncomplicated ABRS is generally not recommended and is not cost effective.[85,86] CT should be performed when complications are suspected or in select patients with history of trauma, surgery, or with comorbid clinical conditions. Although it may not reveal as much bony anatomy, magnetic resonance imaging (MRI) provides excellent soft tissue differentiation and is the best modality for delineating extension of disease into the orbits or intracranial compartments. Both x-ray and ultrasound are of limited utility in the evaluation of sinusitis.

Treatment. Antibiotics are the most frequently recommended medication in the treatment of ARS. They are generally overprescribed and account for approximately 21% of the total antibiotics prescribed for adults and 9% for children.[87,88] Treatment of AVRS should focus on symptom control and to help decrease the potential for conversion to ABRS. Several medications have been demonstrated to be effective in this regard, including analgesics, antipyretics, nasal irrigation, systemic and topical decongestants, topical nasal steroids, and mucolytics. Oral steroids are generally not recommended. In patients with an allergic component, antihistamines may lead to a relief in symptoms.

In those patients with uncomplicated ABRS and mild symptoms (mild pain, fever <101°), an initial observation period of 7 days without antibiotics may be appropriate provided the patient is reliable and there is assurance of follow-up. If the patient's symptoms either worsen or fail to improve after that 7-day period, antibiotics can be initiated. This treatment strategy is supported by randomized controlled trials that demonstrate a high frequency of spontaneous improvement in patients receiving placebo alone versus antibiotics, and is consistent with attempts to minimize the use of unnecessary antibiotics in order to reduce the development of antibiotic resistance.[87,89]

Patients with severe symptoms (moderate-to-severe pain, fever >101°) can be treated with an antibiotic initially. Amoxicillin is generally considered to be the drug of choice and is efficacious, cost effective, and safe. Recommended alternatives for patients with penicillin allergies are trimethoprim-sulfate or a macrolide. Any patients who have been treated with an antibiotic in the past 4 to 6 weeks have an increased likelihood for infection with resistant bacteria and should be prescribed a fluoroquinolone or high-dose amoxicillin-clavulanate.[89]

> Patients with moderate ABRS may be observed for 7 days prior to the initiation of antibiotics.

Complications. A small but significant number of patients with ABRS may experience deleterious sequelae of disease. Complications are generally classified as extracranial and intracranial (Table 5–2, Figures 5–2 and 5–3). Orbital extension is the most common complication of ABRS in both adults and pediatric patients. The Chandler classification system was first introduced in the 1970s and is based

Table 5-2. Complications of Rhinosinusitis

Extracranial Complications		Intracranial Complications
Local inflammation		Meningitis
Anosmia		Extradural abscess
Pott's puffy tumor		Subdural empyema
Orbital extension	Preseptal cellulitis	Intracerebral abscess
	Postseptal cellulitis	Cavernous and sagittal sinus thrombosis
	Subperiosteal abscess	
	Orbital abscess	
	Orbital apex syndrome	
	Retrobulbar abscess	
	Cavernous sinus thrombosis	

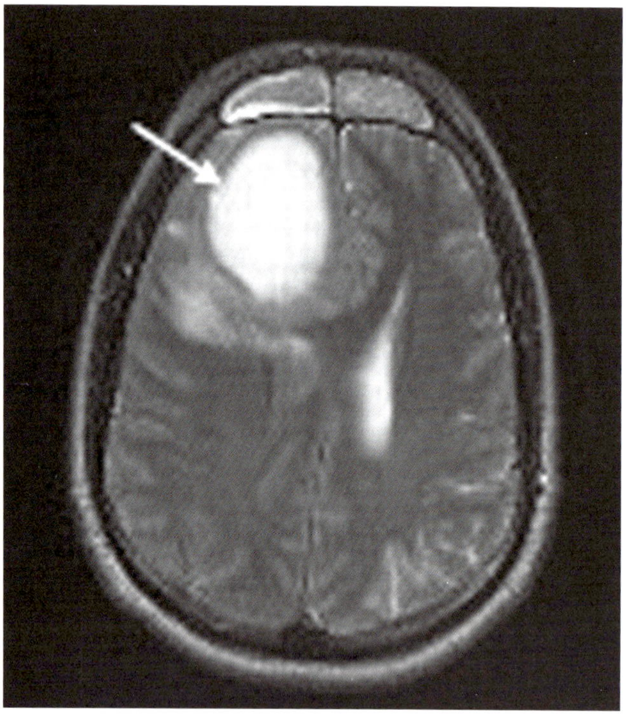

Figure 5–2. Head CT scan demonstrating an intracranial abscess (*arrow*).

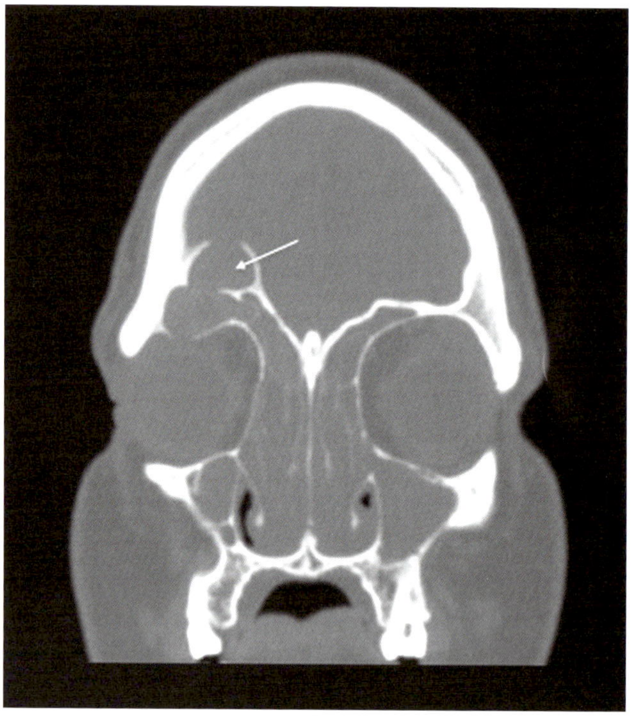

Figure 5–3. Sinus CT scan demonstrating extensive nasal polyposis with a frontal sinus mucocele (*arrow*).

on the pattern of progressive pathogenesis of orbital complications: (1) preseptal cellulitis, (2) postseptal cellulitis, (3) subperiosteal abscess, and (4) orbital abscess.[90] Of note, this classification system omits many of the more advanced orbital complications. Stages 1 and 2 are generally treated medically. Indications for surgical intervention include patients with stage 1 or 2 complications who fail to improve on high-dose antibiotics within the first 24 to 48 hours, any decrease in visual acuity, increasing proptosis or ophthalmoplegia, or abscess as identified on CT. Pediatric patients between the ages of 3 and 6 are at highest risk for complications.[91] The highest risk group for intracranial complications is males during adolescence and young adulthood (10 to 29 years old).

Chronic Rhinosinusitis

Epidemiology. Chronic rhinosinusitis (CRS) is one of the most common chronic conditions reported in the United States, affecting at least 14% of the US population.[92] It causes not only symptoms related directly to the paranasal sinuses, but also negatively impacts quality of life including mood, physical functioning, and social functioning.[93]

Etiology/Pathophysiology. In contrast to ARS, CRS is thought to be more multifactorial in etiology (Table 5–3). The interaction between many systemic factors, local host factors, and environmental factors contribute to paranasal sinus inflammation and their joint contribution to CRS pathophysiology is now increasingly appreciated.[94] Nevertheless, our understanding of the etiology and underlying pathophysiology of CRS remains incomplete.

CRS is generally divided into 2 major categories: chronic rhinosinusitis with nasal polyps (CRSwNP) and chronic sinusitis without nasal polyps (CRSsNP). CRSwNP is characterized by extensive mucosal edema with goblet cell hyperplasia, mononuclear cell infiltration, whereas CRSsNP is often noted to have epithelial damage with very limited neural structures, goblet cell hypoplasia, and eosinophilic cell infiltration. Fibrosis is common in both, but occurs to a greater extent in CRSwNP.[95] A wide variety of

Table 5–3. Pathophysiologic Factors in Chronic Rhinosinusitis

Systemic		Local Host		Environmental
Genetic	Cystic fibrosis	Anatomic	Concha bullosa	Bacterial infection
	Primary ciliary dyskinesia		Septal deviation	Biofilms
Immunodeficiency	HIV		Nasal polyps	Superantigens
	Chemotherapy		Paradoxical middle turbinate	Fungal infection
	IgG/IgA deficiency		Haller cells	Allergy
	X-linked agammaglobulinemia	Iatrogenic	Scarring from previous sinonasal surgery	Environmental pollutants
Autoimmune	Wegener granulomatosis		Trauma	Smoking
	Sarcoidosis	Sinonasal cysts		
	Churg-Strauss syndrome	Mucoceles		
	Other vasculitides	Neoplasms		
Idiopathic	Samter syndrome	Persistent inflammation/osteitis		
Acid reflux		Foreign bodies		

inflammatory mediators are increased in the nasal tissue of patients with CRSsNP and include IL-1, IL-6, IL-8, TNF-α, GM-CSF, ICAM-1, MPO (myeloperoxidase), and ECP (eosinophilic cationic protein).[96–98] Patients with CRSwNP also have increased amounts of these mediators within polypoid tissue, as well as additional inflammatory mediators including RANTES, IL-4 and IL-5, which have been shown to directly activate and increase the survival of eosinophils.[99,100]

Given the prevalence of eosinophilic inflammation in polypoid disease and studies that have demonstrated increased local production of IgE,[101] allergic mechanisms were thought to play a causative role in this disease process. Similarly, bacterial infection was thought to be causative in nonpolypoid disease given the predominance of neutrophil-mediated inflammation. However, it is now better understood that these ideas were oversimplifications and that there is significant overlap between the 2 types of disease. While strongly suspected, a definitive link between allergy and CRS is yet to be established. Allergy is thought to set the stage for the development of CRS due to inflammatory changes stimulated by the production of cytokines, allergic mediators, and neurogenic stimulation.[102,103]

> A definitive link between CRS and allergy has not been established.

Chronic Rhinosinusitis With Nasal Polyposis. CRSwNP refers to nasal polyp disease that arises as a result of paranasal sinus inflammation. It is classified by and may be the result of several different pathologic processes including allergic fungal rhinosinusitis (AFRS), cystic fibrosis (CF), primary ciliary dyskinesia, antrochoanal polyp, eosinophilic mucin rhinosinusitis, aspirin exacerbated respiratory disease (AERD), Churg-Strauss syndrome, and allergy. There are important histopathological differences between many of these variants; however, eosinophilic inflammation is the common denominator.

Nasal polyp disease affects approximately 1% to 4% of Americans with several important variations in terms of geography, race, and age.[104] There is an increased prevalence of nasal polyposis in warm and humid climates where AFRS, which accounts for a significant percentage of cases, is more common.[105] Noneosinophilic disease may be more common in Asian populations.[106] Nasal polyposis of childhood is very rare, which is a key reason why the finding of a nasal polyp in a young child should prompt a close evaluation for underlying conditions such as CF. There is some question about the genetic basis for disease; however, studies have not demonstrated clear heritability via Mendelian genetics.[107]

It is well accepted that inflammation plays an important role in development of nasal polyps. The inflammation of eosinophilic nasal polyps, which constitute the majority of cases, typically features chronic inflammatory cells such as eosinophils, lymphocytes, and increased expression of eosinophil active cytokines such as IL-5, granulocyte-macrophage colony stimulating factors, and chemokines such as RANTES and MCP 3/4. The T cells are the predominant lymphocyte type and may play a role in orchestrating nasal polyp inflammation.[108,109] This idea is supported by the finding that superantigen stimulation of T-cells by *Staphylococcus aureus* enterotoxin B (SEB), which is frequently found in the nasal cavities of CRSwNP patients, is capable of stimulating a pro-inflammatory cytokine cascade.[110]

Several studies have supported the connection between nasal polyps and allergy[111]; however, detailed analysis has been unable to directly correlate nasal polyp disease and allergic rhinitis or skin test positivity.[112,113] This may be explained by the concept of "entopy," which refers to the presence of increased allergen-specific tissue IgE levels in nasal polyps, despite the absence of positive reactions to allergen on skin prick testing and negative levels of serum specific allergen IgE.[114]

The clinical presentation of CRSwNP is highly variable. Symptoms may be similar to that of CRSsNP including nasal obstruction, rhinorrhea, nasal congestion, facial pressure, and postnasal drainage. Hyposmia or smell dysfunction, which may result from obstruction of airflow to the olfactory cleft, is more common in CRSwNP, however by itself it is not reliable enough to make this diagnosis. Symptoms are also typically bilateral due to the general inflammatory state of the paranasal sinuses. The clinical course is similarly variable. Patients may experience months or years or progressive sinonasal symptoms, often after an inciting initial event such as a severe upper respiratory infection. Patients may experience recurrent acute exacerbations of obstructive bacterial sinusitis. Other patients may only experience mild sinonasal symptoms that are alleviated or cured by a single surgery or course of treatment.

> Entopy refers to elevated IgE levels in allergen specific tissues, such as nasal polyps.

Nasal polyps typically appear as smooth round masses with a pale to yellow coloration; however, there may be some variation (Figure 5–4). They may be visible on nasal endoscopy and typically arise from the lateral wall of the middle meatus or sphenoethmoidal recess, although they also may arise lateral to the middle turbinate, and rarely from the nasal septum or olfactory cleft. Nasal endoscopy is a significant tool in diagnosis and surveillance. Grading scales, such as that developed by Lindholdt et al and Johanssen et al, estimate the bulk of nasal polyps in relation to anatomic landmarks within the nose.[115,116] Imaging studies such as noncontrast CT are particularly helpful in differentiating polypoid disease from nonpolypoid lesions such as meningoencephaloceles and malignant lesions. Definitive

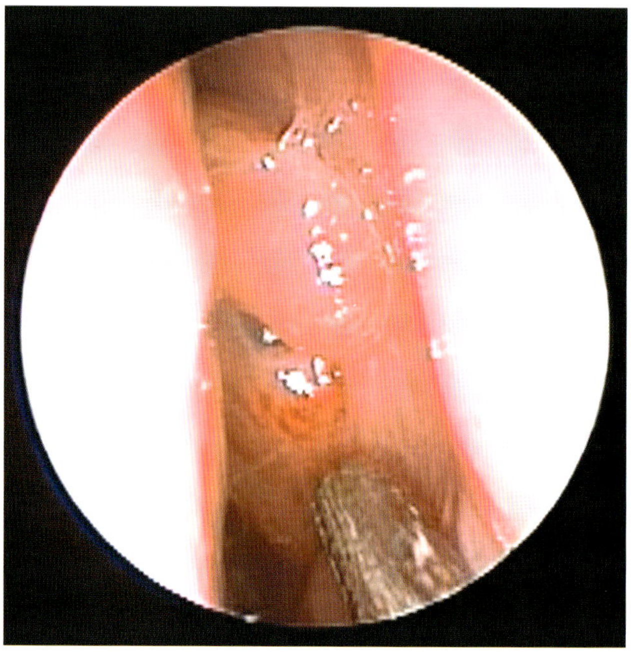

Figure 5–4. Endoscopic view of nasal polyps.

diagnosis relies on histopathologic examination. Nasal polyps are typically divided into 3 different subtypes: (1) "edematous, eosinophilic," (2) fibroinflammatory, and (3) glandular. Edematous, eosinophilic polyps comprise 85% of specimens and may be seen with a wide variety of conditions including AERD, AFRS, Churg-Strauss, and CF[117] (Figure 5–5).

Treatment often relies on management of the underlying pathologic process, such as with CF or avoidance of aspirin in the case of AERD. In terms of nasal polyps specifically, the goal of treatment is to minimize the symptomatic burden of disease and to prevent complications over time while reducing the impact of treatment, including surgery and steroid use. The general variability of CRSwNP lends to similar variability in terms of treatment response. For example, patients with an isolated antrochoanal polyp may be cured with a single surgery, while others with recurrent inflammatory disease may require multiple surgeries.

Diagnosis. The diagnosis of CRS relies on a thorough clinical history and physical examination similar to what is done with ARS (Table 5–4). According to the 2007 Practice Guidelines, diagnosis requires persistent symptomatic inflammation of the sinonasal mucosa for 12 weeks or more. Several validated, sinus-specific questionnaires such as the Sino-Nasal Outcomes Test-22 (SNOT-22) and the Rhinosinusitis Disability Index may be used as adjuncts to assess patient symptoms.[118,119]

The clinical history and physical examination findings may be sufficient alone to make a diagnosis of ABRS, but radiologic imaging is often needed to make a diagnosis of CRS. The Lund-Mackay staging system can be used to stratify patients with CRS based on imaging. A modified version, the Lund-Kennedy grading system, is a more recent update that incorporates the presence of anatomic variants, types of surgery performed, symptom scores, and endoscopic scores in addition to the CT findings.[120] Endoscopic staging systems have been developed and have a relatively high correlation with CT scan findings; however, normal findings on endoscopy does not ensure that the CT scan will be normal.[121]

Treatment. The treatment of CRS aims to reduce symptoms, prevent disease progression and recurrence, and improve quality of life. This is most often achieved with agents that help reduce inflammation and control infection, as well as restore normal mucociliary clearance mechanisms in the paranasal sinuses. Medical treatment is the cornerstone of

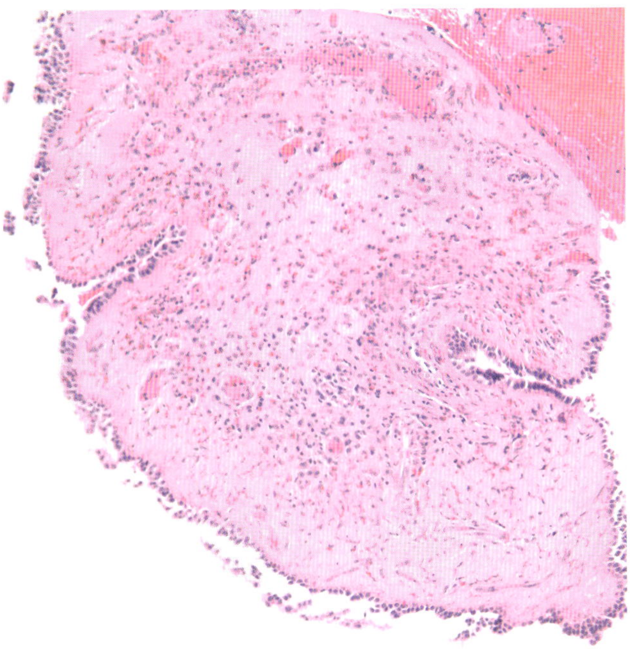

Figure 5–5. Nasal polyp histology demonstrating marked eosinophilia.

Table 5–4. Diagnostic Criteria for Chronic Rhinosinusitis in Adults

Symptom Duration >12 Weeks With:	
Two or more of the following:	Mucopurulent discharge
	Nasal obstruction
	Facial pain/pressure/fullness
	Decreased sense of smell
One or more of the following:	Purulent mucus or edema in the middle meatus or ethmoid region
	Nasal polyps in the nasal cavity or middle meatus
	Radiographic imaging showing inflammation in the paranasal sinuses

Source: Adapted from Rosenfeld RM, Andes D, Bhattacharyya N, et al. Clinical practice guidelines: adult sinusitis 1. *Otolaryngol Head Neck Surg.* 2007;137(suppl 13):S1–S3.

treatment for CRS, the 3 most significant agents of which are corticosteroids, antibiotics, and nasal irrigation. Surgery also plays an important role in some patients (Table 5–5).

Topical corticosteroids are a first-line treatment for CRS, especially for CRSwNP. This is based on several randomized controlled trials.[122] Topical corticosteroids contribute to a maintained reduction in nasal symptoms and medium-sized polyps with continued use, as well as a delay the recurrence of nasal polyps after surgery.[123,124] In contrast, the efficacy of intranasal steroids for nonpolypoid CRS has not been as well demonstrated,[125] One randomized, double-blind, placebo-controlled study on

Table 5-5. Evidence-Based Guidelines for the Treatment of Chronic Rhinosinusitis

Treatment	Recommendation
Topical corticosteroid (spray)	Strong recommendation for routine use
Systemic corticosteroid—CRSwNP	Strong recommendation in short-term management AND in perioperative period
Systemic corticosteroid—CRSsNP	Option in management, not recommended perioperatively
Systemic corticosteroid—AFRS	Recommended in management and in perioperative period
Oral antibacterial therapy (nonmacrolide), <3 weeks' duration	Option
Oral antibacterial therapy (nonmacrolide), >3 weeks' duration	Not recommended
Macrolide antibiotic	Option
Topical antibacterials	Recommendation against for routine CRS
Oral antifungals	Recommendation against for routine CRS
Topical antifungals	Strong recommendation against
Allergy testing and treatment	Option in CRSwNP and CRSsNP (with recommendation for immunotherapy in select patients)
Image-guided surgery	Option
Early postoperative nasal saline irrigation	Recommended
Early postoperative debridement	Recommended
Early postoperative systemic steroids	Option
Early postoperative topical steroids	Recommended
Early postoperative antibiotics	Option
Early postoperative topical decongestants	Not recommended
Early postoperative drug-eluting stents or spacers	Option

Source: Adapted from Orlandi RR, Smith TL, Marple BF, et al. Update on evidence-based reviews with recommendation in adult chronic rhinosinusitis. *Int Forum Allergy Rhinol.* 2014;4:S1–S15.

patients with CRSsNP demonstrated no significant improvement after treatment for 16 weeks.[126] Oral corticosteroids are used frequently used in clinical practice, despite a lack of strong evidence in regard to indication, dose, and duration.[127,128] This form of treatment may be effective in cases of CRSwNP that are refractory to medical treatment or when a rapid, short-term improvement is needed.[129]

Antibiotics may be used to reduce bacterial load, as well as treat acute bacterial exacerbations and refractory cases. The bacteria present in the sinonasal cavities of CRS patients differ from that found in ARS patients, including a greater incidence of anaerobic bacteria, *S. aureus*, and *P. aeruginosa*. Antibiotics are commonly aimed at a mixed population of aerobic and anaerobic bacteria.[130] Typical antibiotics used include amoxicillin-clavulanate, clindamycin, trimethoprim-sulfamethoxazole, or a fluoroquinolone. Duration should typically be 3 weeks or less, with longer courses reserved for refractory cases. Of note, long-term macrolide therapy was the only antibiotic to show efficacy in a blinded, placebo-controlled trial in CRS.[131] The effectiveness of macrolides has been attributed to the drug's anti-inflammatory and immunomodulatory effects, and not to its direct antibacterial effects.[132]

The treatment of methicillin-resistant *Staphylococcus aureus* (MRSA) is of considerable interest given its increased prevalence in CRS patients.[133] In most cases, MRSA is present as a nasal colonizer and thus treatment is reserved for those patients who are symptomatic with nasal purulence or who experience a sudden worsening of symptoms that usually indicates an acute exacerbation. Treatment options for MRSA include intravenous, oral, and topical antibiotics, the choice of which should be based on bacterial sensitivities. The duration of treatment should be based on symptom response and should continue until symptoms are resolved. Even though the use of topical antibiotics has recently grown in popularity,[134] recent evidence-based guidelines recommend against their use.[135]

Intrasinal biofilms may contribute to the high incidence of symptom relapse, surgical failure, and persistent symptoms following ESS.[136–138] The most common biofilm-forming bacteria encountered in sinus infections are *S. aureus*, *P. aeruginosa*, and *H. influenzae*. Biofilms are notoriously difficult to eradicate but are typically treated with topical antibiotics, as well as surgery, mechanical debridement, and surfactants.[139]

Nasal saline irrigation is a well-accepted and recommended part of most treatment regimens. In several randomized controlled trials with CRS patients, it improved symptoms, endoscopic findings, and quality of life.[140] It may both prevent rhinosinusitis and treat active symptoms and is generally safe and well tolerated by patients. Isotonic or hypertonic saline solutions may be used. There are several different irrigation systems commercially available, including Neti pots, Sinuneb, as well as syringe, squeeze bottle, and pump irrigators. Several other therapies may also provide additional relief in select patients, including antihistamines, mucolytics and leukotrienes. The potential of surfactants such as baby shampoo has been demonstrated in small studies, however more comprehensive evaluation is necessary.[141]

Allergy testing and treatment is an important option in treatment; however, its exact role is yet to be determined. It is generally recommended that patients with concomitant allergic rhinitis which is unresponsive to medical therapy or which is significantly affecting quality of life should be evaluated for immunotherapy treatment.

The last significant treatment option is endoscopic sinus surgery (ESS), which was first introduced in the United States in the mid-1980s and has since grown substantially in popularity. Surgical candidates are those patients with evidence of CRS and who are symptomatic despite a trial of medical therapy. The details of ESS are beyond the scope of this chapter, but studies have demonstrated that appropriate candidates who have undergone ESS generally experience improvements in their CRS symptoms,[142,143] with a success rate generally ranging from 80% to the high-90%.[144] Image guidance is now a common adjunct to ESS; however, some have challenged its widespread use.[145] Retrospective and randomized prospective studies have generally been underpowered given the low incidence of complication with ESS, but a more recent meta-analysis concluded that the use of image guidance in select patients might lead to a lower risk of major and total complications compared to non-image–guidance surgery.[146] The timing of surgery relative to medical therapy and patient symptoms, the extent of surgery, and the comparative efficacy of various surgical techniques all require closer evaluation and further evidence. Drug-eluting spacers and stents have been found to be effective as a local drug-delivery platform for a number of different therapeutic agents[147] and their use as a postoperative adjunct is now a subject of closer evaluation.[135]

Balloon sinuplasty was first approved by the FDA in 2005 and may offer a minimally invasive means to open the ostia of the paranasal sinuses without significant mucosal trauma. However, the efficacy, safety, applicability, and economic implications of balloon systems continue to be areas of controversy. The often-cited 2007 CLEAR trial (Clinical Evaluation to Confirm Safety and Efficacy of Sinuplasty in the Paranasal Sinuses) demonstrated a potential for durable ostial patency over a 2-year period with no major complications; however, it was a single-armed, uncontrolled, observational study.[148–150] Based on the current body of medical literature, the efficacy and utility of balloon sinuplasty remains unclear, and randomized controlled trials in this area are needed.[151]

> Allergy testing is generally recommended for patients with CRS and concomitant allergic rhinitis with significant symptoms that are refractory to medical management or affect quality of life.

Fungal Rhinosinusitis

Over the last 30 years, our understanding of the clinical and etiologic role of fungi in sinus disease has grown dramatically. Fungi can cause both acute and chronic rhinosinusitis disorders. Classification is generally based on the clinical, radiologic, and histologic manifestations of the host-pathogen relationship (Table 5–6). Typical classification schemes, such as that published by deShazo et al in 1997 and Chakrabarti et al in 2009, divide disease into noninvasive and invasive subtypes.[152,153] Invasive disease includes acute invasive fungal rhinosinusitis (AIFR), chronic invasive fungal rhinosinusitis (CIFR), and granulomatous invasive fungal rhinosinusitis (GIFR). Noninvasive disease includes localized fungal colonization of the nasal or paranasal sinus mucosa, fungus ball (FB) of the sinus, and allergic fungal rhinosinusitis (AFRS).

Table 5–6. Types of Fungal Rhinosinusitis

Invasive	Acute invasive fungal sinusitis (AIFR)
	Chronic invasive fungal rhinosinusitis (CIFR)
	Granulomatous invasive (indolent) fungal rhinosinusitis
Noninvasive	Fungus ball (mycetoma)
	Allergic fungal rhinosinusitis (AFRS)

Source: Adapted from DeShazo RD, Chapin K, Swain RE. Fungal sinusitis. *N Engl J Med.* 1997;337:254–259.

Invasive Fungal Sinusitis. Invasive fungal sinusitis (IFS) is defined by histopathologic evidence of fungal invasion (hyphal forms) into host sinonasal tissue including the sinus mucosa, submucosa, blood vessels, or bone. Further classification is then based on the host's level of immunocompetence, histologic features of disease, and disease progression. Because the intact immune system typically provides sufficient protection against the incursion of fungal pathogens, IFS typically affects patients with some degree of immunosuppression (with GFIR as the exception). An increase in organ transplant procedures and the increased prevalence of poorly controlled diabetes mellitus throughout the United States has led to a significant increase in the incidence of invasive fungal infections reported in the last 10 years.[154,155]

Acute Invasive Fungal Rhinosinusitis. Acute invasive fungal rhinosinusitis (AIFR) is almost exclusively seen in immunosuppressed patients, specifically with defective neutrophil function such as those with hematologic malignancies, aplastic anemia, insulin-dependent diabetes, AIDS, organ transplantations, or those who are iatrogenically immunosuppressed with chemotherapeutic agents or corticosteroids. In rare cases, disease affecting immunocompetent patients has been reported.[156] The fungi most frequently implicated include *Mucor, Rhizomucor*, and *Absidia*, with several other possible species identified in unusual cases.[157]

AIFR presents similarly to ARS, with symptoms that may include rhinorrhea, headache, nasal congestion, and facial pain. Although fever is not included as a cardinal symptom of ARS, it is a frequent finding in AIFR patients usually in the days preceding diagnosis.[158] The progression of disease can be progressive and rapid with extra-sinus extension by bone erosion, perineural spread, or perivascular extension through communicating vessels in the surrounding bone leading to clinical manifestations such as nasal or palate mucosa necrosis, cranial nerve deficits, regions of facial anesthesia, proptosis, ophthalmoplegia, changes in vision, and mental status changes. Given this level of aggressiveness, early recognition, diagnosis, and treatment of AIFR is especially important. Early detection protocols, such as those that call for neutropenic patients who present with fever of unknown and signs of rhinosinusitis to quickly undergo CT scans and nasal endoscopy, have been shown to significantly reduce the number of surgical treatments required and long-term morbidity of disease.[159] Nasal endoscopy should be utilized early if there is any clinical suspicion for AIFR. Mucosal changes such as pale mucosa that bleeds less than normal tissue or does not elicit a typical painful response in the patient are ominous findings that may signify fungal disease progression.[160] Biopsies of suspicious-appearing mucosa, the middle turbinate, and/or nasal septum can then be used to make a definitive diagnosis. Otolaryngologists should not rely significantly on radiologic findings to make a diagnosis of AIFR as there is a poor correlation between surgical specimens and radiologic extent of disease.[161]

Treatment relies on medical and surgical therapy directed against the offending fungal pathogen. Systemic antifungal therapy such as with amphotericin B deoxycholate, voriconazole, and posaconazole may be used. Of note, several of the newer extended spectrum azoles may offered increased efficacy and decreased side effects as compared to amphotericin, which has typically been the drug of choice in treating AIFR since its introduction in the 1960s.[162] Prophylaxis with antifungal medications may be initiated in very high-risk patients and those with a history of AIFR, but there are concerns with this strategy given the side effect profiles and toxicity of many of these medications.[163] The main goals of surgery are to provide a specimen for histopathologic diagnosis, debride tissue involved with fungus, to remove devitalized tissue, and to monitor the affected sites. Debridement is generally extended until there is healthy bleeding tissue. Prognosis is generally poor.

Chronic and Granulomatous Invasive Fungal Rhinosinusitis and Mycetoma. CIFR and GIFR are less common and generally carry a more favorable prognosis than AIFR. They are considered to be distinct diseases based on histopathologic features and typical causative organisms; however, they are similar to one another in terms of clinical presentation, course, and treatment. CIFR was previously known as "chronic indolent IFS" and was considered to be a slowly progressive form of invasive fungal disease. A typical presentation involves nonspecific sinonasal symptoms that are slowly progressive and refractory to traditional treatment. Certain patients with CIFR, specifically those with poorly controlled diabetes, must be closely monitored for signs of disease progression such as ocular symptoms. The diagnosis is based on histopathologic evidence of submucosal invasion of fungal elements into host tissue. *Aspergillus fumigatus* is the most common pathogen involved, although other more rare types may also be cultured.[164] Nasal endoscopy findings, including mucosal changes, tend to be less dramatic than AIFR; however, nasal polyposis may be an associated finding.[165] There are no pathognomonic radiological findings, but imaging may be particularly helpful for differentiating between CIFR and AFRS. CIFR may be treated successfully with surgery alone[166]; however, the role of systemic antifungals may increase with the introduction of less toxic agents.[167]

Fungal ball (FB) of the paranasal sinus consists of densely tangled, inspissated fungal debris that fills one or more sinuses without invasion into the underlying mucosa. Often referred to as a "mycetoma," the pathogenesis of disease is incompletely understood, however disease more commonly affects female, does not affect children, and has a strong association with prior endodontic treatment of the maxillary teeth.[168–170] FB may cause symptoms of CRS or may be asymptomatic. Symptoms depend on the location of disease and may include facial pain, nasal airway obstruction, purulent rhinorrhea, olfactory sensation of foul odor (cacosmia), and vertex headaches. Unilateral symptoms, prolonged duration of symptoms, and failure to respond to medical therapy may increase suspicion for FB diagnosis.[171] Disease typically affects a single sinus, with less than 10% affecting more than one and the maxillary is the most common involved[169] (Figure 5–6). Characteristic radiologic findings include partial of complete sinus opacification on CT with or without bony erosion, as well as a hypointense signal voice in the area of disease on T2-weighted MRI. Fungal balls are treated with complete surgical removal and thorough irrigation of the involved sinuses. Systemic antifungal therapy is not necessary.

Allergic Fungal Rhinosinusitis

Allergic fungal rhinosinusitis (AFRS) is a noninvasive fungal process that is responsible for approximately 6% to 9% of all types of rhinosinusitis that require surgery.[172] It is due to a hypersensitivity response to the presence of extramucosal sinus fungi that likely involves multiple inflammatory mediators but is primarily a fungal-specific type I hypersensitivity reaction.[173] A large case series from the southwestern United States demonstrated that nearly all AFRS patients are allergic to fungal and nonfungal aeroallergens (based on skin testing or serum specific IgE levels), including to the etiologic mold when it is properly identified (usually dematiaceous fungi).[174,175] Studies have also demonstrated that eosinophilic-derived mediators are far more common than neutrophil-derived mediators in the sinus mucosal specimens of AFRS patients, further emphasizing that the disease is allergic in nature.[176]

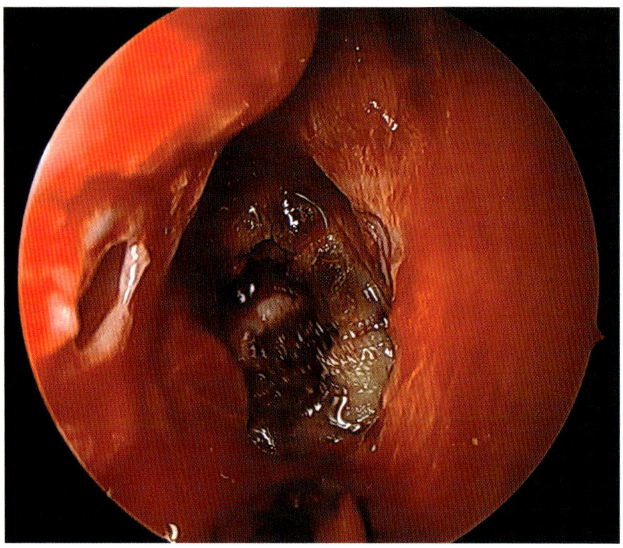

Figure 5-6. Intraoperative photograph of a sphenoid sinus fungal ball.

The pathophysiology of disease is thought to start when an atopic host is exposed to fungi. This leads lead to an inflammatory response and tissue edema as the result of type I and type III allergic reactions. Obstruction of the sinus ostia develops with subsequent stasis within the sinuses, creating an ideal environment for the growth of fungus and resulting in increasing antigenic exposure of the allergic host. The eventual product of this process is allergic mucin, which fills the involved sinuses and is responsible for the hallmark clinical, histologic, and radiographic characteristics of AFRS.

Patients with AFRS generally present with symptoms of CRS and nasal obstruction due to nasal polyps. More significant symptoms such as facial dysmorphia and proptosis may be present in more advanced cases due to the extension of disease into adjacent anatomic spaces. Presentation is often subtle and pain is relatively uncommon. Symptoms are generally unresponsive to antihistamines and intranasal steroids and, while systemic steroids may lead to some relief in symptoms, relapse is typical once the medication course is stopped. There is no consensus regarding diagnostic criteria; however, Bent and Kuhn in 1996 described what is likely the most well-accepted scheme. Diagnostic criteria includes type I hypersensitivity to fungi, nasal polyposis, characteristic radiographic findings including heterogeneous areas of increased signal intensity in affected sinuses (Figure 5–7), eosinophilic mucin without fungal invasion into sinus mucosa, and a positive fungal stain of sinus contents removed at surgery.[177] Of note, total serum IgE is also commonly elevated in AFRS patients, including the presence of specific IgE to *S. aureus*,[178] and it has been suggested that total IgE levels can be used as an indicator of clinical disease activity.

There are no published prospective studies on treatment for AFRS. Surgery is a common first step, the goal of which is to completely remove diseased mucosa and obstructing inspissated allergic mucin, which may appear grossly as a peanut-buttery to viscoelastic material. Inadequate surgery leads to higher relapse rates of disease.[179] Postoperative oral corticosteroids may lead to reduced symptoms and disease recurrence.[180,181] The role of topical antifungals has not yet been comprehensively defined.

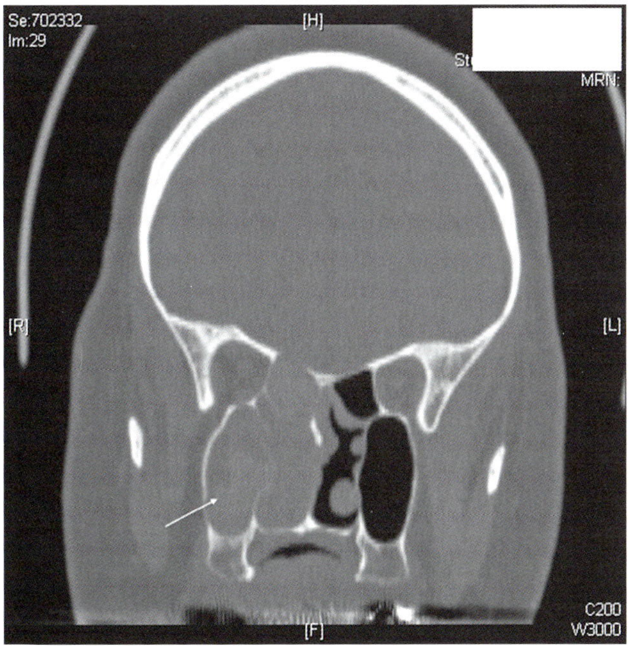

Figure 5-7. Sinus CT scan demonstrating allergic fungal rhinosinusitis (*arrow*). Note the characteristic heterogenous areas of increased signal intensity in the center of the sinus.

Immunotherapy directed against etiologic aeroallergens may also be effective at reducing sinonasal allergic reactivity and thus reducing inflammatory disease burden.[182,183] On the basis of initial studies, a 3- to 5-year duration of immunotherapy is generally recommended, similar to what is recommended for patients with other types of allergic disorders.

> Allergic mucin is responsible for the hallmark clinical, histologic, and radiologic findings of AFRS.

REFERENCES

1. Bosquet J, Khataev N, Cruz AA, et al. Allergic rhinitis and its impact on asthma (ARIA) 2008 update (in collaboration with the World Health Organization, GA(2) LEN and AllerGen). *Allergy.* 2008;63(suppl 86):8–160.
2. Marple BF, Fornadley JA, Patel AA, et al. Keys to successful management of patients with allergic rhinitis: focus on patient confidence, compliance and satisfaction. *Otolaryngol Head Neck Surg.* 2007;136:S107–S124.
3. Pleis JR, Ward BW, Lucas JW. Summary health statistics for U.S. adults: National Health Interview Survey, 2009. National Center for Health Statistics. *Vital Health Stat.* 2010;10(249). http:///www.cdc.gov/nchs/data/series/sr_10/sr10_249.pdf. Accessed November 18, 2014.
4. Bloom B, Cohen RA, Freeman G. Summary health statistics for U.S. children: National Health Interview Survey, 2009. National Center for Health Statistics. *Vital Health Stat.* 2010;10(247). http://www.cdc.gov/nchs/data/series/sr_10/sr10_247.pdf. Accessed November 18, 2014.
5. Settipane RA. Rhinitis: a dose of epidemiological reality. *Allergy Asthma Proc.* 2004;24:147–154.
6. Meltzer EO, Bukstein DA. The economic impact of allergic rhinitis and current guidelines to treatment. *Ann Allergy Asthma Immunol.* 2001;106:S12–S16.
7. Shoenwetter WF, Dupclay L Jr, Appajosyula S, et al. Economic impact and quality-of-life burden of allergic rhinitis. *Curr Med Res Opin.* 2004;20:305–317.
8. Ker J, Hartert TV. The atopic march: what's the evidence? *Ann Allergy Asthma Immunol.* 2009;103:282–289.
9. Bach JF. The effect of infections on susceptibility to autoimmune and allergic diseases. *N Engl J Med.* 2002;347:911–920.
10. Okada H, Kugh C, Feillet H, et al. The "hygeine hypothesis" for autoimmune and allergic diseases: an update. *Clin Exp Immunol.* 2010;160:1–9.
11. Bousquet J, Neukirch F, Bousquet PJ, et al. Severity and impairment of allergic rhinitis in patients consulting in primary care. *J Allergy Clin Immunol.* 2006;117:158–162.
12. Ologe FE, Adebola SO, Dunmade AD, et al. Symptom score for allergic rhinitis. *Otolaryngol Head Neck Surg.* 2013;148(4):557–563.
13. Bresolin D, Shapiro GG, Shapiro PA, et al. Facial characteristics of children who breathe through the mouth. *Pediatrics.* 1984;63:622–625.
14. Salvin RG. Allergy is not a significant cause of nasal polyps. *Arch Otolaryngol Head Neck Surg.* 1992;118:343.
15. Sheikh A, Hurwitz B, Nurmatov U, et al. House dust mite avoidance measures for perennial allergic rhinitis. *Cochrane Database Syst Rev.* 2010:CD001563.
16. Miller JD, Naccara L, Satinover S, et al. Nonwoven in contrast to woven mattress encasings accumulate mite and cat allergen. *J Allergy Clin Immunol.* 2007;120:977–979.
17. Blaiss MS. Safety update regarding intranasal corticosteroids for the treatment of allergic rhinitis. *Allergy Asthma Proc.* 2011;32:413–418.
18. Simons FE, Simon KJ. Histamine and H1-antihistamines: celebrating a century of progress. *J Allergy Clin Immunol.* 2011;128:1139–1150.
19. Meltzer EO. Evaluation of optimal oral antihistamine for patients with allergic rhinitis. *Mayo Clin Proc.* 2005;80:1170–1176.
20. Corren J, Storms W, Bernstein J, Berger W, Nayak A, Sacks H. Effectiveness of azelastine nasal spray compared with oral cetirizine in patients with seasonal allergic rhinitis. *Clin Ther.* 2005;27:543–553.

21. Lee TA, Pickard AS. Meta-analysis of azelastine nasal spray for the treatment of allergic rhinitis. *Pharmacotherapy.* 2007;27:852–859.
22. Carr W, Bernstein J, Lieberman P, et al. A novel intranasal therapy of azelastine with fluticasone for the treatment of allergic rhinitis. *J Allergy Clin Immunol.* 2012;129:1282–1289.
23. Ratner PH, Hampel F, Van Bavel J, et al. Combination of azelastine nasal spray in seasonal allergic rhinitis patients who remain symptomatic after treatment with fexofenadine. *Ann Allergy Asthma Immunol.* 2004;93:154–159.
24. Meltzer EO, Bernstein DI, Prenner BM, et al. Mometasone furoate nasal spray plus oxymetazoline nasal spray: short-term efficacy and safety in seasonal allergic rhinitis. *Am J Rhino Allergy.* 2013;27:102–108.
25. Hermelingermeier KE, Weber RK, Hellmich M, Heubach CP, Mosges R. Nasal irrigation as an adjunctive treatment of allergic rhinitis: a systemic review and meta-analysis. *Am J Rhinol Allergy.* 2012;26:e119–e125.
26. Pullertis T, Praks L, Ristioka V, et al. Comparison of a nasal glucocorticoid, antileukotriene, and a combination of antileukotriene and antihistamine in the treatment of seasonal allergic rhinitis. *J Allergy Clin Immunol.* 2002;109:949–955.
27. Meltzer EO. Intranasal anticholinergic therapy of rhinorrhea. *J Allergy Clin Immunol.* 1992;90(6, pt 2):1055–1064.
28. Casale TB. Anti-immunoglobulin E (omalizumab) therapy in seasonal allergic rhinitis. *Am J Respir Crit Care Med.* 2001;164(8, pt 2):S18–21.
29. Chervinsky P, Casale T, Townley R, et al. Omalizumav, and anti-IgE antibody in the treatment of adults and adolescents with perennial allergic rhinitis. *Ann Allergy Asthma Immunol.* 2003;91:160–167.
30. Corren J. Anti-interleukin-5 antibody theraepy in asthma and allergies. *Curr Opin Allergy Clin Immunol.* 2011;11:565–570.
31. Zhu Z, Stone HF, Thach TQ, Garcia L, Ruegg CL. A novel botulism neurotoxin topical gel: treatment of allergic rhinitis in rats and comparative safety profile. *Am J Rhinol Allergy.* 2012;26:450–454.
32. Roche AM, Wise SK. Subcutaneous immunotherapy. *Int Forum Allergy Rhinol.* 2014;4:S51–54.
33. Dretzke J, MeadowsA, Novielli, et al. Subcutaneous and sublingual immunotherapy for seasonal allergic rhinitis: a systematic review and indirect comparison. *J Allergy Clin Immunol.* 2013;131:1361–1366.
34. Lin SY. Sublinguinal immunotherapy: current concepts for the U.S. practitioner. *Int Forum Allergy Rhinol.* 2014;4:S55–S59.
35. Radulovic S, Wilson D, Calderon M, et al. Systematic review of sublingual immunotherapy (SLIT). *Allergy.* 2011;66:740–752.
36. Creticos PS, Maloney J, Bernstein DI, et al. Randomized controlled trial of ragweed allergy immunotherapy tablets in North American and European adults. *J Allergy Clin Immunol.* 2013;131:1342–1349.
37. Hyander T, Latif L, Petersson-Westin U, et al. Intralymphatic allergic-specific immunotherapy: an effective and safe alternative treatment route for pollen-induced allergic rhinitis. *J Allergy Clin Immunol.* 2013;131:412–420.
38. Chhabra N, Houser SM. Surgery for allergic rhinitis. *Int Forum Allergy Rhinol.* 2014;4:S79–83.
39. Mori S, Fujeida S, Yamada T, et al. Long-term effect of submucous turbinectomy in patients with perennial allergic rhinitis. *Laryngoscope.* 2002;112:865–869.
40. Lin HC, Lin PW, Su CY, et al. Radiofrequency for the treatment of allergic rhinitis refractory to medical therapy. *Laryngoscope.* 2003;113:673–678.
41. Lin HC, Pei-Wen Lin, Friedman M, et al. Long-term results of radiofrequency turbinoplasty for allergic rhinitis refractory to medical therapy. *Arch Otolaryngol Head Neck Surg.* 2010;136(9):892–895.
42. Gunhan K, Unlu H, Yuceturk AV, et al. Intranasal steroids or radiofrequency turbinoplasty in persistent allergic rhinitis: effects on quality of life and objective parameters. *Eur Arch Otorhinolaryngol.* 2011;268:845–850.
43. Kim YH, Kim BJ, Bang KH, Hwang Y, Jang TY. Septoplasty improves life quality related to allergy in patients with septal deviation and allergic rhinitis. *Otolaryngol Head Neck Surg.* 2011;145(6):910–914.
44. Settipane RA, Lieberman P. Update on nonallergic rhinitis. *Ann Allergy Asthma Immunol.* 2001;86(5):494–507.
45. Togias A. Age relationships and clinical features of nonallergic rhinitis. *J Allergy Clin Immunol.* 1990;85:182.
46. Di Lorenzo G, Pacor ML, Amodio E, et al. Differences and similarities between allergic and nonallergic rhinitis in a large sample of adult patients with rhinitis symptoms. *Int Arch Allergy Immunol.* 2011;155:263–270.
47. Bosquet J, Fokkens W, Burney P, et al. Important research questions in allergy and related diseases: nonallergic rhinitis: a GALEN paper. *Allergy.* 2008;63:842–853.
48. Schatz M, Zeiger RS, Chen W, Yang SJ Corrao MA, Quinn VP. The burden of rhinitis in a managed care organization. *Ann Allergy Asthma Immunol.* 2008;101:240–247.
49. Meltzer EO, Nathan R Derebery J, et al. Sleep, quality of life, and productivity impact of nasal symptoms in the United States: findings from the Burden of Rhinitis in America survey. *Allergy Asthma Proc.* 2009;30(3):244–254.
50. Ledford D. Inadequate diagnosis of nonallergic rhinitis: assessing the damage. *Allergy Asthma Proc.* 2003;24:155–162.
51. Liberman P, Meltzer EO, LaForce CF, et al. Two-week comparison study of olopatadine hydrochloride nasal spray 0.6% versus azelastine hydrochloride nasal spray 0.1% in patients with vasomotor rhinitis. *Allergy Asthma Proc.* 2011;32(2):151–158.
52. Banov CH, Lieberman P. Efficacy of azelastine nasal spray in the treatment of vasomotor (perennial nonallergic) rhinitis. *Ann Allergy Asthma Immunol.* 2001;86:28–35.
53. Gehanno P, Deschamps E, Garay E, et al. Vasomotor rhinitis: clinical efficacy of azelastine nasal spray in comparison with placebo. *ORL J Otorhinolaryngol Relat Spec.* 2001;63:76–81.

54. Webb DR, Meltzer EO, Finn AF Jr, et al. Intranasal fluticasone propionate is effective for perennial nonallergic rhinitis with or without eosinophilia. *Ann Allergy Asthma Immunol.* 2002;88:385–390.
55. Tran NP, Vickery J, Blaiss MS. Management of rhinitis: allergic and nonallergic. *Allergy Asthma Immunol Resp.* 2011;3:148–158.
56. Blom HM, Van Rijswij JB, Garrelds IM, Mulder PG, Timmermans, Gerth van Wijk R. Intranasal capsaicin is efficacious in non-allergic, non-infectious perennial rhinitis: a placebo-controlled study. *Clin Exp Allergy.* 1997;27:796–801.
57. Bhargava KB, Shirali GN, Abhyankar US, Gadre KC. Treatment of allergic and vasomotor rhinitis by the local application of different concentrations of silver nitrate. *J Laryngol Otol.* 1992;106:699–701.
58. Fleckenstein J, Raab C, Gleditsch J, et al. Impact of acupuncture on vasomotor rhinitis: a randomized placebo-controlled pilot study. *J Altern Complement Med.* 2009;15:391–398.
59. Rosenfeld RM, Andes D, Bhattacharyya N, et al. Clinical practice guideline: adult sinusitis. *Otolaryngol Head Neck Surg.* 2007;137(suppl 3):S1–31.
60. Anon JB, Jacobs MR, Poole MD, et al. Antimicrobial treatment guidelines for acute bacterial rhinosinusitis. *Otolaryngol Head Neck Surg.* 2004;130(1, suppl):1–45.
61. Pleis J, Ward B, Lucas J. Summary Health Statistics for US Adults: National Health Interview Survey 2009. *Vital and Health Statistics.* 2009;Series 10(249).
62. Murphy NP, Ferguson BJ, Short SO, et al. Health care utilization and cost among adults with chronic rhinosinusitis enrolled in a health maintenance organization. *Otolaryngol Head Neck Surg.* 2002;127(5):367–376.
63. Ray NF, Baraniuk JN, Thamer M, et al. Healthcare expenditures in 1996: contributions of asthma, rhinitis, and other airway disorders. *J Allergy Clin Immunol.* 1999;103:408–414.
64. Anzai Y, Yueh B. Imaging evaluation of sinusitis: diagnostic performance and impact on health outcome. *Neuroimag Clin N Am.* 2003;13:251–263.
65. Bhattacharyya N. Contemporary assessment of the disease burden of sinusitis. *Am J Rhinol Allergy.* 2009;23(4):392–395.
66. Bhattacharyya N. The economic burden and symptom manifestation of chronic rhinosinusitis. *Am J Rhinol.* 2003;17(1):27–32.
67. Brook I. Microbiology of sinusitis. *Proc Am Thorac Soc.* 2011;8(1):90–100.
68. Hendley JO, Gwaltney JM Jr. Mechanisms of transmission of rhinovirus infectious. *Epidemiol Rev.* 1988;10:243–258.
69. Huang WH, Fang SY. High prevalence of antibiotic resistance in isolates from the middle meatus of children and adults with acute rhinosinusitis. *Am J Rhinol.* 2004;18(6):387–391.
70. Slavin RG, Spector SL, Bernstein IL, et al. The diagnosis and management of sinusitis: a practice parameter update. *J Allergy Clin Immunol.* 2005;116(6S):S13–S47.
71. Sokol W. Epidemiology of sinusitis in the primary care setting: results from the 1999–2000 respiratory surveillance program. *Am J Med.* 2001:111(9AS):19–24.
72. Klugman KP, Lonks JR. Hidden epidemic of macrolide-resistant pneumococci. *Emerg Infect Dis.* 2005;11:802–807.
73. Rzesutek M, Wierzbowski A, Hoban DJ, et al. A review of clinical failures associated with macrolide-resistant *Streptococcus pneumoniae. Int J Antimicrob Agents.* 2004;24:95–104.
74. Arroyo-Sanchez A. Nosocomial sinusitis in the intensive care unit: incidence, clinical characteristics and evolution. *Med Intesiva.* 2007;31(4):179–183.
75. Evans FO Jr., Snydnor JB, Moore WE, et al. Sinusitis of maxillary antrum. *N Engl J Med.* 1975;293(15):735–739.
76. Hinni ML, McCaffrey TV, Kasperbauer JL. Early mucosal changes in experiemental sinusitis. *Otolaryngol Head Neck Surg.* 1992;107:537–548.
77. Rudack C, Hauser U, Wagenmann M, Bachert C, Ganzer U. Cytokine pattern in various forms of sinusitis. *Laryngorhinootologie.* 1998;77:34–37.
78. Repka-Ramirez S, Naranch K, Park YJ, Clauw D, Baraniuk JN. Cytokines in nasal lavage fluids from acute sinusitis, allergic rhinitis, and chronic fatigue syndrome subjects. *Allergy Asthma Proc.* 2002;23:185–190.
79. Pearlman AN, Conley B. Review of current guidelines related to the diagnosis and treatment of rhinosinusitis. *Curr Opin Otolaryngol Head Neck Surg.* 2008;16(3):226–230.
80. Williams JW Jr, Simel DL, Roberts L, et al. Clinical evaluation for sinusitis. Making the diagnosis by history and physical examination. *Ann Int Med.* 1992;117:705–710.
81. Benninger MS, Appelbaum PC, Denneny JC, et al. Maxillary sinus puncture and culture in the diagnosis of acute rhinosinusitis: the case for pursuing alternative culture methods. *Otolaryngol Head Neck Surg.* 2002;127:7–12.
82. Hwang PH. A 51-year-old woman with acute onset of facial pressure, rhinorrhea, and tooth pain. Review of acute rhinosinusitis. *JAMA.* 2009;301(17):1798–1807.
83. Batra PS. Radiologic imaging in rhinosinusitis. *Cleve Clin J Med.* 2004;71(11):886–888.
84. Lund VJ, Mackay IS. Staging in rhinosinusitis. *Rhinology.* 1993;31:183–184.
85. Balk EM, Zucker DR, Engeles EA, et al. Strategies for diagnosing and treating suspected acute bacterial sinusitis: a cost-effective analysis. *J Gen Intern Med.* 2001;16:701–711.
86. Fagnan LJ. Acute sinusitis: a cost-effective approach to diagnosis and treatment. *Am Fam Phys.* 1998;58:1795–1802, 805–806.
87. Rosenfeld RM, Singer M, Jones S. Systematic review of antimicrobial therapy in patients with acute rhinosinusitis. *Otolaryngol Head Neck Surg.* 2007;137:S32–45.
88. Sharp JH, Dneman D, Puumala S, et al. Treatment of acute and chronic rhinosinusitis in the United States 1999–2002. *Arch Otolaryngol Head Neck Surg.* 2007;133:260–265.
89. Sinus and Allergy Health Partnership (SAHP). Antimicrobial treatment guidelines for acute bacterial rhinosinusitis. *Otolaryngol Head Neck Surg.* 2004;130:S1–45.

90. Chandley JR, Langenbrunner DJ, Stevens ER. The pathogenesis of orbital complications in acute sinusitis. *Laryngoscope.* 1970;80:1414–1428.
91. Sultesz, Csakanyi Z, Majoros T, et al. Acute bacterial rhinosinusitis and its complications in our pediatric otolaryngological department between 1997 and 2006. *Int J Ped Otorhinolaryngol.* 2009;73:1507–1512.
92. Van Cauwenberge P, Watelet JB. Epidemiology of chronic rhinosinusitis. *Thorax.* 2000;55 (suppl 2):S20–21.
93. Gliklich RE, Metson R. The health impact of chronic rhinosinusitis in patients seeking otolaryngologic care. *Otolaryngol Head Neck Surg.* 1995;113(1):104–109.
94. Patel ZM, Hwang PH. Nonpolypoid rhinosinusitis: pathogenesis, diagnosis, staging, and treatment. In: Johnson JT, Rosen CA, eds. *Bailey's Head and Neck Surgery—Otolaryngology.* 5th ed. Baltimore, MD: Lippincott Williams & Wilkins; 2014:535–549.
95. Berger G, Kattan A, Bernheim J, et al. Polypoid mucosa with eosinophilia and glandular hyperplasia in chronic sinusitis: a histological and immunohistochemical study. *Laryngoscope.* 2002;112:738–745.
96. Rhyoo C, Sanders SP, Leopold DA, et al. Sinus mucosal IL-8 gene expression in chronic rhinosinusitis. *J Allergy Clin Immunol.* 1999;103:395–400.
97. Nonoyama T, Harada T, Shinogi J, et al. Immunohistochemical localization of cytokines and cell adhesion molecules in maxillary sinus mucosa in chronic sinusitis. *Auris Nasis Laynx.* 2000;27:51–58.
98. Rudack C, Stoll W, Bachert C. Cytokines in nasal polyposis, acute and chronic sinusitis. *Am J Rhinol.* 1998;12: 383–388.
99. Bachert C, Gavaert P, van Cauwenberge P. *Staphylococcus aureus* enterotoxins: a key in airway disease? *Allergy.* 2002;57:480–487.
100. Hamilos DL, Leung SY, Huston DP, Kamil A, Wood R, Hamid Q. GM-CSF, IL-5, and RANTES immunoreactivity and mRNA expression in chronic hyperplastic sinusitis with nasal polyposis. *Clin Exper Allergy.* 1998; 28:1145–1152.
101. Bachert C, Gevaert P, Holtappels G, et al. Total and specific IgE in nasal polyps is related to local eosinophilic inflammation. *J Allergy Clin Immunol.* 2001;107:607–614.
102. Benninger MS, Ferguson BJ, Hadley JA, Hamilos DL, et al. Adult chronic rhinosinusitis: definitions, diagnosis, epidemiology, and pathophysiology. *Otolaryngol Head and Neck Surg.* 2003;129:S1–S32.
103. Meltzer EO, Hamilos DL, Hadley JA, Lanza DC, Marple BF, Nicklas RA. Rhinosinusitis: establishing definitions for clinical research and patient care. *Otolaryngol Head Neck Surg.* 2004;131:S1–S62.
104. Larson K, Tos M. The estimated incidence of symptomatic nasal polyps. *Acta Otolarnygol.* 2002;122(2):179–182.
105. Ryan MA. Chronic rhinosinusitis with nasal polyposis. In: Johnson JT, Rosen CA, eds. *Bailey's Head and Neck Surgery—Otolaryngology.* 5th ed. Baltimore, MD: Lippincott Williams & Wilkins; 2014:525–534.
106. Zhang N, Holtappels G, Claeys C, et al. Pattern of inflammation and impact of *Staphylococcus aureus* enterotoxins in nasal polyps from southern China. *Am J Rhinol.* 2006;20:445–450.
107. Cohen NA, Widelitz JS, Chiu AG, et al. Familial aggregation of sinonasal polyps correlates with severity of disease. *Otolaryngol Head Neck Surg.* 2006;134:601–604.
108. Sanchez-Segura A, Brieva JA, Rodriguez C. T lymphocytes that infiltrate nasal polyps have a specialized phenotype and produce a mixed TH1/TH2 pattern of cytokines. *J Allergy Clin Immunol.* 1998;102:953–960.
109. Morinaka S, Nakamura H. Inflammatory cells in nasal mucosa and nasal polyps. *Auris Nasus Larynx.* 2000; 27(1):59–64.
110. Tripathi A, Kern R, Conley DB, et al. Staphylococcal exotoxins and nasal polyposis: analysis of systemic and local responses. *Am J Rhinol.* 2005;19:327–333.
111. Newman LJ, Platts-Mills TA, Phillips CD, et al. Chronic sinusitis/relationship of computed tomographic findings to allergy, asthma, and eosinophilia. *JAMA.* 1994; 271(5):363–367.
112. Fokkens WJ, Lung VJ, Mullol J, et al. European position paper on nasal polyps. *Rhinology.* 2007;45(suppl 20): 1–139.
113. Pearlman AN, Chandra RK, Chang D, et al. Relationships between the severity of chronic rhinosinusitis and nasal polyposis, asthma, and atopy. *Am J Rhinol Allergy.* 2009;23:145–148.
114. Pant H, Ferguson BJ, Macardle PJ. The role of allergy in rhinosinusitis. *Curr Opin Otolaryngol Head Neck Surg.* 2009;17:232–238.
115. Lildholdt T, Rundcrantz H, Bende M, et al. Glucocorticoid treatment for nasal polyps. The use of topical budesonide powder, intramuscular betamethasone, and surgical treatment. *Arch Otolarnygol Head Neck Surg.* 1997;123:595–600.
116. Johansson L, Akerlund A, Holmberg K, et al. Evaluation of methods for endoscopic staging of nasal polyposis. *Acta Otolaryngol.* 2000;120:72–76.
117. Hellquist HB. Nasal polyps update: histopathology. *Allergy Asthma Proc.* 1996;17(5):237–242.
118. Hopkins C, Gillett S, Slack R, et al. Psychometric validation of the 22-item sinonasal outcome test. *Clin Otolaryngol.* 2009;34(5):447–454.
119. Senior BA, Glaze C, Benninger MS. Use of the rhinosinusitis disability index (RDSI) in rhinologic disease. *Am J Rhinol.* 2001;15(1):15–20.
120. Lund VJ, Kennedy DW. Staging for rhinosinusitis. *Otolaryngol Head Neck Surg.* 1997;117(3, pt 2):S35–S40.
121. Casiano RR. Correlation of clinical examination with computer tomography in paranasal sinus disease. *Am J Rhinol.* 1997;11(3):193–196.
122. Fokkens W, Lund V, Mullol J, et al. European position paper on rhinosinusitis and nasal polyps 2007. *Rhinol Suppl.* 2007;20:1–136.
123. Badia L, Lund V. Topical corticosteroids in nasal polyposis. *Drugs.* 2001;61:573–578.
124. Stjarne P, Olsson P, Alenius M. Use of mometasone furoate to prevent polyp relapse after endoscopic sinus surgery. *Arch Otolaryngol Head Neck Surg.* 2009;135(3):296–302.

125. Joe SA, Thambi R, Huang J. A systematic review of the use of intranasal steroids in the treatment of chronic rhinosinusitis. *Otolaryngol Head Neck Surg.* 2008;139(3): 340–347.
126. Parikh A, Scadding GK, Darby Y, et al. Topical corticosteroids in chronic rhinosinusitis: a randomized, double-blind, placebo-controlled trial using fluticasone propionate aqueous nasal spray. *Rhinology.* 2001;39(2): 75–79.
127. Dubin MG, Liu C, Lin SY, et al. American Rhinologic Society member survey on "maximal medical therapy" for chronic rhinosinusitis. *Am J Rhinol.* 2007;21(4):483–488.
128. Lal D, Hwang P. Oral corticosteroid therapy in chronic rhinosinusitis without polyps: a systematic review. *Int Forum Allergy Rhinol.* 2011;1:136–143.
129. Patiar S, Reece P. Oral steroids for nasal polyps. *Cochrane Database Syst Rev.* 2007;CD005232.
130. Finegold SM, Flynn MJ, Rose FV, et al. Bacteriologic findings associated with chronic bacterial maxillary sinusitis in adults. *Clin Infect Dis.* 2002;35:428–433.
131. Kudoh S, Uetake T, Hagiwara K, et al. Clinical effects of low-dose long-term erythromycin chemotherapy on diffuse panbronchiolitis. *Nihon Kyobu Shikkan Gakkai Zasshi.* 197;25:632–654.
132. Harvey RJ, Wallwork BD, Lund VJ. Anti-inflammatory effects of macrolides: applications in chronic rhinosinusitis. *Immunol Allergy Clin North Am.* 2009;29(4):689–703.
133. Brook I, Foote PA, Hausfeld JN. Increase in the frequency of recovery of methicillin-resistant *Staphylococcus aureus* in acute and chronic maxillary sinusitis. *J Med Microbiol.* 2008;57(pt 8):1015–1017.
134. Lim M, Citardi MJ, Leong JL. Topical antimicrobials in the management of chronic rhinosinusitis: a systematic review. *Am J Rhinol.* 2008;22:381–389.
135. Orlandi RR, Smith TL, Marple MF, et al. Updated on evidence-based reviews with recommendations in adult chronic sinusitis. *Int Forum Allergy Rhinol.* 2014;4(suppl 1). S1–15.
136. Suh JD, Ramakrishnan V, Palmer JN. Biofilms. *Otolaryngol Clin North Am.* 2010;43(3):521–530.
137. Hochstim CJ, Masood R, Rice DH. Biofilm and persistent inflammation in endoscopic sinus surgery. *Otolaryngol Head Neck Surg.* 2010;143(5):697–698.
138. Psalis AJ, Weitzel EK, Ha Kr, et al. The effect of bacterial biofilms on post-sinus surgical outcomes. *Am J Rhinol.* 2008;22(1):1–6.
139. Al-Mutairi D, Kilty SJ. Bacterial biofilms and the pathophysiology of chronic rhinosinusitis. *Curr Opin Allergy Clin Immunol.* 2011;11(1):18–23.
140. Harvey R, Hannan SA, Badia L, et al. Nasal saline irrigation for the symptoms of chronic rhinosinusitis. *Cochrane Database Syst Rev.* 2007;(3):CD006394.
141. Chiu AG, Chen B, Plmer JN, et al. Safety evaluation of sinus surfactant solution on respiratory cilia function. *Int Forum Allergy Rhinol.* 2011;1:280–283.
142. Chester AC, Antisdel JL, Sindwani R. Symptom-specific outcomes of endoscopic sinus surgery: a systematic review. *Otolaryngol Head Neck Surg.* 2009;140(5):622–639.
143. Poetker DM, Smith TL. Adult chronic rhinosinusitis: surgical outcomes and the role of endoscopic sinus surgery. *Curr Opin Otolaryngol Head Neck Surg.* 2007;15(1):6–9.
144. Schaitkin B, May M, Shapiro A, et al. Endoscopic sinus surgery: 4-year follow-up on the first 100 patients. *Laryngoscope.* 1993;103(10):117–120.
145. Ramakrishnan VR, Orlandi RR, Citardi MJ, Smith TL, Fried MP, Kingdom TT. The use of image-guided surgery in endoscopic sinus surgery: an evidence-based review with recommendation. *Int Forum Allergy Rhinol.* 2013;3:236–241.
146. Dalgorf DM, Sacks R, Wormald PJ, et al. Image-guidance surgery influences perioperative morbidity from endoscopic sinus surgery: a systematic review and meta-analysis. *Otolaryngol Head Neck Surg.* 2013;149:17–29.
147. Han JK, Marple BF, Smith TL, et al. Effect of steroid-eluting implants on postoperative medical and surgery interventions: an efficacy meta-analysis. *Int Forum Allergy Rhinol.* 2012;2:271–279.
148. Bolger WE, Brown CL, Church CA, et al. Safety and outcomes of balloon catheter sinusotomy: a multicenter 24-week analysis in 115 patients. *Otolaryngol Head Neck Surg.* 2007;137(1):10–20.
149. Kuhn FA, Church CA, Goldberg AN, et al. Balloon catheter sinusotomy: one-year follow-up—outcomes and role in functional endoscopic sinus surgery. *Otolaryngol Head Neck Surg.* 2008;139:S27–37.
150. Weiss RL, Church CA, Kuhn FA, et al. Long-term outcome analysis of balloon catheter sinusotomy: two-year follow-up. *Otolaryngol Head Neck Surg.* 2008;139:S38–46.
151. Batra S, Ryan MW, Sindwani R, et al. Balloon catheter technology in rhinology: reviewing the evidence. *Laryngoscope.* 2011;121(1):226–232.
152. DeShazo RD, Chapin K, Swain RE. Fungal sinusitis. *N Engl J Med.* 1997;337:254–259.
153. Chakrabarti A, Denning DW, Ferguson BJ, et al. Fungal rhinosinusitis: a categorization and definitional schema addressing current controversies. *Laryngoscope.* 2009; 119:1809–1818.
154. Malani PN, Kauffman CA. Prevention and prophylaxis of invasive fungal sinusitis in the immunocompromised patient. *Otolaryngol Clin North Am.* 2000;33(2):301–312.
155. Adelson RT, Marple BF, Ryan MW. Fungal rhinosinusitis. In: Johnson JT, Rosen CA, eds. *Bailey's Head and Neck Surgery—Otolaryngology.* 5th ed. Baltimore, MD: Lippincott Williams & Wilkins; 2014:557–572.
156. DeShazo RD. Syndromes of invasive fungal sinusitis. *Med Mycol.* 2009;47:S309–314.
157. Schell WA. Unusual fungal pathogens in fungal rhinosinusitis. *Otolaryngol Clin North Am.* 2000;33(2):367–371.
158. Gillespie MB, O'Malley BW. An algorithmic approach to the diagnosis and management of invasive fungal rhinosinusitis in the immunocompromised patient. *Otolaryngol Head Neck Surg.* 2002;33(2):323–334.
159. Del Gaudio JM, Clemson LA. An early detection protocol for invasive fungal sinusitis in neutropenic patients successfully reduces extent of disease at presentation and long term morbidity. *Laryngoscope.* 2009;119:180–183.

160. Parikh SL, Venkatranman G, DelGaudio JM. Invasive fungal sinusitis: a 15-year review from a single institution. *Am J Rhinol.* 2004;18(2):75–81.
161. DelGaudio JM, Swain RE, Kingdom TT, et al. Computed tomography findings in patients with invasive fungal sinusitis. *Arch Otolaryngol Head Neck Surg.* 2003;129: 236–240.
162. Herbrecht R, Rajagopala S, Danna R, et al. Comparative survival and cost of antifungal therapy: posaconazole versus standard antifungals in the treatment of refractory invasive aspergillosis. *Curr Med Res Opin.* 2010; 26(10):2457–2464.
163. Sun HY, Singh N. Mucormycosis: it's contemporary face and management strategies. *Lancet Infect Dis.* 2011;11: 301–311.
164. Reddy CE, Gupta AK, Singh P, et al. Imaging of granulomatous and chronic invasive fungal sinusitis: comparison with allergic fungal sinusitis. *Otolaryngol Head Neck Surg.* 2010;143:294–300.
165. Stringer SP, Ryan MW. Chronic invasive fungal rhinosinusitis. *Otolaryngol Clin North Am.* 2000;33:375–387.
166. Li Y, Li Y, Li P, et al. Diagnosis and endoscopic surgery of chronic invasive fungal rhinosinusitis. *Am J Rhinol Allergy.* 2009;23:622–625.
167. Nayaka K, Oshima T, Kudo T, et al. New treatment for invasive fungal sinusitis: 3 cases of chronic invasive fungal sinusitis treated with surgery and voriconazole. *Auris Nasus Larynx.* 2010;37:244–249.
168. Lee TJ, Huang SF, Chang PH. Characteristics of isolated sphenoid sinus aspergilloma: report of twelve cases and literature review. *Ann Otol Rhinol Laryngol.* 2009;118(3): 211–217.
169. Pagella F, Matti E, De Bernardi F, et al. Paranasal sinus fungus ball: diagnoses and management. *Mycoses.* 2007; 50:451–456.
170. Park GY, Kim HY, Min JY, et al. Endodontic treatment: a significant risk factor for the development of maxillary sinus ball. *Clin Exp Otorhinolaryngol.* 2010;3(3):136–140.
171. Nicolai P, Lombadri D, Tomenzoli D, et al. Fungus ball of the paranasal sinuses: experience in 160 patients treated with endoscopic surgery. *Laryngoscope.* 2009;119: 2275–2279.
172. Schubert MS. Allergic fungal sinusitis: pathophysiology, diagnosis and management. *Medical Mycol.* 2009;47 (suppl 1):S324–330.
173. Schubert MS, Hutcheson PS, Graff RJ, et al. HLA-DQB1*03 in allergic fungal sinusitis and other chronic hypertrophic rhinosinusitis disorders. *J Allergy Clin Immunol.* 2004;114:1376–1383.
174. Manning SC, Holman M. Further evidence for allergic pathophysiology in allergic fungal sinusitis. *Laryngoscope.* 1998;108:1485–1496.
175. Manning SC, Mabry RL, Schaefer SD, et al. Evidence of IgE-mediated hypersensitivity in allergic fungal sinusitis. *Laryngoscope.* 1993;103(7):717–721.
176. Feger TA, Rupp NT, Kuhn FA, et al. Local and systemic eosinophil activation in allergic fungal sinusitis. *Ann Allergy Asthma Immunol.* 1997;79(3):221–225.
177. Bent JP, Kuhn FA. Allergic fungal sinusitis/polyposis. *Allergy Asthma Proc.* 1996;17(5):259–258.
178. Clark DW, Wenaas A, Luong A, Citardi MJ, Fakhri S. *Staphylococcus aureus* prevalence I allergic fungal rhinosinusitis vs. other subsets of chronic rhinosinusitis with nasal polyps *Forum Allergy Rhinol.* 2013;3(2):89–93.
179. Kuhn FA, Javer AR. Allergic fungal sinusitis: a four-year follow-up. *Am J Rhinol.* 2000;14:149–156.
180. Marple BF. Allergic fungal rhinosinutis: current theories and management strategies. *Laryngoscope.* 2001;111: 1006–1019.
181. Bent JP, Kuhn FA. Antifungal activity against allergic fungal sinusitis organisms. *Laryngoscope.* 1996;106(11): 1331–1334.
182. Mabry RL, Marple BF, Folker RJ, Mabry CS. Immunotherapy in the treatment of allergic fungal sinusitis: three years' experience. *Otolaryngol Head Neck Surg.* 1998;119:648–651.
183. Marple B, Newcomer M, Scwade N, Mabry R. Natural history of allergic fungal rhinosinusitis: a 4–10-year follow-up. *Otolaryngol Head Neck Surg.* 2002;127:361–366.

6

Asthma, Pulmonary Diseases, and Vocal Cord Dysfunction

Sunit Jariwala, Sumita Sinha, and Deepa Rastogi

ASTHMA

Asthma is a syndrome characterized by lower airway inflammation and reversible bronchial obstruction resulting in different symptoms including cough, a feeling of "tightness in the chest," wheezing, and shortness of breath. It often begins in childhood but can start at any age. Asthmatic symptoms can be limited solely to cough or chest discomfort and many asthmatics never report wheezing. Otolaryngologists frequently encounter patients with asthma due to its strong association with allergic rhinitis, chronic sinusitis, and obstructive sleep apnea.[1] It is important that the otolaryngologist is familiar with these associations, as improvement of these conditions through proper treatment can significantly impact asthma control.

Overview and Epidemiology

During the past 40 years, asthma prevalence has been increasing among children and adults.[2,3] Although asthma can develop at any age, it most commonly starts in childhood.[4] Close to 10% of all children and up to 8% of adults currently carry the diagnosis of asthma in the United States.[5–8] Asthma predominantly affects boys during early childhood. This gender difference equalizes during adolescence. Adult asthma mainly affects women, and typically persists until the end of life.

> Asthma affects 10% of children and 8% of adults in the United States. Boys are more commonly affected during childhood, while more women suffer from asthma during adulthood.

Children of Hispanic and African American ethnicities are disproportionately affected compared to Caucasian children, as evidenced not only by asthma prevalence, but also by disease severity quantified by emergency room visits and hospitalizations.[4,9] For these reasons, asthma is associated with high health care expenditures and results in a substantial loss of school and work days.[8,10,11]

Asthma death rates are higher in African American individuals compared with whites (2.3 compared with 1.3 per 10 000 persons with asthma).[12] Asthma-related death rates are also higher in adults (1.9 per 10 000 persons with asthma) older than 18 years compared with children (0.3 per 10 000 persons with asthma) 17 years or younger.[12] Two-thirds of asthma deaths occur in patients older than 65 years.[2,13]

Pathogenesis

Although the etiology of asthma is still poorly understood, it is increasingly becoming evident that asthma represents the end product of a complex interplay between genetic predisposition and environmental exposures.[14]

In relation to genetics, asthma susceptibility has been associated with single nucleotide polymorphisms (SNPs) in distinct genes (eg, *IL6R, DENND1B, IL33, SMAD3, IL2RB, ORMDL3-GSDMB, GLCCI1*).[15] *ORMDL3-GSDMB* SNPs have been linked to childhood, but not adult, asthma.[15] Furthermore, a *GLCCI1* SNP has been associated with a suboptimal response to inhaled glucocorticoid therapy in asthmatics.[16] In addition, allergies are highly associated with asthma, particularly if allergic sensitization occurs during the first years of life.[17–19]

Environmentally, both asthma and allergy incidence has been associated with environmental factors. One of the most important environmental factors that appears to contribute to the development of asthma and allergies is the reduced microbial exposure during early childhood in the westernized countries. In addition, exposure to airborne irritants (eg, environmental tobacco smoke and air pollution) appears to play an important role.[20–26] Asthma may also result from specific viral respiratory infections (ie, respiratory syncytial virus) during childhood in predisposed children, although high infectious burden (eg, frequent viral infections through siblings or child care facilities) and heavy parasite burden appear to be otherwise inversely related to asthma and allergies (Chapter 2, Hygiene Hypothesis).[27,28]

> Asthma results from a complex interplay between genetic and environmental factors.

Allergens

Several indoor and outdoor allergens, including dust mites, cockroaches, mice, and pet dander as well as windborne plant pollens, have been linked with the initiation of allergen sensitization, which in turn is associated with asthma incidence and severity.[29–32] Exposure to allergens postsensitization is one of the most potent triggers for asthma symptoms and poor disease control.[33] However, the specific allergen and extent of sensitization varies between populations and is frequently related to geographic location. Differences also exist between ethnic groups and are proposed to underlie the disproportionately higher asthma burden borne by African American and Hispanic children.[31]

Air Pollution and Tobacco Smoke

In addition to allergen sensitization, airborne irritants (eg, environmental tobacco smoke) are associated with the onset of asthma among children and ongoing symptoms into adolescence.[21] Children born to mothers who smoked during pregnancy are known to have a smaller cross-sectional area of their airways, and often present earlier with asthma symptoms.[34] Moreover, even low levels of ongoing smoke exposure during childhood are associated with increased airway inflammatory markers in children and reduced lung function.[35,36]

In addition to passive smoke exposure, coal smoke, diesel exhaust particles (DEPs), sulfur dioxide, and nitrogen dioxide are all associated with incident asthma, exacerbations, and diminished lung function.[22,23,25] Regarding the known association between higher asthma incidence and severity, and proximity to highways, DEPs are linked to an increase in airway inflammation.[37] DEPs induce T helper 17 (Th17) cells and thereby increase interleukin-17 (IL-17).[37] Similarly, high ambient ozone levels are associated with asthma morbidity, likely by causing oxidant-driven injury to the airways.[38,39]

> Environmental exposures play a major role in asthma incidence and severity.

Viruses

Several types of viral infections are also linked with asthma exacerbations.[40] Even though rhinovirus is the most common virus associated with asthma exacerbations among all ages, influenza virus is associated with a higher frequency of secondary complications including pneumonia.[41–43] Respiratory syncytial virus (RSV) is associated with the initiation of airway reactivity, particularly among premature babies, and asthma exacerbations in both children and adults.[26,44] Human metapneumovirus has recently been associated with asthma exacerbations and is frequently isolated from the nasal secretions of preschool and school-aged children hospitalized for asthma.[45] Other viruses known to cause poor asthma control and increased emergency department (ED) visits and hospitalizations include parainfluenza virus and adenovirus.[40]

Pathophysiology

The T lymphocytes, mast cells, macrophages, eosinophils, neutrophils, and epithelial cells are key components in the onset and/or progression of the airway inflammation in asthma. Pathologic features of asthmatic airways include denudation of airway epithelium, collagen deposition beneath the basement membrane (subepithelial fibrosis), mast cell degranulation, and the infiltration of eosinophils. In severe persistent and fatal asthma, additional findings include occlusion of the bronchial lumen by mucus, extensive bronchial smooth muscle hyperplasia and hypertrophy, and goblet cell hyperplasia (Figure 6–1).[46]

Inflammatory Cells and Cytokines

There are a number of different cells and cytokines that are known to play a role in the pathogenesis of asthma (Table 6–1). Lymphocytes, specifically $CD4^+$ T helper type 2 (Th2) lymphocytes, are the central effector cells of asthmatic airways. $CD4^+$ Th2 cells secrete cytokines including IL-4, IL-5, IL-9, and IL-13, which collectively promote the growth, activation, and migration of eosinophils, mucous secretion, immunoglobulin E (IgE) production, and expression of adhesion molecules such as Vascular Cell Adhesion Molecule 1 (VCAM-1).[47] The T lymphocytes also produce chemokines (eg, TARC), which contribute to cellular infiltration, while worsening acute and chronic inflammation in asthmatic airways.

Mast cells, which play in a key role in the onset of asthma, release preformed (histamine, tryptase) and newly generated (leukotrienes, prostaglandins, cytokines) mediators that contribute to mucosal inflammation. Mast cells arise in the bone marrow and enter the circulation as $CD34^+$ mononuclear cells that are positive for stem-cell factor and the high-affinity IgE receptor, Fc epsilon receptor 1 (FcεRI).[48] Mast cells travel to mucosal and submucosal sites in the airway and undergo tissue specific maturation. Mast cells also serve as a source of important cytokines (IL-1, IL-2, IL-3, IL-4, IL-5, IL-6, IL-8, IL-16, TNF-alpha, granulocyte-macrophage colony-stimulating factor [GM-CSF]), chemokines (monocyte chemoattractant protein, CCL5), and proteoglycans (eg, heparin).[48]

Macrophages play an important role in the normal host defense through phagocytosis and by generating enzymes and reactive oxygen species. In the airways, alveolar macrophages can also function as antigen-presenting cells, thereby propagating downstream inflammatory responses. In asthmatic patients, macrophages upregulate airway inflammation by producing cytokines (GM-CSF, IL-1, IL-6), lipid mediators, and matrix metalloproteinases.[49]

Eosinophils, which are consistently detected in the sputum of asthmatics, may directly damage airway epithelium through constitutive eosinophil proteins (eg, major basic protein, eosinophil-derived neurotoxin, eosinophil peroxidase, and eosinophil cationic protein). These eosinophil-associated proteins also increase bronchial responsiveness and stimulate the degranulation of mast cells and basophils. Eosinophil function is regulated by specific cytokines; IL-4 mediates eosinophil migration and IL-5 modulates eosinophil survival.[50]

Neutrophils are also involved in the onset and progression of asthma. They contribute to the inflammation of acute asthma exacerbations and chronic severe asthma by producing lipid mediators, reactive oxygen intermediates, and proteases (eg, elastase).[51] Leukotriene B4 (LTB4), IL-8, GM-CSF, and tumor necrosis factor alpha (TNF-alpha) attract neutrophils and reduce neutrophil apoptosis.

Bronchial Epithelium

Bronchial epithelium also serves as a source of pro-inflammatory mediators, and epithelial injury is characteristic of asthma. Bronchial epithelial injury, which exposes the subepithelium to allergens and/or pollutants, is associated with the secretion of inflammatory mediators. Cytokines and chemokines that are constitutively expressed on the bronchial epithelium include IL-1, IL-5, IL-6, IL-8, CCL5, platelet-derived growth factor, and GM-CSF.[52] Other cytokines (IL-2, IL-4, IL-10, IL-16, IL-18, TNF-alpha, eotaxin/CCL11), chemokines (monocyte chemoattractant protein-1 (MCP-1), macrophage inflammatory protein-1 (MIP-1), and leukotrienes (LTC4, LTD4) are secreted following injury. IL-5, GM-CSF, and CCL5 function in eosinophil survival, maturation, and recruitment. IL-8 and GM-CSF induce granulocyte (eg, neutrophil) stimulation and maturation. IL-1 and TNF-alpha are pro-inflammatory

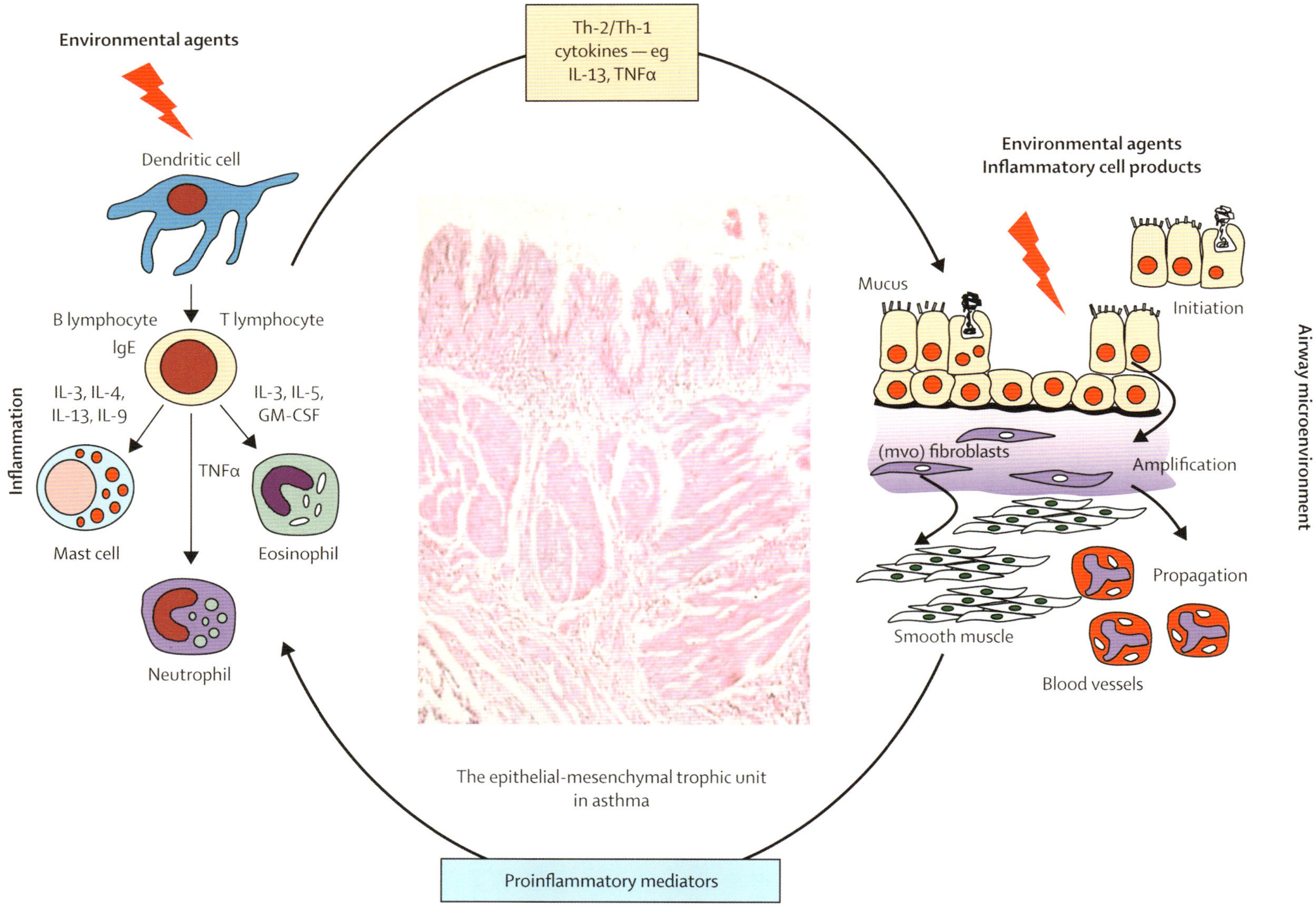

Figure 6-1. Pathophysiologic key factors in asthma. Inflammatory and remodeling responses in asthma with activation of the epithelial mesenchymal trophic unit. Epithelial damage alters the set point for communication between bronchial epithelium and underlying mesenchymal cells, leading to myofibroblast activation, an increase in mesenchymal volume, and induction of structural changes throughout the airway wall. Reprinted with permission from Elsevier. Holgate ST, Polosa R. The mechanisms, diagnosis, and management of severe asthma in adults. *Lancet.* 2006 Aug 26;368(9537):780–793.

Table 6-1. Inflammatory Cells and Mediators in Asthma

Key Cell	Mediator and/or Cytokine Secreted
T lymphocytes	IL-4, IL-5, IL-9, IL-13
Mast cells	Histamine, tryptase, leukotrienes, prostaglandins, IL-1, IL-2, IL-3, IL-4, IL-5, IL-6, IL-8, IL-16, TNF-alpha, granulocyte-macrophage colony stimulating factor (GM-CSF), monocyte chemoattractant protein, CCL5, proteoglycans
Macrophages	GM-CSF, IL-1, IL-6, lipid mediators, matrix metalloproteinases
Eosinophils	IL-4, IL-5
Neutrophils	lipid mediators, reactive oxygen intermediates, proteases

mediators that stimulate B cells and monocytes and upregulate the expression of adhesion molecules.[52]

Inflammatory Mediators

Oxidative stress is another factor that impacts the development of asthma. NADPH oxidase on the plasma membrane of granulocytes and other inflammatory cells is a source of oxygen radicals, which include the hydroxyl group and the superoxide anion. The superoxide anion released by inflammatory cells reacts with nitric oxide, which is synthesized from L-arginine in the presence of nitric oxide synthase (NOS).[53] Nitric oxide induces bronchodilation, vasodilation, and airway mucous secretion; exhaled nitric oxide can be used as a noninvasive marker of airway inflammation. Oxygen radicals may directly damage the airways of asthmatic patients.

Leukotrienes are also key inflammatory mediators in asthma. LTB4 is a neutrophil chemoattractant, whereas LTC4, LTD4, LTE4 are cysteinyl leukotrienes that are smooth muscle contractants. Human airway epithelial cells express the enzymes 5-lipoxygenase (5-LO), 5-lipoxygenase activating protein (FLAP), and LTA4 hydrolase. Cellular expression of 5-LO is restricted to neutrophils, eosinophils, monocytes, macrophages, mast cells, basophils, and human lung parenchyma. Endothelial cells and platelets do not contain 5-LO, but do have LTC4 synthase and LTA4 hydrolase, and can participate in leukotriene production.[54] Leukotriene receptors include at least 3 types of membrane receptors. The BLT receptor is a member of the transmembrane G-protein-coupled receptor family and is activated by the noncysteinyl leukotriene LTB4.[55] The cysteinyl leukotriene receptor 1 (CysLT1) is also a transmembrane G-protein receptor and is expressed in blood monocytes and in the lung with localization to smooth muscle and macrophages.[56] Activation of CysLT1 receptors produces bronchial smooth muscle constriction, plasma leakage, mucus hypersecretion, and eosinophil chemotaxis. The cysteinyl leukotriene receptor 2 (CysLT2) is the third type of membrane receptor. The CysLT2 receptor has the highest affinity for LTC4 and LTD4, and upon activation leads to increased intracellular calcium concentration. This receptor is expressed widely with highest levels in the heart, spleen, peripheral blood leukocytes, and the adrenal gland.

Other Pathogenic Mechanisms

Other mechanisms contributing to asthma include airway remodeling, viral pathogenicity, airway mucus hypersecretion, and neural pathways. Airway remodeling refers to the bronchial smooth muscle thickening and irreversible narrowing of the airways that occurs in chronic asthmatic patients.[57] Patients with asthma show an accelerated rate of decline in their airway function compared to healthy controls. Remodeling may be mediated by endothelins, fibrogenic growth factors (insulin-like growth factor, epidermal growth factor, platelet-derived growth factor, basic fibroblast growth factor, transforming growth factor, vascular endothelial growth factor), matrix metalloproteinases, and IL-13.[57] Viral pathogens also contribute to the pathogenesis of asthma through interactions with bronchial epithelium.[58] Rhinoviruses bind to the adhesion molecule, Intercellular Adhesion Molecule 1 (ICAM-1), which is upregulated in the airways of asthmatic patients, and another adhesion molecule, Vascular Cell Adhesion Molecule 1 (VCAM-1).[59] Infection with the respiratory syncytial virus and rhinovirus can upregulate the pro-inflammatory cytokines IL-6, IL-8, and GM-CSF.

Airway mucous hypersecretion is another asthma-related mechanism. Most of the human mucin genes identified to date are expressed in the human airway and expression of mucin genes in asthmatic patients is stimulated by endotoxin, TNF-alpha, IL-1, IL-4, IL-6, IL-9, and neutrophil elastase. Secretory cell hyperplasia/metaplasia is stimulated by neutrophil elastase, Th2 (IL-4, IL-13) cytokines, exogenous stimuli (endotoxin and ozone), and irritants (tobacco smoke, sulfur dioxide).[60]

The cholinergic nervous system maintains resting bronchial tone, especially in the large airways, and stimulates mucus secretion from submucosal glands and goblet cells. Thermal and mechanical stimuli, cigarette smoke and nicotine, and irritants (eg, formaldehyde, sulfur dioxide) can induce neural depolarization thereby resulting in bronchoconstriction.

Natural History and Clinical Presentation

Asthma With Onset During Childhood

Several birth cohort studies conducted over the past 3 decades have elucidated the natural history of asthma in distinct geographic areas of the world.[61–63] The time of symptom onset and persistence early in life is highly predictive of asthma in later life; approximately 95% of asthmatics may first experience symptoms before the age of 6 years.[2] As reported by the Tucson Children's Respiratory Study, children may be categorized as not wheezing (no wheezing during the first 3 years of life, and no wheezing at 6 years), early transient wheezers (wheezing during the first 3 years of life, but no wheezing at 6 years), late-onset wheezers (no wheezing during the first 3 years of life, but wheezing at 6 years), and persistent wheezers (wheezing in the first 3 years of life, and wheezing at 6 years).[64,65]

> Childhood asthmatics fall into 3 general categories: early transient wheezers, late-onset wheezers, and persistent wheezers.

In the Tucson study, "wheezing" was determined by parents completing a questionnaire that asked whether the child's "chest had ever sounded wheezy or whistling apart from colds."[64] Of the children in the Tucson study, nearly 52% had not wheezed, 20% had early transient wheezing, 15% had late-onset wheezing, and 14% had persistent wheezing. While the category of early transient wheezing is most commonly associated with viral-induced wheeze, the persistent wheeze category is the one that is most severe. Persistent wheezing is associated with atopic sensitization early in life, and with the persistence of symptoms into school age and adolescence. This category is also linked to the early initiation of lung function loss that may begin as early as young adulthood, particularly among those with severe asthma.[61,62] Therefore, it is important to define the risk of persistence of disease into the school-age years. An asthma risk index has been developed to identify those children with wheeze who have a greater chance of symptom persistence and of developing asthma. The risk index is composed of major criteria including eczema, allergen sensitization, and parental history of asthma, and minor criteria including wheezing apart from colds, evidence of food sensitization, and peripheral eosinophilia. The presence of 2 or more major criteria with one or more minor criteria increases the likelihood that childhood wheeze will persist as asthma into the school years and adolescence.

> Diminished pulmonary function in childhood is linked to increased asthma disease burden in adulthood.

Asthma Phenotypes

As mentioned earlier, asthma is a syndrome characterized by airway inflammation and reversible bronchospasm resulting in cough, wheezing, and shortness of breath. Nevertheless, the complex pathogenic mechanisms that lead to asthma may differ significantly between individuals. Recent research has focused on distinguishing between different asthma phenotypes (ie, asthmatics with different pathogenic pathways and contributory factors to their disease). Distinguishing between asthma phenotypes is important because it allows more precise prognosis, choice of treatment and therefore more effective asthma management (Figure 6–2).[15]

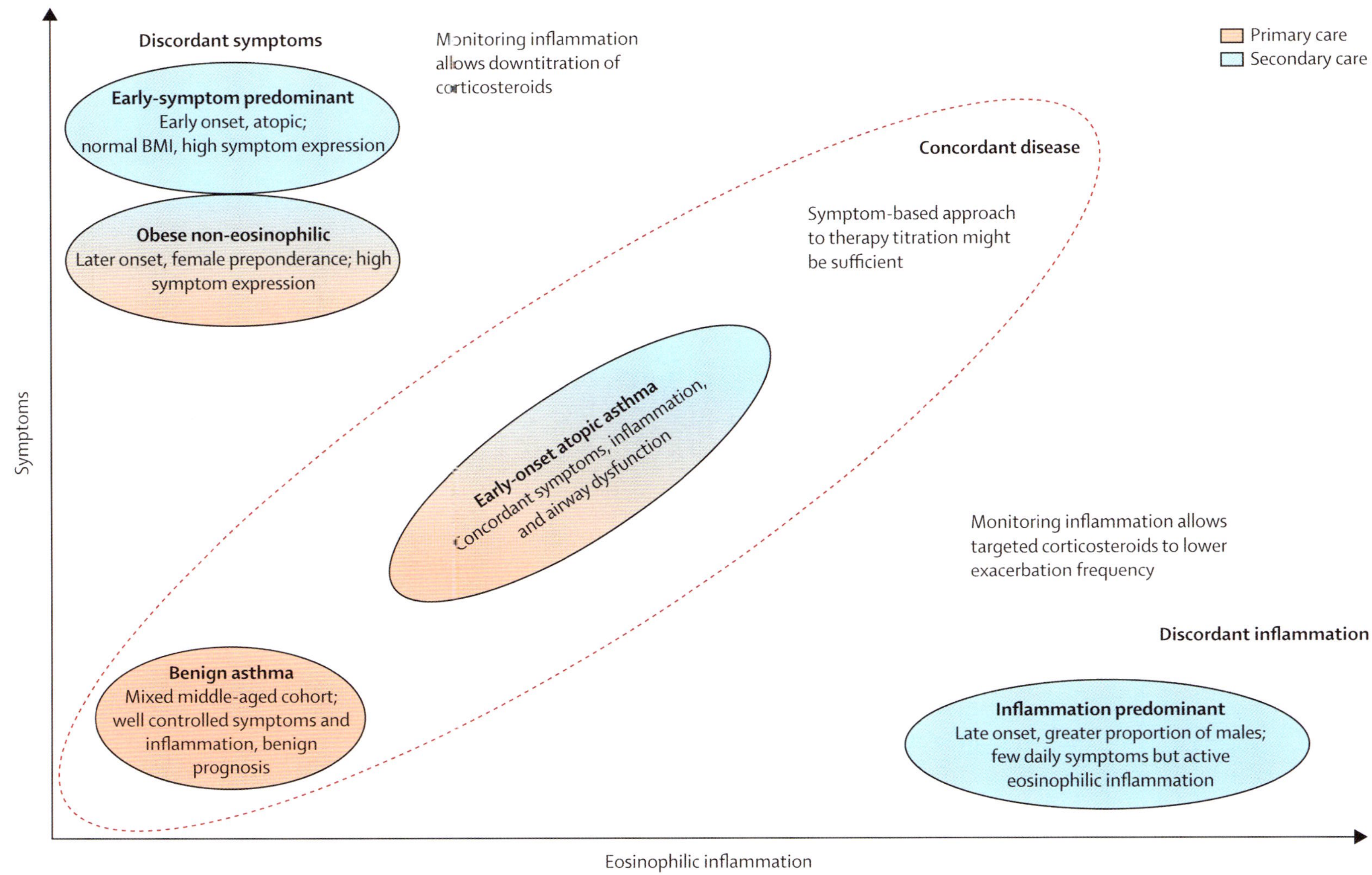

Figure 6–2. Cluster analyses allow differentiation of asthma phenotypes, an aspect that will facilitate an improved understanding of underlying etiologies and, therefore, development of targeted therapies. Reprinted with permission from Elsevier. Martinez FD, Vercelli D. Asthma. *Lancet.* 2013 Oct 19;382(9901):1360–1372.

Beyond the prognostic approach of asthma phenotyping as summarized in Figure 6–2, asthma is also often classified by its main primary trigger (Table 6–2). These triggers play a central role in initiating and maintaining the underlying airway inflammation in sensitized individuals, and in triggering asthma exacerbations.

> Asthma is a heterogeneous disease of chronic airway inflammation and is characterized by distinct clinical phenotypes.

Allergic Asthma. Many allergic asthmatics will not exhibit exacerbations from acute exposures (eg, cats, dust), since these individuals may be persistently exposed to such triggers. The diagnostic evaluation may involve percutaneous skin testing for environmental allergens and/or serum-specific IgE testing. Environmental control, pharmacotherapy including biologics (eg, omalizumab), and/or allergen immunotherapy may be utilized in the management of allergic asthma.

Nonallergic Asthma. Nonallergic asthma presents through symptoms (eg, dyspnea, cough) similar to allergic asthma, but is triggered by nonallergic factors (eg, infections, pollutants, weather changes, strong odors). Most cases of nonallergic asthma may be attributed to infections of the upper and lower respiratory tracts.[66]

Aspirin-Exacerbated Respiratory Disease (AERD). AERD is also known as Samter Triad and is characterized by chronic rhinosinusitis with nasal polyposis, asthma, and aspirin (or other nonsteroidal anti-inflammatory drugs) sensitivity.[67] Interestingly, AERD patients desensitized to aspirin may experience improvement of the underlying upper and lower airway symptoms.

Table 6–2. Asthma Phenotypes Based on Trigger Factors

Allergic asthma
Nonallergic asthma
Aspirin-exacerbated respiratory disease
Exercise-induced bronchospasm
Occupational asthma
Concurrent asthma with chronic obstructive pulmonary disease (COPD)

Exercise-Induced Asthma. Exercise-induced bronchoconstriction (EIB) is characterized by airway narrowing due to physical activity. EIB commonly occurs in asthmatic patients, but may also occur in individuals without a known diagnosis of asthma.[68]

Occupational Asthma. Occupational asthma (OA) is triggered by chemicals or irritants that are present in the workplace. Depending on the frequency and severity of exposures, OA may worsen preexisting asthma or result in newly diagnosed asthma. OA can be divided into 2 (ie, immunologic and nonimmunologic) categories. In immunologic OA, agents such as enzymes, latex, dyes, and dusts, trigger the activation of immune mechanisms. This type of OA typically results from longer periods of exposure. Nonimmunologic OA (ie, irritant-induced asthma or reactive airways dysfunction syndrome) may result from single or multiple episodes of exposure to irritants at high concentrations. In this case, there is often not enough time to develop an immunologic response.[69] Much like the other types of asthma described, the symptoms of OA include coughing, wheezing, and shortness of breath. Generally, symptoms worsen as exposure is increased, and with prolonged periods of exposure, symptoms may become irreversible (reviewed in Chapter 12).

Severe Asthma Phenotypes in Adults. Detailed cluster analysis of persistent asthmatics has recently been performed through the Severe Asthma Research Program cohort, and identified several adult asthma phenotypes.[70] Table 6–3 summarizes the characteristics of the 5 clusters that have been identified based on concomitant clinical characteristics. The distinct asthma phenotypes demonstrate the clinical heterogeneity of this condition, and offer the possibility of targeted therapy.

Comorbid Conditions

Allergic Rhinitis and Eczema. Allergic rhinitis and eczema often predate the onset of childhood asthma, and this progression is recognized as the "atopic march." The presence of aeroallergen and food sen-

Table 6–3. Severe Asthma Phenotypes in Adults

Cluster 1: Mild Allergic Asthma	Early onset; atopic; normal lung function ≤2 controller medications; minimal health care utilization minimal sputum eosinophilia
Cluster 2: Mild-Moderate Allergic Asthma	Most common cluster; early onset; atopic; borderline FEV1 but reverse to normal; ≤2 controller medications; low health care utilization, infrequent need for oral corticosteroids minimal sputum eosinophilia
Cluster 3: More Severe Older Onset Asthma	Older; very late onset; higher BMI (obese); less atopic; slightly decreased FEV1 with some reversibility; frequent need for oral corticosteroids despite ≥3 controller medications including high doses of inhaled corticosteroids sputum eosinophilia
Cluster 4: Severe Variable Allergic Asthma	Early onset; atopic; severely decreased FEV1, but very reversible to near normal; high frequency of symptoms and albuterol use; "variable" with need for frequent oral corticosteroids; high health care utilization sputum eosinophilia
Cluster 5: Severe Fixed Airflow Asthma	Older; longest duration; less atopic; severely decreased FEV1 with less reversibility (COPD similarities); high frequency of symptoms and albuterol use despite oral corticosteroids; high health care utilization; comorbidities Both sputum eosinophilia and neutrophilia

Source: Reprinted with a Creative Commons License from the Korean Association of Internal Medicine. Kim SH. Clinical and pathophysiological characteristics of severe asthma. *Korean J Med.* 2012 Oct;83(4):424–429.

sitization often predicts asthma development.[71] Both allergic rhinitis and eczema frequently coexist with asthma, and impact the recovery of pulmonary function following an exacerbation.[72,73] Improved allergic rhinitis control is associated with good asthma control.[74] Therefore, it is important to promptly diagnose allergic rhinitis in individuals with high asthma morbidity and adequately manage nasal symptoms in order to facilitate the control of asthma symptoms (Table 6–4).

Table 6–4. Common Comorbidities of Asthma

Allergic rhinitis
Eczema
GERD
Obesity
Obstructive sleep apnea
Sinusitis

Gastroesophageal Reflux Disease. Gastroesophageal reflux disease (GERD) is frequently observed among children and adults with asthma and is associated with both asthma incidence and poor control.[75] Some studies have associated GERD with the initiation of wheeze and disease severity in infancy and others have found that adequate GERD management in older children is associated with improved asthma control.[76,77] However, the association between asthma and GERD remains controversial. Although several studies have identified an association between GERD and asthma, particularly in the setting of obesity, others have failed to demonstrate an improvement in asthma symptoms following therapeutic interventions for GERD.[75,77–79] In light of this evidence, we recommend an initial evaluation composed of the elucidation of symptoms and supported by investigations such as pH probe with or without a barium study of the esophagus and stomach. In the setting of a strong suspicion for GERD, a therapeutic trial with antacids (proton pump inhibitors) for 6 to 8 weeks may be warranted.

Obesity. Prospective studies have identified obesity to be an independent risk factor for asthma in children and adults.[80–82] Obese asthmatics have greater disease severity, poor asthma control, and suboptimal response to controller medications including inhaled corticosteroid (ICS) therapy.[83,84] The primary mechanisms underlying the link between asthma and obesity are augmented pulmonary function deficits due to increased systemic inflammation and/or altered pulmonary mechanics, particularly in association with truncal adiposity.[85–87] However, obesity-related asthma appears to be distinct from atopic asthma, with nonatopic systemic inflammation likely mediated by obesity. Given the higher disease burden among obese individuals with asthma, and improvement in asthma morbidity with weight loss, clinicians can manage obesity-related asthma by encouraging weight reduction strategies in conjunction with asthma therapy.[86,88,89]

Obstructive Sleep Apnea. Over the past decade, there has been a growing body of literature surrounding the association between asthma and sleep-disordered breathing (SDB). Obstructive sleep apnea (OSA) is the most common form of SDB observed in children. Children with asthma have a higher prevalence of OSA as compared to their nonasthmatic counterparts. Furthermore, asthma control is directly associated with burden of SDB in children. Although the underlying mechanisms have not been well elucidated, the role of inflammation and that of altered airway architecture have been hypothesized and are being currently investigated. Since obesity is a comorbid condition for both asthma and SDB, there are ongoing studies to better understand the mechanisms that underlie the links between obesity, asthma, and SDB. Similar associations have also been observed in adults.

> Comorbidities are associated with poor asthma control, so their coexistence should be routinely elucidated and managed to facilitate asthma control.

Diagnostic Evaluation

History

Asthma may develop early in life, particularly among those residing in urban neighborhoods, which bear a disproportionately higher disease burden.[7] The clinical evaluation is primarily based on history taking and physical examination. A thorough medical history can help to identify symptoms that are likely due to asthma, to determine asthma severity and control, and identify asthma triggers. In considering a diagnosis of asthma, clinicians should consider the development/onset of symptoms, symptoms that occur or worsen at night, precipitating and/or aggravating factors, medication history, family history, social and occupational history, history of exacerbations, impact of asthma on the patient and family, and assessment of the patient's and family's perception of disease.

Asthma commonly presents with nonspecific symptoms including wheezing, dyspnea, cough, chest tightness, and/or chest pain. Of note, children with asthma are most commonly atopic, and typically present with reversible episodes of cough, wheeze, and shortness of breath between 12 and 18 months of life.[90,91] Wheezing is caused by the vibration of at least one partially obstructed airway. However, patients with severe obstruction may not be able to produce an audible wheeze. When obstruction mainly involves the small airways, asthma may present without wheezing. Furthermore, wheezing may occur in conditions (eg, congestive heart failure, cystic fibrosis, vocal cord dysfunction) other than asthma. Asthma may present with cough alone, especially in the setting of nocturnal asthma or exercise-induced bronchospasm. Asthma may also present with dyspnea, chest tightness, or chest pain; in the appropriate clinical setting, potentially life-threatening conditions (eg, myocardial infarction, pulmonary embolism, aortic dissection) must be considered and excluded. The salient features of an asthma history are summarized in Table 6–5.

Common asthma triggers include allergies, viral infections, household products, dusts, occupational exposures, weather factors (eg, cold air, precipitation, changes in barometric pressure), air pollution, exercise, infection, emotions/stress, rhinitis/

Table 6–5. Important Information to Elicit for an Asthma History

Development/onset of symptoms
Symptoms that occur or worsen at night
Precipitating and/or aggravating factors
Medication history
Family history
Social and occupational history
Exposure to potential environmental triggers
History of exacerbations
Impact of asthma on the patient and family
Assessment of the patient's and family's perception of disease

Table 6–6. Risk Factors for Severe Asthma Exacerbations

Previous severe exacerbations
Hospitalization and/or emergency room visits for asthma within the past year
Use of 2 or more canisters of short-acting beta agonists per month
Difficulty perceiving airway obstruction or the severity of worsening asthma
Low socioeconomic status or inner-city residence
Illicit drug use
Psychosocial disturbances
Comorbidities

sinusitis, GERD, medications, menstrual cycles, and foods.[92] Risk factors for severe asthma exacerbations should be identified and include previous severe exacerbations, hospitalization or emergency room visits for asthma within the past year, use of 2 or more canisters of short-acting beta agonists (SABAs) per month, difficulty perceiving airway obstruction or the severity of worsening asthma, low socioeconomic status or inner-city residence, illicit drug use, psychosocial disturbances, and comorbidities (eg, cardiovascular disease or other chronic lung disease) (Table 6–6).[92]

Physical Examination. On physical examination, the most common sign of severe airway obstruction is wheezing. Upper respiratory signs may include nasal secretions and/or nasal polyps. Chest findings may include wheezing, prolonged expiration, accessory muscle use, or hyperexpansion of the thorax.[93] Cutaneous signs may include eczema. The medical history and physical examination are very important, since there is evidence that asthma is underdiagnosed.

Disease Staging. Once the diagnosis of asthma is confirmed, the clinical evaluation is optimally performed by following the National Heart, Lung, and Blood Institute (NHLBI) asthma guidelines.[90] At the initial evaluation, asthma severity is classified as intermittent or persistent based on symptom frequency and the need for SABA therapy. Daytime symptoms occurring more than 2 times a week and nocturnal symptoms more than 2 nights a month is classified as persistent asthma, for which daily preventative medications are recommended. Among currently available preventive medications, ICS are most potent and effective, and remain the first-line therapy for persistent asthma.[90] After initiating therapy with preventive medications, responsiveness is measured by the ease with which asthma is controlled, irrespective of baseline asthma severity. The same measures of asthma symptom frequency and lung function utilized to classify asthma severity are used to classify control. The preventive regimen is iteratively modified until good asthma control, defined as daytime symptoms less than 2 times a week and nocturnal symptoms less than 2 nights a month, is achieved.

There are a number of standardized questionnaires that can help the clinician to evaluate asthma control in a given patient. For example, the Asthma Control Test (ACT) is a reliable and valid patient-based tool for individuals 12 years or older (Table 6–7).[94] The ACT consists of 5 items (questions assess activity limitation, dyspnea, nocturnal symptoms, use of rescue medication, and overall patient rating of asthma control over the previous 4 weeks) and uses a 5-point scale for each item; an ACT score of 19 or less determines patients with poorly controlled asthma.

Table 6–7. Asthma Control Test (ACT)

1. In the past 4 weeks, how much of the time did your asthma keep you from getting as much done at work, school, or at home?				
1—All of the time	2—Most of the time	3—Some of the time	4—A little of the time	5—None of the time
O	O	O	O	O
2. During the past 4 weeks, how often have you had shortness of breath?				
1—More than once a day	2—Once a day	3—3 to 6 times a week	4—Once or twice a week	5—Not at all
O	O	O	O	O
3. During the past 4 weeks, how often did your asthma symptoms (wheezing, coughing, shortness of breath, chest tightness or pain) wake you up at night or earlier than usual in the morning?				
1—4 or more nights a week	2—2 to 3 nights a week	3—Once a week	4—Once or twice	5—Not at all
O	O	O	O	O
4. During the past 4 weeks, how often have you used your rescue inhaler or nebulizer medication (such as albuterol)?				
1—3 or more times per day	2—1 or 2 times per day	3—2 or 3 times per week	4—Once a week or less	5—Not at all
O	O	O	O	O
5. How would you rate your asthma control during the past 4 weeks?				
1—Not controlled at all	2—Poorly controlled	3—Somewhat controlled	4—Well controlled	5—Completely controlled
O	O	O	O	O

Note. Asthma Control Test © 2002 by QualityMetric Incorporated. All Rights Reserved. Asthma Control Test is a trademark of QualityMetric Incorporated.

Source: Reprinted with permission from Elsevier. Schatz M, Sorkness CA, Li JT, et al. Asthma Control Test: reliability, validity, and responsiveness in patients not previously followed by asthma specialists. *J Allergy Clin Immunol.* 2006 Mar;117(3):549–556.

Laboratory Studies

Spirometry and Peak Expiratory Flow Measurements. Given the importance of preserving pulmonary function, the guidelines also recommend routine pulmonary function testing, which is useful for demonstrating obstruction and assessing reversibility in patients 5 years or older. While infant pulmonary function testing and impulse oscillometry techniques have been developed to allow the evaluation of airway function among infants and preschool children, these are not widely used in the clinical setting.[95,96] Spirometry is performed to measure the degree of airflow obstruction, and the forced expiratory volume in 1 second (FEV1) is the most commonly used measure in the evaluation of asthmatic airflow obstruction. A post-bronchodilator improvement of 12% in the FEV1 suggests significant reversibility of airway obstruction (Figure 6–3). Patients with acute asthma have an obstructive spirometric pattern, which includes reduced FEV1 and FEV1/FVC ratio. Though highly effort dependent and less reproducible than FEV1, peak expiratory flow rates (PEFR) (ie, peak flow) can be very useful for monitoring large airway flow rates. The PEFR can be used to determine the degree of asthma control

Spirometry

		Ref	Pre Meas	Pre % Ref	Post Meas	Post % Ref	Post % Chg
FVC	Liters	3.85	3.71	96	4.16	108	12
FEV1	Liters	3.35	2.33	70	3.14	94	35
FEV1/FVC	%	87	63		75		
FEF25-75%	L/sec	3.80	1.24	33	2.74	72	121
PEF	L/sec	6.92	4.88	71	5.76	83	18
FET100%	Sec		7.87		6.25		-21
FIVC	Liters		3.49		3.68		5
FIF50%	L/sec		4.03		5.31		32
FEF/FIF50			0.44		0.67		51
MVV	L/min						

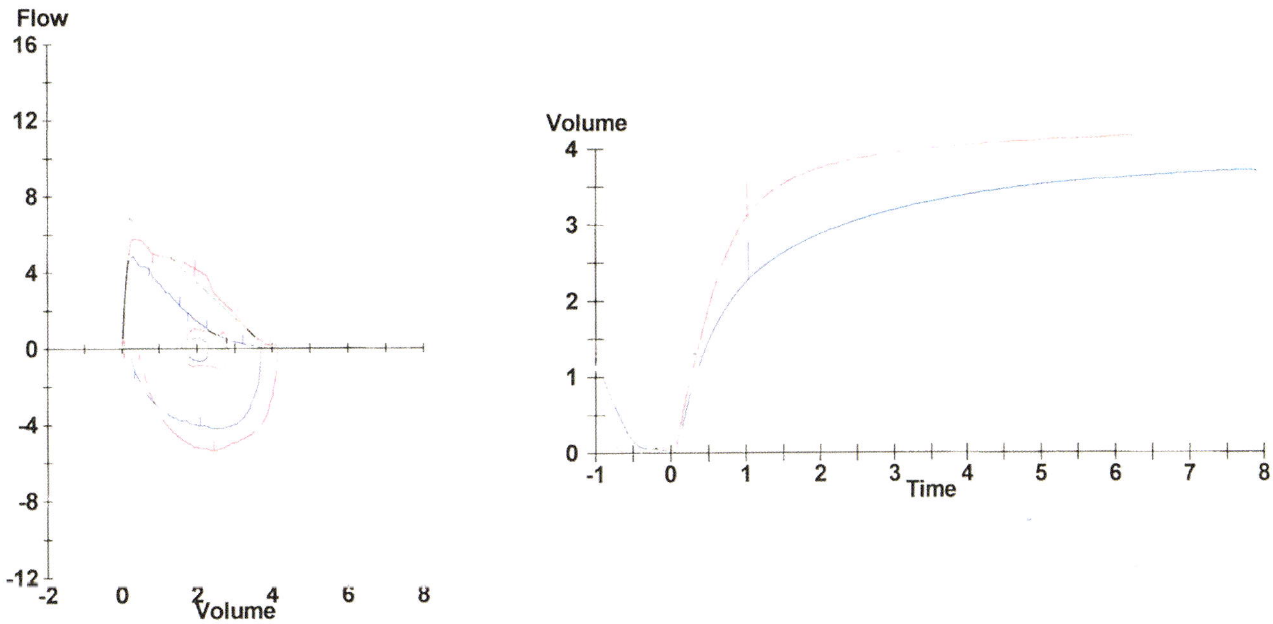

Figure 6-3. A representative spirometry performed on a child with asthma. The black curve is the baseline or pre-bronchodilator effort, and the red curve is the post bronchodilator effort. Concavity to the curve is suggestive of lower airway disease, which corresponds to decrease in FEV_1 and FEV_1/FVC ratio below 80% of predicted. Reversible airway obstruction (asthma) is confirmed by a 35% increase in FEV1 postbronchodilator (70% of normal to 94% of normal).

and can assist a patient in determining the severity of exacerbations. Peak flow rates typically vary 5% throughout the day. As asthma control deteriorates, the normal diurnal variation in airway caliber becomes exaggerated and the values may decrease more than 20% to 30%.[93]

Measurements of Bronchial Hyperreactivity. Bronchial hyperreactivity is a measure of the sensitivity of the airways to provoking agents, and the amount of provoking agent that causes a given reduction in expiratory flow is an indicator of the degree of airway hyperreactivity. Bronchial challenges can be performed with various agents including methacholine (cholinergic agonist), mannitol (osmotic stimulus), histamine or cold air. In direct challenge testing, methacholine (or other agents such as histamine) acts on smooth muscle receptors thereby causing smooth muscle contraction.[97] During indirect challenge testing, mannitol (or other agents such as hypertonic saline) triggers the release of endogenous mediators that cause the airway smooth muscle to contract.[98] Direct challenges are highly sensitive in diagnosing and excluding asthma, while indirect challenges are highly specific in confirming asthma.[99]

In the bronchial challenge, the concentration or dose delivered that results in a predefined reduction in airway flow (usually a 20% decrease in FEV_1) is defined as the provocation concentration (PC20). Methacholine challenge is considered to be positive for bronchial hyperreactivity when the PC20 is <8 to 16 mg/mL.[99] Positive tests are nonspecific, since airway hyperreactivity is also increased in patients with allergic rhinitis, chronic cough, chronic obstructive pulmonary disease, congestive heart failure, and acute viral upper respiratory infections. Bronchoprovocation testing is relatively safe but clinicians need to be aware that there are some risks with the procedure. Patients with airway obstruction less than 70% of predicted and patients taking β-blockers are at higher risk for severe bronchospasm after inhaling methacholine. Relative contraindications include coronary artery disease, stroke, malignant hypertension, and bradycardia.

Radiography and Biomarker Analysis. Other diagnostic measures may include radiography, laboratory (eg, serum), and biomarker analyses. Chest radiography may be performed to evaluate for potential asthma masqueraders (eg, sarcoidosis) and should be performed at least once on every new-onset adult asthmatic. Computed tomography (CT) of the chest or sinuses may be considered in the proper clinical context. For example, CT chest findings are important in the diagnosis and evaluation of allergic bronchopulmonary aspergillosis (ABPA). Total serum IgE is useful in selected asthma patients (eg, those being considered for omalizumab therapy). Biomarkers such as fractional exhaled nitric oxide (FeNO) correlate with airway eosinophilia, and are often increased in steroid-naïve asthmatics as well as severe asthmatics.[100] FeNO measurements are beginning to be used more frequently in the clinical management of asthma. FeNO may be used to predict and evaluate the response to ICS therapy and to assess adherence with these medications.[101] Recent data also suggest that FeNO may predict the risk of future asthma exacerbations and lung function decline.[102] FeNO values may be influenced by several factors (eg, age, height, cigarette smoking, allergen exposure, nitrate consumption, and rhinovirus infection), therefore changes in FeNO values following therapy may be easier to interpret than absolute FeNO values. Periostin is another biomarker of eosinophilic airway inflammation, and may suggest the response to certain biologic therapies (ie, lebrikizumab).[103]

> The diagnostic evaluation for asthma may include pulmonary function testing, bronchoprovocation testing, radiography, laboratory testing, and/or biomarker analyses.

Differential Diagnosis

The differential diagnosis of airway obstruction in adults is summarized in Table 6–8. Wheezing earlier than 1 year of age may not be asthma and should be investigated further for conditions including airway malformations, laryngeal or tracheal web or cyst, laryngo- or tracheomalacia, vascular ring, congenital lung malformations, cystic fibrosis, and primary ciliary dyskinesia. Children born prematurely are at

Table 6–8. Differential Diagnosis of Asthma in Adults

Chronic obstructive pulmonary disease
Congestive heart failure
Bronchiolitis obliterans
Pulmonary embolism
Pulmonary infiltrates with eosinophilia
Drug-induced cough/wheeze
Vocal cord dysfunction
Interstitial lung disease
Foreign bodies
Tracheal and bronchial lesions (eg, tumors)
GERD
Allergic bronchopulmonary aspergillosis
Panic attacks

increased risk for presenting with bronchopulmonary dysplasia (BPD) exacerbations, which present as wheeze, although the inherent pathophysiological changes differ between BPD and asthma. There are several additional conditions that may complicate the diagnosis and/or management of asthma. Among these are GERD, obstructive sleep apnea (OSA), ABPA, obesity, and depression. In the setting of severe or "refractory" asthma, clinicians should consider immunodeficiency, interstitial lung disease, pulmonary infiltration with eosinophilia (PIE) syndromes (ABPA, eosinophilic pneumonia), vasculitis, noncompliance with medications, and the inability to avoid exposure to triggers including occupational asthma (see Table 6–8).

Treatment

The goals of asthma management in children and adults include the reduction of impairment (ie, functional limitations, symptom intensity and frequency) as well as risk (ie, the likelihood of future asthma). It is felt that control of asthma is achieved when there is infrequent (less than 2 days a week) use of inhaled SABA for symptom relief, maintenance of normal activity levels (ie, exercise and school/work), and meeting of the patients' and families' expectations of asthma care (Table 6–9).[90,104]

As detailed in the clinical evaluation section above, following asthma severity classification, there is a step-up and step-down approach to pharmacotherapy. Irrespective of baseline asthma severity, the guidelines recommend ICS to be the first-line preventive regimen. After the initiation or modification of therapy, it is recommended that patients be reassessed every 3 to 4 months to classify control.

One of the most common reasons for poor asthma control is the incorrect technique when using inhalers. Therefore, the inhaler technique should be reviewed at each visit until the patient is fully skilled in the correct use of inhalers. Spacers such as the Aerochamber can greatly facilitate the inhaler use and should be given to all children as well as for adults that have difficulties using the metered dosed inhalers correctly.

Among the subset with suboptimal asthma control despite the appropriate use of ICS, clinicians may increase the ICS dose or add leukotriene antagonists, given their synergistic role with ICS to decrease airway inflammation. Among those who still do not achieve control, the addition of long-acting beta agonist (LABA) therapy is the next step. Clinicians may consider less frequently used regimens including every other day oral corticosteroids, methylxanthines, and immunomodulators including omalizumab (a monoclonal anti-IgE antibody), which has been effective in decreasing asthma symptoms by binding circulating IgE.[105] Allergen immunotherapy may also be considered in the setting of allergic asthma that is adequately controlled.

Since atopy and environmental exposures play a major role in asthma, pharmacotherapy is only one part of asthma management. For optimal asthma control, environmental remediation and removal of triggers (frequently identified by allergy testing) in conjunction with controller medications, are an integral part of achieving adequate asthma control.[106] Potential occupational exposures and/or respiratory irritants (eg, tobacco smoke, strong odors) should also be identified and reduced.

Managing Asthma Flares and Exacerbations

In the acute setting, short-acting beta-receptor agonists (SABA, eg, albuterol) quickly alleviate symptoms associated with minor flares (eg, triggered by exercise, exposure to inhalant allergens etc). SABA medications start to work in 5 minutes and reach their peak effect in 30 minutes. If inhalation through the metered dose inhaler (asthma pump) is difficult, the patient may benefit from inhaling SABA through nebulization of SABA solution, administered through nebulizer machines. If dyspnea persists despite repeated SABA treatments in short intervals, the patient should seek medical attention. Such emergencies are sometimes difficult to recognize, particularly in small children. Use of accessory muscles, unusually rapid breathing, unusually fatigued appearance, and avoidance of physical activity should alert the caregiver to initiate SABA treatment and to rapidly seek medical attention.

In urgent or emergency care or hospital settings, asthma symptoms and signs must be closely monitored and expediently treated. In moderate or severe exacerbations, supplemental oxygen must be administered to correct hypoxemia, and SABA must be administered continuously or repetitively. Additionally,

Table 6-9. Assessment of Asthma Control and Suggested Therapy

Components of Control		Classification of Asthma Control (≥12 years of age): Well Controlled	Not Well Controlled	Very Poorly Controlled
Impairment	Symptoms	≤2 days/week	>2 days/week	Throughout the day
	Nighttime awakenings	≤2×/month	1–3×/week	≥4×/week
	Interference with normal activity	None	Some limitation	Extremely limited
	Short-acting beta-agonist use for symptom control (not prevention of exercise-induced bronchospasm)	≤2 days/week	>2 days/week	Several times per day
	FEV1 or peak flow	>80% predicted/ personal best	60%–80% predicted/ personal best	<60% predicted/ personal best
	Validated questionnaires			
	ATAQ	0	1–2	3–4
	ACQ	≤0.75	≥1.5	N/A
	ACT	≥20	16–19	≤15
Risk	Exacerbations requiring oral systemic corticosteroids	0–1/year	≥2/year	
		Consider severity and interval since last exacerbation		
	Progressive loss of lung function	Evaluation requires long-term follow-up care		
	Treatment-related adverse effects	Medication side effects can vary in intensity from none to very troublesome and worrisome. The level of intensity does not correlate to specific levels of control, but should be considered in the overall assessment of risk.		
Recommended Action for Treatment		Maintain current step	Step up 1 step and re-evaluate in 2–6 weeks	Consider short course of oral systemic corticosteroids
		Regular follow-ups every 1–6 months to maintain control	For side effects, consider alternative treatment options	Step-up 1 to 2 steps and reevaluate in 2 weeks
		Consider step-down if well controlled for at least 3 months		For side effects, consider alternative treatment options

Source: Adapted from Expert Panel Report 3: Guidelines for the Diagnosis and Management of Asthma. National Institutes of Health: National Heart, Lung, and Blood Institute; 2007.

systemic steroids must be administered in order to decrease inflammation in moderate to severe exacerbations or in exacerbations that respond suboptimally to SABA. Oral steroids are usually given for a 3- to 7-day course, and when used for a week or more, are slowly tapered.

A written asthma action plan is very useful for the home management of asthma. This strategy helps patients recognize early indicators of asthma exacerbation, including worsening PEFR and increasing symptoms, and assists them in adjusting medications (eg, short course of oral corticosteroids).

> Components of asthma care include assessing and monitoring asthma severity and control, administering pharmacotherapy (and considering allergen immunotherapy), and controlling the environmental factors that affect asthma.

Summary

In summary, asthma is a common chronic disease that is strongly associated with otolaryngologic conditions such as allergies, chronic rhinitis, sinusitis, and obstructive sleep apnea. As new entities that contribute to disease onset and severity are identified, the development of targeted therapeutic interventions will contribute toward improved asthma control with the ultimate goal of decreasing disease burden and preserving quality of life.

PULMONARY DISEASES

Overview

Pulmonary conditions may be categorized by the specific pathologic site(s) of disease involvement. The lungs include the airways (trachea, bronchi, bronchioles), alveoli, and interstitium. Diseases that predominantly affect the airways include asthma, chronic obstructive pulmonary disease (COPD) (including chronic bronchitis and emphysema), cystic fibrosis, bronchomalacia, and bronchiectasis. Diseases that affect the alveoli include pneumonia, tuberculosis, pulmonary edema (can be a manifestation of congestive heart failure), acute respiratory distress syndrome, lung cancer, and pneumoconiosis (including silicosis, coal worker's pneumoconiosis, asbestosis, berylliosis, byssinosis). Diseases that affect the interstitium include idiopathic interstitial pneumonias (eg, pulmonary fibrosis, nonspecific interstitial pneumonia), hypersensitivity pneumonitis, autoimmune diseases, and sarcoidosis; these diseases may also affect the alveoli. Vascular conditions include pulmonary embolism, chronic thromboembolic pulmonary hypertension, pulmonary arterial hypertension, vasculitis (eg, granulomatosis with polyangiitis otherwise known as Wegener granulomatosis, and eosinophilic granulomatosis with polyangiitis otherwise known as Churg-Strauss syndrome), arteriovenous malformations, and pulmonary veno-occlusive disease. Some of the selected conditions that can mimic asthma or that otolaryngologists may encounter are reviewed in this section.

Clinical Presentations of Selected Pulmonary Diseases

Tracheobronchomalacia

Primary tracheobronchomalacia is typically seen among preschool children, with the highest prevalence among infants, while secondary or acquired tracheobronchomalacia may be seen at any age among children and adults. Malacia is defined as "softening," and typically refers to bone or cartilage. Tracheomalacia (TM) refers to weakened longitudinal elastic fibers of the pars membranacea with impaired cartilage in the trachea.[107] Tracheobronchomalacia (TBM) includes weakening that extends to the bronchi, and this weakening can lead to a less rigid structure that easily collapses. The terms TBM and TM are often used interchangeably. Normally, the intrathoracic trachea slightly increases in diameter during inspiration and slightly decreases in expiration. In TM, the changes in diameter can be significantly and pathologically increased. Excessive narrowing of the intrathoracic trachea during expiration is most notable with forced exhalation, coughing, or during a Valsalva maneuver. This narrowing can lead to collapse of the trachea and subsequent obstructive disease. Extrathoracic TM or cervical TM may also occur, although the collapse is seen on inspiration due to negative pleural pressure. TM can be primary (congenital) or secondary (acquired) (Table 6–10), and most adults have the acquired form of the disease. While the etiology of secondary malacia is related to the underlying disease, which may be extrinsic compression or intrinsic airway defect, the etiology of primary or congenital primary airway malacia is not well known. The most common proposed mechanisms are (1) decreased deposition of calcium on airway cartilages, which explains the higher prevalence among neonates born premature as compared to term neonates, and (2) neurogenic etiology with decreased neural tone of the laryngeal and/or trachealis muscles.

Patients with TM usually present with nonspecific symptoms such as cough, dyspnea, and/or increased sputum production. Inspiratory wheezing or stridor may occur, and may lead to a misdiagnosis of asthma, emphysema, or bronchitis; these conditions may also coexist with TM. If the TM is mild, the patient may be asymptomatic. In some cases, the TM may not be evident unless an infection occurs. Certain clinical situations (anesthesia, progressive hypercapnic respiratory failure) may also bring about TM.

Due to the dynamic nature of TM, plain radiographs usually do not provide much information unless there is a large mass or goiter distorting the trachea. The gold standard for diagnosis is bronchoscopic visualization of dynamic collapse (ie, narrowing of the trachea on expiration). The usual criterion used to define TM is a decrease in diameter of at least 50% on expiration. Dynamic CT with inspiratory and expiratory phases may be useful. Spirometry is not definitive but can support a diagnosis of TM. Typically, an obstructive pattern is seen, with a low FEV1, low peak expiratory flow rate, and rapid decrease in airflow.

Asymptomatic patients do not require treatment. For symptomatic patients, the first step is to optimize treatment of related conditions, such as COPD or asthma. Bronchospasm can cause excessive changes in intrathoracic pressures, thereby worsening collapse. Beyond treating other conditions, some patients improve with stents. Silicone stents are preferred over metal stents due to the ease of removal and fewer complications. Tracheostomy may benefit some patients as the tube may bypass the weakened

Table 6–10. Causes of Tracheomalacia

Primary (congenital)	Secondary (acquired)
Genetic Idiopathic "giant trachea" or Mounier-Kuhn Syndrome	Post-traumatic • Postintubation • Post-tracheostomy • External chest trauma • Post-lung transplantation Emphysema Chronic infection/bronchitis Chronic inflammation (eg, relapsing polychondritis) Chronic external compression of the trachea • Malignancy • Benign tumors • Cysts • Abscesses • Aortic aneurysm • Vascular rings

segment. Noninvasive positive pressure can be used in acute situations.

Chronic Obstructive Pulmonary Disease

COPD is characterized as a disease of the airways with airflow limitation that is not fully reversible, whereas asthma may be fully reversible.[108] COPD may refer to emphysema, chronic bronchitis, or chronic obstructive asthma. Morbidity associated with COPD is significant as this condition is responsible for a large number of hospital admissions and ambulatory care visits. Risk factors for developing COPD include smoking (amount and duration worsen disease severity), biomass smoke exposure, and occupational exposures (eg, diesel exhaust).[108] Genetic causes are uncommon, although alpha-1 antitrypsin (AAT) deficiency can lead to early emphysema. AAT deficiency should be suspected in patients who are young (less than 45 years of age), minimal or nonsmokers, have a basilar predominance of emphysema, or have a personal or family history of liver disease.

The most common symptoms of COPD are dyspnea, cough, and increased sputum production. Patients may also complain of wheezing, chest tightness, and exertional dyspnea. Physical examination may be normal early in the disease, whereas patients with more advanced disease may have wheezing, decreased breath sounds, crackles, and/or distant heart sounds. With severe disease, the patient may have an increased antero-posterior diameter of the thorax or "barrel-shaped" chest. Laboratory testing is not particularly helpful in diagnosing COPD, but may be useful in excluding other causes of dyspnea. The most important tests in diagnosing COPD are pre-bronchodilator and post-bronchodilator spirometry, which can document persistent obstruction. Typically, a ratio of FEV1/FVC of <0.70 L is used to define obstructive disease in adults.[108] Lung volumes and diffusing capacity are additional pulmonary function tests that can add information about air trapping, hyperinflation, and degree of emphysema. Although imaging is not necessary for the diagnosis of COPD, radiography may demonstrate bullae, hyperinflation, and/or a flattened diaphragm in severe disease. Computed tomography (CT) scanning is more sensitive and specific than radiography, and is usually obtained in certain situations (acute illness such as pneumonia, considering alternative diagnoses or lung volume reduction surgery).

Smoking cessation is vital to the successful management of COPD and is the initial step in treatment. Other nonpharmacologic interventions include timely immunizations (most importantly influenza and pneumococcal vaccine), continuous oxygen therapy if there is exertional or resting hypoxemia ($SaO_2 \leq 88\%$ or $PaO_2 \leq 55$ mm Hg), and pulmonary rehabilitation for symptomatic patients with severe COPD.[109] Medications include long-acting inhaled bronchodilators (beta-agonists, anticholinergics), inhaled corticosteroids, and combination inhaled therapies.

Bronchiectasis

Bronchiectasis is characterized by dilation or stretching of the bronchi, and is a chronic disease characterized by cough, daily sputum production, and susceptibility to lower respiratory tract infections. It is important to recognize that bronchiectasis may be misdiagnosed as asthma due to a similar presentation, but the treatment is quite different. Bronchiectasis has distinct etiologies (Table 6–11), one of which is cystic fibrosis (CF).[110] The prevalence of bronchiectasis in the United States appears to be increasing, and is more common in older patients (peak age 80 to 84) and in women.[111]

The typical presentation includes chronic cough with daily mucopurulent sputum production lasting for months to years, although patients may also present with chronic cough without sputum production. Patients may complain of repeated episodes of "bronchitis" requiring antibiotics. A retrospective chart review of 103 bronchiectasis patients revealed the following symptom frequency: cough (98%), daily sputum production (78%), dyspnea (62%), rhinosinusitis (73%), hemoptysis (27%), and recurrent pleurisy (20%).[112] On physical examination, crackles were most common (75%) along with wheezing (22%), while only 2% had clubbing. Patients with an "acute exacerbation" of bronchiectasis usually have an increase in sputum production with a change in consistency and color, fatigue, dyspnea, and/or pleuritic chest pain.

For patients with bronchiectasis, studies should include laboratory testing, pulmonary function

Table 6-11. Recognized Causes of Bronchiectasis

Postinfective	Severe pneumonia, tuberculosis, pertussis, measles
Impaired mucociliary clearance	Cystic fibrosis, primary ciliary dyskinesia, Young syndrome
Immune deficiency	Common variable immune deficiency, specific polysaccharide antibody deficiency, secondary immunodeficiency (chronic lymphocytic leukemia), HIV infection
Exaggerated immune response	Allergic bronchopulmonary aspergillosis, graft-versus-host-disease, inflammatory bowel disease (ulcerative colitis and Crohn disease)
Congenital abnormalities of the bronchial wall	Mounier-Kuhn syndrome, Williams-Campbell syndrome, Marfan syndrome
Inflammatory pneumonitis	Aspiration of gastric contents, smoke inhalation
Fibrosis (traction bronchiectasis)	Sarcoidosis, idiopathic pulmonary fibrosis
Mechanical obstruction	Foreign body, tumor, extrinsic compression
Miscellaneous conditions	Mycobacterium avium complex infection (Lady Windermere syndrome), connective tissue diseases (rheumatoid arthritis, systemic lupus erythematosus, Sjogren syndrome), pulmonary sequestration, yellow nail syndrome, infertility (primary ciliary dyskinesia, cystic fibrosis), diffuse panbronchiolitis, alpha-1 antitrypsin deficiency

Source: Reprinted with due diligence from Wolters Kluwer Health, Inc. Zoumot Z, Wilson R. Respiratory infection in noncystic fibrosis bronchiectasis. *Curr Opin Infect Dis.* 2010; 23(2):165–170.

testing, and imaging. Laboratory testing includes a complete blood cell count with differential, CF sweat testing, cystic fibrosis transmembrane regulator (CFTR) genetic mutation analysis, serum immunoglobulin levels (IgA, IgG, IgE, and IgM), antinuclear antibody, rheumatoid factor, anticyclic citrullinated peptide (anti-CCP) antibody, SSA/SSB antibodies, *Aspergillus*-specific IgE and precipitins, and sputum microscopy with culture. Obstructive disease (reduced FEV1, reduced or normal FVC, and reduced FEV1/FVC ratio) is usually seen in bronchiectasis. Chest radiography may show linear atelectasis, thickened airways, or irregular opacities, although the chest radiograph is sometimes normal.[113] Chest CT has become the gold standard for diagnosis as irregularities of the airways are easily seen in cross section. Characteristic CT findings include airway dilatation, lack of tapering of the airway toward the periphery, and bronchial wall thickening. Mucopurulent plugs may be seen in affected airways and cysts may be seen in severe disease.

Treatment of the underlying disease (if known) should be initiated; however, therapy commonly prevents progression of disease rather than cure. It is important to obtain a sputum sample, which will determine the choice of antibiotic regimen when needed for an acute exacerbation. The bacterial flora in bronchiectasis patients differs from that of a typical pneumonia or bronchitis. Gram-negative bacteria such as *Hemophilus influenzae* and *Pseudomonas aeruginosa* are most commonly found.[112,114] Gram-positive bacteria are less common but include *Streptococcus pneumoniae* and *Staphylococcus aureus*. Antibiotics are usually reserved for acute exacerbations; however, macrolide therapy has been shown to reduce the frequency of exacerbations when given chronically.[115] Influenza vaccine and pneumococcal vaccine should be administered to all patients. Immunoglobulin replacement therapy (intravenous or subcutaneous) should be given to any patients with documented immunoglobulin deficiency. Airway clearance techniques or chest physiotherapy with postural drainage should be administered to clear secretions and loosen mucus plugs. Bronchodilators and ICS are not indicated unless there is concomitant asthma or wheezing noted. Systemic corticosteroids are typically used only for patients with wheezing or those with ABPA, since the side effects cause more risks than benefits in most bronchiectasis patients. Despite medical therapy, some patients continue to have persistent symptoms and recurrent exacerbations. For those patients with localized bronchiectasis (one lobe or segment), surgical resection of the bronchiectatic lung can lessen symptoms and decrease exacerbations. Surgical resection may also be required to control massive hemoptysis. Double lung transplantation is the only definitive surgical treatment for patients with diffuse bronchiectasis.

Allergic Bronchopulmonary Aspergillosis

ABPA is a hypersensitivity reaction to noninvasive, bronchial-colonizing *Aspergillus* species, which primarily occurs in nonimmunocompromised patients with asthma or cystic fibrosis. ABPA most commonly occurs in adults between the ages of 20 and 40 years, and rarely affects pediatric patients.[116] Patients with refractory asthma, peripheral eosinophilia, and centrally located bronchiectasis should arouse suspicion for ABPA. The diagnostic criteria for ABPA in patients with asthma are shown in Table 6–12. ABPA may complicate CF, and occurs in about 2% to 15% of these patients.[117] Common findings that are seen in CF patients who develop ABPA include clinical deterioration (eg, increased cough, wheezing, sputum) not attributable to another etiology, immediate cutaneous reactivity (and/or positive serum-specific IgE) to *Aspergillus*, increased total serum IgE concentration >417 kU/L (1000 ng/mL), serum precipitating antibodies to *A fumigatus*, and abnormal chest radiograph (eg, pulmonary infiltrates, change from earlier films, mucus plugging).[118] All patients with ABPA should be started on glucocorticoids. There are no data for dose or duration, although a common

Table 6–12. ABPA Diagnostic Criteria in Patients With Asthma

Criteria for ABPA-Central Bronchiectasis	Minimal Essential Criteria
1. Asthma	Yes
2. Central bronchiectasis	Yes
3. Immediate cutaneous reactivity to *Aspergillus*	Yes
4. Total serum IgE concentration > 417 kU/L (1000 ng/mL)	Yes
5. Increased serum IgE-*A fumigatus* and/or IgG-*A fumigatus*	Yes
6. CXR infiltrates	No
7. Serum precipitating antibodies to *A fumigatus*	No
Criteria for the Diagnosis of ABPA-Seropositive	**Minimal Essential Criteria**
1. Asthma	Yes
2. Immediate cutaneous reactivity to *Aspergillus*	Yes
3. Total serum IgE concentration > 417 kU/L (1000 ng/mL)	Yes
4. Increased serum IgE-*A fumigatus* and/or IgG-*A fumigatus*	Yes
5. CXR infiltrates	No

Source: Reprinted with permission from Elsevier. Greenberger PA. Allergic bronchopulmonary aspergillosis. *J Allergy Clin Immunol*. 2002;110:685–692.

protocol is prednisolone 0.5 mg/kg/d for 2 weeks followed by slow taper over several weeks to months. Omalizumab may be beneficial in patients with CF and ABPA.[119]

Cystic Fibrosis

Cystic fibrosis (CF) has historically been thought to be a pediatric disease and can be mistaken for asthma. However, with improved life expectancy, there are increasing numbers of young adults living with CF. CF is caused by mutations in the cystic fibrosis transmembrane regulator (CFTR) gene that is located on the long arm of chromosome 7. CF is the most common autosomal recessive condition in the United States and is more common in Caucasians. The most common mutation is homozygous ΔF508, but there are over 1950 other known CFTR mutations; these variants are subdivided based on their effects on the degree of residual CFTR function.[120–122] CFTR is a protein that regulates chloride secretion and sodium absorption and is found in all exocrine glands. CFTR defects may result in thick secretions in the respiratory system, pancreas, intestines, and reproductive tract. Due to the numerous distinct mutations, CF may manifest differently among individuals, ranging from mild to very severe disease. There is substantial variability in disease phenotype between these genetic variants, which may range from presentation of disease in utero with meconium ileus to presentation in mid-adulthood with nasal polyps and without substantial respiratory morbidity. Phenotypic manifestations also differ among children and adults. Infants and children usually present with respiratory symptoms, meconium ileus, or failure to thrive.[123] In a study on patients diagnosed with CF as adults, the most common presentations included recurrent sinopulmonary infections (usually due to *P. aeruginosa*), pulmonary symptoms with gastrointestinal disease, and male infertility.[124] There is some overlap between CF and asthma, and patients with CF can exhibit wheezing and have concomitant asthma. Obstruction and bronchial hyperreactivity can also be seen on pulmonary function testing with CF.[125] Suspicion for CF should be raised in a patient with unexplained bronchiectasis, chronic sinopulmonary infections, recurrent bouts of pancreatitis, or male infertility. Diagnosis can be made by sweat chloride testing (>60 mmol/L), but there is a 5% chance of false-negative results and the tests need to be repeated. Confirmation of the diagnosis is made by genotyping for CFTR mutations.

Eosinophilic Granulomatosis With Polyangiitis (Churg-Strauss Syndrome)

Eosinophilic granulomatosis with polyangiitis (EGPA), previously known as Churg-Strauss syndrome or allergic granulomatosis and angiitis, is a rare disease that affects multiple organ systems. The features of EGPA may combine vasculitis, chronic rhinosinusitis, asthma, eosinophilia, and the involvement of other organ systems (eg, cardiac, renal, gastrointestinal, peripheral nervous system). It is important to recognize this disease as the management approach differs from asthma. The lung and the skin are the most commonly affected organs. EGPA is classified as an antineutrophil cytoplasmic antibody (ANCA) vasculitis affecting small and medium-sized vessels, although only 30% to 40% of patients are positive for ANCA. Most patients have antibodies directed against myeloperoxidase that cause a perinuclear staining pattern in the ANCA test (p-ANCA). Diagnosis can be difficult due to the phasic nature of the disease. A typical presentation is an adult with new onset asthma with concomitant allergic rhinitis and sinusitis. Over 90% of patients with EGPA have asthma. The patient may then develop hypereosinophilia, usually associated with tissue infiltration (pulmonary or gastrointestinal), and may then progress to vasculitis. This progression from asthma to vasculitis may not happen for several months to years.

Diagnostic criteria for EGPA include asthma, peripheral blood eosinophilia greater than 10%, evidence for vasculitis, neuropathy, paranasal sinus abnormality, and pulmonary infiltrates. The "gold standard" for diagnosis is surgical lung biopsy with the classic findings of eosinophilic pneumonia, granulomatous inflammation, and vasculitis. Initial therapy for EGPA includes corticosteroids; a typical regimen is prednisone 0.5 to 1 mg/kg/day. Additional immunosuppressive agents such as cyclophosphamide or azathioprine may be required in refractory disease. EGPA may be masked in patients with severe asthma on chronic corticosteroids. Such patients should be monitored carefully for symptoms of EGPA with tapering steroid doses.

PARADOXIC VOCAL FOLD MOVEMENT DISORDER

Paradoxic vocal fold movement disorder (PVFMD) is a disorder that is commonly misdiagnosed as asthma. Patients with PVFMD suffer from an involuntary closure of the vocal cords during respiration. The nonspecific term *vocal cord dysfunction* is slowly falling out of favor since vocal cord dysfunction can also refer to vocal cord lesions or vocal cord paralysis. Other terms that are used interchangeably with PVFMD include paradoxical vocal cord motion, laryngeal dyskinesia, periodic occurrence of laryngeal obstruction, paroxysmal laryngospasm, functional stridor, and irritable larynx syndrome. Patients with PVFMD are commonly misdiagnosed with asthma, allergies, or upper airway obstruction and may receive many unnecessary medications and treatments including intubation and tracheostomy.

Normally, the true vocal folds abduct on inspiration and slightly adduct on expiration. PVFMD can occur during inspiration, expiration, or both. The vocal folds can adduct suddenly, while leaving only a small aperture posteriorly. This condition can cause dyspnea, throat tightness, or even a choking sensation (Tables 6–13 and 6–14).[126] Patients may also complain of more difficulty getting air in than out. The sensation of dyspnea may lead to anxiety or panic in some patients and perpetuate the abnormal vocal fold movement. Other symptoms include chest tightness or pain, dysphagia, aphonia or dysphonia, neck or chest retractions, fatigue or throat clearing during episodes. Dyspnea associated with PVFMD rapidly appears and may rapidly dissipate compared to other causes of dyspnea such as asthma. Physical examination during an episode may reveal a high-pitched inspiratory sound or stridor heard in the tracheal area as opposed to end-expiratory wheezing heard in the chest. Patients with PVFMD have normal oxygenation even during an acute episode and both pulse oximetry and arterial blood gas should be normal.[127] Patients with PVFMD are sometimes mistakenly diagnosed with asthma; however, the 2 conditions frequently coexist. In a group of refractory asthmatic patients, PVFMD occurred alone in 10%, whereas 30% had both asthma and PVFMD.[128,129]

PVFMD was initially described as "hysteric croup" in the 1800s and linked to psychologic disorders. Since then, numerous studies continue to show an association with psychogenic causes. One study found that 45/48 cases of PVFMD had psychologic diagnoses.[130] The most common diagnosis was conversion disorder (52%), 13% had depression or dysthymia, and 10% had factitious disorder. Another study of 95 patients hospitalized for PFVMD found that 73% had a psychiatric diagnosis.[131] Other stressors such as physical or sexual abuse, depression, and post-traumatic stress disorder have been associated with PVFMD.[132]

However, PVFMD is not always psychogenic in nature. Irritant-associated PVFMD can be due to numerous causes including gastroesophageal reflux, laryngopharyngeal reflux, and rhinitis/sinusitis. Another common trigger for PVFMD is exercise or exertion, and this has been noted especially in highly competitive athletes. A study of 370 developmental or elite athletes, found 5% to have PVFMD and 30% to have exercise-induced bronchospasm.[133] In athletes, PVFMD may be mistakenly diagnosed as exercise-induced bronchospasm. Exercise-induced bronchospasm is similar to asthma in that it causes a peripheral expiratory wheeze. However, PVFMD usually begins soon after starting exercise and resolves within 5 minutes of cessation whereas exercise-induced bronchospasm develops after 5 to 10 minutes of exercise and peaks 5 to 20 minutes after stopping. Pre- and postexercise spirometry can be used to definitively diagnose exercise-induced bronchospasm. PVFMD and exercise-induced bronchospasm may coexist, and in such cases, it is important to find evidence for both.

There are no definitive laboratory or radiologic tests for the diagnosis of PVFMD. The "gold standard" for diagnosis is direct laryngoscopy while the patient is symptomatic. The patient should be asked to sequentially phonate, breathe, pant, and take deep breaths to best assess vocal fold movement. Greater than 50% closure of the vocal folds during inspiration is sufficient for diagnosis; however, the cords may appear normal if the patient is not experiencing an acute episode. Pulmonary function testing is also not usually diagnostic but can provide supplementary evidence. The most likely abnormality on spirometry is a flattening or truncation of the inspiratory limb of the flow-volume loop. In addition to flattening, a sawtooth pattern may appear in the inspiratory limb during an acute episode.

Table 6-13. Approach to the Patient With Possible Vocal Cord Dysfunction

1. Clinical History and Physical Examination
   a. Questions regarding symptoms
      i. Do you have more trouble getting air in or getting air out?
      ii. Do you feel any tightness?
      iii. If so, where is the tightness located (throat, upper chest, lower chest)?
      iv. Do you hear any noises when you breathe in?
      v. When symptoms start, do you generally cough?
      vi. Do you ever lose your voice or have a change in the way your voice sounds?
      vii. Do you have numbness or tingling in your hands, feet, or lips during episodes?
      viii. Do you ever feel lightheaded or dizzy?
      ix. Have you ever passed out or felt as though you were going to pass out?
      x. Do symptoms come on rapidly?
      xi. Do symptoms resolve rapidly?
      xii. Do asthma medications help?
      xiii. Does use of your asthma inhalers sometimes make symptoms worse?
   b. Assessing for potential risk factors or laryngopharyngeal irritants
      i. GERD/LPR
      ii. Postnasal drip because of upper airway inflammatory conditions
      iii. Psychological factors
   c. Physical examination
      i. Rule out upper airway obstruction from an organic cause
      ii. Look for signs of upper airway inflammation or allergic rhinitis
      iii. Look for signs of acute VCD: stridor, tachypnea, hoarseness or dysphonia, cough, tugging of the neck or upper chest muscles, and a look of anxiety or even distress
   d. Response to treatment
      i. During an acute episode, no improvement or even worsening with inhaled medications
      ii. During chronic management, lack of response to escalating asthma therapy including corticosteroids
2. Pulmonary Function Testing
   a. Inspiratory loop that is often poorly reproducible and truncated, sawtoothed, or irregular
   b. FEF50 (forced expiratory flow at 50% of the exhaled vital capacity)/FIF50 (forced inspiratory flow at 50% of the inhaled vital capacity) greater than 1
   c. If FEV1 (FEV in first second of expiration) is reduced, FEV1/FVC (forced vital capacity) ratio is normal
   d. Normal lung volumes
3. Measure of Oxygenation and Ventilation During Episodes
   a. Pulse oximetry normal
   b. Normal oxygen tension measured on arterial blood gas (PaO_2 (partial pressure of oxygen, arterial))
   c. Normal alveolar-arterial (A-a) gradient
   d. Reduced arterial PCO_2 (partial pressure of carbon dioxide) because of hyperventilation
4. Flexible Laryngoscopy
   a. Paradoxic adduction of vocal cords during exhalation
   b. Inappropriate adduction of vocal cords during exhalation
   c. Secondary evidence of postnasal drip/GERD/LPR (edema and erythema of the glottis or periglottic region)

Source: Reprinted with permission from Elsevier. Hoyte FCL. Vocal cord dysfunction. *Immunol Allergy Clin N Am.* 2013;33(1):1–22.

Table 6-14. Important Aspects of the Clinical History in a Patient With Vocal Cord Dysfunction

Symptoms of VCD	Throat or upper chest tightness
	Shortness of breath or dyspnea
	Sensation of choking or suffocation
	More difficulty getting air in than out
	Cough
	Lightheadedness or dizziness
	Heavy sensation of the extremities
	Perioral or extremity numbness or tingling
	Rapid onset and rapid resolution of these symptoms
Signs of VCD	Tachypnea or hyperventilation
	Stridor
	Neck or chest retractions
	Pallor, but no cyanosis
	Hoarseness or dysphonia
	Lack of relief, and sometimes worsening, from asthma inhalers
Risk factors for VCD	Upper airway inflammation (allergic or nonallergic rhinitis, chronic sinusitis, or recurrent upper respiratory infections)
	GERD
	Previous traumatic event involving breathing (eg, suffocation, near-drowning, witness a severe asthma attack)
	Severe emotional stress
	Female gender
	Playing a wind instrument
	Competitive athletics

Source: Reprinted with permission from Elsevier. Hoyte FCL. Vocal cord dysfunction. *Immunol Allergy Clin N Am.* 2013;33(1):1–22.

Another measure that can be helpful is the FEF50/FIF50 ratio, which is normally less than or equal to 1. As the inspiratory effort is decreased in PVFMD, the ratio will become greater than 1. Results must be interpreted with caution if the patient has comorbid asthma because the expiratory effort will be affected and the ratio may be normal.

Treatment for an acute episode of PVFMD is directed at relieving the airway obstruction. The patient should be reassured that he/she is not in a life-threatening situation and that oxygenation is normal despite symptoms. Reassurance alone may alleviate acute airway symptoms.[134] Certain maneuvers such as panting, sniffing, or pursed-lip breathing can also terminate an attack. Medications are sometimes required, and benzodiazepines have been used effectively to treat episodes. In the outpatient setting, it is important to address comorbidities (ie, gastroesophageal reflux disease or sinusitis) and any psychological factors that may be either aggravating or causing PVFMD. Educating the patient on normal laryngeal anatomy and what occurs to the vocal cords during PVFMD can help to elucidate the diagnosis and symptoms. Referral to a speech-language pathologist is essential in managing PVFMD. The patient will learn about throat relaxation and breathing techniques to relieve symptoms and abort acute attacks.

Acknowledgments. This chapter's authors would like to thank Ms. Tulsi Desai for assisting with the preparation of this chapter.

REFERENCES

1. Worldwide variation in prevalence of symptoms of asthma, allergic rhinoconjunctivitis, and atopic eczema: ISAAC. The International Study of Asthma and Allergies in Childhood (ISAAC) Steering Committee. *Lancet*. 1998;351(9111):1225–1232.
2. de Nijs SB, Venekamp LN, Bel EH. Adult-onset asthma: is it really different? *Eur Respir Rev*. 2013;22(127):44–52.
3. Asher MI, Montefort S, Björkstén B, et al. Worldwide time trends in the prevalence of symptoms of asthma, allergic rhinoconjunctivitis, and eczema in childhood: ISAAC Phases One and Three repeat multicountry cross-sectional surveys. *Lancet*. 2006;368(9537):733–743.
4. Bloom B, Jones LI, Freeman G. Summary health statistics for U.S. children: National Health Interview Survey, 2012. *Vital Health Stat*. 2013;10(258):1–81.
5. Akinbami LJ. *The State of Childhood Asthma, US, 1980–2005. Advance Data from Vital and Health Statistics 381*. Hyattsville, MD: Centers for Disease Control and Prevention, National Center for Health Statistics; 2006.
6. Akinbami LJ, Moorman JE, Bailey C, et al. *Trends in Asthma Prevalence, Health Care Use, and Mortality in the United States, 2001–2010*. NCHS data brief, no 94. Hyattsville, MD: National Center for Health Statistics; 2012.
7. Akinbami LJ, Moorman JE, Garbe PL, Sondik EJ. Status of childhood asthma in the United States, 1980–2007. *Pediatrics*. 2009;123(suppl 3):S131–145.
8. Asthma in the U.S. Centers for Disease Control and Prevention website. http://www.cdc.gov/vitalsigns/asthma/. Published May 3, 2011. Accessed May 28, 2015.
9. Akinbami LJ, Rhodes JC, Lara M. Racial and ethnic differences in asthma diagnosis among children who wheeze. *Pediatrics*. 2005;115(5):1254–1260.
10. Pearson WS, Goates SA, Harrykissoon SD, Miller SA. State-based Medicaid costs for pediatric asthma emergency department visits. *Prev Chronic Dis*. 2014;11(140139).
11. Szefler SJ, Zeiger RS, Haselkorn T, Mink DR, Kamath TV, Fish JE, Chipps BE. Economic burden of impairment in children with severe or difficult-to-treat asthma. *Ann Allergy Asthma Immunol*. 2011;107(2):110–119.
12. Moorman JE AL, Bailey CM, Zahran HS, King ME, Johnson CA, Liu X. National surveillance of asthma: United States, 2001–2010. *Vital Health Stat 3*. 2012 Nov;35:1–67.
13. Bauer BA, Reed CE, Yunginger JW, Wollan PC, Silverstein MD. Incidence and outcomes of asthma in the elderly. A population-based study in Rochester, Minnesota. *Chest*. 1997;111(2):303–310.
14. von Mutius E. Gene-environment interactions in asthma. *J Allergy Clin Immunol*. 2009;123(1):3–11.
15. Martinez FD, Vercelli D. Asthma. *Lancet*. 2013;382(9901):1360–1372.
16. Tantisira KG, Lasky-Su J, Harada M, et al. Genomewide association between GLCCI1 and response to glucocorticoid therapy in asthma. *N Engl J Med*. 2011;365(13):1173–1183.
17. Illi S, von Mutius E, Lau S, Niggemann B, Gruber C, Wahn U. Perennial allergen sensitisation early in life and chronic asthma in children: a birth cohort study. *Lancet*. 2006;368(9537):763–770.
18. Jackson DJ, Evans MD, Gangnon RE, et al. Evidence for a causal relationship between allergic sensitization and rhinovirus wheezing in early life. *Am J Respir Crit Care Med*. 2012;185(3):281–285.
19. Jackson DJ, Gangnon RE, Evans MD, et al. Wheezing rhinovirus illnesses in early life predict asthma development in high-risk children. *Am J Respir Crit Care Med*. 2008;178(7):667–672.
20. von Mutius E. 99th Dahlem conference on infection, inflammation and chronic inflammatory disorders: farm lifestyles and the hygiene hypothesis. *Clin Exp Immunol*. 2010;160(1):130–135.
21. Thacher JD, Gruzieva O, Pershagen G, et al. Pre- and postnatal exposure to parental smoking and allergic disease through adolescence. *Pediatrics*. 2014;134(3):428–434.
22. Qian Z, He Q, Kong L, et al. Respiratory responses to diverse indoor combustion air pollution sources. *Indoor Air*. 2007;17(2):135–142.
23. Patel MM, Chillrud SN, Correa JC, et al. Traffic-related particulate matter and acute respiratory symptoms among New York City area adolescents. *Environ Health Perspect*. 2010;118(9):1338–1343.
24. Brown MS, Sarnat SE, DeMuth KA, et al. Residential proximity to a major roadway is associated with features of asthma control in children. *PloS One*. 2012;7(5):e37044.
25. Sarnat SE, Raysoni AU, Li WW, et al. Air pollution and acute respiratory response in a panel of asthmatic children along the U.S.-Mexico border. *Environ Health Perspect*. 2012;120(3):437–444.
26. Zomer-Kooijker K, van der Ent CK, Ermers MJ, et al. Increased risk of wheeze and decreased lung function after respiratory syncytial virus infection. *PLos One*. 2014;9(1):e87162.
27. Ball TM, Castro-Rodriguez JA, Griffith KA, Holberg CJ, Martinez FD, Wright AL. Siblings, day-care attendance, and the risk of asthma and wheezing during childhood. *N Engl J Med*. 2000;343(8):538–543.

28. Yazdanbakhsh M, Kremsner PG, van Ree R. Allergy, parasites, and the hygiene hypothesis. *Science*. 2002; 296(5567):490–494.
29. Miller RL, Chew GL, Bell CA, et al. Prenatal exposure, maternal sensitization, and sensitization in utero to indoor allergens in an inner-city cohort. *Am J Respir Crit Care Med*. 2001;164(6):995–1001.
30. Gaffin JM, Kanchongkittiphon W, Phipatanakul W. Perinatal and early childhood environmental factors influencing allergic asthma immunopathogenesis. *Int Immunopharmacol*. 2014;22(1):21–30.
31. Rastogi D, Reddy M, Neugebauer R. Comparison of patterns of allergen sensitization among inner-city Hispanic and African American children with asthma. *Ann Allergy Asthma Immunol*. 2006;97(5):636–642.
32. Chiu CY, Huang YL, Tsai MH, et al. Sensitization to food and inhalant allergens in relation to atopic diseases in early childhood: a birth cohort study. *PloS One*. 2014;9(7):e102809.
33. Gent JF, Kezik JM, Hill ME, Tsai E, Li DW, Leaderer BP. Household mold and dust allergens: exposure, sensitization and childhood asthma morbidity. *Environ Res*. 2012;118:86–93.
34. Cunningham J, Dockery DW, Speizer FE. Maternal smoking during pregnancy as a predictor of lung function in children. *Am J Epidemiol*. 1994;139(12):1139–1152.
35. Gill R, Krishnan S, Dozor AJ. Low-level environmental tobacco smoke exposure and inflammatory biomarkers in children with asthma. *J Asthma*. 2014;51(4):355–359.
36. Valsamis C, Krishnan S, Dozor AJ. The effects of low-level environmental tobacco smoke exposure on pulmonary function tests in preschool children with asthma. *J Asthma*. 2014;51(7):685–690.
37. Brandt EB, Kovacic MB, Lee GB, et al. Diesel exhaust particle induction of IL-17A contributes to severe asthma. *J Allergy Clin Immmunol*. 2013;132(5):1194–1204.
38. Delfino RJ, Wu J, Tjoa T, Gullesserian SK, Nickerson B, Gillen DL. Asthma morbidity and ambient air pollution: effect modification by residential traffic-related air pollution. *Epidemiology*. 2014;25(1):48–57.
39. Kheirbek I, Wheeler K, Walters S, Kass D, Matte T. PM2.5 and ozone health impacts and disparities in New York City: sensitivity to spatial and temporal resolution. *Air Qual Atmos Health*. 2013;6(2):473–486.
40. Moser S, Peroni DG, Comberiati P, Piacentini GL. Asthma and viruses: is there a relationship? *Front Biosci*. 2014;6:46–54.
41. Midulla F, Nicolai A, Ferrara M, et al. Recurrent wheezing 36 months after bronchiolitis is associated with rhinovirus infections and blood eosinophilia. *Acta Paediatr*. 2014;103(10):1094–1099.
42. Saraya T, Kurai D, Ishii H, et al. Epidemiology of virus-induced asthma exacerbations: with special reference to the role of human rhinovirus. *Front Microbiol*. 2014;5:226.
43. Neuzil KM, Wright PF, Mitchel EF Jr, Griffin MR. The burden of influenza illness in children with asthma and other chronic medical conditions. *J Pediatr*. 2000;137(6):856–864.
44. Lotz MT, Moore ML, Peebles RS Jr. Respiratory syncytial virus and reactive airway disease. *Curr Top Microbiol Immunol*. 2013;372:105–118.
45. Schuster JE, Williams JV. Human metapneumovirus. *Pediatr Rev*. 2013;34(12):558–565.
46. Holgate ST, Polosa R. The mechanisms, diagnosis, and management of severe asthma in adults. *Lancet*. 2006; 368(9537):780–793.
47. Ricci M, Matucci A, Rossi O. [Bronchial asthma: pathogenetic mechanisms and genetic aspects]. *Recenti Prog Med*. 1997;88(11):530–540.
48. Gao YD, Cao J, Li P, Huang G, Yang J. Th2 cytokine-primed airway smooth muscle cells induce mast cell chemotaxis via secretion of ATP. *J Asthma*. 2014;51(10): 997–1003.
49. Bang BR, Chun E, Shim EJ, et al. Alveolar macrophages modulate allergic inflammation in a murine model of asthma. *Exp Mol Med*. 2011;43(5):275–280.
50. Silberstein DS, David JR. The regulation of human eosinophil function by cytokines. *Immunol Today*. 1987; 8(12):380–385.
51. Nakagome K, Nagata M. Pathogenesis of airway inflammation in bronchial asthma. *Auris Nasus Larynx*. 2011; 38(5):555–563.
52. Renauld JC. New insights into the role of cytokines in asthma. *J Clin Pathol*. 2001;54(8):577–589.
53. Scott JA, Grasemann H. Arginine metabolism in asthma. *Immunol Allergy Clin North Am*. 2014;34(4):767–775.
54. Shin K, Hwang JJ, Kwon BI, Kheradmand F, Corry DB, Lee SH. Leukotriene enhanced allergic lung inflammation through induction of chemokine production. *Clin Exp Med*. 2014. [Epub ahead of print].
55. Back M, Bu DX, Branstrom R, Sheikine Y, Yan ZQ, Hansson GK. Leukotriene B4 signaling through NF-kappaB-dependent BLT1 receptors on vascular smooth muscle cells in atherosclerosis and intimal hyperplasia. *Proc Natl Acad Sci USA*. 2005;102(48):17501–17506.
56. Theron AJ, Steel HC, Tintinger GR, Gravett CM, Anderson R, Feldman C. Cysteinyl leukotriene receptor-1 antagonists as modulators of innate immune cell function. *J Immunol Res*. 2014;2014:608930.
57. Mehrotra AK, Henderson WR, Jr. The role of leukotrienes in airway remodeling. *Curr Mol Med*. 2009;9(3):383–391.
58. Royce SG, Patel KP, Samuel CS. Characterization of a novel model incorporating airway epithelial damage and related fibrosis to the pathogenesis of asthma. *Lab Invest*. 2014;94(12):1326–1339.
59. Traub S, Nikonova A, Carruthers A, et al. An anti-human ICAM-1 antibody inhibits rhinovirus-induced exacerbations of lung inflammation. *PLoS Pathogens*. 2013;9(8):e1003520.
60. Voynow JA, Young LR, Wang Y, Horger T, Rose MC, Fischer BM. Neutrophil elastase increases MUC5AC mRNA and protein expression in respiratory epithelial cells. *Am J Physiol*. 1999;276(5, pt 1):L835–843.
61. Taussig LM, Wright AL, Holberg CJ, Halonen M, Morgan WJ, Martinez FD. Tucson Children's Respiratory

Study: 1980 to present. *J Allergy Clin Immunol*. 2003;111(4):661–675; quiz 676.
62. Phelan PD, Robertson CF, Olinsky A. The Melbourne Asthma Study: 1964–1999. *J Allergy Clin Immunol*. 2002;109(2):189–194.
63. Keil T, Kulig M, Simpson A, et al. European birth cohort studies on asthma and atopic diseases: I. Comparison of study designs—a GALEN initiative. *Allergy*. 2006;61(2):221–228.
64. Martinez FD, Wright AL, Taussig LM, Holberg CJ, Halonen M, Morgan WJ. Asthma and wheezing in the first six years of life. The Group Health Medical Associates. *N Engl J Med*. 1995;332(3):133–138.
65. Stein RT, Martinez FD. Asthma phenotypes in childhood: lessons from an epidemiological approach. *Paediatr Respir Rev*. 2004;5(2):155–161.
66. Hurwitz SH. Nonallergic asthma; differential diagnosis and treatment. *Calif Med*. 1955;83(2):61–67.
67. Lee RU, Stevenson DD. Aspirin-exacerbated respiratory disease: evaluation and management. *Allergy Asthma Immunol Res*. 2011;3(1):3–10.
68. Krafczyk MA, Asplund CA. Exercise-induced bronchoconstriction: diagnosis and management. *Am Fam Physician*. 2011;84(4):427–434.
69. Beckett WS. Occupational respiratory diseases. *N Engl J Med*. 2000;342(6):406–413.
70. Moore WC, Meyers DA, Wenzel SE, et al. Identification of asthma phenotypes using cluster analysis in the Severe Asthma Research Program. *Am J Respir Crit Care Med*. 2010;181(4):315–323.
71. Castro-Rodríguez JA, Holberg CJ, Wright AL, Martinez FD. A clinical index to define risk of asthma in young children with recurrent wheezing. *Am J Resp Crit Care Med*. 2000;162(4, pt 1):1403–1406.
72. Esteban CA, Klein RB, Kopel SJ, et al. Underdiagnosed and undertreated allergic rhinitis in urban school-aged children with asthma. *Pediatr Allergy Immunol Pulmonol*. 2014;27(2):75–81.
73. Yilmaz O, Bakirtas A, Ertoy Karagol HI, Topal E, Demirsoy MS. Allergic rhinitis may impact the recovery of pulmonary function tests after moderate/severe asthma exacerbation in children. *Allergy*. 2014;69(5):652–657.
74. Boulay ME, Morin A, Laprise C, Boulet LP. Asthma and rhinitis: what is the relationship? *Curr Opin Allergy Clin Immunol*. 2012;12(5):449–454.
75. Balson BM, Kravitz EK, McGeady SJ. Diagnosis and treatment of gastroesophageal reflux in children and adolescents with severe asthma. *Ann Allergy Asthma Immunol*. 1998;81(2):159–164.
76. Valet RS, Carroll KN, Gebretsadik T, et al. Gastroesophageal reflux disease increases infant acute respiratory illness severity, but not childhood asthma. *Pediatr Allergy Immunol Pulmonol*. 2014;27(1):30–33.
77. Khoshoo V, Le T, Haydel RM, Jr., Landry L, Nelson C. Role of gastroesophageal reflux in older children with persistent asthma. *Chest*. 2003;123(4):1008–1013.
78. Gunnbjörnsdóttir MI, Omenaas E, Gíslason T, et al. Obesity and nocturnal gastro-oesophageal reflux are related to onset of asthma and respiratory symptoms. *Eur Resp J*. 2004;24(1):116–121.
79. Blake K, Teague WG. Gastroesophageal reflux disease and childhood asthma. *Curr Opin Pulm Med*. 2013;19(1):24–29.
80. Chinn S, Rona RJ. Obesity and asthma in children. *Am J Respir Crit Care Med*. 2004;170(1):95; author reply 95–96.
81. Figueroa-Munoz JI, Chinn S, Rona RJ. Association between obesity and asthma in 4–11 year old children in the UK. *Thorax*. 2001;56(2):133–137.
82. Beuther DA, Sutherland ER. Overweight, obesity, and incident asthma: a meta-analysis of prospective epidemiologic studies. *Am J Respir Crit Care Med*. 2007;175(7):661–666.
83. Belamarich PF, Luder E, Kattan M, et al. Do obese inner-city children with asthma have more symptoms than nonobese children with asthma? *Pediatrics*. 2000;106(6):1436–1441.
84. Forno E, Lescher R, Strunk R, Weiss S, Fuhlbrigge A, Celedón JC. Decreased response to inhaled steroids in overweight and obese asthmatic children. *J Allergy Clin Immunol*. 2011;127(3):741–749.
85. Vo P, Makker K, Matta-Arroyo E, Hall CB, Arens R, Rastogi D. The association of overweight and obesity with spirometric values in minority children referred for asthma evaluation. *J Asthma*. 2013;50(1):56–63.
86. Rastogi D, Canfield S, Andrade A, et al. Obesity-associated asthma in children: A distinct entity. *Chest*. 2012;141(4):895–905.
87. Rastogi D, Bhalani K, Hall CB, Isasi CR. Association of pulmonary function with adiposity and metabolic abnormalities in urban minority adolescents. *Ann Amer Thor Soc*. 2014;11(5):744–752.
88. Nagel G, Koenig W, Rapp K, Wabitsch M, Zoellner I, Weiland SK. Associations of adipokines with asthma, rhinoconjunctivitis, and eczema in German schoolchildren. *Pediatr Allergy Immunol*. 2009;20(1):81–88.
89. Jensen ME, Gibson PG, Collins CE, Hilton JM, Wood LG. Diet-induced weight loss in obese children with asthma: a randomized controlled trial. *Clin Exp Allergy*. 2013;43(7):775–784.
90. *Expert Panel Report 3: Guidelines for the Diagnosis and Management of Asthma*. Bethesda, MD: National Institutes of Health, National Heart, Lung, and Blood Institute; 2007.
91. Lemanske RF Jr, Busse WW. Asthma: clinical expression and molecular mechanisms. *J Allergy Clin Immmunol*. 2010;125(2, suppl 2):S95–S102.
92. Ritz T, Bobb C, Griffiths C. Predicting asthma control: the role of psychological triggers. *Allergy Asthma Proc*. 2014;35(5):390–397.
93. van Erp N, Little P, Stuart B, et al. Influence of lung function on course of disease and response to antibiotic therapy in adult primary care patients with acute cough: a post hoc analysis of patients enrolled in a prospective multicentre study. *NPJ Prim Care Respir Med*. 2014;24:14067.

94. Schatz M, Sorkness CA, Li JT, et al. Asthma Control Test: reliability, validity, and responsiveness in patients not previously followed by asthma specialists. *J Allergy Clin Immunol*. 2006;117(3):549–556.
95. Bickel S, Popler J, Lesnick B, Eid N. Impulse oscillometry: interpretation and practical applications. *Chest*. 2014;146(3):841–847.
96. Rosenfeld M, Allen J, Arets BH, et al. An official American Thoracic Society workshop report: optimal lung function tests for monitoring cystic fibrosis, bronchopulmonary dysplasia, and recurrent wheezing in children less than 6 years of age. *Ann Am Thorac Soc*. 2013;10(2):S1–S11.
97. Mazi A, Lands LC. Effect of lowering methacholine challenge test cutoff in children. *Ann Allergy Asthma Immunol*. 2014;113(4):393–397.
98. Johnson JD, Theurer WM. A stepwise approach to the interpretation of pulmonary function tests. *Am Fam Physician*. 2014;89(5):359–366.
99. Cockcroft DW. Direct challenge tests: Airway hyperresponsiveness in asthma: its measurement and clinical significance. *Chest*. 2010;138(2, suppl):18S–24S.
100. Silkoff PE, Lent AM, Busacker AA, et al. Exhaled nitric oxide identifies the persistent eosinophilic phenotype in severe refractory asthma. *J Allergy Clin Immunol*. 2005; 116(6):1249–1255.
101. Bjermer L, Alving K, Diamant Z, et al. Current evidence and future research needs for FeNO measurement in respiratory diseases. *Respir Med*. 2014;108(6): 830–841.
102. Harkins MS, Fiato KL, Iwamoto GK. Exhaled nitric oxide predicts asthma exacerbation. *J Asthma*. 2004;41(4): 471–476.
103. Corren J, Lemanske RF, Hanania NA, et al. Lebrikizumab treatment in adults with asthma. *N Engl J Med*. 2011;365(12):1088–1098.
104. Papiris SA, Manali ED, Kolilekas L, Triantafillidou C, Tsangaris I. Acute severe asthma: new approaches to assessment and treatment. *Drugs*. 2009;69(17):2363–2391.
105. Busse WW, Morgan WJ, Gergen PJ, et al. Randomized trial of omalizumab (anti-IgE) for asthma in inner-city children. *N Engl J Med*. 2011;364(11):1005–1015.
106. Wright LS, Phipatanakul W. Environmental remediation in the treatment of allergy and asthma: latest updates. *Curr Allergy Asthma Rep*. 2014;14(3):419.
107. Carden KA, Boiselle PM, Waltz DA, Ernst A. Tracheomalacia and tracheobronchomalacia in children and adults: an in-depth review. *Chest*. 2005;127(3):984–1005.
108. Celli BR, MacNee W, Force AET. Standards for the diagnosis and treatment of patients with COPD: a summary of the ATS/ERS position paper. *Eur Respir J*. 2004;23(6): 932–946.
109. Qaseem A, Wilt TJ, Weinberger SE, et al. Diagnosis and management of stable chronic obstructive pulmonary disease: a clinical practice guideline update from the American College of Physicians, American College of Chest Physicians, American Thoracic Society, and European Respiratory Society. *Ann Intern Med*. 2011;155(3): 179–191.
110. Zoumot Z, Wilson R. Respiratory infection in noncystic fibrosis bronchiectasis. *Curr Opin Infect Dis*. 2010;23(2): 165–170.
111. Seitz AE, Olivier KN, Adjemian J, Holland SM, Prevots R. Trends in bronchiectasis among medicare beneficiaries in the United States, 2000 to 2007. *Chest*. 2012;142(2): 432–439.
112. King PT, Holdsworth SR, Freezer NJ, Villanueva E, Holmes PW. Microbiologic follow-up study in adult bronchiectasis. *Respir Med*. 2007;101(8):1633–1638.
113. Aronchick JM, Miller WT, Jr. Bronchiectasis. *J Thorac Imaging*. 1995;10(4):255–267.
114. King PT, Holdsworth SR, Freezer NJ, Villanueva E, Holmes PW. Characterisation of the onset and presenting clinical features of adult bronchiectasis. *Respir Med*. 2006;100(12):2183–2189.
115. Wong C, Jayaram L, Karalus N, et al. Azithromycin for prevention of exacerbations in non-cystic fibrosis bronchiectasis (EMBRACE): a randomised, double-blind, placebo-controlled trial. *Lancet*. 2012;380(9842): 660–667.
116. Shah A, Panjabi C. Allergic aspergillosis of the respiratory tract. *Eur Respir Rev*. 2014;23(131):8–29.
117. Stevens DA, Moss RB, Kurup VP, et al. Allergic bronchopulmonary aspergillosis in cystic fibrosis—state of the art: Cystic Fibrosis Foundation Consensus Conference. *Clin Infect Dis*. 2003;37 (suppl 3):S225–S264.
118. Greenberger PA. Allergic bronchopulmonary aspergillosis. *J Allergy Clin Immunol*. 2002;110(5):685–692.
119. Lehmann S, Pfannenstiel C, Friedrichs F, Kroger K, Wagner N, Tenbrock K. Omalizumab: a new treatment option for allergic bronchopulmonary aspergillosis in patients with cystic fibrosis. *Ther Adv Respir Dis*. 2014; 8(5):141–149.
120. Fanen P, Wohlhuter-Haddad A, Hinzpeter A. Genetics of cystic fibrosis: CFTR mutation classifications toward genotype-based CF therapies. *Int J Biochem Cell Biol*. 2014;52:94–102.
121. O'Sullivan BP, Freedman SD. Cystic fibrosis. *Lancet*. 2009;373(9678):1891–1904.
122. Rogan MP, Stoltz DA, Hornick DB. Cystic fibrosis transmembrane conductance regulator intracellular processing, trafficking, and opportunities for mutation-specific treatment. *Chest*. 2011;139(6):1480–1490.
123. Accurso FJ, Sontag MK, Wagener JS. Complications associated with symptomatic diagnosis in infants with cystic fibrosis. *J Pediatr*. 2005;147(3, suppl):S37–S41.
124. Gilljam M, Ellis L, Corey M, Zielenski J, Durie P, Tullis DE. Clinical manifestations of cystic fibrosis among patients with diagnosis in adulthood. *Chest*. 2004;126(4): 1215–1224.
125. Conway SP, Watson A. Nebulised bronchodilators, corticosteroids, and rhDNase in adult patients with cystic fibrosis. *Thorax*. 1997;52(suppl 2):S64–S68.
126. Hoyte FC. Vocal cord dysfunction. *Immunol Allergy Clin North Am*. 2013;33(1):1–22.

127. Nolan PK, Chrysler M, Phillips G, Goodman D, Rusakow LS. Pulse oximetry coupled with spirometry in the emergency department helps differentiate an asthma exacerbation from possible vocal cord dysfunction. *Pediatr Pulmonol*. 2007;42(7):605–609.
128. Corren J, Newman KB. Vocal cord dysfunction mimicking bronchial asthma. *Postgrad Med*. 1992;92(6):153–156.
129. Newman KB DS. Vocal Cord Dysfunction: masquerader of asthma. *D Semin Respir Crit Care Med*. 1994;15:161–167.
130. Lacy TJ, McManis SE. Psychogenic stridor. *Gen Hosp Psychiatry*. 1994;16(3):213–223.
131. Newman KB, Mason UG, 3rd, Schmaling KB. Clinical features of vocal cord dysfunction. *Am J Respir Crit Care Medicine*. 1995;152(4, pt 1):1382–1386.
132. Mathers-Schmidt BA. Paradoxical vocal fold motion: a tutorial on a complex disorder and the speech-language pathologist's role. *Am J Speech Lang Pathol*. 2001;10: 111–125.
133. Rundell KW, Spiering BA. Inspiratory stridor in elite athletes. *Chest*. 2003;123(2):468–474.
134. Morris MJ AP, Perkins PJ. Vocal cord dysfunction: etiologies and treatment. *Clin Pulmonary Med*. 2006;13(2): 73–86.

7

Urticaria and Angioedema

Luz Fonacier and Mark Davis-Lorton

INTRODUCTION

Urticaria is a common condition, occurring both in adults and children, although less frequently in the latter. The lifetime prevalence rate of urticaria is 8.8% for all types of urticaria and the lifetime prevalence for chronic urticaria is 1.8%.[1] The incidence in children varies from 2% to 8% in those living in Scandinavian countries to as high as 23.5% in India. Angioedema —swelling of the lips, eyes, cheeks, and tongue—can also coexist in adults and children with urticaria.

Patients with recurrent angioedema without associated urticaria should be evaluated for ACE inhibitor associated angioedema, hereditary angioedema (HAE), or acquired C1 inhibitor deficiency (AAE). The management of these patients is substantially different from patients with chronic idiopathic urticaria (CIU). This chapter focuses on the diagnosis, and management of angioedema and urticaria that may be encountered by otolaryngologists.

URTICARIA

Definition

Acute urticaria and angioedema is differentiated from CIU and angioedema by the duration of symptoms. Acute urticaria and angioedema occurs for less than 6 weeks and is often, but not always, related to mast cell and basophil activation. Chronic urticaria and angioedema occurs for at least 6 weeks (either continuously or intermittently) and is less likely to be associated with an underlying cause. The associated angioedema in these patients may occur independently of the urticaria.

> Acute urticaria and angioedema are defined as hives and swelling present for less than 6 weeks in duration. Chronic urticaria and angioedema are defined as hives and swelling present for at least 6 weeks in duration (continuously or intermittently).

ACUTE URTICARIA

Diagnosis

Acute urticaria and angioedema are often associated with a specific cause or trigger which includes physical factors (eg, cold, pressure, heat, or solar radiation), allergens (eg, food, medication, latex), toxins (eg, scombroid fish), and infections.[2,3] In most cases, the specific trigger of the symptoms can be elicited through a detailed history.

Diagnostic tests include skin testing or laboratory evaluation for food allergens or aeroallergens. Testing for specific food allergens should be supported by the history that is compatible with an IgE-mediated pathogenesis. Skin testing involves application of an allergen extract onto the skin which is then pricked by a sharp device allowing the extract to enter the epidermis where it can encounter mast cells. This can lead to the release of histamine, forming a characteristic urticarial lesion with a wheal and flare if the individual is allergic to the extract (reviewed in Chapter 3). Skin testing should be performed after resolution of an acute episode of hives. The patient must also be off H1 antihistamines for several days, based on the half-life of the specific medication, to avoid obtaining a false-negative skin test result. Even if associated with a viral or other infectious illness,[4,5] extensive evaluation for the specific pathogens (or antiviral therapy) is usually not indicated (Table 7–1).

> Acute urticaria and angioedema are often associated with a specific trigger such as physical factors (eg, cold, pressure, heat, or solar radiation), allergens (eg, food, medication, latex), toxins (eg, scombroid fish) or infections.

Management of Acute Urticaria

Management of acute urticaria includes identification of specific triggers as suggested by a careful history, and focused diagnostic testing combined with symptomatic treatment. Medications thought to be causing urticaria or angioedema should be withheld to see if symptoms resolve. If testing for the relevant food allergen is positive, the culprit foods should also be avoided and an autoinjectable epinephrine should be prescribed and the patient educated on its use.

Antihistamines

H1 antihistamines are the first-line therapy for acute urticaria. First-generation antihistamines (eg, diphenhydramine, hydroxyzine), although more rapidly acting, may be associated with sedation and impaired motor skills, but it may be useful in cases where urticaria interferes with sleep. Nonsedating or low sedating, also known as "second- or third-generation" antihistamines (eg, loratadine, desloratadine, fexofenedine, cetirizine, levocetirizine) have limited transfer across the blood-brain barrier and are therefore less sedating than first-generation antihistamines. The low-sedating antihistamines have all been shown to be effective for urticaria. The differences among antihistamines are summarized in Table 7–2.

More potent antihistamines, such as doxepin, may also be effective for patients who fail conventional (or higher) doses of US Food and Drug

Table 7–1. Causes and Diagnostic Test for Acute Urticaria and Angioedema

Cause	Diagnostic Test
Physical urticaria	See separate table
Food allergies (IgE mediated)	Skin prick test or specific IgE in the blood
Contact urticaria (eg, plant, animal)	Challenge if appropriate
Medications (eg, opiates, ACE inhibitors, NSAIDS)	Skin test if available (eg, penicillin skin test) Challenge if appropriate
Papular urticaria due to insect bite (eg, scabies, fleas)	Skin scraping for scabies
Infection (eg, Parvovirus B-19, Epstein-Barr virus)	Serology if available and appropriate
Food toxin (eg, scombroid)	No specific test available; diagnosis by history

Table 7–2. Characteristics of Low-Sedating or Second- and Third-Generation H1 Antihistamines

Drug	Adult Dose	Pediatric Dose	Pregnancy Category	Metabolism Excretion	Dosage in Kidney and Hepatic Failure
Cetirizine (Zyrtec)	10 mg OD	6 mo–6 yr: 2.5–5 mg >6 yr: 5 mg OD	B	Kidney	K: 5 mg OD H: 5 mg OD
Levocetirizine (Xyzal)	5 mg OD	6 mo–5 yr: 1.25 mg 6–11 yr: 2.5 mg	B	Kidney	K: 2.5 mg OD to EOD H: none
Fexofenadine (Allegra)	180 mg OD	6–11 yr: 30 mg BID	C	Kidney	K: 60 mg OD H: none
Desloratadine (Clarinex)	5 mg OD	6 mo: 2 mg OD 12 yr: 5 mg OD	C	Liver	K: 5 mg EOD H: 5 mg EOD
Loratadine (Claritin)	10 mg OD	2–5 yr: 5 mg OD	B	Liver	K: 10 mg EOD H: 10 mg EOD

Note. K = kidney; *H* = hepatic; *OD* = once a day, *EOD* = every other day.

Administration (FDA)–approved antihistamines. In patients with severe acute urticaria and angioedema not responding to H1-antihistamines, a trial of a brief course of oral corticosteroids may be considered. A randomized, controlled study in adults showed that the time to resolution of acute urticaria was decreased with the addition of oral corticosteroids to antihistamines in an emergency department.[6]

If associated with other signs and symptoms such as wheezing, cough, vomiting, diarrhea, dizziness, loss of consciousness, or changes in blood pressure or heart rate, the diagnosis of anaphylaxis must be considered and epinephrine would be the drug of choice. The otolaryngologist may be asked to evaluate for the presence of laryngeal swelling.

CHRONIC URTICARIA (CU)

Clinical Characteristics

Chronic urticaria are hives that persist for at least 6 weeks. The prevalence of CU in the general population has been estimated to range from 0.5% to 5%, with most studies showing an increased prevalence in females.[7,8] No underlying cause is found in more than 60% of CU, and it is termed *chronic idiopathic urticaria*. About 40% to 50% of patients have both urticaria and angioedema occurring simultaneously or separately, another 40% to 50% have urticaria alone, and 10% to 20% have angioedema alone.[8,9] Patients with angioedema without concomitant urticaria may need further evaluation for C1inhibitor deficiency and this will be discussed in a separate section of this chapter. If the patient is taking an ACE inhibitor, discontinuation of this drug may be necessary as the differential diagnosis for angioedema without urticaria also includes ACE inhibitor-associated angioedema.

> Most cases of chronic urticaria and angioedema do not have an identifiable cause or trigger.

Diagnosis

In the evaluation of a patient with CU, one should remember that most cases of CU do not have an identifiable cause. Foods, drugs, or other allergens, though common causes of acute urticaria, are rarely associated with CU. Recurrent acute urticaria from medication or food would resolve once the trigger is removed. Although chronic infectious processes (eg, hepatitis B and C, Epstein-Barr virus, herpes simplex virus, and helminthic parasitic infections) have been reported in the literature as causes of CU, their incidence in cases of CIU is not well established.

In addition, there are no convincing data that associate occult infections such as *Helicobacter pylori*, chronic sinusitis, or cutaneous fungal infections[10,11] with CU. Chronic urticaria may present as an initial clinical manifestation of an underlying systemic illness such as a specific complement component deficiency, cryoglobulinemia (eg, associated with hepatitis C, chronic lymphocytic leukemia), serum sickness, connective tissue diseases (eg, systemic lupus erythematous, juvenile rheumatoid arthritis), hypothyroidism, hyperthyroidism, neoplasms (eg, lymphoreticular malignancy and lymphoproliferative disorders), and other endocrine disorders (eg, ovarian tumors).

Diagnostic Tests

Autoantibody Tests. The presence of autoantibodies that are associated with urticaria has prompted the term *autoantibody associated urticaria*. These autoantibodies include antibodies to thyroid peroxidase, thyroglobulin,[12,13] rheumatoid factor, anti-dsDNA, anti-SSA/SSB, ENA profile, anti-cardiolipin, anti-beta 2-glycoprotein 1, anti-myeloperoxidase, anti-proteinase-3, anti-smooth muscle, and ANA. The presence of these autoantibodies, however, does not carry any etiologic, therapeutic, or prognostic value. Serological testing for these autoantibodies is therefore not warranted unless the history and associated symptoms (eg, joint pains, myalgias, heat or cold intolerance) suggest the presence of an underlying systemic illness.

Up to 50% of CU patients have autoantibodies to FcεRIα, a component of the high-affinity IgE receptor, whereas 10% of CU patients have autoantibodies to the IgE molecule. It has been suggested that cross-linking of mast cell IgE receptors by an IgG antibody to the FcεRIα subunit results in the release of bioactive mediators such as histamine.[14–16] The autologous serum skin test (ASST) and the autologous plasma skin test (APST) have been proposed as screening tests to identify patients with autoantibody associated urticaria. This involves injection of the patient's own serum or plasma into their skin and observing for a wheal and flare reaction. There are also commercial in vitro assays that can measure basophil histamine release from the patient's serum. The ASST, APST, and basophil histamine release assay, however, cannot identify the distinct subgroup involved on the IgE molecule. Because these tests do not influence the management of CU, current evidence does not support the routine use of these tests in CU.

Inhalants, Foods, and/or Other Laboratory Testing. The history and physical exam findings should guide the diagnostic testing in patients with CU. Patients with an unremarkable history do not need to undergo skin or in vitro IgE testing to inhalants and/or foods. They also do not require extensive laboratory testing. Laboratory abnormalities identified in routine testing do not usually lead to changes in management and are not associated with improved patient care outcomes.[17]

If, however, the history or physical exam is suggestive of an underlying systemic process (eg, joint pains, photosensitivity, or malar rash), limited and targeted testing is warranted (eg, ANA). In rare instances, limited and selective testing may be done if an underlying condition may not be discernible by history or physical examination findings, or to provide "reassurance" for the patient and family members. Although the utility of performing these tests routinely for CU patients has not been established, the Practice Parameters Task Force on the Diagnosis and Management of Acute and Chronic Urticaria: 2014 Update states that a limited panel of routine laboratory tests can be considered for patients with CU without atypical features (eg, complete blood count with differential, erythrocyte sedimentation rate, liver enzymes, and thyroid-stimulating hormone).[18]

Treatment of Chronic Urticaria

H1 Antihistamines

Both first- and second-generation H1-antihistamines have been shown to be safe and effective for the treatment of acute and chronic urticaria, and remain the first-line agents for patients with CU. Second-generation H1-antihistamines are equally effective as first-generation antihistamines[19–23] with fewer side effects and are preferred for long-term treatment and dose escalation in CU. Daily dosing of antihistamines is more effective than intermittent dosing in improving a patient's quality of life.[24]

Many CU patients, however, continue to have hives with conventional, FDA-approved doses of second-generation antihistamines. Higher doses of second-generation antihistamines are commonly given and may be more efficacious, although data are limited and conflicting for certain agents (Figure 7–1).

> The first-line treatment of chronic urticaria and angioedema is use of second-generation H1-antihistamines.

H2-Antihistamines

The addition of H2-antihistamines to H1-antihistamines has been reported to be more effective compared to H1-antihistamines alone. Most studies demonstrating efficacy have used cimetidine, which may affect the metabolism of first-generation antihistamines by increasing their concentration. Since these agents are well tolerated, this treatment option may be considered.

Leukotriene Modifiers

Several randomized controlled studies have shown efficacy of leukotriene receptor antagonists in CU. Since they are generally well tolerated, they may be used in patients with unsatisfactory responses to second-generation H1-antihistamines. Most studies show that thc benefit of leukotriene receptor antagonists may take weeks to occur after its initiation. Leukotriene receptor antagonists may be beneficial in nonsteroidal anti-inflammatory drug (NSAID)-exacerbated CIU,[25] some physical urticarias (eg, cold urticarial,[26] delayed pressure urticaria), and angioedema.[27]

Antidepressants With H1 and H2 Antagonist Activity

Doxepin, a tricyclic antidepressant, is a potent H1 and H2 antagonist. In vitro studies show that it is 775 times more potent than diphenhydramine in antagonizing the H1 receptor.[28] It has both sedating

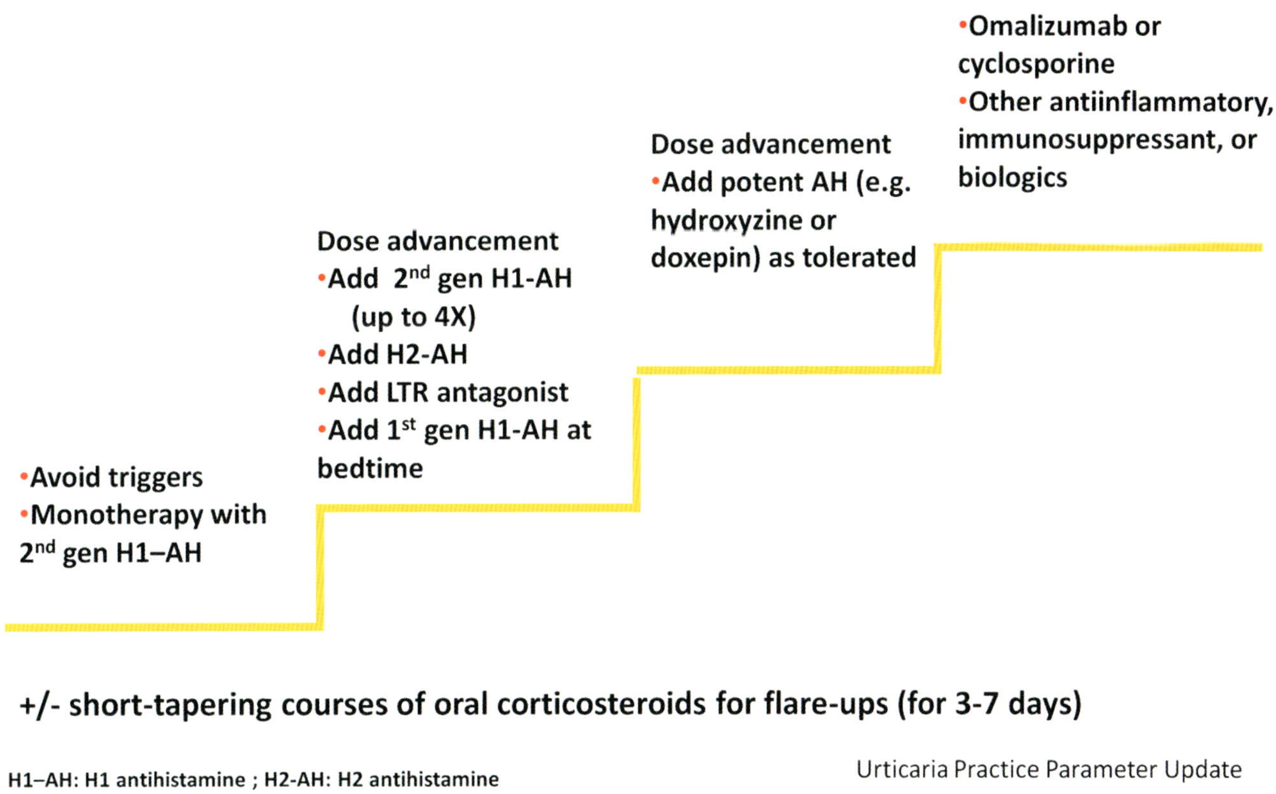

Figure 7-1. Treatment algorithm for severe refractory chronic urticaria.

and prominent anticholinergic properties. Because of its long half-life of 13 hours and sedating properties,[29] Doxepin is given preferably at bedtime.

Omalizumab

In March 2014, the FDA approved omalizumab (Xolair) for the treatment of CU in adults and adolescents (12 years of age and above) who remain symptomatic despite H1-antihistamine treatment. Until then, H1-antihistamines were the only FDA-approved therapy for CU in the United States.

Omalizumab is a recombinant humanized monoclonal antibody that binds to free IgE and inhibits binding of IgE to FcεRI, the high-affinity IgE receptor. Omalizumab reduces the number of FcεRI receptors on the surface of mast cells and basophils.[30]

Two phase III studies, ASTERIA I and II, that involved CIU patients not responding to approved doses of H1-antihistamines, found that omalizumab 300 mg and 150 mg significantly improved symptoms of itch and hives. Patients noted rapid relief of itching and, in many cases, complete resolution of urticaria symptoms. Quality of life was also significantly improved for patients treated with omalizumab 300 mg.[31,32] Recurrence of urticaria/angioedema was seen in the majority of patients after discontinuation of omalizumab.

Omalizumab is administered as a subcutaneous injection on a regular basis under supervision in a physician's office. Because it is a costly medication, insurance coverage may be limited.

Anaphylaxis has been reported in patients receiving omalizumab. The reaction can occur after the first dose, or after several doses. It may also occur immediately after an injection or few days later. For patients who are receiving omalizumab, it is therefore important to prescribe self-injectable epinephrine and educate them about its proper use.

Systemic Corticosteroids

Systemic corticosteroids are frequently used in CU patients refractory to H1- antihistamine treatment. Although there are conflicting studies regarding its efficacy, short-term use (eg, 1 to 3 weeks duration) may be required to control CU until other therapies can achieve control. Long-term use in CU patients should be avoided because of its serious adverse effects such as weight gain, fluid retention, mood changes, insomnia, risk of infection, hyperglycemia, osteoporosis, risk of fracture, avascular necrosis, cataracts, and adrenal suppression.

Calcineurin Inhibitors

The efficacy of cyclosporine for refractory CU has been observed in multiple randomized, double-blinded, controlled trials.[33–35] Cyclosporine down-regulates Th1 responses and T-cell-dependent antibody generation by B lymphocytes, thus inhibiting the release of histamine and other mediators from mast cells and basophils.[36] The cyclosporine dose used in these trials was initially 4 to 5 mg/kg followed by a tapering regimen. Side effects of cyclosporine include renal dysfunction, tremor, hirsuitism, hypertension, gum hyperplasia, and an increased risk of developing infection or cancer (in particular, lymphoma and skin cancer). Drug-drug interactions also need to be considered before prescribing cyclosporine to patients since other drugs may affect the metabolism of cyclosporine. These medications include amphotericin B, cimetidine, ciprofloxacin, colchicine, fenofibrate, gemfibrozil, gentamicin, ketoconazole, melphalan, some nonsteroidal anti-inflammatory agents, ranitidine, tobramycin, trimethoprim with sulfamethoxazole, and vancomycin. Periodic and regular clinical and laboratory monitoring is also required to monitor for systemic side effects.

Alternative Therapies

Up to 50% of CU patients may not achieve satisfactory control with antihistamine therapy alone,[37] so other agents with immunosuppressant or immunomodulatory activity have been used, such as dapsone, sulfasalazine, hydroxychloroquine, and colchicine. There is limited evidence on the efficacy of these medications for CU, and laboratory monitoring is often required due to the risk of systemic side effects.

Dapsone. Case reports and case series suggest the benefit of dapsone in CIU, idiopathic angioedema, delayed pressure urticaria and angioedema, and urticarial vasculitis.[38–40] The side effects of dapsone include anemia, peripheral neuropathy, rash, gastrointestinal complaints, hepatotoxicity, and, rarely, methemoglobinemia, blood dyscrasias, or the syndrome of drug rash with eosinophilia and systemic symptoms (DRESS). It is recommended to obtain a glucose-6-phosphate dehydrogenase (G6PD) level prior to initiation of dapsone as G6PD-deficient patients have an increased risk of severe hemolysis. Ongoing laboratory monitoring for anemia and hepatotoxicity is recommended.

Sulfasalazine. Sulfasalazine decreases prostaglandin D2 synthesis and histamine release from activated mast cells. Case reports and case series have also suggested efficacy of sulfasalazine in patients with CU and delayed pressure urticaria and angioedema[41,42] Side effects include nausea, vomiting, dyspepsia, anorexia, and headache. Laboratory monitoring for hematologic abnormalities, proteinuria, and hepatotoxicity is recommended.

Hydroxychloroquine. There are limited data available on the use of hydroxychloroquine in CU. It is, however, generally well tolerated though the risk of retinopathy is the most worrisome side effect. This occurrence is rare and usually develops in patients who have used the drug for more than 5 years and with dosages greater than 6.5 mg/kg/day. The American Academy of Ophthalmology recommends a baseline ocular examination within the first year of therapy and annual screening after 5 years of therapy.[43]

Other Agents. Other agents that have been used in CU include colchicine, tacrolimus, mycophenolate, sirolimus, tumor necrosis factor inhibitors (etanercept and infliximab), anakinra, rituximab, phototherapy, attenuated androgens, anticoagulants, NSAIDs, beta-agonists, cyclophosphamide, gold, plasmapheresis, stanozolol, cromolyn, theophylline, and nifedipine. There are limited data on the efficacy of these drugs. The data on the role of allergen immunotherapy, herbal therapies, vitamins, supplements, and acupuncture in CU are even more limited. There is also limited evidence to support the role of "pseudoallergens" (artificial preservatives, dyes, naturally occurring histamine, aromatic compounds in certain foods, wine, tomatoes, and spice; phenols such as *p*-hydroxybenzoic acid, citrus and orange oil, and salicylates) in CU.

> Recalcitrant chronic urticaria and angioedema can be treated with higher doses of H1-antihistamines, omalizumab, H2-antihistamines, leukotriene modifiers, or other immunomodulating drugs.

PHYSICAL URTICARIA

Urticaria triggered exclusively by specific physical causes (eg, heat, cold, pressure, light or vibration) is considered to be a distinct entity. However, physical urticaria commonly occurs concomitantly with CIU, and these patients may be less likely to respond to conventional treatment.[44,45] Delayed pressure urticaria and angioedema have been described in up to 30% of patients with CU.[46]

Dermatographism is the most common physical urticaria. Cholinergic urticaria accounts for approximately 5% of all CU cases but 30% of all physical urticaria cases.[47] The other physical urticaria/angioedema syndromes such as cold urticaria, solar urticaria, vibratory angioedema, and aquagenic urticaria are less common.[45] However, because the face and neck area are commonly exposed to cold air and UV light, cold and solar urticaria may be encountered in an ENT practice.

Dermographism

Individuals with dermographism (also known as dermatographism, dermographia, and dermatographia) develop a prompt wheal and flare response when pressure is applied to the skin. The wheal and flare reaction can be elicited by stroking the skin with a firm object, such as a tongue blade. Most patients have mild symptoms and do not seek medical attention. Interestingly, there is one case report of familial dermographism on the face.[48] Treatment is focused on avoidance measures, skin hydration (to reduce skin pruritus), and antihistamines for symptomatic relief. Both first- and second-generation H1 antihistamines have been shown to improve the urticaria.[49,50] More severe cases may require alternative therapies like UV-B light therapy which has been reported to be effective in dermatographism.[51]

Delayed Pressure Urticaria and Angioedema

Patients with delayed pressure urticaria develop erythematous and painful swelling within 4 to 6 hours (but can be as long as 12 to 24 hours) after pressure stimuli. Patients may also report associated symptoms of arthralgias, malaise, fever, rigors, and lassitude.[52] Elevation in erythrocyte sedimentation rate has also been reported.[53] Diagnosis of delayed pressure urticaria and angioedema is confirmed by a challenge with a 15-pound (6.8 kg) weight suspended from the patient's shoulder for 10 or 15 minutes. A painful wheal will develop at the site between 2 to 12 hours after the pressure stimulus; however, it is typically observed between 4 and 6.5 hours.[54] Similar to other physical urticarias, avoidance of the trigger is critical in the management of delayed pressure urticaria and angioedema because conventional doses of antihistamines are usually insufficiently effective. Common provoking factors include working with power or hand tools, sitting on a bench, or wearing constricting garments. Delayed pressure urticaria and angioedema is often very difficult to treat and may require higher doses of antihistamines (cetirizine 30 mg/day)[55] and short courses of systemic corticosteroids. The use of montelukast, sulfasalazine, chloroquine, dapsone, intravenous gamma globulin, tranexamic acid, and anti-TNF alpha[55–61] has also been reported in the medical literature.

Cholinergic Urticaria

Cholinergic urticaria appears as pruritic "pinpoint" (1 to 3 mm), hives surrounded by a large flare. It is triggered by an increase in core body temperature from activities like exercise, sweating, emotional factors, and hot baths or showers. Although most cases of cholinergic urticaria are mild, some patients may develop generalized urticaria, angioedema, bronchospasm, and hypotension. Diagnosis includes provocative testing to raise the core body temperature (eg, exercise and hot water immersion) or methacholine intradermal challenge. The negative predictive value of the methacholine intradermal challenge is low so a negative test cannot rule out a diagnosis of cholinergic urticaria.

Treatment includes avoidance of the precipitating factors and regular use of antihistamines. For patients who are poorly responsive to antihistamines, the use of ketotifen, danazol, and omalizumab has provided some efficacy.[62–64] Patients with severe episodes of cholinergic urticaria and systemic symptoms are advised to carry self-injectable epinephrine and be well educated on its use.

Cold Urticaria

Patients with cold urticaria develop pruritus, skin erythema, and swelling after exposure to a cold stimulus. Symptoms are typically confined to cold-exposed areas and are maximal during the rewarming of the exposed skin. Patients may therefore develop urticaria on the face in winter or on cold windy days because of the skin exposure to cold. Lip swelling or pharyngeal symptoms may also develop when ingesting cold foods or beverages.[65] Patients with cold urticaria may have systemic reactions associated with prolonged and systemic cold exposure (eg, swimming in cold water). Headache, dyspnea, hypotension, and fatalities due to subsequent drowning have been reported.[66]

Cold urticaria has been classified into familial or acquired syndromes; the latter further subdivided into primary or secondary acquired cold urticaria. Primary acquired cold urticaria is the most common form and may resolve spontaneously, with a mean duration of symptoms of 4 to 9 years.[67,68] Secondary acquired cold urticaria are associated with underlying disorders such as cryoglobulinemia, leukocytoclastic vasculitis, syphilis, rubeola, hepatitis, respiratory syncytial virus, infectious mononucleosis, medications (eg, penicillin, oral contraceptives, ACE inhibitors, griseofulvin), and malignancy.[68]

Diagnosis of both primary and secondary acquired cold urticaria is confirmed with a positive provocative cold test. This is performed by applying a cold stimulus (eg, ice cube) on the patient's skin (usually the volar aspect of the forearm) for 5 minutes and then observing for a wheal and flare reaction during rewarming of the skin. If the ice cube test is positive at 5 minutes, a cold stimulation time test can help to determine the severity of the reaction. If the cold stimulation test is positive at 5 minutes, it is repeated at 1-minute decrements to determine the minimum time needed to induce a wheal. If the ice cube test is negative at 5 minutes, it is repeated at 1-minute increments up to 10 minutes to determine the minimum time needed to induce a wheal.[64,66] The ice cube needs to be reexposed to different areas of the skin. Up to 20% of patients may have a negative ice cube test.[67] Another diagnostic test is the "hand immersion test" where the hand is immersed in a 10°C water bath for 5 minutes and observed for urticaria during rewarming. This, however, carries a greater risk of systemic reactions.

Management of acquired cold urticaria includes avoidance measures. Patients with a cold stimulation test time of less than 3 minutes[64] and those with laryngeal symptoms with exposure to cold food or drink[69] are at a higher risk of developing systemic symptoms. Antihistamines may be effective in suppressing the cutaneous symptoms but must not be relied upon to suppress systemic symptoms. Epinephrine self-injectors must be prescribed. Other medications with published efficacy for cold urticaria include cyproheptadine, doxepin, combinations of cyproheptadine or hydroxyzine with cimetidine, ketotifen, montelukast, and cetirizine with zafirlukast.[70,71] Induction of tolerance by gradual immersion of extremities into cold water at regular intervals until the urticaria ceases has also been reported.[72] However, daily cold exposure is necessary to maintain cold tolerance. For patients requiring surgery, such as in an ENT practice, the general recommendation is to increase operating room temperatures and to prewarm all fluids and blood products to prevent cold-induced symptoms.

Solar Urticaria

Solar urticaria is a relatively rare condition but may be important to the ENT physician because the face is commonly exposed to sunlight. Individuals with solar urticaria develop erythema, pruritus, and urticaria within 1 to 3 minutes of skin exposure to sunlight. The severity and duration of symptoms may vary with the intensity and duration of light exposure. The urticaria typically resolves within 30 minutes after removal from sun exposure and rarely persists after 24 hours. Systemic manifestation of diaphoresis, dyspnea, headache, and loss of consciousness have been described.[73] Various wavelengths of light including UVB (280 to 320 nm), UVA (320 to 400 nm), visible light (400 to 600 nm), and even infrared (>600 nm) radiation have been reported to trigger solar urticaria. The diagnosis is confirmed with photo-testing to various wavelengths of light with the most common wavelength lying in the UVA and visible range. Avoidance of the triggering wavelengths of light is key to the management of patients with solar urticaria. Broad-spectrum sunscreens are often prescribed but are generally limited in benefit as most patients are sensitive to wavelengths in the visible range which the majority of sunscreens do not filter. H1-antihistamines have variable efficacy. Skin exposed to natural sunlight on a regular basis may become less reactive than skin routinely covered from the sun.[74] Desensitization to light with broadband UVB, narrowband UVB, UVA, and visible light therapy have been reported.[75] Methoxypsoralen taken prior to UVA irradiation may lead to a more durable response, but maintenance treatment is necessary. and it is associated with risks of burns and skin cancer.[76] Case reports of sucessful treatment with plasmapheresis, plasmapheresis and PUVA, cyclosporin A, intravenous immunoglobulin,[77,78] and omalizumab[79] have also been reported. Table 7–3 summarizes the physical urticaria and angioedema syndromes including the diagnostic tests and their treatment.

ANGIOEDEMA

Definition

Angioedema is characterized by sudden, pronounced, non-pitting, erythematous or skin-colored swelling of the lower dermis, frequently the underlying mucous membranes, and pain rather than itch, which may take multiple days to resolve[80] (Figure 7–2). Angioedema is the clinical manifestation of a number of pathophysiologic processes which can include mast cell degranulation and bradykinin associated swelling. Over the last few years, understanding of the underlying pathophysiology and the number of new therapeutic modalities for angioedema has expanded greatly. Otolaryngological management of potentially life-threatening angioedema of the upper aerodigestive tract can be enhanced through a thorough understanding of the underlying pathophysiology of the swelling; a complete differential diagnosis; knowledge of the clinical factors that predict the need for intervention; appropriate laboratory evaluation; and an appropriate

Table 7–3. Physical Urticaria and Angioedema Syndromes

Type	Challenge Procedure	First-Line Treatment	Other Treatment
Dermographism	Stroke skin with tongue blade	95.8% responsive to H1-AH	
Delayed pressure	15 lbs (6.8 kg) hung on shoulder for 10–15 min	Very poor response to H1-AH	Steroids, sulfasalazine, danazole, dapsone, NSAIDs
Cold	Ice cube test on forearm for 5 min	Cyproheptadine Doxepin	B2 sympathomimetics, aminophylline Induction of tolerance Epinephrine self-injector
Cholinergic	Methacholine intradermal or partial immersion in 42°C water	Cetirizine Ketotifen Hydroxyzine	Danazole Induction of tolerance Epinephrine self-injector if severe
Solar	Exposure to specific wavelengths	Poor response Chlorpheniramine Hydroxyzine	Induction of tolerance (PUVA) highly effective Cyclosporine
Aquagenic	Water compress 35° for 30 min	H1-AH	Barrier creams, SSRI, ultraviolet therapy
Vibratory	Vortex on forearm	Hydroxyzine Fexofenadine	Induction of tolerance
Exercise-induced	Treadmill Food identification if relevant	Avoidance	Epinephrine self-injector

H1-AH: H1 Antihistamines

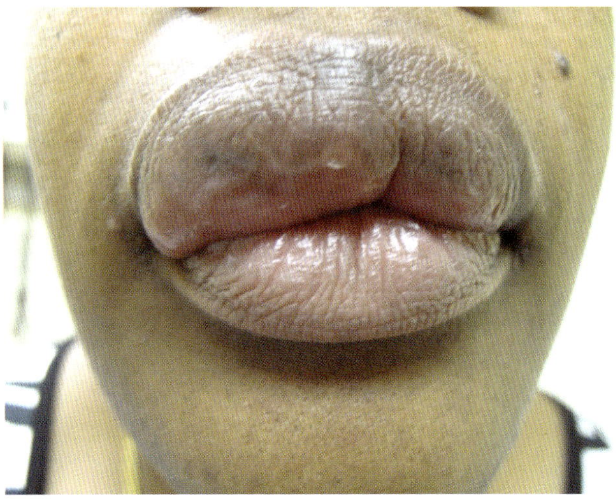

Figure 7–2. Lip angioedema.

approach to acute or recurring head and neck swelling.

Classification

A recent, international position paper on the classification system of angioedema divided the problem into hereditary and acquired forms. The hereditary forms were further subdivided into those patients with a genetic C1 esterase inhibitor (C1-INH) deficiency, termed hereditary angioedema (HAE) with C1-INH deficiency (C1-INH-HAE), and those with normal C1-INH. Those with normal C1-INH were further subdivided into those with factor XII mutation, termed HAE with factor XII mutation (FXII-

HAE) and those without the mutation, termed HAE of unknown origin (U-HAE). Because the prevalence of factor XII mutation is very low in the United States, this group will be referred to here as HAE with normal C1 inhibitor (HAE with NL-C1-INH). The acquired form of angioedema was separated into those with C-INH deficiency (onset of disease at >40 years with no family history, termed *acquired angioedema* [AAE] with C1-INH deficiency, C1-INH-AAE); those taking angiotensin-converting enzyme inhibitor (ACEi) medications with no other cause of angioedema (ACEi-AAE), and those with no identifiable cause. The last group of AAE angioedema patients was further classified by response to antihistamines into idiopathic histaminergic (IH-AAE) and idiopathic nonhistaminergic (InH-AAE).[81]

The major mediators of angioedema are histamine and bradykinin, and knowledge of their pathophysiologic effects is important for understanding the clinical disease manifestations and is essential for the selection of appropriate therapy. Angioedema may be acute or recurrent. Acute angioedema frequently occurs as an allergic or pseudoallergic response to food, insect sting, medication, latex, autoimmune disease, or other environmental allergens that are commonly accompanied by wheals (when angioedema occurs with wheals, the disease process is referred to as urticaria with angioedema) and, often, with a constellation of other symptoms that can qualify as anaphylaxis. Acute angioedema that is responsive to antihistamines is called *histaminergic*, and the release of histamine from cutaneous mast cells and/or basophils after an inciting stimulus suggests allergy. Clinical evaluation should include a laboratory assessment to try to confirm specific IgE to the suspected cause.

Pathogenesis

Mast cells located in the deep dermis, subcutaneous or submucosal tissues, when stimulated to degranulate, precipitate angioedematous swelling. Mast cells located in the upper dermis play an integral part in the complex pathogenesis of urticaria.

Bradykinin is an oligopeptide with 9 amino acids and is a potent vasodilator. By binding to the bradykinin B2 receptor (B2R), bradykinin induces nitric oxide production by endothelial cells and subsequent relaxation of smooth muscle cells. This smooth muscle cell relaxation leads to vasodilatation, increased permeability of the vascular wall, and fluid third spacing.[82] Nussberger et al demonstrated that bradykinin levels were elevated in HAE and AAE patients and were highest during angioedematous attacks; and the infusion of C- INH lowered bradykinin levels.[83] Angioedema, when caused by bradykinin, is not responsive to antihistamines, corticosteroids, or epinephrine. Although "bradykinin-mediated" angioedema is frequently substituted for "nonhistaminergic," other vasoactive mediators like cystenyl leukotrienes, platelet-activating factor, and prostaglandins should be considered as possible etiological causes in some patients with drug-related angioedema that is not responsive to antihistamines.[81] C1-INH-HAE, ACEi-AAE, C1-INH-AAE are mediated by bradykinin activity, and HAE with NL-C1-INH and InH-HAE may also share this causative agent.[82–84]

Genetics

C1-INH-HAE is caused by mutations in the SERPIN 1 gene that either decrease the production of C1-INH (HAE-C1-INH type 1) or produce functionally defective C1-INH (HAE-C1-INH type 2). C1-INH, a serine protease inhibitor, inhibits the C1r and C1s components of the complement pathway and factor XIa, factor XIIa, and kallikrein in the contact and coagulation systems. Without inhibition of these contact proteins, during acute attacks, uncontrolled formation of plasma kallikrein cleaves high molecular weight kininogen to produce bradykinin leading to angioedema. The inheritance of C1-INH-HAE, which affects approximately 6000 to 10 000 people in the United States, follows an autosomal dominant pattern; however, 25% of patients develop the disease de novo with no family history of the disease.

Clinical/Laboratory Characteristics

Differences in clinical and laboratory findings of the individual will guide the correct diagnosis of the specific type of angioedema[85] (Table 7–4).

Erythema marginatum is a prominent prodromal symptom that presents as a nonpruritic, nonraised, serpentine erythematous rash on the trunk,

Table 7-4. Clinical and Laboratory Characteristics of Different Types of Recurrent Angioedema Without Urticaria

	C1-INH-HAE	HAE With NL-C1-INH	Histamine AE	Nonhistamine AE	C1-INH AAE	ACEi-AAE
Tongue angioedema	+	++	++	++	++	+++
Laryngeal angioedema	+++	+++	+	+	+++	+++
Peripheral angioedema	+++	+++	+	+	++	+/−
Gastrointestinal angioedema	+++	+	+/−	+/−	++	+/−
Onset <6 h	+	+	+++	++	+	++
Duration >48 h	+++	+++	+	+	+++	++
Family with AE	+++ (75%)	+++	—	—	—	—
C1-INH function <50% normal	100%	—	—	—	100%	—
C1-INH antigen <50% normal	85%	—	—	—	85%	—
C4 antigen <12 mg/dL	>90%	Occasional	Occasional	Occasional	>90%	Occasional
C1Q antigen <50 normal	Occasional	0	0	0	>70%	0

Source: Adapted from Cicardi M and Zanichelli A. Diagnosing angioedema, *Immuno Allergy Clin N Amer.* 2013;33:449–456.

arms, and legs which commonly spares the face. Other prodromal symptoms include tingling, itching, warmth, or burning at the affected site; increase fatigue, hunger, abdominal bloating, or gassiness.[86] Patients will normally develop symptoms in childhood or adolescence. Although swelling can occur without an inciting event, triggers for acute attacks in HAE-C1-INH can include trauma, infection, menstruation, estrogen-containing birth control pills, mental stress, and dental work. It is very important to be aware that approximately 17% of dental surgeries in C1-INH-HAE who do not receive C1-INH prophylaxis result in angioedema. Lip swelling progressing to facial swelling, tongue edema, and laryngeal swelling with upper airway obstruction has been seen following dental surgery, as well as laryngeal edema without lip or facial swelling.[87] Since 50% of HAE-C1-INH patients develop laryngeal swelling at some point in their lifetime,[88] the otolaryngology community needs to be keenly aware of this disease process as effective lifesaving therapy is now available to treat angioedema in these patients.

> Angioedema without urticaria primarily occurs secondary to bradykinin-mediated mechanisms.

Treatment

In the United States, 4 medications have been approved by the FDA for the treatment of acute attacks in adolescent and adults with C1-INH-

HAE since 2009. The first to be FDA approved was a plasma-derived C-1-INH (Berinert, CSL Behring) dosed at 20 U/Kg given intravenously by slow infusion for the approved indication of acute abdominal, facial, or laryngeal attacks of HAE in adult and adolescent patients. In a randomized, placebo-controlled trial of 125 patients, the time to symptom relief in acute attacks was significantly shortened at this dose when compared to placebo.[89] The concern over viral transmission from human blood products have been addressed by an addition of a heat treatment step followed by chromogenic separation and nanofiltration which has successfully prevented viral transmission.[90] The first recombinant C1-INH product (rhC1INH), Ruconest (Salix Pharmaceuticals), purified from the milk of genetically modified rabbits, was evaluated for safety and efficacy in 75 patients randomized (3:2) to receive rhC1INH ($n = 44$) or a saline placebo ($n = 31$). Statistically significant differences between rhC1-INH and placebo were seen in this study in the visual analog scale (VAS) assessments when examining the median time to the beginning of symptom relief at the primary attack location. Median time to the beginning of symptom relief was 75 minutes for the rhC1-INH patients vs 303 minutes for the controls ($p = 0.003$) using the VAS assessment. Median time to minimal symptoms using the VAS was 240 minutes in the medication treatment group and 362 minutes for the placebo group ($p = 0.005$). Statistical significance was not reached for these measures when evaluating with the Treatment Effect Questionnaire (TEQ). In this study, RhC1INH was dosed at 50 IU/kg to a maximum of 4200 IU/treatment.[91] Because rhC1-INH is made from rabbits' milk, patients allergic to rabbits should not receive this medication (Table 7–5).

Ecallantide (Kalbitor, Dyax Corp.) is a recombinant protein produced in the yeast *Pichia pastoris* and is a potent inhibitor of the plasma enzyme, kallikrein. By blocking kallikrein's binding site, bradykinin cannot be liberated from high molecular weight kininogen. Two double-blind, placebo-controlled trials (EDEMA 3 and EDEMA4) involving 143 unique patients clearly demonstrated that subcutaneously

Table 7–5. Medication Used to Treat Hereditary Angioedema

Medications Commonly Used to Treat HAE in the United States	Indication	Usual Adult Dose (Range)	Mechanism of Action
Ecallantide (Kalbitor, Dyax)	Acute attacks	3, 1 cc 10 mg subcutaneous injections (30 mg)	Inhibits plasma kallekrein
Icatibant (Firazyr, Shire)	Acute attacks	30 mg subcutaneous injection	Bradykinin B2 receptor antagonist
Plasma-derived C1 esterase inhibitor (Berinert, CSL Behring)	Acute attacks	20 IU per kg IVP	Inhibits plasma kallikrein, factor XIa and XIIa, MASP (mannose binding lectin serine protease) 1 and 2, plasmin, and C1r and s
Recombinant C1 esterase inhibitor (Ruconest, Valeant)	Acute attacks	50 IU per kg IVP (>84 kg–4200 IU)	Inhibits plasma kallikrein, factor XIa and XIIa, MASP 1 and 2, plasmin, and C1r and s
Plasma-derived C1 esterase inhibitor (Cinryze, Shire)	Long-term prophylaxis	1000 IU IVP every 3–4 days	Inhibits plasma kallikrein, factor XIa and XIIa, MASP 1 and 2, plasmin, and C1r and s
Danazol (Danocrine, Sanofi-Synthelabo)	Long-term prophylaxis	200 mg/day (50 mg/wk–200 mg/day)	

administered drug was highly effect in mitigating HAE-C1-INH attacks in adults and children.[92–94] Because of possible hypersensitivity reactions including anaphylaxis, ecallantide must be administered by a health care professional, although this is a very rare complication.

Another medication approved for the acute symptomatic treatment of HAE-C1-INH, Icatibant (Firazyr, Shire Plc.) works by selectively blocking the bradykinin B2 receptor and is approved for self-administration in appropriately trained patients. Two separate, more recent, phase III multicenter, double-blind, placebo-controlled trials demonstrated that it significantly reduced the median time to the onset of symptom relief when compared to placebo (2 vs 19.8 h; $p < 0.001$) in one, and an older HAE treatment, tranexamic acid (2 vs 12 h, $p > 0.0001$) in the other.[95,96]

Placebo-controlled clinical trials have shown plasma-derived C1 inhibitor, attenuated androgens, and antifibrinolytic agents to be effective in long-term prophylaxis of hereditary angioedematous events.[97–100] In the United States, the 2 medications approved for prophylaxis by the FDA are the attenuated androgen, danazol (*Danocrine*), and the human, plasma-derived nanofiltered C1-inhibitor protein (*Cinryze*). In a 2012 study, 126 patients receiving human, plasma-derived nanofiltered C1-inhibitor protein (*Cinryze*) intravenously at a dose of 1000 units every 3 to 7 days experienced a 93.7% reduction in acute angioedematous attacks.Attenuated androgens have also been shown to be effective. [101] However, significant adverse events have prompted multiple guidelines to recommend using danazol at a maximum dose of 200 mg/day.[102,103]

> New treatments for acute swelling for hereditary angioedema include C1 inhibitor protein, kallikrein inhibitors, and bradykinin receptor blockers.

HAE with Normal C1 Inhibitor Levels

HAE with normal C1 inhibitor levels (formerly type III HAE) was initially described by Bork and Binkley in the early part of the 21st century. An international consensus group paper recently clarified its diagnostic criteria. The diagnosis of HAE with normal C1-inhibitor (NL-C1-INH) is made in a patient with a history of recurrent angioedema in the absence of concomitant hives or concomitant use of a medication known to cause angioedema; documented normal or near normal C4, C1-INH and C1-INH function; plus either a demonstrated factor XII mutation associated with the disease or a positive family history; and documented evidence of lack of efficacy of chronic high-dose antihistamine therapy (cetirizine at 40 mg/day or equivalent for at least 1 month or interval expected to be associated with 3 or more attacks of angioedema).[104] Because of the diagnostic challenge of the lack of a validated confirmatory diagnostic test, some of the features that may help distinguish HAE with NL-C1-INH from other forms of HAE include (Table 7–6)

Table 7-6. Diagnostic Criteria for Hereditary Angioedema with Normal C1-Inhibitor Levels

Hx of recurrent angioedema in the absence of hives	
No use of a medication known to cause angioedema	
Normal or near normal C4, C1-INH and C1-INH function blood tests	
Either:	A demonstrated factor XII mutation associated with the disease **or**
	A positive family history and documented evidence of lack of efficacy of chronic high-dose antihistamine therapy (cetirizine at 40 mg/day or equivalent for at least 1 month or interval expected to be associated with three or more attacks of angioedema)

- More than 90% of patients experience their first symptoms during or after their second decade of life[105]
- The predilection for facial, tongue, and oropharyngeal swelling[105]
- Female predominance in patients with factor XII mutation[106–108]
- Erythema marginatum has not been identified as a prodromal symptom
- Unique to this subtype, some patients may hemorrhage into angioedematous areas[105]

No controlled studies on therapeutic options for acute or prophylactic treatment for HAE with NL-C1-INH have been published. However, case reports and case series have reported efficacy in treating acute angioedema with icatibant and ecallantide and these drugs have been effective in managing acute angioedema in this group of patients.[107–111] Despite the fact that C1-INH levels are normal in C1-INH with NL C1-INH, as the name implies, C1-INH infusions have been effectively used in multiple case reports to manage their angioedematous attacks though some patients have failed to respond.[107,108,112,113]

ACE Inhibitor Angioedema

The most common cause of angioedema in adults that most practioners as well as otolaryngologists will encounter, is ACEi induced acute angioedema.[114,115] Angioedema occurs in approximately 0.1% to 0.7% of those treated with an ACEi.[116] Aside from converting angiotensinogen to angiotensin, ACE functions along with aminopeptidase P (APP), membrane metallo-endopeptidase (MME, also called neutral endopeptidase, NEP), and dipeptidyl peptidase IV (DPP) to degrade bradykinin into inactive metabolites. ACEi blocking of the degradation of bradykinin is postulated as a causative factor in the development of angioedema in patients taking ACEi[117] (Figure 7–3).

Some risk factors for angioedema in ACEi-AAE patients include African American ethnicity, history of a drug rash, seasonal allergies, history of ACEi-induced cough, smoking, female gender, and chronic heart failure.[116,118] Interestingly, multiple genetic abnormalities in APP production have been identified and associated with increase rates of angioedema in patients taking ACEi.[119] These genetic abnormalities seem to be present more frequently in African American patients and female patients[120] (Table 7–7).

> Angiotensin-converting enzyme inhibitor (ACEi) medications are the most common cause of head and neck angioedema. Though most common in the first 6 weeks of ACEi therapy, angioedema from these medications may occur years to decades after their initiation.

Acquired Angioedema With C1-Inhibitor Deficiency

C1-INH-AAE is a rare form of C1-INH deficiency associated with B-cell lymphoproliferative diseases (lymphomas, monoclonal gammopathies, and myeloma), solid tumor cancers, and connective tissue diseases (mainly systemic lupus erythematosus).[121–123] Patients present similarly to those with C1-INH-HAE. However, the age of onset of angioedema is normally greater than 40 years, there is no family history of angioedema, and there is no C1-INH gene mutation. This disease is thought to be caused by the direct consumption of C1 and C1-INH by the associated tumor or by autoantibodies to C1-INH.[124] The predominant sites of angioedema in these patients include the face, tongue, uvula, and upper airway.[125] C1-INH antigen, C4 and C1-INH functional levels in C1-INH-AAE are similar to those found in C1-INH-HAE patients, but a majority of C1-INH-AAE patients will also have low C1Q levels.[126]

Assessment of Patients With Angioedema

When assessing a patient with angioedema, the following clinical factors should be documented: timing of onset, the presence or absence of urticaria, the exact location and extent of the swelling, precipitating factors, the patient's age, drug history, and family

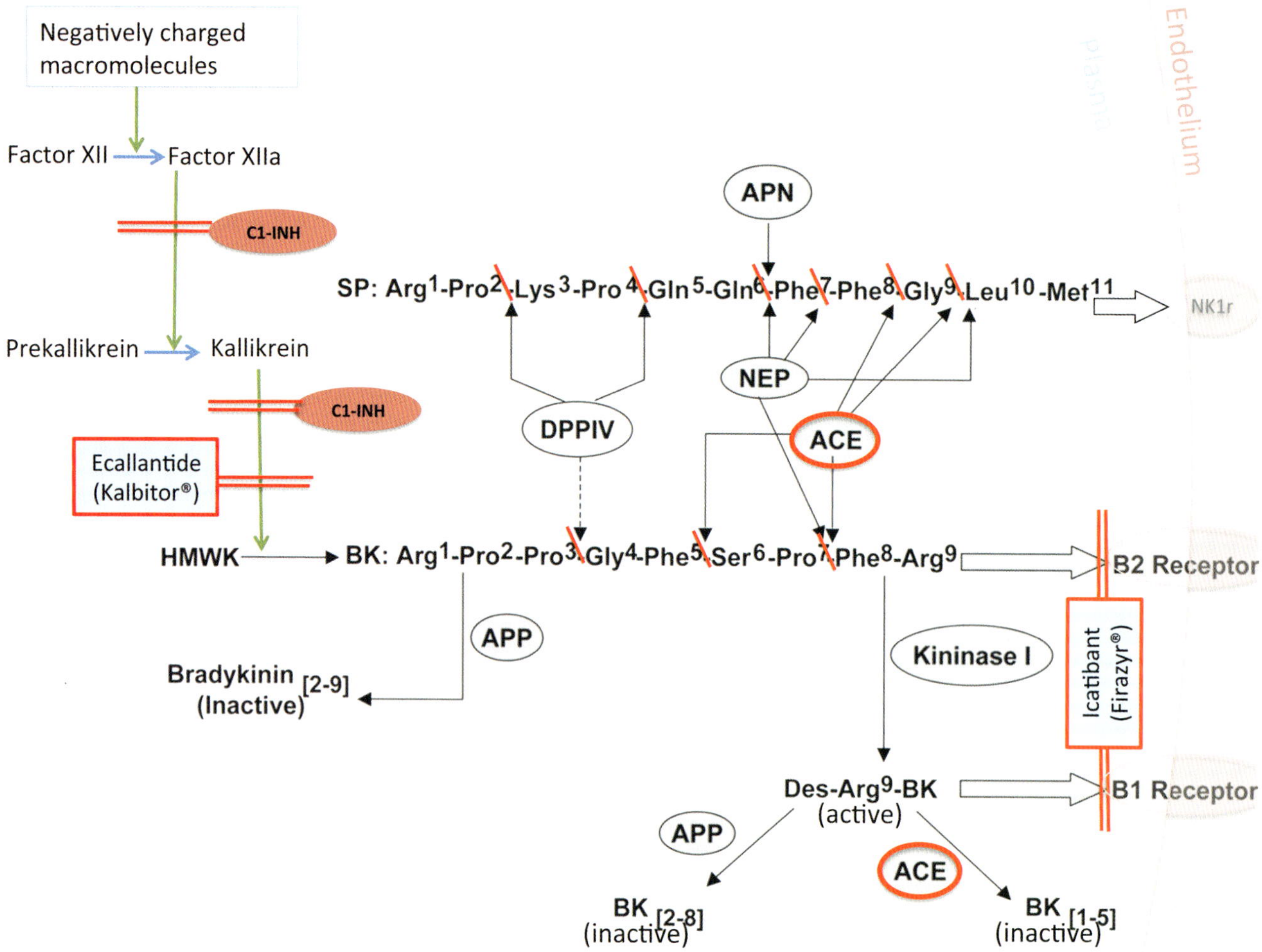

Figure 7-3. Mechanism of bradykinin mediated angioedema. Bradykinin (BK, center) is a 9-amino acid spanning peptide with potent vasodilatory effects through binding to Bradykinin-1 (B1) and Bradykinin-2 (B2) receptors on the endothelium. Bradykinin synthesis and metabolism are held in balance by a number of enzymes. Angiotensin Converting Enzyme (ACE) is an important metabolizer of bradykinin, leading to its inactivation. It should be noted that ACE also breaks down and inactivates Substance P (SP), another potent vasodilator produced in response to certain inflammations or injuries. Through the inhibition of ACE by ACE-inhibitors, bradykinin degradation depends on other enzymes, such as Neutral Endopeptidase (NEP), Aminopeptidase P (APP) and Dipeptidyl Peptidase IV (DPPIV). When these enzyme's capacities are exceeded, elevated bradykinin levels may cause excessive vasodilation, leading to plasma extravasation and angioedema. C1-inhibitor (C1-INH) is another enzyme regulating bradykinin levels in plasma by inhibiting its production from High Molecular Weight Kininogen (HMWK). C1-INH deficiency may thus lead to an overproduction of bradykinin and subsequent angioedema. Icatibant and Ecallantide (blue boxes) are recently developed medicines used in the treatment of HAE. Icatibant has also been shown to be effective in ACEi induced angioedema. Modified with permission from Wolters Kluwer Health, Inc. Byrd JB, Touzin K, Sile S, Gainer JV, Yu C, Nadeau J, Adam A, Brown NJ. Dipeptidyl peptidase IV in angiotensin-converting enzyme inhibitor associated angioedema. *Hypertension*. 2008 Jan;51(1):141–147.

Table 7–7. Risk Factors for ACE Inhibitor-Induced Angioedema

African American ethnicity
Seasonal allergies
History of ACEi-induced cough
Smoking
Female gender
Chronic heart failure
History of drug rash

history of angioedema. A thorough understanding of differences in clinical and laboratory characteristics (see Table 7–4), alternative diagnoses (Table 7–8), and an algorithmic approach to the acute management (Figure 7–4, Table 7–5) will aid the otolaryngologist in providing optimal initial and follow-up care for the angioedematous patient. In addition, Ishoo et al have recommended a staging system for classification and prediction of upper airway risk in angioedema.[127] For stage I manifesting as facial or lip edema and stage II manifesting as soft palate edema, home monitoring or admission is acceptable. For stage III manifesting as lingual edema and stage IV manifesting as laryngeal edema, intensive care monitoring is recommended.

Table 7–8. Differential Diagnosis of Head and Neck Angioedema

	Cause	Clinical Keys
Common	Urticaria	Pruritus
	Anaphylaxis	Hypotension
	Trauma	Hx of trauma, bruising
	Dermatitis	Pruritus, association with contactant
	Cellulitis	Erythema, pain, redness
	Oncotic edema	Low albumin, eyelids and face, worse in the morning, pitting
Uncommon/rare	Gleich syndrome	Episodic angioedema with marked eosinophilia
	Melkerson-Rosenthal syndrome	Intermittent, persistent lip and check swelling, fissured tongue, and Bell palsy
	Superior vena cava syndrome	Chest tumor-associated, plethoric facies, engorged neck veins
	Muckle-Wells syndrome	Periodic episodes of fever, rash, joint swelling, conjunctivitis, progressive hearing loss
	Asher syndrome	Blepharochalasis, double upper lip, euthyroid goiter (10%)
	NERDS syndrome	Eosinophilia with para-articular nodules, rheumatism, xerosis, urticaria, and angioedema (primarily of the hands and feet)

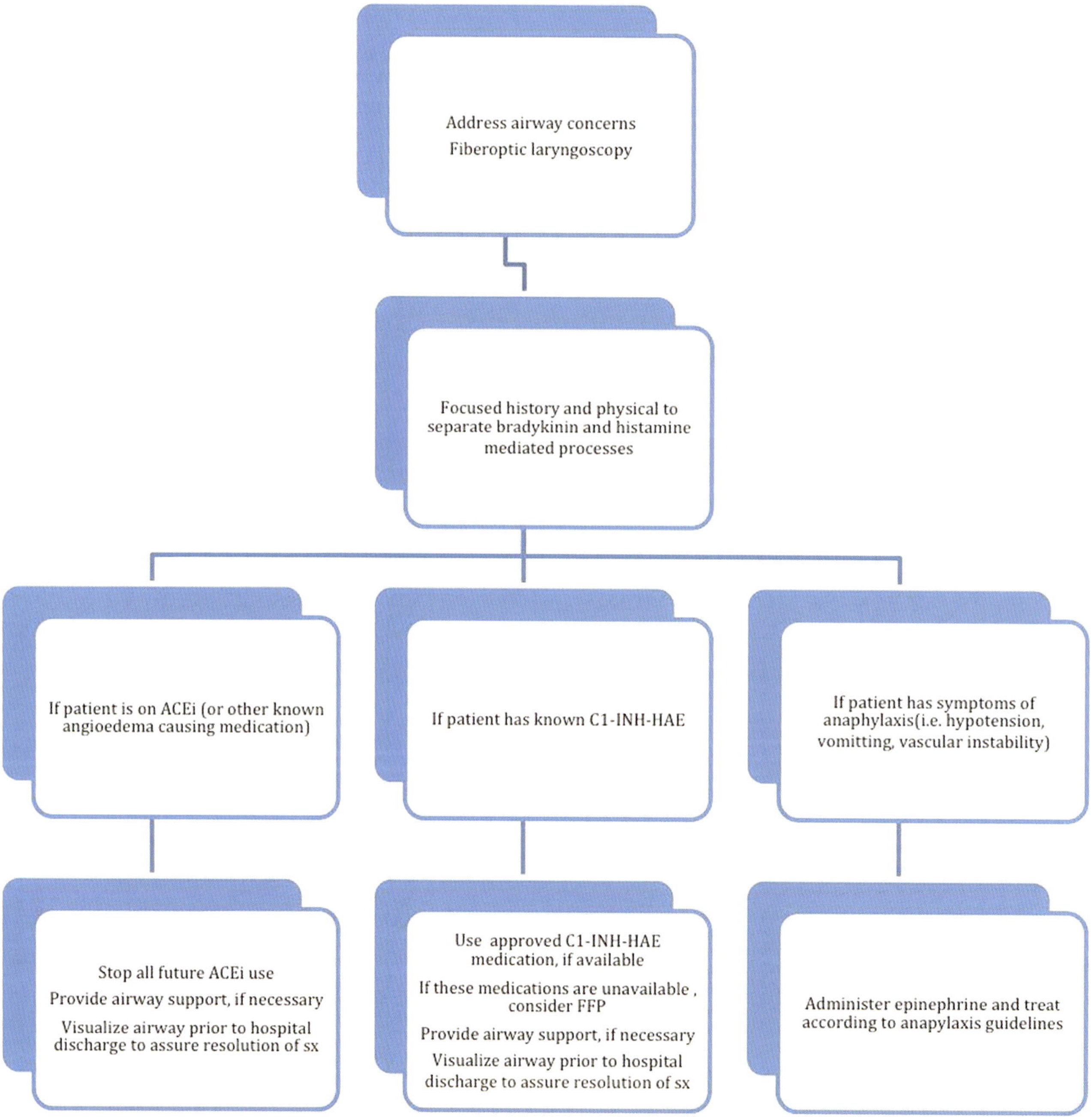

Figure 7-4. Algorithm for ENT evaluation and management of laryngeal edema.

REFERENCES

1. Zuberbier T, Balke M, Worm M, Edenharter G, Maurer M. Epidemiology of urticaria: a representative cross-sectional population survey. *Clin Experiment Dermatol*, 2010;35:869–873.
2. Sackesen C, Sekerel BE, Orhan F, et al. The etiology of different forms of urticaria in childhood. *Pediatr Dermatol*. 2004;21(2):102–108.
3. Sakurai M, Oba M, Matsumoto K, et al. Acute infectious urticaria: clinical and laboratory analysis in nineteen patients. *J Dermatol*. 2000;27(2):87–93.
4. Pruksachatkunakorn C, Apichartpiyakul N, Kanjanaratanakorn K. Parvovirus B19 infection in children with acute illness and rash. *Pediatr Dermatol*. 2006;23(3): 216–218.
5. Cribier B. Urticaria and hepatitis. *Clin Rev Allergy Immunol*. 2006;30(1):25–29.
6. Pollack CV, Jr, Romano TJ. Outpatient management of acute urticaria: the role of prednisone. *Ann Emerg Med*. 1995;26(5):547–551.
7. Gaig P, Olona M, Muñoz Lejarazu D, et al. Epidemiology of urticaria in Spain. *J Investig Allergol Clin Immunol*. 2004;14(3):214–220.
8. Vazquez Nava F, Almeida Arvizu VM, Sánchez Nuncio HR, et al. Prevalence and potential triggering factors of chronic urticaria and angioedema in an urban area of northeastern Mexico. *Rev Alerg Mex*. 2004;51(5):181–188.
9. Champion RH, Roberts SO, Carpenter RG, et al. Urticaria and angio-oedema. A review of 554 patients. *Br J Dermatol*. 1969;81(8):588–597.
10. Ozkaya-Bayazit E, Demir K, Ozgüroğlu E, et al. *Helicobacter pylori* eradication in patients with chronic urticaria. *Arch Dermatol*. 1998;134(9):1165–1166.
11. Schnyder B, Helbling A, Pichler WJ. Chronic idiopathic urticaria: natural course and association with *Helicobacter pylori* infection. *Int Arch Allergy Immunol*. 1999; 119(1):60–63.
12. Leznoff A, Sussman GL. Syndrome of idiopathic chronic urticaria and angioedema with thyroid autoimmunity: a study of 90 patients. *J Allergy Clin Immunol*. 1989;84(1): 66–71.
13. Levy Y, Segal N, Weintrob N, et al. Chronic urticaria: association with thyroid autoimmunity. *Arch Dis Child*. 2003;88(6):517–519.
14. Ferrer M, Kinet JP, Kaplan AP. Comparative studies of functional and binding assays for IgG anti- Fc(epsilon) RIalpha (alpha-subunit) in chronic urticaria. *J Allergy Clin Immunol*. 1998;101(5):672–676.
15. Tong LJ, Balakrishnan G, Kochan JP, et al. Assessment of autoimmunity in patients with chronic urticaria. *J Allergy Clin Immunol*. 1997;99(4):461–465.
16. Puccetti A, Bason C, Simeoni S, et al. In chronic idiopathic urticaria autoantibodies against Fc epsilonRII/ CD23 induce histamine release via eosinophil activation. *Clin Exp Allergy*. 2005;35(12):1599–1607.
17. Tarbox JA, Gutta RC, Radojicic C, et al. Utility of routine laboratory testing in management of chronic urticaria/ angioedema. *Ann Allergy Asthma Immunol*. 2011;107(3): 239–243.
18. Bernstein JA, Lang DM, Khan DA, et al. The diagnosis and management of acute and chronic urticaria: 2014 update. *J Allergy Clin Immunol*. May 2014;33(5)2070–2077.
19. Ortonne JP, Grob JJ, Auquier P, et al. Efficacy and safety of desloratadine in adults with chronic idiopathic urticaria: a randomized, double-blind, placebo-controlled, multicenter trial. *Am J Clin Dermatol*. 2007;8(1):37–42.
20. Monroe EW. Relative efficacy and safety of loratadine, hydroxyzine, and placebo in chronic idiopathic urticaria and atopic dermatitis. *Clin Ther*. 1992;14(1):17–21.
21. Breneman DL. Cetirizine versus hydroxyzine and placebo in chronic idiopathic urticaria. *Ann Pharmacother*. 1996;30(10):1075–1079.
22. Kapp A, Pichler WJ. Levocetirizine is an effective treatment in patients suffering from chronic idiopathic urticaria: a randomized, double-blind, placebo-controlled, parallel, multicenter study. *Int J Dermatol*. 2006;45(4):469–474.
23. Kaplan AP, Spector SL, Meeves S, et al. Once-daily fexofenadine treatment for chronic idiopathic urticaria: a multicenter, randomized, double-blind, placebo-controlled study. *Ann Allergy Asthma Immunol*. 2005;94(6):662–669.
24. Grob JJ, Auquier P, Dreyfus I, et al. How to prescribe antihistamines for chronic idiopathic urticaria: desloratadine daily vs PRN and quality of life. *Allergy*. 2009 April;64(4):605–612.
25. Pacor ML, Di Lorenzo G, Corrocher R. Efficacy of leukotriene receptor antagonist in chronic urticaria. A double-blind, placebo-controlled comparison of treatment with montelukast and cetirizine in patients with chronic urticaria with intolerance to food additive and/ or acetylsalicylic acid. *Clin Exp Allergy*. 2001;31(10): 1607–1614.
26. Hani N, Hartmann K, Casper C, et al. Improvement of cold urticaria by treatment with the leukotriene receptor antagonist montelukast. *Acta Derm Venereol*. 2000; 80(3):229.
27. Nettis E, Colanardi MC, Soccio AL, et al. Desloratadine in combination with montelukast suppresses the dermographometer challenge test papule, and is effective in the treatment of delayed pressure urticaria: a randomized, doubleblind, placebo-controlled study. *Br J Dermatol*. 2006;155(6):1279–1282.
28. Richelson E. Tricyclic antidepressants and histamine H1 receptors. *Mayo Clin Proc*. 1979;54(10):669–674.
29. Simons FE. Advances in H1-antihistamines. *N Engl J Med*. 2004;351(21):2203–2217.
30. Holgate S, Casale T, Wenzel S, et al. The anti-inflammatory effects of omalizumab confirm the central role of IgE in allergic inflammation. *J Allergy Clin Immunol*. 2005;115(3):459–465.
31. Maurer M, Rosén K, Hsieh HJ, et al. Omalizumab for the treatment of chronic idiopathic or spontaneous urticaria. *NEJM*. 2013;368(10):924–935.

32. Kaplan A, Ledford D, Ashby M, et al. Omalizumab in patients with symptomatic chronic idiopathic/spontaneous urticaria despite standard combination therapy. *J Allergy Clin Immunol.* 2013;132(1):101–109.
33. Grattan CE, O'Donnell BF, Francis DM, et al. Randomized double-blind study of cyclosporin in chronic "idiopathic" urticaria. *Br J Dermatol.* 2000;143(2):365–372.
34. Baskan EB, Tunali S, Turker T, et al. Comparison of short- and long-term cyclosporine A therapy in chronic idiopathic urticaria. *J Dermatolog Treat.* 2004;15(3):164–168.
35. Vena GA, Cassano N, Colombo D, et al. Cyclosporine in chronic idiopathic urticaria: a double-blind, randomized, placebocontrolled trial. *J Am Acad Dermatol.* 2006; 55(4):705–709.
36. Madan V, Griffiths CE. Systemic ciclosporin and tacrolimus in dermatology. *Dermatol Ther.* 2007;20(4):239–250.
37. Humphreys F, Hunter JA. The characteristics of urticaria in 390 patients. *Br J Dermatol.* 1998;138(4):635–638.
38. Cassano N, D'Argento V, Filotico R, et al. Low-dose dapsone in chronic idiopathic urticaria: preliminary results of an open study. *Acta Derm Venereol.* 2005;85(3):254–255.
39. Dayani A, Gould DJ, Campbell S. Delayed pressure urticaria: treatment with dapsone. *J Dermatolog Treat.* 1992;3: 61–62.
40. Muramatsu C, Tanabe E. Urticarial vasculitis: response to dapsone and colchicine. *J Am Acad Dermatol.* 1985; 13(6):1055.
41. Jaffer AM. Sulfasalazine in the treatment of corticosteroid-dependent chronic idiopathic urticaria. *J Allergy Clin Immunol.* 1991;88(6):964–965.
42. Hartmann K, Hani N, Hinrichs R, et al. Successful sulfasalazine treatment of severe chronic idiopathic urticaria associated with pressure urticaria. *Acta Derm Venereol.* 2001;81(1):71.
43. Marmor MF, Kellner U, Lai TY, et al. Revised recommendations on screening for chloroquine and hydroxychloroquine retinopathy. *Ophthalmology.* 2011;118(2): 415–422.
44. Orfan NA, Kolski GB. Physical urticarias. *Ann Allergy.* 1993;71(3):205–212; quiz 212–215.
45. Kontou-Fili K, Borici-Mazi R, Kapp A, et al. Physical urticaria: classification and diagnostic guidelines. An EAACI position paper. *Allergy.* 1997;52(5):504–513.
46. Barlow RJ, Warburton F, Watson K, et al. Diagnosis and incidence of delayed pressure urticaria in patients with chronic urticaria. *J Am Acad Dermatol.* 1993;29(6):954–958.
47. Zuberbier T, Althaus C, Chantraine-Hess S, et al. Prevalence of cholinergic urticaria in young adults. *J Am Acad Dermatol.* 1994;31(6):978–981.
48. Jedele KB, Michels VV. Familial dermographism. *Am J Med Genet.* 1991;39(2):201–203.
49. Breathnach SM, Allen R, Ward AM, et al. Symptomatic dermographism: natural history, clinical features laboratory investigations and response to therapy. *Clin Exp Dermatol.* 1983;8(5):463–476.
50. Juhlin L, de Vos C, Rihoux JP. Inhibiting effect of cetirizine on histamine-induced and 48/80-induced wheals and flares, experimental dermographism, and cold-induced urticaria. *J Allergy Clin Immunol.* 1987;80(4): 599–602.
51. Johnsson M, Falk ES, Volden G. UVB treatment of factitious urticaria. *Photodermatology.* 1987;4(6):302–304.
52. Dover JS, Black AK, Ward AM, et al. Delayed pressure urticaria. Clinical features, laboratory investigations, and response to therapy of 44 patients. *J Am Acad Dermatol.* 1988;18(6):1289–1298.
53. Lawlor F, Black AK, Ward AM, et al. Delayed pressure urticaria, objective evaluation of a variable disease using a dermographometer and assessment of treatment using colchicine. *Br J Dermatol.* 1989;120(3):403–408.
54. Sussman GL, Harvey RP, Schocket AL. Delayed pressure urticaria. *J Allergy Clin Immunol.* 1982;70(5):337–342.
55. Kontou-Fili K, Maniatakou G, Demaka P, et al. Therapeutic effects of cetirizine in delayed pressure urticaria. Part 1. Effects on weight tests and skin-window cytology. *Ann Allergy.* 1990;65(6):517–519.
56. Berkun Y, Shalit M. Successful treatment of delayed pressure urticaria with montelukast. *Allergy.* 2000;55(2): 203–204.
57. Engler RJ, Squire E, Benson P. Chronic sulfasalazine therapy in the treatment of delayed pressure urticaria and angioedema. *Ann Allergy Asthma Immunol.* 1995; 74(2):155–159.
58. Kulthanan K, Thumpimukvatana N. Positive impact of chloroquine on delayed pressure urticaria. *J Drugs Dermatol.* 2007;6(4):445–446.
59. Dawn G, Urcelay M, Ah-Weng A, et al. Effect of high-dose intravenous immunoglobulin in delayed pressure urticaria. *Br J Dermatol.* 2003;149(4):836–840.
60. Shedden C, Highet AS. Delayed pressure urticaria controlled by tranexamic acid. *Clin Exp Dermatol.* 2006; 31(2):295–296.
61. Magerl M, Philipp S, Manasterski M, et al. Successful treatment of delayed pressure urticaria with anti-TNF-alpha. *J Allergy Clin Immunol.* 2007;119(3):752–754.
62. McClean SP, Arreaza EE, Lett-Brown MA, et al. Refractory cholinergic urticaria successfully treated with ketotifen. *J Allergy Clin Immunol.* 1989;83(4):738–741.
63. La Shell MS, England RW. Severe refractory cholinergic urticaria treated with danazol. *J Drugs Dermatol.* 2006; 5(7):664–667.
64. Metz M, Bergmann P, Zuberbier T, et al. Successful treatment of cholinergic urticaria with anti-immunoglobulin E therapy. *Allergy.* 2008;63(2):247–249.
65. Wanderer AA. Cold urticaria syndromes: historical background, diagnostic classification, clinical and laboratory characteristics, pathogenesis, and management. *J Allergy Clin Immunol.* 1990;85(6):965–981.
66. Gorevic PD, Kaplan AP. The physical urticarias. *Int J Dermatol.* 1980;19(8):417–435.
67. Wanderer AA, Grandel KE, Wasserman SI, et al. Clinical characteristics of cold-induced systemic reactions in acquired cold urticaria syndromes: recommendations for prevention of this complication and a proposal for a

diagnostic classification of cold urticaria. *J Allergy Clin Immunol*. 1986;78(3, pt 1):417–423.
68. Neittaanmaki H. Cold urticaria. Clinical findings in 220 patients. *J Am Acad Dermatol*. 1985;13(4):636–644.
69. Mathelier-Fusade P, Aïssaoui M, Bakhos D, et al. Clinical predictive factors of severity in cold urticaria. *Arch Dermatol*. 1998;134(1):106–107.
70. Wanderer AA, St Pierre JP, Ellis EF. Primary acquired cold urticaria. Double-blind comparative study of treatment with cyproheptadine, chlorpheniramine, and placebo. *Arch Dermatol*. 1977;113(10):1375–1377.
71. Neittaanmaki H, Myohanen T, Fraki JE. Comparison of cinnarizine, cyproheptadine, doxepin, and hydroxyzine in treatment of idiopathic cold urticaria: usefulness of doxepin. *J Am Acad Dermatol*. 1984;11(3):483–489.
72. Bentley-Phillips CB, Black AK, Greaves MW. Induced tolerance in cold urticaria caused by cold evoked histamine release. *Lancet*. 1976;2(7976):63–66.
73. Uetsu N, Miyauchi-Hashimoto H, Okamoto H, et al. The clinical and photobiological characteristics of solar urticaria in 40 patients. *Br J Dermatol*. 2000;142(1):32–38.
74. Blum HF, West RJ. Studies of an urticarial response to blue and violet light in man. *J Clin Invest*. 1937;16:261–267.
75. Kalimo K, Jansen C. Severe solar urticaria: active and passive action spectra and hyposensitizing effect of different UV modalities. *Photodermatology*. 1986;3(3):194–195.
76. Roelandts R. Pre-PUVA UVA desensitization for solar urticaria. *Photodermatology*. 1985;2(3):174–176.
77. Duschet P, Leyen P, Schwarz T, et al. Solar urticaria: treatment by plasmapheresis. *J Am Acad Dermatol*. 1986; 15(4, pt 1):712–713.
78. Edstrom DW, Ros AM. Cyclosporin A therapy for severe solar urticaria. *Photodermatol Photoimmunol Photomed*. 1997;13(1–2):61–63.
79. Chong MH, Aquino M, Davis-Lorton M, et al. A successful treatment of solar urticaria with Omalizumab. *Ann Allergy Asthma Immunol*. 2014;113(5):A15.
80. Zuberbier T, Aberer W, Asero R, et al. The EAACI/GA(2) LEN/EDF/WAO Guideline for the definition, classification, diagnosis, and management of urticaria: the 2013 revision and update. *Allergy*. 2014;69(7):868–887.
81. Cicardi M, Aberer W, Banerji A, et al. Classification, diagnosis, and approach to treatment for angioedema: consensus report from the Hereditary Angioedema International Working Group. *Allergy*. 2014;69(5):602–616.
82. Bauer V, Sotnikova R. Nitric oxide—the endothelium-derived relaxing factor and its role in endothelial functions. *Gen Physiol Biophys*. 2010;29(4):319–340.
83. Nussberger J, Cugno M, Amstutz C, Cicardi M, Pellacani A, Agostoni A. Plasma bradykinin in angio-oedema. *Lancet*. 1998;351(9117):1693–1697.
84. Nussberger J, Cugno M, Cicardi M. Bradykinin-mediated angioedema. *N Engl J Med*. 2002;347(8):621–622.
85. Cicardi M, Zanichelli A. Diagnosing angioedema. *Immunol Allergy Clin North Am*. 2013;33(4):449–456.
86. Prematta MJ, Kemp JG, Gibbs JG, Mende C, Rhoads C, Craig TJ. Frequency, timing, and type of prodromal symptoms associated with hereditary angioedema attacks. *Allergy Asthma Proc*. 2009;30(5):506–511.
87. Bork K, Barnstedt SE. Laryngeal edema and death from asphyxiation after tooth extraction in four patients with hereditary angioedema. *J Am Dental Assoc*. 2003; 134(8):1088–1094.
88. Bork K, Barnstedt SE. Treatment of 193 episodes of laryngeal edema with C1 inhibitor concentrate in patients with hereditary angioedema. *Arch Intern Med*. 2001;161(5):714–718.
89. Craig TJ, Levy RJ, Wasserman RL, et al. Efficacy of human C1 esterase inhibitor concentrate compared with placebo in acute hereditary angioedema attacks. *J Allergy Clin Immunol*. 2009;124(4):801–808.
90. Cicardi M, Zingale L. How do we treat patients with hereditary angioedema. *Transfus Apher Sci*. 2003;29(3): 221–227.
91. Riedl MA, Bernstein JA, Li H, et al. Recombinant human C1-esterase inhibitor relieves symptoms of hereditary angioedema attacks: phase 3, randomized, placebo-controlled trial. *Ann Allergy Asthma Immunol*. 2014; 112(2):163–169 e1.
92. Cicardi M, Levy RJ, McNeil DL, et al. Ecallantide for the treatment of acute attacks in hereditary angioedema. *N Engl J Med*. 2010;363(6):523–531.
93. Levy RJ, Lumry WR, McNeil DL, et al. EDEMA4: a phase 3, double-blind study of subcutaneous ecallantide treatment for acute attacks of hereditary angioedema. *Ann Allergy Asthma Immunol*. 2010;104(6):523–529.
94. MacGinnitie AJ, Davis-Lorton M, Stolz LE, Tachdjian R. Use of ecallantide in pediatric hereditary angioedema. *Pediatrics*. 2013;132(2):e490–e497.
95. Cicardi M, Banerji A, Bracho F, et al. Icatibant, a new bradykinin-receptor antagonist, in hereditary angioedema. *N Engl J Med*. 2010;363(6):532–541.
96. Lumry WR, Li HH, Levy RJ, et al. Randomized placebo-controlled trial of the bradykinin B(2) receptor antagonist icatibant for the treatment of acute attacks of hereditary angioedema: the FAST-3 trial. *Ann Allergy Asthma Immunol*. 2011;107(6):529–537.
97. Bowen T, Cicardi M, Farkas H, et al. 2010 International consensus algorithm for the diagnosis, therapy and management of hereditary angioedema. *Allergy Asthma Clin Immunol*. 2010;6:24.
98. Blomne G. Treatment of hereditary angioneurotic edema with transexamic acid: a random double-blind cross-over study. *Acta Med Scand*. 1972;192:808–809.
99. Gelfand JA, Sherins RJ, Alling DW, Frank MM. Treatment of hereditary angioedema with danazol: reversal of clinical and biochemical abnormalities. *N Engl J Med*. 1976;295:1444–1448.
100. Zuraw BL, Busse PJ, White M, et al. Nanofiltered C1 inhibitor concentrate for the treatment of hereditary angioedema. *N Engl J Med*. 2010;363: 513–522.
101. Bork K, Bygum A, Hardt J. Benefits and risks of danazol in hereditary angioedema: a long term survey of 118 patients. *Ann Allergy Asthma Immunol*. 2008;100;153–161.

102. Cicardi M, Bork K, Caballero T, et al, on behalf of HAWK (Hereditary Angioedema International Working Group). Evidence-based recommendations for the therepeutic management of andioedema owing to hereditary C1 inhibitor deficiency: consensus report of an International Working Group. *Allergy*. 2012;67:147–157.
103. Zuraw BL, Banerji A, Bernstein JA, et al. US Hereditary Angioedema Association Medical Advisory Board 2013 recommendations for the management of hereditary angioedema due to C1 inhibitor deficiency. *J Allergy Clin Immunol: In Practice*. 2013;1:458–467.
104. Zuraw BL, Bork K, Binkley KE, et al. Hereditary angioedema with normal C1 inhibitor function: consensus of an international expert panel. *Allergy Asthma Proc*. 2012; 33(suppl 1):S145–S156.
105. Bork K, Gul D, Hardt J, Dewald G. Hereditary angioedema with normal C1 inhibitor: clinical symptoms and course. *Am J Med*. 2007;120(11):987–992.
106. Bork K. Diagnosis and treatment of hereditary angioedema with normal C1 inhibitor. *Allergy Asthma Clin Immunol*. 2010;6(1):15.
107. Marcos C, Lopez Lera A, Varela S, Linares T, Alvarez-Eire MG, Lopez-Trascasa M. Clinical, biochemical, and genetic characterization of type III hereditary angioedema in 13 Northwest Spanish families. *Ann Allergy Asthma Immunol*. 2012;109(3):195–200, e2.
108. Vitrat-Hincky V, Gompel A, Dumestre-Perard C, et al. Type III hereditary angio-oedema: clinical and biological features in a French cohort. *Allergy*. 2010;65(10): 1331–1336.
109. Boccon-Gibod I, Bouillet L. Safety and efficacy of icatibant self-administration for acute hereditary angioedema. *Clin Exp Immunol*. 2012;168(3):303–307.
110. Bouillet L, Boccon-Gibod I, Ponard D, et al. Bradykinin receptor 2 antagonist (icatibant) for hereditary angioedema type III attacks. *Ann Allergy Asthma Immunol*. 2009;103(5):448.
111. Cronin JA, Maples KM. Treatment of an acute attack of type III hereditary angioedema with ecallantide. *Ann Allergy Asthma Immunol*. 2012;108(1):61–62.
112. Bork K, Wulff K, Hardt J, Witzke G, Staubach P. Hereditary angioedema caused by missense mutations in the factor XII gene: clinical features, trigger factors, and therapy. *J Allergy Clin Immunol*. 2009;124(1):129–134.
113. Bouillet L, Ponard D, Rousset H, Cichon S, Drouet C. A case of hereditary angio-oedema type III presenting with C1-inhibitor cleavage and a missense mutation in the F12 gene. *Br J Dermatol*. 2007;156(5):1063–1065.
114. Brown NJ, Snowden M, Griffin MR. Recurrent angiotensin-converting enzyme inhibitor--associated angioedema. *JAMA*. 1997;278(3):232–233.
115. Kaplan AP. Angioedema. *World Allergy Org J*. 2008;1(6): 103–113.
116. Miller DR, Oliveria SA, Berlowitz DR, Fincke BG, Stang P, Lillienfeld DE. Angioedema incidence in US veterans initiating angiotensin-converting enzyme inhibitors. *Hypertension*. 2008;51(6):1624–1630.
117. Mahmoudpour SH, Leusink M, van der Putten L, et al. Pharmacogenetics of ACE inhibitor-induced angioedema and cough: a systematic review and meta-analysis. *Pharmacogenomics*. 2013;14(3):249–260.
118. Kostis JB, Kim HJ, Rusnak J, et al. Incidence and characteristics of angioedema associated with enalapril. *Arch Internal Med*. 2005;165(14):1637–1642.
119. Pare G, Kubo M, Byrd JB, et al. Genetic variants associated with angiotensin-converting enzyme inhibitor-associated angioedema. *Pharmacogenetics and genomics*. 2013;23(9):470–478.
120. Woodard-Grice AV, Lucisano AC, Byrd JB, Stone ER, Simmons WH, Brown NJ. Sex-dependent and race-dependent association of XPNPEP2 C-2399A polymorphism with angiotensin-converting enzyme inhibitor-associated angioedema. *Pharmacogenet Genomics*. 2010;20(9):532–536.
121. Castelli R, Deliliers DL, Zingale LC, Pogliani EM, Cicardi M. Lymphoproliferative disease and acquired C1 inhibitor deficiency. *Haematologica*. 2007;92(5):716–718.
122. Hauptmann G, Petitjean F, Lang JM, Oberling F. Acquired C1 inhibitor deficiency in a case of lymphosarcoma of the spleen. Reversal of complement abnormalities after splenectomy. *Clin Exp Immunol*. 1979;37(3):523–531.
123. Lam DH, Levy NB, Nickerson JM, Gruenberg DA, Lansigan F. Acquired angioedema and marginal zone lymphoma. *J Clin Oncol*. 2012;30(16):e151–e153.
124. Jackson J, Feighery C. Autoantibody-mediated acquired deficiency of C1 inhibitor. *N Engl J Med*. 1988;318(2): 122–123.
125. Zingale LC, Castelli R, Zanichelli A, Cicardi M. Acquired deficiency of the inhibitor of the first complement component: presentation, diagnosis, course, and conventional management. *Immunol Allergy Clin North Am*. 2006;26(4):669–690.
126. Breitbart SI, Bielory L. Acquired angioedema: autoantibody associations and C1q utility as a diagnostic tool. *Allergy Asthma Proc*. 2010;31(5):428–434.
127. Ishoo E, Shah UK, Grillone GA, Stram JR, Fuleihan NS. Predicting airway risk in angioedema: staging system based on presentation. *Otolaryngol Head Neck Surg*. 1999; 121(3):263–268.

8

Drug Hypersensitivity

Juliane A. Pichler, Marco D. Caversaccio, and Werner J. Pichler

INTRODUCTION

Drug-induced adverse reactions are common. Rawlings and Edwards have proposed classifying them into type A and type B reactions.[1] Type A reactions are those with predictable side effects due to the pharmacological actions of the drug. An example would be sleepiness caused by first-generation antihistamines, when they bind to H1-receptors in the brain. Type B reactions occur only in individuals with an "idiosyncratic" predisposition. They comprise about one-sixth of all adverse reactions, and the majority of such type B reactions are drug hypersensitivity reactions. The idiosyncrasy can be due to a genetic difference, which results in a less active or absent enzyme or receptor expression.[2] This may cause an altered/diminished metabolism and thus trigger an immune response to the drug. Genetic analyses and the linkage of specific gene products to drug metabolism or antigen presentation suggest that some of these idiosyncratic reactions may be predictable.[3]

Drug hypersensitivity reactions fall into 3 categories, *allergic* (immune-mediated), *pharmacological* (pharmacological interaction with specific immune receptors [HLA, TCR] [p-i concept]), and *nonallergic* ("pseudo-allergic") hypersensitivity reactions.

RISK FACTORS FOR DRUG HYPERSENSITIVITY

Any drug can elicit a hypersensitivity reaction, but the incidence between different drugs varies widely. The drugs most frequently responsible are antibiotics, anti-inflammatory drugs, anti-epileptics, occasionally diuretics, proton pump inhibitors, muscle relaxants, and antiviral drugs. The risk of sensitization or immune stimulation and the severity of clinical symptoms depend on many factors, including the type of drug, dosage, duration of treatment, and patient immunogenetic makeup, such as human leukocyte antigen (HLA) type[2] (Table 8–1). Patient pharmacogenetic makeup (eg, variability of cytochrome P450-related enzymes) is occasionally related to drug hypersensitivity reactions, since slower metabolism may result in higher plasma drug levels and more side effects.[3] In addition, an individual's state of immune activation is also important. For example, activation of the immune system due to a generalized viral infection (Epstein-Barr virus [EBV] or HIV) predisposes to the development of predominantly T-cell–mediated drug hypersensitivity responses. Pseudo-allergic reactions to nonsteroidal anti-inflammatory drugs (NSAIDs) may be related to the intensity of eosinophilic inflammation

Table 8–1. Risk Factors for Drug Hypersensitivity

Previous drug hypersensitivity (to the same drug or drug class)
Type of drug: antibiotics (beta-lactam antibiotics), antiviral drugs (abacavir and nevirapine), anti-epileptics (carbamazepine, lamotrigine, phenytoin, etc)
High dose and longer duration of treatment
Immunogenetic predisposition (eg, HLA-B*57:01 for abacavir)[2,19]
Pharmacogenetic predisposition (phenytoin levels increased in CYP2C9*3 carriers)
Immune activation:
Generalized viral infection (EBV, HIV)
Ongoing drug hypersensitivity reaction
Active autoimmune disease
Underlying eosinophilic inflammation in NSAID intolerance
Epicutaneous application (eg, antibiotics)

in the upper and lower respiratory tract. Some reactions are more common in females. Epicutaneous application of a drug clearly increases the risk of immune-mediated sensitization compared to oral or parenteral treatment. Atopy is normally not associated with a higher risk of drug hypersensitivity, but an atopic predisposition was found to prolong the detectability of drug-specific IgE in the serum.[4]

TIME OF APPEARANCE

Drug hypersensitivity reactions can have many different clinical presentations, some of which can be severe and even fatal.[5] Drug hypersensitivity has become a major imitator of other diseases, taking over the role previously held by syphilis. The most common allergic reactions affect the skin and are observed in about 2% to 3% of hospitalized patients,[5–7] but elevation of liver enzymes and eosinophilia are also common in more severe forms. From a clinical point of view, the time of appearance of clinical drug hypersensitivity is helpful to distinguish different forms of this condition (Figure 8–1).

In already sensitized individuals, IgE-mediated reactions tend to appear rapidly, normally within minutes to 1 hour after drug intake. However, the sensitization and development of IgE antibodies to the drug (or drug metabolite) must have occurred previously in a nonclinically apparent form. In this situation, the drug causes a silent sensitization during the initial treatment and, upon reexposure, a sudden anaphylactic reaction occurs. On the other hand, delayed appearing drug hypersensitivity reactions (mostly T-cell mediated) appear later and often become manifest *during* the initial treatment, which may last for many days. At the beginning of treatment, only a few T-cells are able to react with the drug, and no symptoms appear. Clinical symptoms such as maculopapular rashes appear only after expansion of drug-specific T-cell clones and their migration into the tissue. This explains the typical time interval between start of treatment and appearance of a rash (eg, from amoxicillin or quinolone, usually at day 9 or 10). However, after reexposure to the same drug, symptoms of these T-cell reactions may appear rather rapidly (within 2 to 48 hours), depending on the preexisting numbers of drug-reactive (primed) T cells and the drug dosage.

Most pseudo-allergic reactions occur rapidly, within 15 minutes to 1 to 2 hours after oral drug intake, depending on previous food intake. They do not require previous sensitization but are highly dose dependent.

MECHANISMS OF DRUG STIMULATION OF THE IMMUNE SYSTEM

To understand drug hypersensitivity, it is essential to know that there are at least 3 different ways that drugs can stimulate the immune system:

1. *Allergic/immune reactions*, which are based on formation of a hapten (drug)-carrier antigenic complex, and stimulation of innate and adaptive immunity, resulting in a *complete* immune response.
2. *Pharmacological interaction with an immune receptor* (p-i concept) involves selective stimulations of T cells, driven by drug binding to a TCR (T-cell receptor) or HLA molecules.[8] The activation of dendritic cells is not a requirement.[8,9] This type

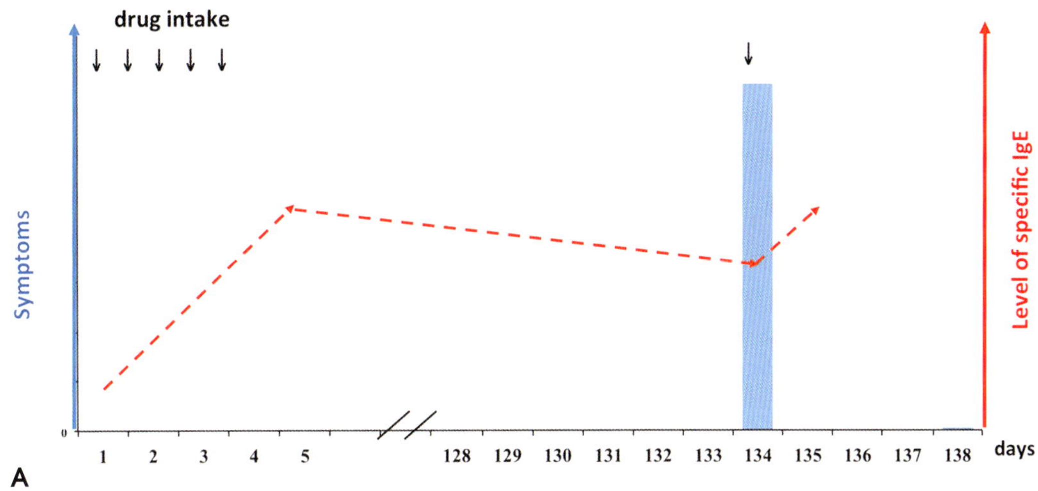

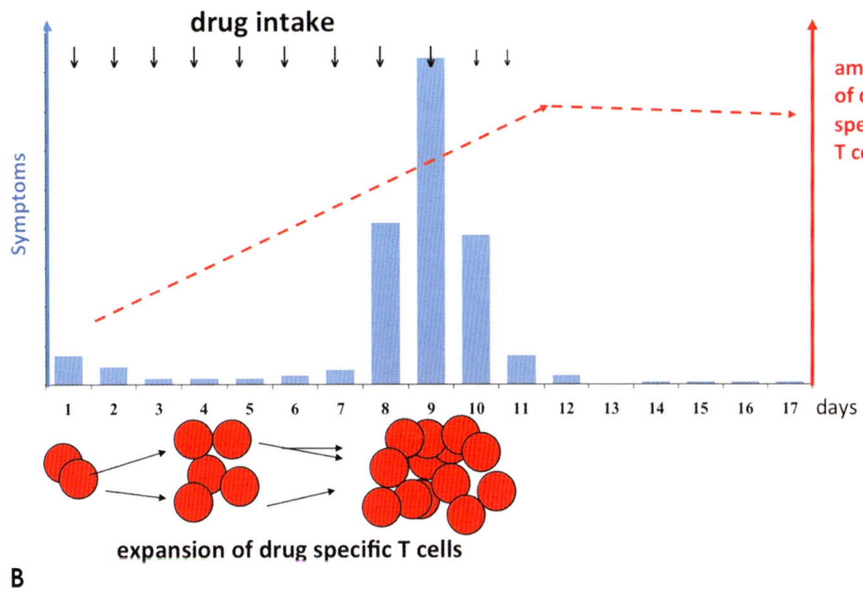

Figure 8–1. Kinetics of immunoglobulin E (IgE) and T-cell–mediated reactions. **A.** Immediate (IgE mediated) type: a sensitization phase, which was asymptomatic, meaning that the gradual increase of drug specific IgE went along with an adaptation (similar to a desensitization). Only after an interruption of drug exposure and new exposure, acute symptoms emerge, mostly within 1 hour. **B.** Delayed (T-cell mediated) type hypersensitivity: it develops upon continuous treatment over days. During this time period the drug specific T cells expand and reach the tissue causing symptoms. Sensitization can persist for many years.

of immune stimulation may be peculiar to small molecules such as drugs and may result in an immune response and a clinical picture similar to a graft-vs-host (GVH) reaction.[9]

3. *Nonallergic hypersensitivity ("pseudo-allergic" reactions).* In these reactions, neither drug-specific T cells nor B cells (immunoglobulins) can be detected, and their pathogenetic mechanism is unclear. They may represent a different form of drug-dependent stimulation of inflammatory effector cells, such as mast cells, basophils, eosinophils, or neutrophils. The clinical picture imitates the end phase of an allergic reaction, explaining the term *pseudo-allergy*.

The Immune (Allergic) Pathway: Hapten and Prohapten Mechanism

This mechanism is the classical explanation for drug hypersensitivity.[10] The drug (or drug metabolite) is too small to stimulate the immune system by itself. However, it can act as a hapten, meaning that the drug or metabolite binds via covalent bonds to a carrier protein, and the complex acquires antigenic features.[11] This hapten mechanism is experimentally well established and has been extensively studied in allergic conditions such as contact dermatitis.[11,12] It is dependent on the ability of the hapten to stimulate both *innate* (eg, dendritic cells) as well as *adaptive* immunity (specific T and B cells/antibodies) in order to produce a specific immune response to the hapten.

The innate inflammatory response involves the triggering of pattern recognition receptors either by direct chemical interaction with such receptors or by induction of endogenous activators. This induces the expression of CD40 or other costimulatory molecules on the dendritic cells.[12] Whether and where the stimulation of innate immunity by haptens takes place in systemic drug hypersensitivity is unknown.

The adaptive immune response is triggered by newly formed hapten-carrier complexes. Carrier proteins usually consist of soluble autologous (eg, albumin, transferrin) or cell-bound proteins (eg, integrins, selectins) to which the drug covalently binds. This causes stimulation of both B-cell and T-cell immunity directed against the "neo-antigen" (Figure 8–2).[13] Since many different proteins may

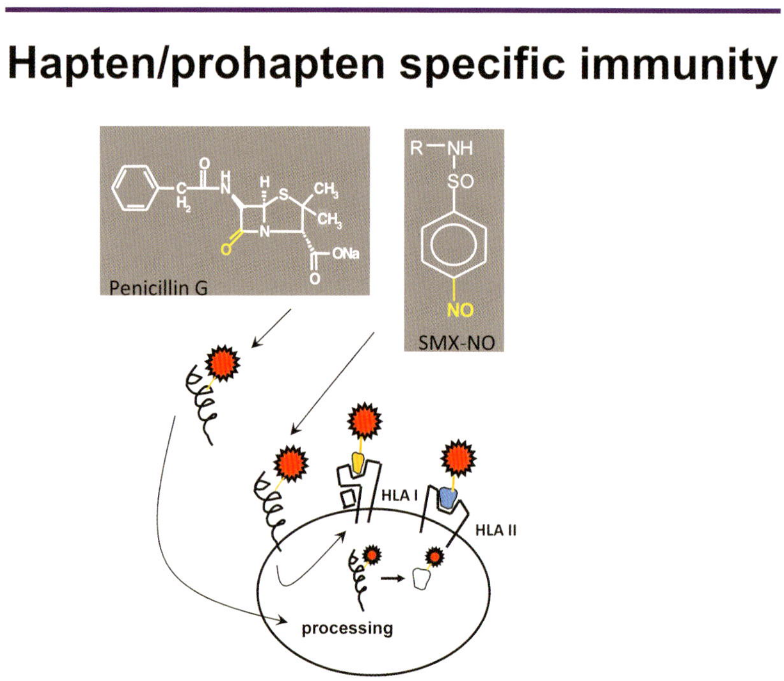

Figure 8-2. Hapten and prohapten mechanisms. Haptens are chemically reactive molecules able to bind covalently to certain amino acids like lysine or cysteine in proteins (eg, penicillin G). Other drugs are prohaptens requiring metabolic activation to become haptens. The metabolism leads to the formation of a chemically reactive compound (eg, sulfamethoxazole (SMX) is converted to the chemically reactive form SMX-NO). The target protein for haptens can be soluble or cell bound. The hapten-carrier complex can be recognized by immunoglobulins, or after processing and presentation on the HLA on antigen-presenting cells (APCs) by drug-specific T cells. Thus, based on the chemical reactivity of haptens many distinct antigenic epitopes are generated, which can elicit both humoral and cellular immune responses.

bind to a drug, the clinical picture elicited by the immune response to these neo-antigens may also be very heterogeneous. Penicillin G and other penicillins are typical haptens, which bind covalently to ε-amino groups on lysine residues in soluble or cell-bound proteins.[13]

Some drugs are pro-haptens gaining the ability to bind covalently only after metabolism. Sulfamethoxazole is a prototype of a pro-hapten.[14] It is metabolized by cytochrome p450 2C9, which produces sulfamethoxazole-hydroxylamine. This latter compound can be detected in tissues and in urine. It is easily transformed by oxidation to the highly reactive sulfamethoxazole-nitroso (SMX-NO) compound (see Figure 8–2). SMX-NO is chemically highly reactive and binds covalently to cysteines within proteins/peptides, forming neoantigens. The clinical picture elicited by pro-haptens can be as variable as the one elicited by haptens.

The *Pharmacological Pathway* (p-i Concept): Drug Binding to Specific Immune Receptors

Drugs may also stimulate the immune system by binding to immune receptors, namely HLA molecules or T-cell receptors (TCRs).[8,15] These immune receptors are highly polymorphic. One estimates that there are more than 10^{11} different TCRs per individual and more than 10 000 different HLA-class I and more than 3000 class II alleles in the human population (http://www.allelefrequencies.net/hla6006a.asp). Thus, the chances are high that a certain drug may bind to some part of these receptors with high affinity. This binding of drugs to proteins functioning as immune receptors is *noncovalent* and due to van der Waals forces, hydrogen bonds, and electrostatic interactions. Such interactions are common but in most instances the drug-protein interaction occurs without a functional consequence (eg, the binding occurs on irrelevant sites of the protein [HLA or TCR] and/or the binding may be too labile to elicit a functional consequence).[8] However, occasionally a drug will interact with a region of the immune receptor (peptide binding site of HLA proteins or TCR), which then stimulates a specific immune system (T cells). This interaction is termed the *pharmacological interaction of drugs with immune receptors* (p-i concept, Figure 8–3).[8,16,17]

It is important to understand that according to the p-i-concept, the drug binds to the *receptor-structure* (HLA or TCR protein) and not to a peptide, as a hapten does. This phenomenon has *not* been described for B-cell stimulation. The ensuing T-cell stimulation is *not* a "classical" immune reaction to an altered protein. It is a pharmacological activation of immune cells, which imitates an immune reaction. This p-i reaction is probably the explanation for most delayed, severe generalized T-cell–mediated drug reactions such as maculopapular or bullous exanthem, hepatitis, and nephritis (see Figure 8–3).

In this type of mechanism, drugs can bind either to the TCR (p-i TCR) or to HLA receptors (p-i HLA).[8]

p-i T-Cell Receptor

Drugs can fit into some of the innumerable different TCRs. Some of these interactions may occur at "crucial" sites and can lead to stimulation of T cells. As shown for sulfamethoxazole, the drug can directly interact with the CDR3 regions of TCR (which usually interacts with the peptide-HLA complex),[16] and then stimulate TCR triggered signals. Alternatively the drug can bind to the CDR2 region and causes an allogeneic alteration of the TCR which can interact more strongly with the HLA-peptide complex.[17] In both forms of p-i TCR, an additional interaction with HLA-molecules is required for full T-cell stimulation.

It is assumed that this TCR-mediated stimulation by a small molecule is possible because the reactive T cells are already preactivated and thus have a lower threshold of reactivity than resting T cells. This type of preactivation may be caused by cytokine secretion during a massive immune stimulation such as generalized herpes or HIV infection. Similarly, other forms of increased immunity such as exacerbations of autoimmune diseases and other drug hypersensitivity reactions are known risk factors for the development of drug hypersensitivity reactions (see Table 8–1). This preactivation of the immune system is probably necessary for a p-i TCR reaction, but not for a p-i HLA reaction.

p-i HLA

In this type of reaction, the drug binds directly to the HLA molecule (p-i HLA). It may bind preferentially (or exclusively) to a specific HLA-allele. This explains the high association of certain drug

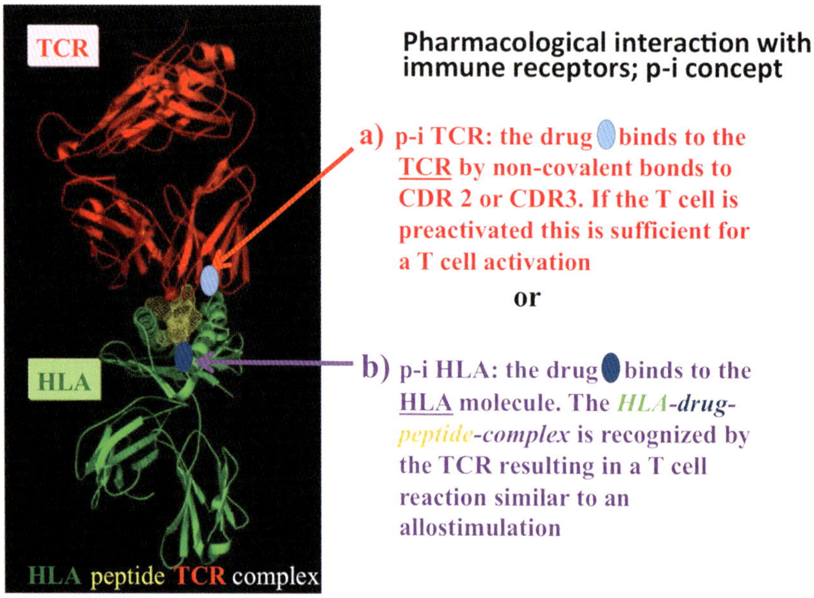

Figure 8–3. The p-i-concept (pharmacological interaction with immune receptors). Drugs are often designed to fit into certain proteins/enzymes to block their function. Some drugs may happen to bind aberrantly into some of the available T-cell receptors or HLA molecules. Under certain conditions (see text) this drug-immune receptor interaction may lead to a T-cell stimulation: (a) p-i TCR: The drug (shown for sulfamethoxazole) binds to the CDR3 or CDR2 region of a unique TCR: Such an interaction may result in TCR stimulation when contact to HLA-peptide complex is provided.[8] Often preactivation of T cells is needed. (b) p-i HLA: the drug happens to bind noncovalently to the peptide binding groove of an peculiar HLA molecule. This results in (i) formation of an altered drug-HLA-peptide complex, which stimulates T cells like an allo-antigen[8,9] (ii) or it induces an exchange of peptide presented, as a peptide binding site is occupied by the drug and thus an altered peptide is presented: as the "altered" peptide is new, it is stimulatory.[22–24]

hypersensitivity reactions with certain HLA-alleles that is seen in reactions to drugs such as abacavir (Table 8–2).[2,18–20]

Two functional consequences of p-i HLA have been described: The drug binding to HLA changes the appearance of the self HLA-molecule so it resembles a foreign HLA molecule.[9] This alteration of the crucial self-determining molecule elicits a strong allo-immune response.[9] In fact, the altered HLA-drug peptide complex stimulates T cells in a rather unusual way, without involving dendritic cell stimulation.[9] This scenario, documented experimentally for abacavir allergy, helps explain why some symptoms of drug hypersensitivity are similar to GVH immune reactions.[21]

Another result of drug binding to the HLA molecule is an alteration in its peptide binding ability. In the case of abacavir, instead of the usual peptides that normally bind to HLA-B*57:01, now other peptides that normally bind only to another HLA (eg, HLA-B*58:01), can also bind to the abacavir-altered HLA-B*57:01.[22–24] This phenomenon is termed *altered peptide repertoire* and may lead to autoimmunity or allo-reactivity. It is important to note that in spite of the "abnormal" T-cell stimulation induced by p-i, the resultant T-cell activations are "normal," with

Table 8-2. Associations Between Some Severe Delayed-Type Drug Hypersensitivity Reactions and Specific HLA Alleles[2,18–20]

Causative Drug	HLA	Hypersensitivity Reactions	Ethnicity	Odds Ratio (95% CI)
Abacavir	B*57:01	Abacavir hypersensitivity	Caucasian	117 (29–481)
Allopurinol	B*58:01	SJS/TEN/DRESS	Asian	74.18 (26.95–204.14)
Allopurinol	B*58:01	SJS/TEN/DRESS	Non-Asian	101.45 (44.98–228.82)
Carbamazepine	B*15:02	SJS/TEN	Han Chinese	115.32 (18.17–732.13)
Carbamazepine	B*15:11	SJS/TEN	Japanese, Korean	16.3 (4.76–55.61)
Carbamazepine	A*31:01	SJS/TEN	European	4.4 (1.1–17.3)
Carbamazepine	A*31:01	DRESS	European	57.6 (11.0–340)
Dapsone	B*13:01	DRESS	Mainland China, Han Chinese	20.53 (11.55–36.48)
Lamotrigine	B*15:02	SJS/TEN	Han Chinese	3.59 (1.15–11.22)
Flucloxacillin	B*57:01	Hepatitis	European/Caucasian	80,6 (22.8–284.9)

Note. DRESS = drug reaction with eosinophilia and systemic symptoms; *SJS* = Stevens-Johnson syndrome; *TEN* = toxic epidermal necrolysis; *CI* = confidence interval.

typical secretion of cytokines or target cell–directed cytotoxicity.

The p-i concept has radically changed our understanding of drug-induced hypersensitivity reactions and explains some unusual features of drug hypersensitivity that are not explained by the hapten mechanism. The p-i concept explains the occurrence of symptoms after the first encounter with a drug without a prior sensitization phase, or the lack of a memory response in weak drug stimulations, where the limited drug stimulation of T cells may suffice to cause some symptoms (a transient rash) but no memory response. Also the higher risk of drug hypersensitivity in generalized viral infections may be linked to the p-i concept, as T-cell stimulation by a drug depends on prior T-cell activation.[17]

Table 8–2 shows some relevant HLA associations of several severe, CD8-mediated drug hypersensitivity reactions.[2,18–20] These associations have been found mainly with HLA-class I alleles and are specific for a certain drug. Of note is that the relevant differences of associations correspond to the frequency of an allele in certain ethnic groups (eg, the HLA-allele B*15:02 is common in the Chinese/East Asian population and strikingly associated with carbamazepine-induced SJS/TEN). In European and Japanese populations, HLA-B*15:02 is almost absent, and 50% to 60% of these carbamazepine-allergic patients carry HLA-A*31:01.[18,25]

For some alleles, the association is rather unique for one allele (abacavir and HLA-B*57:01). But for other HLA-associated drug hypersensitivity reactions the association is not absolute: Only about 60% of European patients with allopurinol-induced SJS/TEN carry HLA-B*58:01.

The frequent association of certain HLA-alleles with hypersensitivity reactions to particular drugs not only leads to a better understanding of drug hypersensitivity, but is already being used to prevent such side effects. Reactions to carbamazepine can be avoided by typing Southeast Asian patients for HLA-*B15:02, and in Europe and the United States, severe abacavir drug reactions have been greatly reduced, by pre-drug treatment HLA typing.[26,27]

Pseudo-Allergy (Non-Immune-Mediated Drug Hypersensitivity)

There is a third, distinct mechanism of drug hypersensitivity whose possibly heterogeneous mechanisms are less well understood, and are termed *nonallergic* drug hypersensitivity, *drug intolerance* or *pseudo-allergy*.[28] The effector cells of this type of inflammation, such as eosinophils, basophils, or mast cells (and possibly neutrophils) seem to be directly activated by certain drugs, without evidence of drug-specific IgE or T cells. However, in vitro, these drugs do not induce mediator release from basophils or mast cells.

Pseudo-allergic reactions are at least as frequent as IgE-mediated reactions to drugs. They can be elicited by many different drugs, but some drugs seem to elicit them more often (Table 8–3). The main elicitors of pseudo-allergic reactions are NSAIDs but many other drugs (radiocontrast media, muscle relaxants, quinolones and vancomycin) may cause them as well, often with rapidly appearing skin symptoms.[29,30] In the case of pseudo-allergic reactions to NSAIDs, some of the side effects can be explained by known pharmacological activities such as blockade of prostaglandin (PG) synthesis and a shift to increased leukotriene (LT) synthesis. However many symptoms of "pseudo-allergy" are not explained by this pharmacological action on PG synthesis.[31] Some might be due to a recently described receptor ("MRGPRX2", Mas-Related G-Protein Coupled Receptor Member X2), which was found to be crucial for IgE-independent, direct mast cells stimulation by fluoroquinolone antibiotics and neuromuscular blocking agents (NMBA).[32]

The majority of these reactions are mild and not dangerous, but some cause anaphylaxis and can be lethal, even at the first encounter with the drug. They may appear as rapidly as true IgE-mediated allergies/anaphylaxis (5 to 30 minutes after drug intake). These reactions are clearly dose dependent and often require higher doses to elicit clinical symptoms than IgE-mediated reactions. The typical initial symptoms of early anaphylaxis, namely palmar and/or plantar itch, may be less common in pseudo-allergy than in IgE-mediated anaphylaxis. High serum tryptase levels 1 to 4 hours after an anaphylactic reaction due to pseudo-allergy confirm that mast cell degranulation has occurred. In other pseudo-allergic reactions, other inflammatory cells such as eosinophils, are stimulated.

A common feature of some of these pseudo-allergic reactions seems to be an ongoing, often eosinophilic inflammation in the affected patient. As a result, many of these patients also experience similar, but milder symptoms of affected organs in the absence of drug exposure (rhinosinusitis/asthma or chronic urticaria). This underlying inflam-

Table 8–3. Common Causes of Allergic and "Pseudoallergic" Drug Reactions

Drugs Involved in IgE-Mediated Allergies[a]	Drugs Causing Pseudoallergic Reactions[a]
Foreign proteins (chimeric antibodies)	(Radio)contrast media[b]
Immunoglobulin preparations (containing IgA in IgA-deficient patients)	Plasma expanders
β-lactam antibiotics	NSAID: acetylsalicylic acid, diclofenac, mefenamic acid, ibuprofen
Penicillins, cephalosporins	Pyrazolones
Pyrazolones	Quinolones
Quinolones	Muscle relaxants
Muscle relaxants	
(Radio)contrast media	

Note. IgE, immunoglobulin E; *NSAID*, nonsteroidal anti-inflammatory drug.
[a]Not complete; only main groups mentioned.
[b]Some reactions appear to be IgE mediated.

mation seems to be important for the drug sensitivity, because the drug intolerance is reduced if the inflammatory symptoms are controlled.

understanding whether immune, p-i, or pseudo-allergic stimulations are involved is very important.

CLASSIFICATION OF DRUG HYPERSENSITIVITY REACTIONS BASED ON CLINICAL PRESENTATION

Drug hypersensitivity reactions are complex and result in different symptoms and diseases. To account for this heterogeneity and to explain the various clinical pictures, Gell and Coombs classified drug hypersensitivity as well as other immune reactions in 4 categories (types I to IV reactions).[33] Pichler has revised and extended this classification to take into account the heterogeneity of T-cell functions[34] (Figure 8–4).

For many years, the Gell and Coombs classification has been a useful tool to help understand drug allergy and its underlying immune pathological mechanisms. It is still a valuable tool but has various drawbacks, and one should be aware of its limitations:

- The Gell and Coombs classification is based on the immune/hapten concept. It does not explain pseudo-allergic reactions, and it does not explain the different clinic observed with p-i TCR or p-i HLA.
- A specific clinical picture is not exclusively linked to a single type of Gell and Coombs reaction. Urticaria may be caused by mast cell degranulation following IgE cross-linking by a hapten-carrier complex (type I), or complement activation (C3a, C5a) in the setting of immune complex disease (type III), or may be due to an undefined "pseudo-allergic" mechanism. Similarly, a maculopapular rash may be due to a p-i or a hapten-based immune stimulation of T cells. Since the type of stimulation (immune, p-i or pseudo-allergic) may predict multiple aspects of the clinical course including the risk of cross-reactivity with other drugs, the association with HLA alleles, the advice for avoidance strategies, and the treatment of drug hypersensitivity,

IgE-Mediated Reactions (Anaphylactic Reactions, Type I)

As outlined in Figure 8–2, a drug acting as a hapten can modify soluble and cell-bound proteins. This hapten-protein complex induces a *humoral* immune response that involves T and B cell activation. B cells mature into Ig-secreting plasma cells upon contact with the hapten-protein complex, provided they obtain help by stimulated T cells, which recognize processed hapten-protein fragments. The interaction occurs through a CD40–CD40L interaction and requires several T-cell derived cytokines (IL-4, IL-13, IL-5 or IFN-gamma). The type of cytokine secreted by the T cells determines the type of immunoglobulin (IgG, IgA or IgE) that is produced. When there is a second contact with the drug, a hapten-carrier complex is formed again, which then interacts with the preformed antibodies and elicits symptoms. For humoral immune responses, the drug binds to Ig receptors on B cells as an *unprocessed hapten-protein* complex, and to the TCR on T cells as a *processed hapten-peptide* fragment. The development of a complete immune response strongly indicates that the drug can act as a hapten, which stably binds to a protein. An important exception to this rule is anaphylaxis on first exposure (see box below).

The sensitization phase and development of drug-specific immunity is normally clinically inapparent and symptoms only appear after a second drug exposure. If drug-specific IgE molecules had been previously induced, they bind to FcεI receptors (FcεRI) on mast cells and basophils. Since the drug/hapten is normally too small to cross-link 2 cell surface, IgE molecules, the cross-linking is achieved by a protein, to which the drug/hapten binds at 2 distinct sites. This hapten-protein complex is big enough to cross-link 2 adjacent IgE molecules and to induce mast cell degranulation.

The IgE system is optimized to react to small amounts of antigens. It achieves this extraordinary sensitivity by the ubiquitous presence of mast cells containing high-affinity FcεRI, to which allergen/drug-specific IgE is bound. Very small amounts of

	Type I	Type II	Type III	Type IV a	Type IV b	Type IV c	Type IV d
Immune reactant	IgE	IgG	IgG	IIFNγ, TNFα (T_H1 cells)	IL-5, IL-4/ IL-13 (T_H2 cells)	perforin/ granzymeB, granulysin (CTL)	CXCL-8. GM-CSF, (T-cells)
Antigen	Soluble antigen	Cell- or matrix-associated antigen	Soluble antigen	Peptide and hapten-peptide antigen presented by HLA calass I or II or p-i stimulations (p-i TCR and p-i HLA)			
Effector	Mast-cell activation	FcR^+ cells (phagocytes, NK cells)	FcR^+ cells Complement	Macrophage activation	Eosinophils	T cells	Neutrophils
Example of hypersen-sitivity reaction	Allergic rhinitis, asthma, systemic anaphylaxis	Some drug allergies (e.g., penicillin)	Serum sickness, Arthus reaction	Tuberculin reaction, contact dermatitis (with IVc)	Chronic asthma, chronic allergic rhinitis Maculopap. exanthem with eosinoph.	Contact dermatitis Maculopap. & bullous exanthema Hepatitis	AGEP Behçet disease

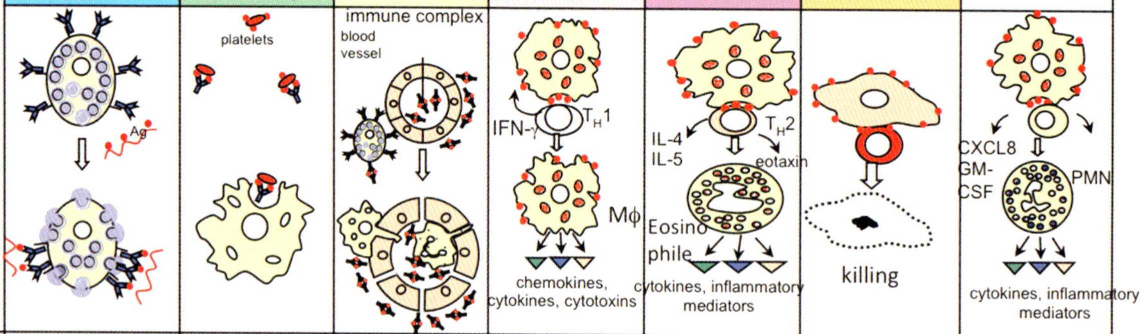

Figure 8-4. Revised Gell and Coombs classification of drug reactions. Drugs can elicit all types of immune reactions. Although all reactions are T-cell regulated, the effector functions are either predominantly antibody-mediated (type I–III) or rely more on T-cell/cytokine-dependent functions (type IVa–IVd). Type I reactions are IgE-mediated. Cross-linking IgE molecules on high-affinity IgE receptors (Fcε-RI) on mast cells and basophilic granulocytes leads to degranulation and release of mediators, which cause a variety of symptoms (vasodilatation, increased permeability, bronchoconstriction, itch). Type II and III reactions are IgG mediated: type II cause cell destruction due to complement activation by membrane fixed immunoglobulins or interaction with Fcγ receptor-bearing killer cells (cell dyscrasia). Type III reactions do also involve complement deposition and activation in small vessels and recruitment of neutrophilic granulocytes via Fcγ receptor interaction. The local vascular inflammation leads to vasculitis and serum sickness like symptoms. Type IVa correspond to Th1 reactions with high IFN-γ/TNF-α secretion and involves monocyte/macrophage activation. Often, one can see also a CD8 cell recruitment (type IVc reaction). Type IVb reactions correspond to eosinophilic inflammation and to a Th2 response with high IL-4/IL-5/IL-13 secretion; they are often associated with an IgE-mediated type I reaction. Type IVc: the cytotoxic reactions rely on cytotoxic T cells (both CD4 and CD8 cells) themselves as effector cells. They seem to occur in all drug-related delayed hypersensitivity reactions. Type IVd reactions correspond to a T-cell-dependent, sterile neutrophilic inflammatory process. They are clearly distinct from the rapid influx of polymorphonuclear leukocytes in bacterial infections and seem to be related to high CXCL-8/granulocyte-macrophage colony-stimulating factor (GM-CSF) production by T cells (and tissue cells). The role of IL-17 in IVd reactions is not yet defined. Adapted from Pichler WJ. Immune mechanism of drug hypersensitivity. *Immunol Allergy Clin North Am.* 2004;24:373–397.

Anaphylaxis on first exposure:

Many anaphylactic reactions to radiocontrast dyes, muscle relaxants, and many other drugs occur at the first drug encounter. How do these drug-reactive IgE antibodies develop? Most of these reactions occur against intravenous drugs, which are given rapidly and in a rather high concentrations. The affected patient may have previously developed IgE antibodies against drug "A," which also cross-reacts with high concentrations of drug "B." Drug "A" and drug "B" may only be minimally structurally related (eg, have a common cationic ammonium). Some generated IgE antibodies react preferentially with this cationic ammonium and recognize it also in "B," if high concentrations of B are provided. The high drug concentration partially compensates for the low affinity of the IgE to the cross-reactive compound. How cross-linking of IgE on mast cells by rather small compounds which are not known to bind covalently to proteins is achieved is unclear. However, it is clear that even the first dose of a drug can provoke an anaphylactic reaction.

a drug are sufficient to interact and stimulate these receptor-bound IgE molecules, as shown by the fact that systemic reactions can occur even with relatively low-dose drug allergen skin testing. After cross-linking the FcεRI, various mediators (histamine, tryptase, leukotrienes, prostaglandins, tumor necrosis factor-α [TNF-α], platelet activating factor, etc.) are released, which induce the typical allergic symptoms. IgE-mediated symptoms were once considered not to be dose independent, because such small amounts of allergen could cause severe reactions. However, further diminishing the dose, as is done during desensitization procedures, demonstrates that these reactions *are* clearly dose dependent.

A clinically important exception is the phenomenon of *anaphylaxis at first exposure* (see the box). This occurs if IgE antibodies previously developed against a different substance are able to cross-react with the new drug. As the new drug is given rapidly and in high amounts (intravenously), it may bind to mast cell bound IgE even if the IgE avidity is low. This type of cross-reactivity helps explain the puzzling observation that many anaphylactic reactions to intravenous drugs such as radiocontrast dyes, muscle relaxants, and cephalosporins, occur at the *first encounter* with the drug, without any prior drug exposure.

Clinical Aspects of Anaphylaxis

Anaphylaxis is a serious allergic reaction that is rapid in onset and may cause death.[35] Drugs are a main cause of anaphylaxis, and the most frequent cause of *fatal* anaphylaxis (60% of anaphylaxis fatalities are due to drugs).[36] It typically involves several organs and causes a number of symptoms including an itchy rash, throat swelling, and low blood pressure. In already sensitized individuals the reaction can start within seconds to minutes after parenteral administration, and minutes after oral intake (Figure 8–5). Anaphylactic shock occurs often within 2 to 15 minutes, and asphyxia due to laryngeal edema may occur within 10 to 60 minutes.[37] During the infusion the patient may begin to complain about warmth along the vein, local itch, and malaise. Often palmar, plantar, genital, or axillary itch is the initial symptom, which along with patient anxiety, should be appreciated as important alarm signals, since they often herald a possibly severe, anaphylactic reaction. Within minutes the skin becomes red, often starting with the upper thorax, neck, and face, and then spreading to the whole body. In the next 20 to 60 minutes an urticarial rash may appear, together with swelling (angioedema) of the periorbital, perioral, and sometimes genital areas. Asphyxia may account for 60% of anaphylaxis-related deaths, and laryngeal swelling should be suspected if the voice becomes hoarse, and the patient has difficulty speaking and swallowing due to tongue swelling.[38] Patients may also complain of chest tightness and dyspnea, signs of acute bronchospasm. Some patients develop gastrointestinal symptoms (nausea, cramps, vomiting, and fecal incontinence). The full syndrome of cardiac and/or bronchial, cutaneous, and/or GI involvement results in anaphylactic shock, which is lethal in about 1% of cases. Hypotension may occur, either due to heightened permeability

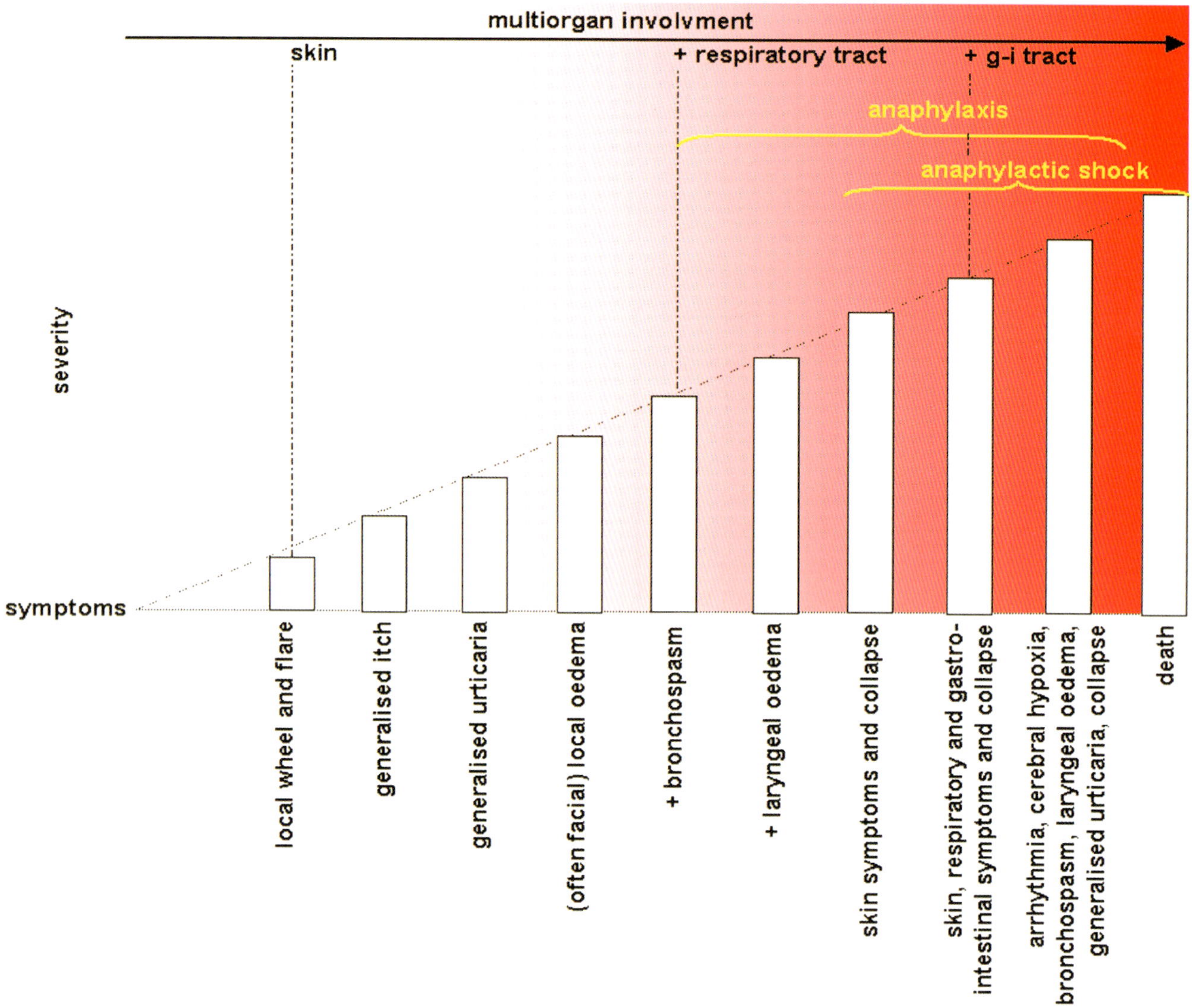

Figure 8–5. Anaphylaxis. Symptoms of IgE-mediated allergy; from wheal and flare to fulminant anaphylaxis and anaphylactic shock. Reprinted with permission from Karger S, Pichler WJ. *Drug Hypersensitivity*. Basel, Switzerland: S. Karger AG; 2007.

of small vessels and subsequent shift of volume into the extravascular space or, faster and more dangerously, because of cardiac arrhythmia. Sudden cardiac arrest may be the only symptom of anaphylaxis. Cardiac arrest may appear extremely rapidly (just after starting the infusion) and even without (before) other signs appearing; urticaria and swelling may follow later.

Risk factors for a severe episode are a fulminant appearance of symptoms, preexisting (untreated) asthma, underlying mastocytosis, treatment with β-blocking agents (which makes adrenaline/epinephrine less effective), and use of ACE inhibitors, which increase and prolong bradykinin-related symptoms like swelling, since bradykinin degradation is blocked by ACE inhibitors. Older age is a risk for anaphylaxis-associated myocardial infarction or cerebral hypoxia/damage. Anaphylactic shock is a severe event, and survivors are often left with some cognitive or intellectual impairment.

The acute symptoms of anaphylaxis normally last 2 to 3 hours, but surveillance for 6 to 24 hours is strongly recommended. About 20% of patients with severe anaphylaxis develop a second attack (urticaria, bronchospasm) 3 to 6 hours after the first attack, due to renewed mediator release. Table 8–3 summarizes the main drugs causing anaphylaxis.

Most IgE-mediated allergies to drugs are less severe, and often general redness, diffuse urticaria, or angioedema are the only symptoms. These reactions occur normally in the first hour after drug exposure but can occur later, if the oral absorption of the drug is slow. The symptoms last for hours, and swelling from angioedema may last for days.

It is important to be aware that *any IgE-mediated drug allergy can be potentially life threatening.* Mild symptoms might simply be due to a relatively low dose, and higher doses or more rapid administration (IV) may cause more severe reactions. In addition, each drug exposure may further boost the IgE response. Pretreatment with anti-H1 blockers and corticosteroids may attenuate mild reactions but do not prevent severe reactions.

Patients developing anaphylaxis should receive adrenaline (epinephrine) intramuscularly (thigh) as soon as possible (0.3 to 0.5 mg intramuscularly [IM]), preferentially before full-blown symptoms begin: *do not hesitate, there is no contraindication to IM adrenalin in anaphylaxis. The sooner the better.* Administer corticosteroids and begin intravenous infusion. If no improvement occurs within 2 to 3 minutes, repeat adrenaline.

Clinical Descriptions of Pseudo-Allergic Reactions

The most frequent cause of pseudo-allergic reactions is NSAIDs.[31] In the majority of these reactions no drug-specific IgE-antibodies (or T-cell reactions) can be identified. Moreover, other drugs with the similar ability to block prostaglandin-synthesis elicit similar reactions, although the structure of these drugs is different. This makes a specific immune reaction unlikely, since antibody and T-cell reactions and their cross-reactivity are highly dependent on structural similarity.

Clinically, there is a distinction between reactions with primarily respiratory symptoms (AERD [aspirin-exacerbated respiratory disease], (previously termed Widal disease in Europe and Samter Triad in the United States) and those with primarily cutaneous symptoms (AECD [aspirin-exacerbated cutaneous disease]).[39,40] In a small subgroup of patients NSAIDs may cause both bronchial and cutaneous symptoms, and patients may even develop fatal anaphylactic shock.[31]

AERD

AERD is a common and important clinical entity.[31,39] Patients with both nasal polyposis/rhinosinusitis *and* asthma have a high incidence of intolerance reactions to NSAID (60%), while only about 15% of patients with only severe asthma (without polyposis) exhibit NSAID sensitivity. AERD develops mainly in the third/fourth decades and is slightly more prevalent in females (female:male ratio 3:2). It is an acquired disease, and sensitive patients often report previous tolerance of NSAIDs. In most patients a careful analysis (history and inflammatory markers) reveals symptoms of progressive eosinophilic inflammation of the respiratory mucosa, often starting with nasal polyps and rhinosinusitis. Occasionally, the rhinorrhea and mild asthma might have been ignored for years. After a few years, more severe asthma develops. Systemic eosinophilia is often present (>0.7 G/l) that increases with time and correlates with more extensive inflammation of upper and lower respiratory tract. The eosinophilic inflammation may not only involve the bronchi, but also the middle ear and the larynx and some patients develop generalized pruritus.[41]

Clinical Manifestations

Within minutes (3 to 20 minutes) of oral intake of NSAIDs patients develop rhinorrhea, nasal blockade, flushing, conjunctivitis, and bronchospasm. Asthma is often severe, and occasionally life threatening. Reactions occur after low or medium doses (often <100 mg) of acetylsalicylic acid (ASA), diclofenac, ibuprofen, or mefenamic acid. Some highly sensitive patients can even react to high doses of paracetamol/acetaminophen (>1 g), which is only a weak prostaglandin synthesis inhibitor. Some patients report persistent worsening of nasal and asthma symptoms after the first NSAID reaction, even though they strictly avoid NSAIDs.

Patients with AERD require continuous treatment. While the asthma is often well controlled by high-dose inhaled corticosteroids, the treatment of recurring rhinosinusitis and nasal polyps is more difficult. Histologically, the pathology is due to eosinophilic inflammation, which typically responds well to corticosteroids. However, often topical application is not sufficient and systemic steroids are required, because the inflamed area cannot be reached by topical application. Surgical polypectomy often brings only *transient* relief, and the polyposis and rhinosinusitis recur within weeks to months, particularly if the corticosteroid dose is reduced.[31] Effective treatment requires a well-coordinated therapeutic regimen that balances systemic corticosteroid side effects and disease control. Continued anti-inflammatory treatment is important not only for diminishing symptoms but also to reduce the degree of NSAID intolerance.[42] The leukotriene receptor antagonist montelukast is helpful for asthma symptoms in 30% to 50% of AERD patients with nonallergic asthma, but its efficacy is actually independent of aspirin intolerance.[43] Azathioprine, methotrexate, and omalizumab have been used successfully in some patients, but none of these are considered a consistently efficacious, established treatment.[31] Mepolizumab (anti IL-5 antibodies) and other new monoclonal antibodies may prove to be effective in the severe asthma forms of AERD.[44,45]

AECD. Another form of NSAID intolerance/pseudoallergy occurs on the skin.[40] Many of these patients start with chronic idiopathic urticaria (CIU) and after NSAID intake, develop acute generalized urticaria, often in association with angioedema in the perioral, periorbital, or genital regions. Some patients with AECD may develop anaphylaxis and anaphylactic shock. After the initial NSAID triggered attack, the baseline cutaneous symptoms often become more severe (with angioedema), even without any further NSAID intake. Provocation tests reveal that AECD patients require higher doses of ASA to elicit urticaria (mostly >300 mg) than patients with AERD, who may react to 5 to 100 mg ASA. CIU is associated with cutaneous inflammation so it seems that AECD, like AERD, is also a chronic inflammatory process, which in these cases occurs in the skin.[46] A minority of patients deny having prior CIU and develop urticaria, angioedema, and even anaphylaxis, only after NSAID intake. Both AERD and AECD are chronic diseases that often last between 10 and >20 years, but they may become less symptomatic with age.[31]

IgG-Mediated Reactions (Cytotoxic Mechanism, Type II)

Type II and type III reactions are due primarily to complement-fixing IgG antibodies (IgG_1, IgG_3), and occasionally to IgM. They both result in the formation of immune complexes and the interaction with complement and Fcγ receptor-bearing cells (macrophages, natural killer cells, neutrophilic granulocytes, and platelets), but the target structures and physiological consequences of these 2 types of reactions are different.

In type II reactions, either the antibody is directed against cell structures on the membrane, or immune complex activation occurs on the cell surface. Both events can lead to cell destruction or sequestration. Affected target cells include erythrocytes, leukocytes, platelets, and probably hematopoietic precursor cells in the bone marrow. The mechanism of type II reaction is not as clear as originally thought, since a clear hapten-specific immune reaction often cannot be documented.[47,48]

Clinical Picture of Type II Reactions

Hemolytic Anemia. *Hemolytic anemia* can be caused by reactions to penicillin and its derivatives, cephalosporins, levodopa, methyldopa, quinidine, and some anti-inflammatory drugs (Table 8–4). The clinical symptoms of hemolytic anemia are insidious and may be restricted to symptoms of anemia (fatigue, pallor, shortness of breath, tachycardia) and jaundice with dark urine. Laboratory investigation may reveal reduced erythrocyte and hemoglobin levels, increased reticulocytes, and positive direct and (if the drug is present during the test) indirect Coombs tests. Unconjugated bilirubin levels are elevated and haptoglobulin is decreased. Urinary hemoglobin and hemosiderin are increased.

Thrombocytopenia. *Thrombocytopenia* is a relatively common side effect of drug treatment.[49] Drug-induced immune thrombocytopenia is a challenging clinical problem that is under-recognized, difficult

Table 8–4. Drugs Causing Immune-Mediated Blood Cell Dyscrasias

Hemolytic Anemia	Thrombocytopenia	Neutropenia
Cephalosporin+ (cefotetan, ceftriaxone)	**Heparin**	**Clonazepam**
Penicillin and piperacillin	**Abciximab**	**Methimazole**
Levodopa	**Tirofiban**	**Propylthiouracil**
Methyldopa	Beta-lactam antibiotics	**Metamizole/dipyrone**
Quinine	Sulfanilamide antibiotics (trimethoprim/ sulfamethoxazole)	Levamisole
Various NSAID	Quinine, quinidine	Carbimazole
Oxaliplatin and cisplatin	Influenza vaccine	Ibuprofen
(rare: beta-interferon, pristinamycine, hydralazine)	Citalopram	Indometacin
	Various NSAID	Sulfopyridine, sulfasalacin
	(rare: quinolones, pantoprazol)*	Sulfamethoxazole
		Pantoprazole, omeprazole
		Procainamide
		Gold salts
		Ticlopidine

Note. + bold, relatively frequent.

*A comprehensive list is given at http://www.ouhsc.edu/platelets

to diagnose, and associated with severe bleeding complications. Different drugs cause different types of antiplatelet sensitivity. It may be caused by classic drug-dependent antiplatelet antibodies (eg, quinine), haptens (eg, penicillin), fiban-dependent antibodies (eg, tirofiban), monoclonal antibodies (eg, abciximab), autoantibody formation (eg, gold), or immune complex formation (eg, heparin) (see Table 8–4). Drug-induced immune thrombocytopenia usually develops after 5 to 8 days of exposure to the sensitizing medication or after a single exposure in a patient previously exposed to the same drug. Patients often present with widespread petechial hemorrhages in the skin and buccal mucosa, sometimes accompanied by urinary tract or gastrointestinal bleeding. Intracranial hemorrhage is rare but has been reported. In these cases, drugs that interfere with coagulation, such as ASA should be avoided. After discontinuing the culprit medication, platelet counts usually return to normal within 3 to 5 days.

A special, intermediate form between type II and III reactions is *heparin-induced thrombocytopenia* (HIT).[49] Platelets have low-affinity Fc-receptors (Fcγ-RIIa) that can bind immune complexes, causing platelet activation. Heparin is a high-molecular-weight, sulfated, linear polysaccharide that inhibits blood coagulation by activating regulatory proteins such as anti-thrombin III. About 50% of patients anticoagulated with heparin for more than 7 days produce antibodies that recognize complexes consisting of heparin and platelet factor 4 (PF), a CXC chemokine normally stored in platelet alpha granules. When a patient with such an antibody is given heparin, heparin–PF4 complexes are formed. These complexes react with antibodies to form immune complexes, which bind to the FcIgG-RIIa receptors on platelets, leading to platelet activation, additional PF4 release, and eventually platelet destruction. Thrombocytopenia occurs in about 5% of patients given heparin and is rarely severe enough to cause bleeding. However, about 10% of affected patients experience *paradoxical thrombosis* that can be life threatening.

Neutropenia. Neutropenia can occur in association with various analgesics, psychotropics, anticonvulsants, antithyroid drugs, antihistaminics, antirheumatics, GI drugs, antimicrobials, cardiovascular drugs, and, as expected, with chemotherapy drugs (see Table 8–4).[50] Immune-mediated mechanisms are associated with some drugs such as penicillins which act as haptens inducing antibody formation against neutrophils. Clozapine accelerates apoptosis of neutrophils, and propylthiouracil causes complement mediated destruction of neutrophils. Drugs such as beta-lactam antibiotics, carbamazepine, and valproate have a dose-dependent inhibition of granulopoiesis. Drugs with direct toxic effects on myeloid precursors include ticlopidine, busulfan, ethosuximide, and chlorpromazine. Methimazole may act by direct toxicity or by immune-mediated destruction of granulocytes and granulocyte precursor cells. Rituximab, an anti-CD20 antibody, used in the treatment of B-cell lymphoproliferative disorders and in benign autoimmune disorders, can induce neutropenia that is typically of delayed onset.

Treatment of drug-induced neutropenia includes withdrawing the drug, antibiotic coverage when appropriate, and administration of recombinant human granulocyte colony-stimulating factor (rhG-CSF). The use of CSFs can reduce the duration of neutropenia, the frequency of infection, and possibly mortality, particularly in patients with profound neutropenia. Mortality, although lower than in the past, remains about 5%.[50]

IgG-Mediated Reactions (Immune Complex Deposition, Type III)

Immune complex formation is common during a normal immune response and does not necessarily cause symptoms. Immune complexes can also be formed during drug treatment, either if the drug forms a hapten-carrier complex and gives rise to a humoral immune reaction or if the drug is a protein that elicits an immune reaction (eg, antibodies against variable or constant parts of therapeutic antibodies). Such immune complexes will normally be rapidly cleared by binding to immunoglobulin receptors (Fcγ-RI) or complement receptors (CR1) on reticuloendothelial cells. No symptoms arise, but higher drug concentrations might be needed for effective therapeutic response because of the lowered drug levels.

Why immune complex–related symptoms and disease develop is not clear. Potential mechanisms include very high immune complex levels; a deficiency of some complement components, with a subsequent decreased capacity to eliminate immune complexes; or an aberrant Fcγ-R function.[51,52] Type III reactions involve complement activation, probably activation of Fcγ-R bearing neutrophils and may present as *small-vessel vasculitis and/or serum sickness*. Antibodies are generated within 4 to 10 days which react with the antigen forming soluble circulating immune complexes. Complement (C1q)-containing immune complexes are deposited in the postcapillary venules and attract leukocytes by interacting with their Fcγ-RIII which then release proteolytic enzymes that mediate tissue damage.

Serum sickness can be elicited by nonprotein or protein drugs.[53,54] Hypersensitivity vasculitis has a reported incidence of 10 to 30 cases per million people per year. Cefaclor is most frequently reported to cause serum sickness followed by trimethoprim-sulfamethoxazole, cephalexin, amoxicillin, NSAIDs, and diuretics. The use of biological agents appears to be a more frequent cause of vasculitis: but most cases appear to be mild and restricted to cutaneous lesions.[53]

Clinical Picture of Type III Reactions

The main symptoms of *immune complex disease* are arthralgia, myalgia, fever, and vasculitis. Cutaneous symptoms include purple, red spots, usually on the legs ("palpable purpura"), also termed Henoch-Schönlein purpura. Lesions may coalesce to form plaques that occasionally ulcerate. The gastrointestinal tract, the kidneys, and joints (arthritis) may be involved. The prognosis is good when there is no involvement of internal organs. Histology can reveal IgA-containing immune complexes, and the histology of kidney lesions is in fact identical to IgA nephropathy.

T-Cell-Mediated, Delayed Drug Hypersensitivity Reactions

T cells can orchestrate different forms of inflammation.[34] To account for this heterogeneity the type IV reaction was further subclassified into IVa–IVd reactions, as shown in Figure 8–4. This subclassification considers the distinct cytokine production by T cells and emphasizes the participation of different effector cells such as monocytes (IVa), eosinophils (IVb), or neutrophils (IVd), which cause the inflammation and tissue damage. It is important to be aware that most clinical manifestations of type IV reactions are due to a combined effect. For example, in contact dermatitis, type IVa and IVc reactions occur together.

Type IVa Reactions

Type IVa reactions are due to *Th1-type* immune reactions. Th1-type T cells activate macrophages by secreting large amounts of interferon-γ (IFN-γ), drive the production of complement-fixing antibody isotypes that are involved in type II and III reactions (IgG_1, IgG_3), and are costimulatory for pro-inflammatory responses (TNF, IL-12) and CD8 T-cell responses. The T cells promote these reactions by secretion of IFN-γ and possibly other cytokines (TNF-α, IL-18). Examples of this type of monocyte activation are positive skin test reactions to the purified protein derivative (PPD) of tuberculin, or granuloma formation in sarcoidosis.

Type IVb Reactions

Type IVb are due to *Th2-type* immune reactions. Th2 T cells secrete the cytokines IL-4, IL-13, and IL-5, which promote B-cell production of IgE and IgG_4, macrophage deactivation, and mast cell and eosinophil responses. The high production of the Th2 cytokine IL-5 leads to *eosinophilic inflammation*, which is the characteristic inflammatory cell type in many drug hypersensitivity reactions. There is a link between type IVb reactions and type I reactions, since the Th2 cytokines, IL-4/IL-13 are required for IgE production. In vivo correlates of type IVb reactions include eosinophil-rich maculopapular exanthem (MPE), infestations with nematodes, or allergic inflammation of the bronchi or nasal mucosa (asthma and rhinitis).

Type IVc Reactions

T cells are also important effector cells. They migrate into tissues and kill tissue cells such as keratinocytes or hepatocytes using a mechanism that involves perforin/granzyme B, granulysin, and the Fas ligand.[55,56] Cytotoxic mechanisms play an important role in all forms of delayed drug-induced reactions like exanthems, nephritis, and hepatitis. The clinical picture is determined by the strength of cytotoxic reaction (amount of drug-specific cytotoxic T cells and tissue destruction); it is stronger if cytotoxic CD8 versus cytotoxic CD4 cells are involved and the involvement of other types of T-cell effector mechanisms (types IVa, IVb, or IVd) will recruit other inflammatory cell types. Type IVc reactions are most likely relevant for the tissue damage seen in bullous skin reactions like Stevens-Johnson syndrome (SJS) and TEN, where activated $CD8^+$ T cells and NK cells kill keratinocytes but are also involved in drug-induced hepatitis or nephritis.[57]

Type IVd Reactions

T cells can induce sterile neutrophilic inflammation. A typical example would be acute generalized exanthematous pustulosis (AGEP). In this disease, CXCL8 (also termed IL-8) and granulocyte-macrophage colony-stimulating factor (GM-CSF)–producing T cells recruit neutrophilic leukocytes via CXCL8 release, and prevent their apoptosis via GM-CSF release.[58] In addition to AGEP, this type of T-cell reaction is also involved in Behçet disease, pustular psoriasis, and possibly Sweet syndrome.[59] The role of IL-17–related cytokines is not yet clarified.

Clinical Picture of T-Cell–Mediated Drug Hypersensitivity Reactions

Maculopapular Exanthem (MPE): A Combined Type IVb and IVc Reaction. The most frequent manifestations of drug allergies are delayed-appearing *cutaneous reactions* ("drug rash"). They include a broad spectrum of clinical and distinct histopathological features which appear more than 6 hours to 10 days after drug intake (Figure 8–6).

MPE is the most frequent drug hypersensitivity reaction, affecting 2% to 8% of hospitalized patients, especially after treatment with β-lactams, quinolones, sulfamethoxazole, diuretics, and many other drugs.[7] In most cases it appears 8 to 11 days after the start of treatment, but may even occur 1 to 3 days after the drug treatment was stopped (see Figure 8–1). In previously sensitized individuals it can appear on the first day of treatment and is clearly dose dependent.

Immunohistology reveals drug-specific CD4 cell infiltration in perivascular areas of the dermis.[60] The

TYPE IV a	TYPE IV b	TYPE IV c	TYPE IV d
Th1	Th2	Cytotoxic T cells	T cells
IFN-γ, TNF-α	IL-5, IL-4, IL-13, eotaxin	Perforin, granzyme B, FasL	CXCL-8, GM-CFS IL-17?
Monocyte, Macrophage	Eosinophilic inflammation	Cytotoxic T cells	Neutrophils
Tuberculin skin test, Contact dermatitis	Maculopapular exanthem with eosinophilia	Contact dermatitis bullous & maculo-papular exanthema	Pustular exanthema

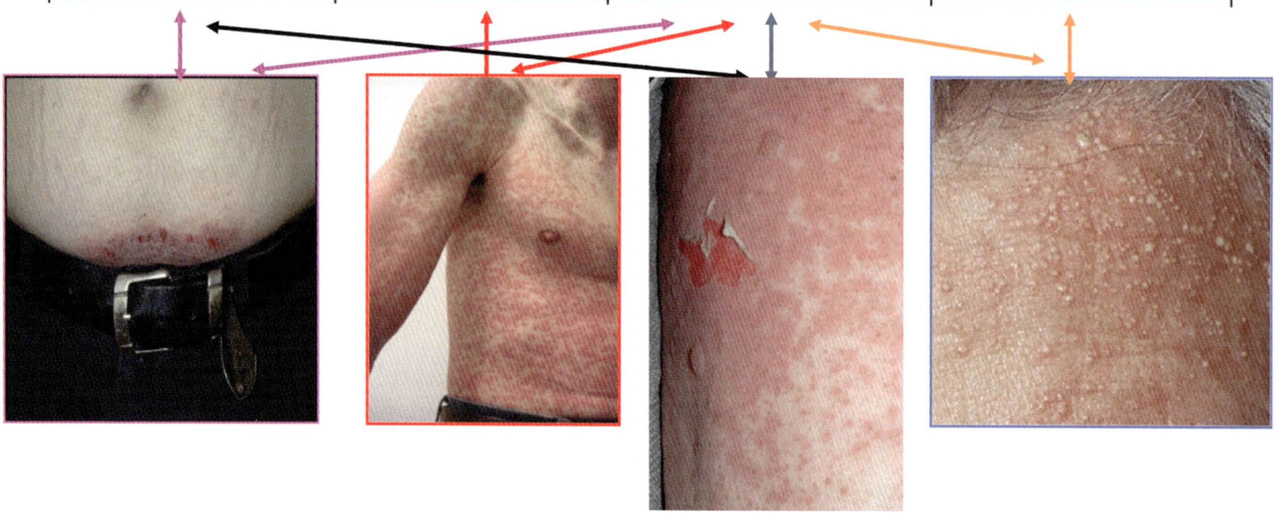

Figure 8–6. Clinical picture and histology of various exanthematous drug eruptions.

infiltrating CD4 T cells express type 1 (IFN-γ) and type 2 (IL-4, IL-5) cytokines, and are also cytotoxic (perforin/granzymeB^{+}). Some T cells progress into the dermoepidermal junction zone and epidermis, where they cause hydropic degeneration of keratinocytes (spongiotic dermatitis). The cytokine IL-5 is often also detectable in the serum, and tissue and blood eosinophilia can be found.[61] The recruitment of eosinophils is also enhanced by expression of the chemokines, eotaxins 1 and 2 (CCL11, CCL24) and RANTES (CCL5) in MPE lesions.

Most maculopapular exanthems, particularly if caused by β-lactams or quinolones like gemifloxacin, are rather mild, and treatment with an emollient cream, and possibly topical corticosteroids, or systemic antihistamines to treat pruritus is sufficient. Some patients can continue treatment without worsening. The exanthem often heals with desquamation within 2 to 10 days after stopping the incriminated drug. It is unlikely that SJS/TEN will develop from MPE as the cells involved are different, but prolonged treatment may lead to expansion of co-stimulated cytotoxic CD8^{+} T cells as well. At that point, confluence of the papules with formation of bullae on the heavily inflamed skin may appear. In addition, the patient may complain of malaise and fever, and liver function tests indicate hepatitis (more than three-fold increase of transaminase levels). Eosinophilia (>0.5 G/l) and activated CD8 cells are found in the blood.[60] This finding illustrates that even "mild" drug hypersensitivity reactions are *systemic diseases*, and that cutaneous manifestations are the major but not the only symptom.

Acute Generalized Exanthematous Pustulosis (AGEP). Acute generalized exanthematous pustulosis (AGEP) is a rare disease (about 1/100 000 treatments) with an estimated incidence equal to severe bullous skin diseases (SJS and TEN combined).[62] It is caused by drugs in more than 90% of cases (Table 8–5). Its clinical hallmark is the rapid appearance of multiple disseminated, *sterile* pustules in the skin (see Figure 8–6), often 2 to 5 days after starting treatment. Patients have fever and massive leukocytosis in the blood, sometimes with eosinophilia, but no involvement of mucous membranes. Epicutaneous patch test reactions can cause a similar pustular reaction locally (see Figure 8–6).

Immunohistology of the acute lesion reveals an initial T-cell migration into the epidermis. The T cells are cytotoxic, kill keratinocytes, and form vesicles.[58] They also express CXCL-8 and GM-CSF, thereby recruiting neutrophilic granulocytes, which transform the vesicles into pustules. AGEP is therefore a combination of IVc and IVd reactions. The condition is fatal in less than 2% of cases, mainly in older people. Healing occurs within 5 days after stopping the drug.

Bullous Exanthems, SJS, and Toxic Epidermal Necrolysis. The most severe bullous skin reactions involve formation of bullae and are termed SJS or TEN.[57,63] TEN and SJS are rare (about 1/1 000 000 for TEN, and about 1/100 000 for SJS). They are the milder and more severe form of the same disease; SJS has less than 10% skin detachment, while TEN has more than 30% skin detachment. They are graded using the SCORTEN scale, in which age, underlying disease, and the amount of maximal skin detachment are the most important prognostic factors.[64] According to the European study group of severe cutaneous drug reactions, SJS has a mortality of about 13%, and TEN of about 39% (64). There is an intermediate form with 10% to 30% skin detachment, termed SJS/TEN overlap syndrome, which has a lethality of about 21%.

SJS/TEN differs from a distinct syndrome, erythema exudativum multiforme, which is mainly caused by viral infections, is often recurrent, and affects younger persons (mean age 24 years). The main causes for SJS/TEN are drugs (see Table 8–5), and these vary in frequency between different regions based on genetic and ethnic background differences.[65] Important risk factors are HIV infection (low CD4, high CD8 counts), renal disease, and active systemic autoimmune diseases. SJS/TEN can also be caused by GVH,[21] an observation that reinforces the concept that drug hypersensitivity reactions are similar to alloimmune responses.[9] Most reactions start within the first 5 weeks of

Table 8-5. Drugs Eliciting Severe Cutaneous or Systemic, Delayed Appearing Reactions

Acute Generalized Exanthematous Pustulosis (AGEP)	Stevens-Johnson Syndrome (SJS) and Toxic Epidermal Necrolysis (TEN)	Drug Rash With Eosinophilia and Systemic Symptoms (DRESS)†
Aminopenicillins	**Allopurinol***	**Carbamazepine***
Cephalosporins	**Phenytoin***	**Phenytoin***
Pristinamycin	**Carbamazepin***	**Lamotrigin**
Celecoxib	Lamotrigin	Minocyclin
Quinolone	Cotrimoxazole (SMX)	Allopurinol*
Diltiazem	Nevirapine	Dapsone*
Terbinafin	Barbiturate	Sulfasalazin
Macrolides	NSAID (oxicams)	Cotrimoxazole (SMX)
		Vancomycin
		Abacavir*†

Note. List incomplete: the most frequent elicitors are given in bold.

*The type of reaction might be determined by the presence of a certain HLA-allele.

†Abacavir-induced systemic reactions are classified outside of DRESS; they often lack eosinophilia and preferentially affect the respiratory and gastrointestinal tract.

treatment (mean onset of symptoms at about 17 days).

SJS/TEN can develop quite rapidly. Initially a macular, purple-red exanthem may appear, which can become painful, which is an ominous sign. Within 12 to 24 hours, bullae develop, and the Nikolsky sign is positive (Table 8–6, danger signs). Stopping drug treatment at this stage of SJS may prevent further progression to an even more severe reaction (TEN). Mucous membranes (mouth, genitalia) are involved with blister formation, as well as a purulent keratoconjunctivitis with formation of synechiae, which require intensive ocular care to avoid permanent eye damage.

In biopsies of TEN lesions, many dead keratinocytes are found, but there is little cellular infiltration. However, the bullae may be filled by cytotoxic CD8 T cells, expressing CD56 and αβ-TCRs, which kill via granulysin and perforin/granzyme B, but not via the Fas-mediated pathway at this stage of the disease.[56] Newer data underline the role of granulysin in cell damage, and attempts to neutralize this molecule are under way.

Systemic Drug Reactions—Severe Drug Hypersensitivity Syndromes. Some drugs are known to cause severe systemic disease with fever, lymphadenopathy, massive hepatitis, and various types of exanthems (see Table 8–5). A few patients develop colitis, pancreatitis, or interstitial lung disease.[66,67] Over 70% have a marked eosinophilia (often >1500 cells/l), and activated lymphocytes are often found in the circulation, similar to acute EBV infections.[65] This syndrome has many names. The most frequently used are drug (induced) hypersensitivity syndrome (DHS or DiHS) or drug rash with eosinophilia and systemic symptoms (DRESS). Importantly, the symptoms can begin up to 10 weeks after starting treatment, often beginning after a dose increase, and may then persist and recur for many weeks, *even after cessation of the culprit drug*. The clinical picture resembles a generalized viral infection (eg, acute Epstein-Barr virus infection), but it is distinguished by the prominent eosinophilia. Many patients have facial swelling, and some have signs of a capillary leak syndrome, similar to patients experiencing a cytokine release syndrome, and various cytokines are massively increased in the serum of these patients.[68] Because the clinical picture is quite dramatic and since the disease tends to persist in spite of stopping drug treatment, many patients are not diagnosed correctly or in a timely manner. However, any physicians that prescribe anticonvulsants must be familiar with this syndrome, since it occurs in about 1 in 3000 treated patients. The mortality is about 10%, and some patients require emergency liver transplantation.[69]

Patients with DHS/DRESS have increased numbers of circulating activated T cells. These cells are stimulated by the p-i mechanism and secrete large amounts of TNF-α, IL-5 and IFN-γ.[69] A peculiar feature of this syndrome is its long-lasting clinical course despite withdrawal of the causative drug. There may also be persistent intolerance to other, chemically distinct drugs, leading to flare-up reactions to previously tolerated, usually innocuous drugs (eg, acetaminophen) weeks to months after stopping the initial drug therapy, further adding to the diagnostic confusion. Treatment often requires high doses of corticosteroids, particularly if the hepatitis is severe.

It has been shown that in many patients with this syndrome, human herpes virus type 6 DNA can be found in the circulation during the third or fourth week of the disease, followed by a rising IgM anti-

Table 8-6. Danger Signs in Drug-Induced Exanthems

Clinical findings	Extent and type of exanthem: infiltration, bullae, pustules
	Skin pain
	Positive Nikolsky sign
	Involvement of mucous membranes
	Systemic symptoms like malaise, fever, lymphadenopathy, hepatosplenomegaly, conjunctivitis
Laboratory findings	Eosinophilia (>1000/μL[a])
	Atypical activated lymphocytes in the circulation (>2%[a])
	Liver enzymes (ALAT, ASAT, gamma-GT, AP) (increase >2.5–3x[a])

[a]The cutoff values of the laboratory parameters are estimated and are not based on prospective studies; severe reactions can also develop in the absence of these signs. Additional investigations depend on clinical signs: liver, kidney, lung, pancreas involvement.

body titer to human herpes virus 6.[70] Other reports document reactivation of cytomegalovirus infection. Thus, similar to HIV where T-cell activation can also enhance virus production, the drug-induced massive immune stimulation may somehow reactivate these latent lymphotropic herpes viruses which subsequently replicate and possibly contribute to the chronic course and persistent drug intolerance in affected patients.

Many drugs can induce isolated hepatitis and some can cause an isolated (interstitial) nephritis (penicillins, proton pump inhibitors, quinolones, and disulfiram).[71,72] More rare are interstitial lung diseases (furadantin), pancreatitis, isolated fever, or eosinophilia as the only symptom of a drug allergy. In drug-induced interstitial nephritis eosinophils can sometimes be detected in the urine even in the absence of blood eosinophilia.

Multiple Drug Hypersensitivity Syndrome and Flare-Up Reactions. Multiple drug hypersensitivity (MDH) syndrome is seen in some patients who develop immunologically mediated adverse effects to multiple different drugs. It is distinct from "multiple drug intolerance" caused by NSAID, or cross-reactivity due to structural similarity. It should be used only for well-documented, repeated *immune*-mediated reactions to structurally unrelated drugs.[73]

In our experience, about 10% of patients with well-documented, severe drug hypersensitivity reactions (documented with positive skin and/or lymphocyte transformation tests) have multiple drug allergies.[74] Actually, many patients with MDH begin with DRESS/DiHS and remain permanently hyperreactive.[73,75] Affected patients continue to have activated T cells in their circulation for months/years after the initial clinical manifestation, similar to what is seen in chronic herpes virus infections or chronic GVH reactions. For example, a patient first develops DRESS from phenytoin, then requires antibiotic treatment and within months develops additional hypersensitivities to amoxicillin (MPE), and then to sulfamethoxazole (erythrodermia). These are primarily T-cell–mediated reactions, but occasionally agranulocytosis or cholestatic hepatitis develop, where the pathological mechanism is still unclear.

Multiple delayed hypersensitivity syndrome should be differentiated from *flare-up reactions*.[73] In patients with systemic drug allergies, the T-cell immune system is massively activated, similar to what is seen in acute viral infections (see Table 8–1). As in the latter, these patients seem to have an increased tendency to react to new drugs and might develop a flare-up of an ongoing or just diminishing rash when a new drug is given. Skin testing with the second drug is usually negative, and the second drug is well tolerated when given at a later time as the costimulatory conditions are no longer present. This illustrates the fact that an ongoing *drug hypersensitivity reaction is by itself a risk factor for the development of further drug allergies.* Stopping treatment, or reducing the immune activation by a short treatment course with corticosteroids may reduce these flare-up reactions. Some flare-up reactions result in the development of an actual new drug hypersensitivity.

DIAGNOSIS OF DRUG HYPERSENSITIVITY

The diagnosis of drug hypersensitivity requires asking 3 questions: first, is it truly drug hypersensitivity? Second, which immune mechanism is involved? Third, which is the causative drug? Drug hypersensitivity symptoms can be extremely heterogeneous. Given the extensive use of drugs, a drug hypersensitivity reaction should always be included in the differential diagnosis, particularly in patients presenting with *"bizarre" symptoms* or in patients with *eosinophilia*. But some of the above-described skin exanthems are rather typical for drug hypersensitivity and easy to recognize.

Clinical Diagnosis

Drug hypersensitivity is often suspected if a "rash" appears. Differential diagnosis of this rash includes viral exanthems, occasionally other infections, food allergy, and a GVH reaction. Pruritus, blood eosinophilia, and recent administration of a new drug argue for an allergic reaction. Quite commonly, the symptoms might be due to the combined effects of a viral infection and drug treatment, since both augment immune reactivity, while each factor alone only rarely causes the symptoms. This situation is particularly frequent in children. Often they are mistakenly treated with amoxicillin for a viral infection and develop a rash, but can later tolerate the drug by itself in the absence of a concomitant viral infection.[76]

Since drug hypersensitivity is an iatrogenic disease, it is important to document the severity of the presumed reaction.[34] This may determine whether the drug can be given again, and may help avoid the use of more expensive or more harmful alternative drugs. Physicians should be aware of the danger signs (see Table 8–6) and the most important elicitors of severe reactions (see Table 8–5). Special attention should be paid to the type and extent of skin symptoms (photo is helpful), the involvement of mucosal areas, lymph node enlargement, fever, and subjective symptoms like malaise, as this could indicate involvement of internal organs (SJS/TEN and DRESS). A painful skin and a positive Nikolsky sign might herald a severe bullous skin reaction (SJS/TEN). Some patients have no skin involvement but develop an isolated drug-allergic hepatitis or interstitial nephritis.

It is important to consider the underlying mechanisms for drug hypersensitivity, since distinct diagnostic steps might be required. For example, while in hapten and p-i reactions structural similarity between drugs determines cross-reactivity, NSAID intolerance (AERD, AECD) involves many structurally different NSAIDs, all of which have similar pharmacological activity (cyclo-oxygenase inhibition). In current clinical practice, determining which of these mechanisms are involved is difficult and based mainly on experience and the clinical picture. For instance, can the drug elicit a combination of immune mechanisms (eg, IgE *and* T-cell reactions together)? If so, it would argue for a hapten mechanism. Alternatively, is the drug known to preferentially elicit pseudo-allergic symptoms, like NSAID?

Timing of symptoms is important in making a correct diagnosis. Immediate reactions start less than 1 hour after drug intake and are usually IgE mediated or pseudo-allergic. Typical symptoms are urticaria and anaphylaxis. Delayed reactions start mostly more than 24 hours after drug intake and are mostly not IgE mediated, but involve T-cell orchestrated inflammation or (rarely) IgG-mediated reactions. In highly sensitized individuals, symptoms from T-cell activation can arise as early as 2 to 4 hours after drug intake—the more drug-specific precursor T cells are present, the more rapidly symptoms can appear.

Laboratory Investigation

Laboratory investigation can also help to document the severity of the reaction (see Table 8–6). In more severe *acute reactions,* tryptase levels should be measured to confirm mast cell involvement, optimally between 1 and 4 hours after the peak of the reaction. The analysis should be repeated later (>1 day) to rule out a constitutively elevated tryptase level (such is seen in mastocytosis). Such measurements are particularly important if anaphylaxis is suspected during anesthesia, as elevated levels can support the diagnosis of anaphylaxis. Of note, individual levels of tryptase are rather constant. An increase by 2.5 to 3-fold (eg, 3.1 to 9.2 microg/ml) during a suspected anaphylactic event may be sufficient confirmation, even if the level is still in the normal range (<11.4 microg/ml).

In delayed reactions, a differential blood count may reveal activated lymphocytes in the circulation as sign of a general massive immune stimulation. Eosinophilia is observed in up to 40% of patients with MPE, in 20% to 30% with AGEP and in more than 70% in DRESS. Measurements of liver enzymes (ALAT, ASAT, ALP, and γGT) should be done (1) in patients with extensive skin involvement, (2) in patients with severe malaise, or (3) if drugs known to cause DRESS or hepatitis/cholestasis are involved. A transient mild hepatitis is not rare and seems to occur in about 25% of patients with more severe MPE.[60] Depending on the symptoms, other tests may also be indicated (creatinine, urinary analysis). C-reactive protein (CRP) may be elevated (eg, in drug-induced interstitial lung or kidney diseases). However, it is important to be aware that CRP levels can be normal even in severe hypersensitivity reactions like DRESS. Many patients with rash may have no systemic symptoms and just complain of itching. The degree of sensitization in such patients may be low, and skin testing is often negative.

Identifying the Culprit Drug

The identification of the cause of a drug reaction is based primarily on clinical history. Important questions to ask include: which drugs were taken, and what was the timing; was the drug dose recently increased; were there any co-medications and could they interfere with the metabolism of the suspect drug; were the drugs tolerated previously or were other drugs tolerated that are known to cause similar effects; is the underlying disease known to be associated with drug allergies; has the patient experienced similar reactions previously without or with other drugs. Books listing side effects, websites (eg, http://www.pneumotox.com) and pharmaceutical companies can provide information about the known side effects of a drug. In many instances, the combination of the clinical history and using external sources may allow a reasonably conclusive connection between the symptoms and drug intake. However, many patients are taking several drugs and the history alone may be insufficient. In these cases additional tests may be helpful, although many of these are not well validated.

Currently, most of the *in vivo* (skin test) and *in vitro* tests for drug allergy diagnosis have been difficult to standardize. Although drug allergy is common, it only occurs rarely for any individual drug. Any single drug may elicit different symptoms, requiring different types of tests. Direct provocation tests, which could confirm the drug allergy, are usually not performed for ethical reasons. For some tests, living cells are needed rather than serum, which requires a greater logistical effort. In spite of these obstacles, skin testing can be useful, but 2 general rules are important to keep in mind. First, test results can only supplement the clinical history. More importantly, the sensitivity of the tests is generally low, while the specificity is high, so a positive test may be meaningful, while a negative test cannot rule out a drug allergy.[77,78]

Immediate Reactions

For investigating immediate reactions, both percutaneous and intradermal tests are available. A penicillin test reagent (Pre-pen) is commercially available and widely used.[79] This reagent consists of the repetitive determinants of the major allergenic metabolite of penicillin (penicilloyl) bound to a poly-L-lysine carrier. It is able to cross-link 2 FcεRI-bound penicillin-specific IgE molecules and trigger mast cell degranulation in the skin. It is not suitable for detecting delayed (T-cell) reactions. Penicillin may also bind to carrier proteins by their thiol structure (minor allergenic components); mixtures of these minor determinants (MDM) are not commercially available in the United States. It is important to include the native drugs (eg, amoxicillin) in the test reagents as well (5 mg/mL for i.d. tests). The amoxicillin i.d. test is more sensitive than standard Pre-pen, if the IgE is against the side chain and not the beta lactam core structure and can also serve to detect delayed reactions (reading at 24 and 48 hours). To detect a possible cross-reactivity to other beta lactam antibiotics, one can also include skin tests to cephalosporins (eg, 7.5 mg/mL cefuroxime for i.d. test) or monobactams and carbapenems.[80] The sensitivity of the penicillin skin tests is somewhat controversial. Older studies from the United States suggested a sensitivity of greater than 95%; but more recent studies from Spain found only 70%.[79]

Reactivity to other drugs can be tested as well, both by prick or intradermal tests.[80] It is important to be aware that each test and test concentration is standardized, because false-positive reactions (eg, to quinolones) can occur. It is essential to test control individuals as well. More detailed information about test procedures and concentrations is available elsewhere.[80,81]

In vitro tests for immediate reactions include the determination of drug-specific IgE. However, availability of such tests is very limited and the sensitivity of commercial assays for drug-specific IgE appears to be rather low. Moreover, specific IgE to drugs disappear rather rapidly from the circulation (often in 12 months), while skin test reactivity persists longer. Various read-out systems for basophil degranulation/activation tests have been proposed to be usable for drug hypersensitivity diagnosis (eg, Flow-Cast). Sensitivity for IgE-mediated reactions is reported to be about 40%.

Delayed Reactions

In Europe it is common to perform epicutaneous (patch) tests for diagnosing delayed T-cell reactions to some drugs.[78] The overall sensitivity is considered to be less than 50% and depends on the disease, often negative in macular and delayed appearing urticarial exanthems, but is more useful in severe MPE, DiHS/DRESS, and AGEP. It can also be used in SJS/TEN, and skin testing is *not* dangerous in these patients.[78]

The lymphocyte transformation test (LTT) relies on the activation and proliferation of T cells cultured in the presence of the drug.[82] Reactivity can be measured by ^{3}H-thymidine incorporation after 5- to 6-day culture, or by ELISPOT, CSFE staining, or CD69 upregulation. LTT is cumbersome, but a clearly positive response can be clinically useful. The sensitivity of LTT depends on the mechanism of the drug hypersensitivity and is greater than 90% for DiHS/DRESS, but only 20% to 30% for SJS/TEN, where cytotoxic T-cell reactions dominate over those T cells, whose activation can be measured by lymphocyte proliferation in vitro. LTT can be positive for drugs that sensitize either by the hapten mechanism or by the p-i mechanism.

Provocation tests are considered to be the gold standard for the diagnosis, and they are useful, if no ethical contraindications exist.[83] However, they are also limited in their meaning, as cofactors that were present in the acute reaction might be missing during the time of provocation. As a result, a positive provocation test is more reliable than a negative provocation, and the role of cofactors, dosage, and underlying disease should be considered (see Table 8–1). Provocation tests are not standardized for delayed reactions, and the dose needed to elicit symptoms will often not be reached in provocation tests. Provocation tests are the only way to prove the involvement of a certain drug in pseudo-allergy, where neither IgE nor T cell is involved. It is widely used in AERD and AECD and may be combined with desensitization (see below).

Of great clinical value is the challenge with an alternative drug: such challenge tests with alternatives are imperative in pseudo-allergy to NSAID, since a whole group of important drugs are prohibited from being used for further treatment and the patient may need an alternative for pain treatment: The alternatives are mainly acetaminophen or selective Cox2 inhibitors like etoricoxib or celecoxib, if opioids are to be avoided. Challenges begin with 25% to 50% of the normal single dose, and increase at 30-minute intervals. Reactions are rare, mostly mild, and often occur only at very high doses.

There is no single gold standard for the diagnosis of drug hypersensitivity, not even the provocation test. The best approach seems to be a combination of carefully taken history, understanding the mechanism and cofactors leading to drug hypersensitivity, skin and in vitro tests. Therefore, only rarely a provocation test is needed to make a reliable diagnosis, a fact that should be emphasized to the patient. Patients with assumed drug hypersensitivity should be given a precise information ("an allergy passport") regarding their specific adverse reaction: causative drug, dose used, route of exposure, clinical symptoms, mode of allergy proof (skin tests, provocation, history), lists of cross-reactive drugs, recommended alternative (with dose in challenge test), and other tolerated drugs.

TREATMENT OF DRUG ALLERGIES

Drug hypersensitivity is an *iatrogenic disease* and optimal management is essential. The therapy of drug hypersensitivity diseases is dependent on the symptoms and ranges from the usual treatment of anaphylaxis to acute liver transplantation. Stopping the possible culprit drugs and avoiding the relevant drug and its structural homologues in the future, until clarity is achieved, should be possible in most circumstances and might reduce the development of more severe symptoms. In some milder skin reactions, such as a nonbullous exanthem due to sulfamethoxazole in HIV-positive patients, which is probably due to p-i TCR,[17] experience has shown that the continuation of treatment may be possible. In severe reactions, like DRESS or SJS/TEN, where different organs are involved, an interdisciplinary approach and therapy are often necessary (eg, ophthalmic care in SJS/TEN).

Desensitization

Under certain circumstances a drug that causes allergic or "pseudo-allergic" side effects is essential for treatment, for example, certain cytostatic drugs (eg, cisplatin) or monoclonal antibodies in cancer treatments.[84] To allow treatment in spite of previous side effects, desensitization may be attempted. Most desensitization protocols are done for hypersensitivity reactions involving mast cell degranulation (IgE or non-IgE mediated), and the procedure is best established for penicillin, NSAIDs, and some monoclonal antibodies.[84] There are reports on desensitization of delayed appearing drug hypersensitivity, but experience is still rather limited.

The starting dose for desensitization is determined by the dose the patient tolerated in skin testing (immediate reading). This dose generally translates to 1:10 000 of the therapeutic dose. The treatment involves administering a low dose of drug, with gradual dose escalation every 15 to 30 minutes (usually via IV application), until the therapeutic dose is reached. This produces a transient adaptation of the immune system to the specific drug, but the underlying immune sensitization persists. Desensitization reduces sensitivity only to the drug used in the protocol and is not suppressive of reactions to unrelated drugs, as demonstrated by persisting immediate skin tests and in vitro basophil activation tests. Desensitization does not lead to an increase of serum levels of the mast cell-specific molecule tryptase.

Mild urticaria occurs rather frequently during drug desensitization but does not require stopping the procedure. Treating the symptoms (usually just with antihistamines), reducing the infusion speed, and lowering the next desensitization dose are usually all that is required.

If treatment is discontinued for more than 48 hours, the patient will once more be at risk of developing anaphylaxis and the full desensitization protocol must be repeated (eg, before each chemotherapy course).

In skin test negative cases, where allergy appears very unlikely, *graded drug challenges* are often used. As any form of drug hypersensitivity is a dose-dependent event, the treatment is started with 1/100 or 1/20 of the standard dose, so any reaction that occurs will be milder. The dose is increased stepwise (double or triple) every 30 to 60 minutes. The full dose may be achieved in 1 day and can be continued during subsequent days.

ASA Desensitization

Aspirin (acetylsalicylic acid, ASA) desensitization is a widely used procedure which has different goals: (1) amelioration of chronic rhinosinusitis with nasal polyposis that is refractory to topical corticosteroids and other therapies; (2) the need for aspirin-antiplatelet therapy due to cardiovascular risk factors or confirmed cardiovascular disease; or (3) the need for NSAIDs to treat chronic inflammatory conditions, such as arthritis.

The efficacy and usefulness of ASA desensitization in AERD for these indications are still controversial. It is highly successful if its goal is to allow continuous ASA treatment for patients with cardiac disease, which mostly require only a 100- to 300-mg daily dose of ASA.[85,86] If its goal is to diminish the symptoms of rhinosinusitis and nasal polyposis in patients with AERD, the treatment requires a higher dose (mostly >325–650 mg ASA/day), and the effect may just be a relief of nasal obstruction.[87] Moreover, as pain therapy with an NSAID like ibuprofen or diclofenac also requires higher doses, other unwanted side effects like gastric ulcers and gastrointestinal bleeding frequently appear. Other reasons to stop ASA therapy are elective surgery or pregnancy.

A protocol for ASA desensitization of AERD patients is shown in Table 8–7.[87] The patients should have an FEV1 >70%, are normally on anti-inflammatory treatment for their respiratory disease (topical corticosteroids), and also receive anti-leukotriene therapy (montelukast, 10 mg/day in adults or zafirlukast, 20 mg/2×/day in adults). The starting dose may be 40-mg ASA, but patients with baseline FEV1 of <80% of predicted value, or who have a history of emergency visits for acute asthma, should start with 20 mg. Subsequent doses are given at 3-hour intervals, since symptoms often develop only after 2 hours. Once the patient develops symptoms, the same dose has to be repeated. Once the reaction has subsided, the protocol can be continued until the dose of 325 mg is reached. After having reached the 325 mg dose, it is very unlikely that the patient will develop symptoms at 650 mg, so the further dose increase can be done at home. It takes 3 months to see effects of this therapy on rhinosinusitis/nasal polyposis symptoms. If the ASA intake is interrupted, a restart at a lower dose is possible if the break is no longer than 5 days. Beyond 5 days, the full desensitization

Table 8-7. ASA (Acetylsalicylic Acid, Aspirin) Desensitization for AERD

Time	Day 1	Day 2	Day 3	Day 4
8 AM	40 mg	320 mg	320 mg	320 mg
11 AM	80 mg			
2 AM	160 mg		320 mg	320 mg

Note. The procedure is normally done over 2 days; maintenance doses are 320 mg bid or 640 mg once a day. The goal is amelioration of symptoms and transient tolerance of ASA. For details of procedure, see text.

process is needed again. The NSAID tolerance lasts only as long as the patient remains on ASA. Patients who tolerate 100 mg/day ASA cannot take higher doses of ASA or NSAID (eg, for pain therapy).

REFERENCES

1. Rawlins MD, Thompson JW. Pathogenesis of adverse drug reactions. In: Davies DM, ed. *Textbook of Adverse Drug Reactions*. New York, NY: Oxford University Press; 1981:11.
2. Pavlos R, Mallal S, Phillips E. HLA and pharmacogenetics of drug hypersensitivity. *Pharmacogenomics*. 2012 Aug;13(11):1285–1306. doi:10.2217.
3. Chung WH, Chang WC, Lee YS, et al. Taiwan Severe Cutaneous Adverse Reaction Consortium; Japan Pharmacogenomics Data Science Consortium. Genetic variants associated with phenytoin-related severe cutaneous adverse reactions. *JAMA*. 2014 Aug 6;312(5):525–534.
4. Manfredi M, Severino M, Testi S, et al. Detection of specific IgE to quinolones. *J Allergy Clin Immunol*. 2004;113: 155–160.
5. Lazarou J, Pomeranz BH, Corey P. Incidence of adverse drug reactions in hospitalized patients: a meta-analysis of prospective studies. *JAMA*. 1998;279:1200–1205.
6. Hunziker T, Kunzi UP, Braunschweig S, et al. Comprehensive hospital drug monitoring (CHDM): adverse skin reactions, a 20-year survey. *Allergy*. 1997; 52:388–393.
7. Fiszenson-Albala F, Auzerie V, Mahe E, et al. A 6-month prospective survey of cutaneous drug reactions in a hospital setting. *Br J Dermatol*. 2003;149(5):1018–1022.
8. Pichler WJ, Watkins S. Interaction of small molecules with specific immune receptors: the p-i concept and its consequences. *Curr Immunol Rev*. 2014;10:7–18.
9. Adam J, Wuillemin N, Watkins S, et al. Abacavir induced T cell reactivity from drug naïve individuals shares features of allo-immune responses. *PLoS One*. 2014 Apr 21; 9(4):e95339.
10. Landsteiner K, Jacobs J. Studies on the sensitization of animals with simple chemical compounds, *J Exp Med*. 1936;64:625–639.
11. Martin S, Weltzien HU. T cell recognition of haptens, a molecular view. *Int Arch Allergy Immunol*. 1994;104:10–16.
12. Esser PR, Wölfle U, Dürr C, et al. Contact sensitizers induce skin inflammation via ROS production and hyaluronic acid degradation. *PLoS One*. 2012;7(7):e41340.
13. Whitaker P, Meng X, Lavergne SN, et al. Mass spectrometric characterization of circulating and functional antigens derived from piperacillin in patients with cystic fibrosis. *J Immunol*. 2011 Jul 1;187(1):200–211.
14. Naisbitt DJ, Farrell J, Gordon SF, et al. Covalent binding of the nitroso metabolite of sulfamethoxazole leads to toxicity and major histocompatibility complex-restricted antigen presentation. *Mol Pharmacol*. 2002;62(3):628–637.
15. Adam J, Pichler WJ, Yerly D. Delayed drug hypersensitivity: models of T-cell stimulation. *Br J Clin Pharmacol*. 2011;71:701–707.
16. Watkins S, Pichler WJ. Activating interactions of sulfanilamides with T cell receptors. *Open J Immunol*. 2013; 3/3:139–157. http://dx.doi.org/10.4236/oji.2013.33019.
17. Watkins S, Pichler WJ. Sulfamethoxazole induces a switch mechanism in T cell receptors containing TCRVβ20-1, altering peptHLA recognition. *PLoS One*. 2013 Oct 7; 8(10):e76211. doi:10.1371/journal.pone.0076211.
18. Chung WH, Hung SI, Hong HS, et al. Medical genetics: a marker for Stevens-Johnson syndrome. *Nature*. 2004; 428:486.
19. Mallal S, Nolan D, Witt C, et al. Association between presence of HLA-B*5701, HLA-DR7, and HLA-DQ3 and hypersensitivity to HIV-1 reverse-transcriptase inhibitor abacavir. *Lancet*. 2002;359:727–732.
20. Hung SI, Chung WH, Liou LB, et al. HLA-B*5801 allele as a genetic marker for severe cutaneous adverse reactions caused by allopurinol. *Proc Natl Acad Sci USA*. 2005; 102:4134–4139.
21. Azukizawa H, Itami S. Animal models of toxic epidermal necrolysis. In: Pichler WJ, ed. *Drug Hypersensitivity*. Basel, Switzerland: Karger; 2007:129–139.
22. Illing PT, Vivian JP, Dudek NL, et al. Immune self-reactivity triggered by drug-modified HLA-peptide repertoire. *Nature*. 2012;486:554–558.
23. Ostrov DA, Grant BJ, Pompeu YA, et al. Drug hypersensitivity caused by alteration of the MHC-presented self-peptide repertoire. *Proc Natl Acad Sci USA*. 2012;109: 9959–9964.
24. Norcross MA, Luo S, Lu L, et al. Abacavir induces loading of novel self-peptides into HLA-B*57: 01: an autoimmune model for HLA-associated drug hypersensitivity. *AIDS*. 2012;26:F21–F29.
25. McCormack M, Alfirevic A, Bourgeois S, et al. HLA-A*3101 and carbamazepine-induced hypersensitivity reactions in Europeans. *N Engl J Med*. 2011 Mar 24;364(12): 1134–1143.
26. Mallal S, Phillips E, Carosi G, et al. PREDICT-1 Study Team. HLA-B*5701 screening for hypersensitivity to abacavir. *N Engl J Med*. 2008; 358(6):568–579.
27. Chen P, Lin JJ, Lu CS, et al. Taiwan SJS Consortium. Carbamazepine-induced toxic effects and HLA-B*1502 screening in Taiwan. *N Engl J Med*. 2011 Mar 24;364(12): 1126–1133.
28. Wang H, Wang HS, Liu ZP. Agents that induce pseudo-allergic reaction. *Drug Discov Ther*. 2011 Oct;5(5):211–219.
29. Kelesidis T, Fleisher J, Tsiodras S. Anaphylactoid reaction considered ciprofloxacin related: a case report and literature review. *Clin Ther*. 2010 Mar;32(3):515–526. doi:10.1016/j.clinthera.2010.03.002. Review.
30. Polk RE, Healy DP, Schwartz LB, Rock DT, Garson ML, Roller K. Vancomycin and the red-man syndrome: pharmacodynamics of histamine release. *J Infect Dis*. 1988 Mar;157(3):502–507.
31. Kowalski ML, Asero R, Bavbek S, et al. Classification and practical approach to the diagnosis and management

of hypersensitivity to nonsteroidal anti-inflammatory drugs. *Allergy*. 2013 Oct;68(10):1219–1232.
32. McNeil BD, Pundir P, Meeker S, et al. Identification of a mast-cell-specific receptor crucial for pseudo-allergic drug reactions. *Nature*. 2015 Mar 12;519(7542):237–241. doi:10.1038/nature14022.
33. Coombs RR, Gell PG. Classification of allergic reactions responsible for clinical hypersensitivity and disease. In: Gell PG, ed. *Clinical Aspects of Immunology*. New York, NY: Oxford University Press; 1976:575.
34. Pichler WJ. Delayed drug hypersensitivity reactions. *Ann Intern Med*. 2003;139:683–693.
35. Simons FE, Ardusso LR, Bilò MB, et al. International consensus on (ICON) anaphylaxis. *World Allergy Organ J*. 2014 May 30;7(1):9.
36. Liew WK, Williamson E, Tang ML. Anaphylaxis fatalities and admissions in Australia. *J Allergy Clin Immunol*. 2009 Feb;123(2):434–442. doi:10.1016/j.jaci.2008.10.049.
37. Pumphrey RS. Lessons for management of anaphylaxis from a study of fatal reactions. *Clin Exp Allergy*. 2000 Aug;30(8):1144–1150. Review. PubMed PMID: 10931122.
38. Jerschow E, Lin RY, Scaperotti MM, McGinn AP. Fatal anaphylaxis in the United States, 1999–2010: temporal patterns and demographic associations. *J Allergy Clin Immunol*. 2014;134:1318–1328.
39. Nabavi M, Esmaeilzadeh H, Arshi S, et al. Aspirin hypersensitivity in patients with chronic rhinosinusitis and nasal polyposis: frequency and contributing factors. *Am J Rhinol Allergy*. 2014 May–Jun;28(3):239–243. doi:10.2500/ajra.2014.28.4034.
40. Sánchez-Borges M, Caballero-Fonseca F, Capriles-Hulett A, González-Aveledo L. Aspirin-exacerbated cutaneous disease (AECD) is a distinct subphenotype of chronic spontaneous urticaria [published online September 29, 2014]. *J Eur Acad Dermatol Venereol*. doi:10.1111/jdv.12658. PubMed PMID:25263736.
41. Caversaccio M, Häusler R, Helbling A. Otologic manifestations in Samter's syndrome [published online October 16, 2008]. *ORL J Otorhinolaryngol Relat Spec*. 2009;71(1):6–10. doi:10.1159/000163218.
42. Kim S, Choi IS, Kim YJ, et al. Airway responsiveness to inhaled aspirin is influenced by airway hyperresponsiveness in asthmatic patients. *Korean J Intern Med*. 2010 Sep;25(3):309–316.
43. Mastalerz L, Nizankowska E, Sanak M, et al. Clinical and genetic features underlying the response of patients with bronchial asthma to treatment with a leukotriene receptor antagonist. *Eur J Clin Invest*. 2002 Dec;32(12):949–955.
44. Bel EH, Wenzel SE, Thompson PJ, et al. SIRIUS Investigators. Oral glucocorticoid-sparing effect of mepolizumab in eosinophilic asthma. *N Engl J Med*. 2014 Sep 25; 371(13):1189–1197.
45. Ortega HG, Liu MC, Pavord ID, et al. MENSA Investigators. Mepolizumab treatment in patients with severe eosinophilic asthma. *N Engl J Med*. 2014 Sep 25;371(13): 1198–1207.
46. Caproni M, Giomi B, Melani L, et al. Cellular infiltrate and related cytokines, chemokines, chemokine receptors and adhesion molecules in chronic autoimmune urticaria: comparison between spontaneous and autologous serum skin test induced wheal. *Int J Immunopathol Pharmacol*. 2006 Jul–Sep;19(3):507–515.
47. Aster RH. Drug-induced immune thrombocytopenia: an overview of pathogenesis. *Semin Hematol*. 1999;36:2–6.
48. Arndt PA, Garratty G. The changing spectrum of drug-induced immune hemolytic anemia. *Semin Hematol*. 2005; 42:137–144.
49. Greinacher A, Warkentin TE. Recognition, treatment, and prevention of heparin-induced thrombocytopenia: review and up-date. *Thromb Res*. 2006;118:165–176.
50. Mintzer DM, Billet SN, Chmielewski L. Drug-induced hematologic syndromes. *Adv Hematol*. 2009;2009:495863. doi:10.1155/2009/495863.
51. Stokol T, O'Donnell P, Xiao L, et al. C1q governs deposition of circulating immune complexes and leukocyte Fc gamma receptors mediate subsequent neutrophil recruitment. *J Exp Med*. 2004;200:835–846.
52. Aitman TJ, Dong R, Vyse TJ, et al. Copy number polymorphism in Fcgr3 predisposes to glomerulonephritis in rats and humans. *Nature*. 2006;439:851–855.
53. Hansel TT, Kropshofer H, Singer T, Mitchell JA, George AJ. The safety and side effects of monoclonal antibodies. *Nat Rev Drug Discov*. 2010 Apr;9(4):325–338. doi:10.1038/nrd3003.
54. Zhang Z, Xiang Y, Wang B, et al. Intestinal mucosal permeability of children with cefaclor-associated serum sickness-like reactions. *Eur J Pediatr*. 2013 Apr;172(4):537–543.
55. Schnyder B, Frutig K, Mauri-Hellweg D, et al. T-cell-mediated cytotoxicity against keratinocytes in sulfamethoxazol-induced skin reaction. *Clin Exp Allergy*. 1998; 28:1412–1417.
56. Chung WH, Hung SI, Yang JY, et al. Granulysin is a key mediator for disseminated keratinocyte death in Stevens-Johnson syndrome and toxic epidermal necrolysis. *Nat Med*. 2008 Dec;14(12):1343–1350.
57. Nassif A, Bensussan A, Dorothee G, et al. Drug specific cytotoxic T-cells in the skin lesions of a patient with toxic epidermal necrolysis. *J Invest Dermatol*. 2002;118:728–733.
58. Britschgi M, Steiner UC, Schmid S, et al. T-cell involvement in drug-induced acute generalized exanthematous pustulosis. *J Clin Invest*. 2001;107:1433–1441.
59. Keller M, Spanou Z, Schaerli P, et al. T cell-regulated neutrophilic inflammation in autoinflammatory diseases. *J Immunol*. 2005;175:7678–7686.
60. Hari Y, Frutig-Schnyder, Hurni M., et al. T cell involvement in cutaneous drug eruptions. *Clin Exp Allergy*. 2001; 31:1398–1408.
61. Hari Y, Urwyler A, Hurni M, et al. Distinct serum cytokine levels in drug- and measles-induced exanthem. *Int Arch Allergy Immunol*. 1999;120:225–229.
62. Roujeau J, Bioulac-Sage P, Bourseau C. Acute generalized exanthematous pustulosis: analysis of 63 cases. *Arch Dermatol*. 1991;127:1333–1338.
63. Roujeau JC. The spectrum of Stevens-Johnson syndrome and toxic epidermal necrolysis: a clinical classification. *J Invest Dermatol*. 1994 Jun;102(6):28S–30S. Review.

64. Sekula P, Liss Y, Davidovici B, et al. Evaluation of SCORTEN on a cohort of patients with Stevens-Johnson syndrome and toxic epidermal necrolysis included in the RegiSCAR study. *J Burn Care Res.* 2011 Mar–Apr;32(2): 237–245.
65. Mockenhaupt M, Viboud C, Dunant A, et al. Stevens-Johnson syndrome and toxic epidermal necrolysis: assessment of medication risks with emphasis on recently marketed drugs. The EuroSCAR-study. *J Invest Dermatol.* 2008 Jan;128(1):35–44.
66. Ben m'rad M, Leclerc-Mercier S, Blanche P, et al. Drug-induced hypersensitivity syndrome: clinical and biologic disease patterns in 24 patients. *Medicine (Baltimore).* 2009 May;88(3):131–140.
67. Pavlos R, Mallal S, Ostrov D, Pompeu Y, Phillips E. Fever, rash, and systemic symptoms: understanding the role of virus and HLA in severe cutaneous drug allergy. *J Allergy Clin Immunol Pract.* 2014 Jan–Feb;2(1):21–33. doi:10.1016/j.jaip.2013.11.005. Review.
68. Pichler WJ. Drug hypersensitivity reactions: classification and relationship to T cell activation. In: Pichler WJ, ed. *Drug Hypersensitivity*, Basel, Switzerland: Karger; 2007: 168–189.
69. Mennicke M, Zawodniak A, Keller M, et al. Fulminant liver failure after vancomycin in a sulfasalazine induced DRESS syndrome: fatal recurrence after liver transplantation. *AJT.* 2009;9:2197–2202.
70. Kano Y, Horie C, Inaoka M, Tadashi I, Mizukawa Y, Shiohara T. Herpes zoster in patients with drug-induced hypersensitivity syndrome/DRESS. *Acta Derm Venereol.* 2012; 92(2):206–207.
71. Kleiner DE, Chalasani NP, Lee WM, et al. Drug-Induced Liver Injury Network (DILIN). Hepatic histological findings in suspected drug-induced liver injury: systematic evaluation and clinical associations [published online December 18, 2013]. *Hepatology.* 2014 Feb;59(2):661–670. doi:10.1002/hep.26709.
72. Keller M, Spanou Z, Pichler WJ. Drug induced interstitial nephritis. In: Pichler WJ, ed. *Drug hypersensitivity*. Basel, Swizerland: Karger; 2007:295–305.
73. Pichler WJ, Dauber B, Kawabata T. Drug hypersensitivity: flare-up reactions, cross-reactivity and multiple drug hypersensitivity. *J Dermatol.* 2011;38:216–221.
74. Gex-Collet C, Helbling A, Pichler WJ. Multiple drug hypersensitivity—proof of multiple drug hypersensitivity by patch and lymphocyte transformation tests. *J Invest Allergol Clin Immunol.* 2005;15:293–296.
75. Daubner B, Groux-Keller M, Hausmann OV, et al. Multiple drug hypersensitivity: normal Treg cell function but enhanced in vivo activation of drug-specific T cells. *Allergy.* 2012 Jan;67(1):58–66. doi:10.1111/j.1398-995.2011.02720.x.
76. Caubet JC, Kaiser L, Lemaître B, Fellay B, Gervaix A, Eigenmann PA. The role of penicillin in benign skin rashes in childhood: a prospective study based on drug rechallenge. *J Allergy Clin Immunol.* 2011 Jan;127(1):218–222. doi:10.1016/j.jaci.2010.08.025.
77. Brockow K, Romano A, Blanca M, et al. General considerations for skin test procedures in the diagnosis of drug hypersensitivity. *Allergy.* 2002;57:45–51.
78. Barbaud A. Skin testing and patch testing in non-IgE-mediated drug allergy. *Curr Allergy Asthma Rep.* 2014 Jun;14(6):442. doi:10.1007/s11882-014-0442-8.
79. Torres MJ, Blanca M. The complex clinical picture of beta-lactam hypersensitivity: penicillins, cephalosporins, monobactams, carbapenems, and clavams. *Med Clin North Am.* 2010 Jul;94(4):805–820, xii. doi:10.1016/j.mcna.2010.04.006. Review.
80. Empedrad R, Darter AL, Earl HS, Gruchalla RS. Nonirritating intradermal skin test concentrations for commonly prescribed antibiotics. *J Allergy Clin Immunol.* 2003 Sep;112(3):629–630.
81. Brockow K, Garvey LH, Aberer W, et al. ENDA/EAACI Drug Allergy Interest Group. Skin test concentrations for systemically administered drugs—an ENDA/EAACI Drug Allergy Interest Group position paper. *Allergy.* 2013 Jun;68(6):702–712. doi:10.1111/all.12142.
82. Pichler WJ, Tilch J. The lymphocyte transformation test in the diagnosis of drug hypersensitivity. *Allergy.* 2004;59:809–820.
83. Aberer W, Bircher A, Romano A, et al. European Network for Drug Allergy (ENDA); EAACI interest group on drug hypersensitivity. Drug provocation testing in the diagnosis of drug hypersensitivity reactions: general considerations. *Allergy.* 2003 Sep;58(9):854–863.
84. Castells Guitart MC. Rapid drug desensitization for hypersensitivity reactions to chemotherapy and monoclonal antibodies in the 21st century. *J Investig Allergol Clin Immunol.* 2014;24(2):72–79; quiz 2 p following 79. Review. PubMed PMID:24834769.
85. Fruth K, Pogorzelski B, Schmidtmann I, et al. Low-dose aspirin desensitization in individuals with aspirin-exacerbated respiratory disease. *Allergy.* 2013;68(5):659–665.
86. Fajt ML, Petrov AA. Outpatient aspirin desensitization for patients with aspirin hypersensitivity and cardiac disease. *Crit Pathw Cardiol.* 2011 Mar;10(1):17–21.
87. Hope AP, Woessner KA, Simon RA, Stevenson DD. Rational approach to aspirin dosing during oral challenges and desensitization of patients with aspirin-exacerbated respiratory disease. *J Allergy Clin Immunol.* 2009 Feb; 123(2):406–410.

9

Anaphylaxis and Mast Cell Disorders

Gabriele S. de Vos and Marianne Frieri

INTRODUCTION

Anaphylaxis is a serious systemic hypersensitivity reaction involving vital organ systems (respiratory or circulatory) with a fatality rate of 0.7% to 2%.[1,2] Otolaryngologists may encounter anaphylaxis at any unpredictable time (eg, as a result of an allergic reaction to anesthetic drugs during surgery, allergen immunotherapy, or less commonly allergy skin testing in outpatient settings). Otolaryngologists may also be confronted with some of the most life-threatening cases of anaphylaxis when called to assess anaphylactic patients with swelling of the upper airways and pending asphyxia. Prompt recognition and treatment of anaphylaxis are crucial to prevent respiratory or circulatory failure and death.

EPIDEMIOLOGY

The lifetime prevalence of anaphylaxis from all possible causes has been estimated to be between 0.05% and 2% with increasing occurrence and recognition in recent years.[3–6] Atopic individuals are at increased risk of anaphylaxis from food, radiocontrast media, insect venoms, or latex. In contrast, medication-induced anaphylaxis equally affects atopic and non-atopic people.[7] In general, anaphylaxis is thought to be underrecognized because of the varying symptoms with which it may present.

> The lifetime prevalence of anaphylaxis is estimated at 0.05% to 2%. Death may occur in up to 2% of anaphylaxis cases.

DEFINITION AND DIAGNOSIS

Presenting symptoms of anaphylaxis may vary widely and can range from isolated hypotension to more generalized manifestations with hives, bronchospasm, diarrhea, and vomiting (Table 9–1).[4,7] In 2005 the US National Institute of Allergy and Infectious Disease and Food Allergy and Anaphylaxis Network convened an expert panel that suggested a uniform definition of anaphylaxis based on the presence of certain diagnostic criteria (Table 9–2).[8] These criteria were shown to reliably predict the presence or absence of anaphylaxis.[8,9] The main purpose of establishing a clear diagnosis of anaphylaxis is to enable rapid initiation of appropriate treatment, including the immediate injection of epinephrine to prevent progression to a life-threatening situation.[10]

CLINICAL MANIFESTATIONS

Time Course

At the onset of an acute allergic reaction it is generally not possible to predict if the reaction will evolve

Table 9–1. Common Signs and Symptoms of Anaphylaxis and Their Prevalence

Skin	
Urticaria and/or angioedema	85%–90%
Flushing	45%–55%
Pruritus without rash	2%–5%
Respiratory Symptoms (50%–70%)	
Dyspnea, wheeze	45%–50%
Upper airway angioedema	50%–60%
Rhinitis	15%–20%
Cardiovascular	
Dizziness, syncope, hypotension	30%–35%
Gastrointestinal	
Nausea, vomiting, diarrhea, cramping pain	25%–30%
Other	
Headache	5%–8%
Substernal pain	4%–6%
Seizure	1%–2%

Source: Reprinted with permission from Elsevier. Lieberman P, Nicklas RA, Oppenheimer J, et al. The diagnosis and management of anaphylaxis practice parameter: 2010 update. *J Allergy Clin Immunol.* Sep 2010;126(3):477–480, e471–442.

into anaphylaxis with life-threatening symptoms or instead remain mild and resolve spontaneously. Anaphylaxis typically reaches its peak symptoms within minutes to a few hours. The more rapidly it evolves, the more severe it typically is. Spontaneous involution usually occurs within hours. In 5% to 20% of cases, a second "flare" of anaphylaxis may occur 6 to 10 hours after the initial reaction had already resolved or significantly improved ("biphasic anaphylaxis"). Rarely, such biphasic reactions may occur >24 hours and up to 72 hours after the initial anaphylactic event. Similarly, there are rare cases of protracted anaphylaxis that can last several days.[11] Both biphasic and protracted anaphylaxis likely occur because of massive release of inflammatory mediators during the initial reaction that then cause the late or prolonged systemic inflammation.

Table 9–2. Diagnostic Criteria of Anaphylaxis

Anaphylaxis is Highly Likely When Any One of the Following Three Criteria is Fulfilled:

1. Acute onset of an illness (minutes to several hours) with involvement of the skin, mucosal tissue, or both (eg, generalized hives, pruritus or flushing, swollen lips-tongue-uvula)

and at least one of the following:

A. Respiratory compromise (eg, dyspnea, wheeze-bronchospasm, stridor, reduced PEF, hypoxemia)

B. Reduced BP or associated symptoms of end-organ dysfunction (eg, hypotension, collapse, syncope, incontinence)

2. Two or more of the following that occur rapidly after exposure to a *likely* allergen for that patient (minutes to several hours):

A. Involvement of the skin-mucosal tissue (eg, generalized hives, itch-flush, swollen lips-tongue-uvula)

B. Respiratory compromise (eg, dyspnea, wheeze-bronchospasm, stridor, hypoxemia)

C. Reduced BP or associated symptoms (eg, hypotension, collapse, syncope, incontinence)

D. Persistent gastrointestinal symptoms (eg, crampy abdominal pain, vomiting)

3. Reduced BP after exposure to a *known* allergen for that patient (minutes to several hours):

A. Infants and children—Low systolic BP (age specific) or greater than 30% decrease in systolic BP

B. Adults—Systolic BP of less than 90 mm Hg or greater than 30% decrease from that person's baseline

*Low systolic blood pressure for children is defined as:

- Less than 70 mm Hg from 1 month to 1 year
- Less than (70 mm Hg + (2 × age)) from 1 to 10 years
- Less than 90 mm Hg from 11 to 17 years (like adults)

Note. PEF = peak expiratory flow rate; *BP* = blood pressure.

Source: Reprinted with permission from Elsevier. Sampson HA, Munoz-Furlong A, Campbell RL, et al. Second symposium on the definition and management of anaphylaxis: summary report—Second National Institute of Allergy and Infectious Disease/Food Allergy and Anaphylaxis Network symposium. *J Allergy Clin Immunol.* Feb 2006;117(2):391–397.

Time course of anaphylaxis:

- In most cases, unpredictable at onset of allergic reaction
- Predisposing factor for severe course: reexposure to allergen that has previously caused anaphylaxis, exposure to large amounts of allergen, mast cell disorders
- Biphasic course in 5% to 20% with a second anaphylactic flare 6 to 10 hours after first reaction, rarely more than 24 hours
- Rare: protracted anaphylaxis (days to weeks)

Differential Diagnosis of Anaphylaxis

Most anaphylaxis episodes are accompanied by characteristic allergic skin symptoms (eg, pruritus, urticaria, angioedema, or flushing), facilitating the diagnosis. However, in about 10% to 20% of cases, skin symptoms may be absent, fleeting, or unrecognized, making the diagnosis of anaphylaxis more difficult. Table 9–3 lists the most common differential diagnoses of anaphylaxis.[12] In clinical practice, the most common differential diagnosis of severe anaphylaxis with isolated hypotension and loss of consciousness in a previously healthy patient, is vasovagal syncope. As opposed to anaphylaxis, in vasovagal episodes the patient's skin is typically clammy, cool, and pale. The patient may report "feeling weak" or "feeling not so good." These signs should prompt the health provider to immediately put the patient in reclined position with raised legs to ensure blood flow to the brain, possibly preventing impending loss of consciousness and subsequent falls with potential injuries. The patient's pulse rate is typically slow, and the patient may feel faint due to sometimes profoundly decreased blood pressure. Once sufficient blood flow to the brain has returned, the patient regains consciousness. Supportive measures (ie, oxygen supplementation and atropine for prolonged vasovagal episodes) are rarely needed, since recovery is usually rapid. The patient should remain in a reclined position until the blood pressure has returned to normal. In patients who are needle-phobic or have a history of vasovagal syncope, it is

Table 9-3. Differential Diagnosis of Anaphylaxis

Common Disorders
Acute asthma[a]
Acute generalized urticaria[a]
Acute angioedema
Vasovagal syncope (faint)
Panic attack/acute anxiety attack
Aspiration of a foreign body
Cardiovascular events (myocardial infarction,[a] pulmonary embolus)
Neurologic events (seizure, cerebrovascular event)
Postprandial Syndromes
Scombroid fish poisoning
Monosodium glutamate
Sulfites
Food poisoning
Flush Syndromes
Perimenopause
Carcinoid syndrome
Autonomic epilepsy
Medullary carcinoma of the thyroid
Other Nonorganic Disease
Vocal cord dysfunction
Hyperventilation
Psychosomatic episode
Shock
Hypovolemic
Cardiogenic
Distributive[b]
Septic
Other
Nonallergic angioedema (hereditary angioedema types I, II, and III, ACE inhibitor-associated angioedema)
Systemic capillary leak syndrome
Red man syndrome (vancomycin)
Pheochromocytoma (paradoxical response)

Note. ACE inhibitors: angiotensin-converting enzyme inhibitors.

[a]Acute asthma symptoms, acute generalized urticaria, or myocardial infarction symptoms can also occur during an anaphylactic episode.

[b]In anaphylaxis, shock is distributive and hypovolemic. Distributive shock may be due to anaphylaxis or to spinal cord injury.

Source: Reprinted with permission from Elsevier. Simons FECC.[12]

prudent to perform skin testing and blood drawing while they are recumbent.

> The most common diagnosis for a sudden drop of blood pressure and syncope in an outpatient setting is vasovagal syncope.

It should be noted that even though anaphylaxis is typically accompanied by tachycardia (in contrast to vasovagal syncope), in rare circumstances patients may present with bradycardia or normal heart rate, similar to vasovagal syncope. This may be the result of an intrinsic cardioinhibitory reflex with increased vagal tone (Bezold-Jarisch reflex), conduction defects, or concomitant effects of antisympathetic drugs (eg, beta-receptor antagonists).

Otherwise, syncope in an outpatient setting may also be caused by hypoglycemia (patients with diabetes mellitus on antiglycemic medicines) and less commonly due to cardiovascular events or other causes.

PATHOPHYSIOLOGY

Anaphylaxis can result from "immunologic" or "nonimmunologic" mechanisms, though overlaps may occur (Figure 9–1). Clinically, both forms are indistinguishable, and they are both treated in the same way.

Immunologic Mechanisms

Immunologic mechanisms account for the vast majority of anaphylaxis and refer to any mechanism that involves antigen-specific recognition of an allergen. IgE-mediated reactions are the most common and best-characterized type of immunologic reactions in anaphylaxis and represent the most common mechanism for most anaphylactic events.[7] Far less common are immune-complex or complement-mediated reactions (eg, when antigen binds to IgG, thereby creating immune complexes and activating

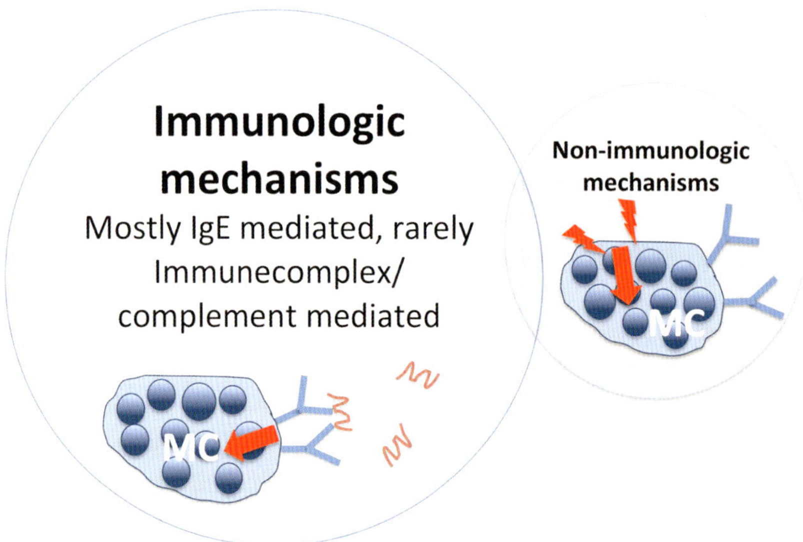

Figure 9–1. *Left:* Immunologic mechanisms of mast cell activation and degranulation. Most common are IgE-mediated reactions. Allergen binds to IgE on the surface of mast cells, causing activating signals to the mast cell (MC). *Right:* In nonimmunologic reactions the trigger for mast cell degranulation does not use IgE or other antigen-specific receptor.

the complement system that in turn can activate mast cells).

> Anaphylaxis may occur as a result of immunologic reactions (most commonly IgE mediated, eg, to food or drugs) or nonimmunologic reactions (eg, vancomycin, muscle relaxants, or radiocontrast media).

IgE-Mediated Reactions

Typical examples of IgE-mediated anaphylaxis are food allergies and many medication allergies (eg, beta-lactam antibiotics). In these IgE-mediated reactions, the allergen (eg, food or drugs metabolites) binds to IgE on a mast cell and cross-links allergen/IgE complexes on the mast cell surface, inducing mast cell activation and degranulation. Once the mast cell is activated, it releases preformed mediators from its granules into the surrounding environment. These mediators include histamine, tryptase, and cytokines. Histamine then binds to its peripheral histamine receptors. Table 9–4 lists the different histamine receptors and histamine effects.[13] Histamine and inflammatory mediators recruit and activate other immune cells (eg, eosinophils) that in turn release additional inflammatory mediators, propagating the allergic reaction.

Table 9–4. Distribution of Histamine Receptors and Their Effects

	H1	H2	H3	H4	Function (Physiologic or Pathologic)
Sensory nerve endings	++		+		Mediates itching and pain
Smooth muscle (vasculature, airways, GI tract)	+++	+	(+)		Direct vasodilation (flushing/rashes, drop of blood pressure)/axonal reflex Bronchoconstriction Diarrhea/vomiting
Endothelial cells	+++				Edema/wheals (hives)
Uterus (bladder)	+	+			Contraction of uterus and bladder
Heart	(+)	+	(+)		Direct tachycardia and ventricular contractility
CNS	+++	+	++	(+)	**H_1 > H_2:** role in sleep/wake cycle, food intake, thermal regulation, emotions, aggressive behavior, locomotion, memory, learning **H_3:** presynaptic receptor that leads to decreased release of histamine, dopamine, serotonin, noradrenaline, acetylcholine
Neutrophils, eosinophils, monocytes	+	+	+	+	Inflammation
T and B cells, hepatocytes, chondrocytes	+	+			Inflammation
Bone marrow (hematopoietic cells)				++	Differentiation of (pro)myeloblasts
Stomach (parietal cells)		+++			Gastric acid secretion (and pepsin, intrinsic factor)

Other Immunologically Mediated Reactions

IgG-mediated and immune complex–mediated reactions have been proposed to explain some drug-induced anaphylaxis when IgE could not be identified or if IgE binding appears unlikely (eg, anaphylaxis to omalizumab, an anti-IgE antibody, or allergic reactions to protamine).[14,15] During such reactions, multiple factors may lead to mast cell degranulation, including complement products able to induce mast cell activation through complement receptors on mast cells.

Nonimmunologic Anaphylaxis

Nonimmunologic mechanisms are also sometimes referred to as "anaphylactoid" or "pseudoallergic" reactions. Nonimmunologic-mediated anaphylaxis is typical for radiocontrast media and neuromuscular blocking agents that can trigger mast cell degranulation without involving IgE.[16] However, many other intrinsic and extrinsic factors are known to trigger mast cell degranulation, even though most of them typically trigger mild allergic reactions in susceptible individuals and not anaphylaxis (Table 9–5). However, they can act as contributors or amplifiers in anaphylaxis (see below). The exact mechanisms through which these substances activate mast cells are poorly understood. Patients with systemic mastocytosis or mast cell activation syndrome may report enhanced susceptibility to the effects of many of these substances.

Table 9–5. Substances Able to Induce Histamine Release From Mast Cells Through Nonimmunologic Mechanisms

Intrinsic: Substance P, "histamine-releasing factors" from lymphocytes, neutrophils, platelets, macrophages, eosinophils, IL-1, IL-3, IL-8, GM-CSF, connective tissue–activating peptide (CTAPIII), complement-derived anaphylotoxins (eg, in immune complex deposition due to blood transfusion, IVIG)
Emotional stress
Physical stimuli (eg, heat, **cold**, friction, exercise, sunlight)
Extrinsic:
Radiographic contrast dyes (iodine containing)
Muscle relaxants (eg, d-Tubocurarine)
Vancomycin
Opiates and opioids: heroine, morphine, codeine, etc
Amphotericin B
Ethanol
Gallium
Dextromethorphan, polymyxin B, quinine, reserpine, scopolamine
Bacterial toxins
Insect and snake venoms
Biologic polypeptides (eg, strawberry, jellyfish)
Spicy food
Polymeric eye drops (containing dextran)
In vitro: Compound 48/80

Note. Anaphylaxis may occur when exposed to radiocontrast dyes, muscle relaxants, rapid vancomycin infusion, or cold-exposure in susceptible individuals (**bold**). The other listed factors typically cause milder forms of allergic reactions (eg, urticaria) or may act as amplifiers of anaphylaxis.

TRIGGERS OF ANAPHYLAXIS

Overview of Causative Factors

Drugs, and less commonly insect venoms, are the most prevalent causative agents in adults while food-induced anaphylaxis is more common in children. A recent analysis of the US National Mortality Database from 1999 to 2010 revealed that drug allergy was by far the most commonly diagnosed cause of fatal anaphylaxis (58%) as opposed to venom allergy (15.2%), food allergy (6.7%), or unspecified triggers (19.3%).[17] Table 9–6 lists the most common causes of anaphylaxis. Beyond the more common triggers of anaphylaxis mentioned in this chapter, it is important to realize that any food (including food additives and nutritional supplements), drugs (including inactive drug ingredients), contact agents, or airborne substances, can act as allergens and must be carefully evaluated if the cause is otherwise unclear.

Table 9-6. Most Common Triggers and Cofactors of Anaphylaxis

Food Allergy
• Peanut, tree nuts, shellfish, fish, sesame seed, milk, egg • Pollen-associated food allergens: fruit, vegetables, herbs, or spices
Drug Allergy
• Beta-lactam antibiotics, other antibiotics, NSAIDs, opioids, muscle relaxants, anesthetics, chemotherapy drugs (eg, taxenes, platins), biologic agents (rituximab, cetuximab, infliximab, omalizumab) • Allergen immunotherapy
Insect Venom
• Wasps, bees, yellow jackets, hornets, etc • Fire ants
Inhalants (uncommon)
• Animal dander, dust, pollen, airborne latex, airborne food allergens
Uncommon Causes
• Physical causes such as cold-induced anaphylaxis, heat, sunlight • Seminal fluid in women • Mast cell disorders systemic mastocytosis or mast cell activation syndrome
Factors That Can Act as Cotriggers for Anaphylaxis
1. Exercise (eg, certain food may trigger allergic reaction only when ingested before or immediately after physical exertion but are tolerated otherwise—"exercise-induced anaphylaxis") 2. Coexisting infections (eg, patients receiving allergy immunotherapy may be more likely to have a systemic allergic reaction while having a cold or viral syndrome) 3. Mast cell disorders (systemic mastocytosis or mast cell activation syndrome) 4. Alcohol consumption

Foods

Peanuts, tree nuts, and shellfish are among the most common food allergies in many westernized societies. Death from food allergies occurs most commonly among teenagers and young adults with known food allergies, probably because of more frequent risk-taking behaviors.

Depending on the nutritional culture of a country, other foods may be more prevalent allergens. For example, chickpea allergy may be more prevalent than peanut sensitization in some Asian societies, while peach allergy is a common cause of anaphylaxis in Italy.[18,19]

Drugs

For drug-induced anaphylaxis, antibiotics are the most common cause, followed by nonsteroidal anti-inflammatory drugs (NSAIDs). Penicillin allergy is the most common antibiotic allergy. However, most patients reporting a history of penicillin allergy can tolerate penicillin. The reason for penicillin tolerance in a previously reported penicillin-allergic patient may be loss of IgE-mediated allergy over time as well as an initial erroneous diagnosis of penicillin allergy (eg, by confounding a viral exanthema/urticaria with allergic urticaria during a childhood infection). Penicillin skin testing can help estimating the risk of anaphylaxis to both penicillin and related cephalosporins in a given patient (Chapter 8). NSAID hypersensitivity is most commonly caused by non-IgE–mediated mechanisms and is commonly associated with asthma exacerbations and urticaria. However, among patients experiencing anaphylaxis to an NSAID, IgE-mediated mechanisms are more common. Such patients are allergic only to the specific culprit NSAID but may tolerate other NSAIDs.

A rather rare cause of drug-induced anaphylaxis is omalizumab (Xolair). Omalizumab, an injectable, recombinant, humanized anti-IgE antibody is used in the treatment of asthma and chronic urticaria. It may also be effective in allergic fungal sinusitis and allergic bronchopulmonary aspergillosis.[20,21] Anaphylaxis may occur in up to 0.2% of patients receiving omalizumab, mostly after the first injection. Therefore, injections must be given by a health-care provider, and the patient should be advised to remain in the office for 2 hours after the first 3 injections (due to some reports of delayed anaphylaxis) and for 30 minutes after subsequent injections and to carry an epinephrine autoinjector in case of delayed, out-of-office anaphylaxis.

Intraoperative Anaphylaxis and Latex

In 60% to 70% of cases, intraoperative anaphylaxis is caused by neuromuscular blocking agents (muscle relaxants). This is complicated by the fact that some other drugs used during anesthesia may cross-react with muscle relaxants, such as pentolinium, neostigmine, morphine, or acetylcholine (Table 9–7).[7]

In contrast, latex allergy may account for only up to 17% of intraoperative anaphylaxis. Latex allergy is particularly common among health-care workers and other occupationally exposed persons, as well as among children with spina bifida or genitourinary abnormalities due to frequent contact with latex during surgical procedures.[7,22] Latex-allergic patients typically report pruritus and skin rashes upon contact with latex products. Systemic reactions may occur when latex is introduced into tissues during medical procedures or when latex powder becomes airborne and is inhaled by highly sensitive individuals. To support the diagnosis of latex allergy, serum can be tested for specific IgE against *Hevea brasiliensis*, the source plant of latex. Skin test may also help to confirm the diagnosis, but no standardized extract is currently available in the United States.

Table 9–7. Causes of Intraoperative Anaphylaxis

- Neuromuscular blocking agents (muscle relaxants) 60% to 70%; the majority are non-IgE mediated, but severe anaphylaxis is more commonly caused by IgE-mediated reactions
- Latex 17%, IgE mediated
- Barbiturates (eg, thiopental) and propofol uncommon, mostly IgE mediated, but non-IgE–mediated reactions can also occur
- Narcotics/opioids: common cause for non-IgE–mediated urticaria and flushing, rare cause of anaphylaxis
- Antibiotics: eg, beta-lactam antibiotics (penicillin), IgE mediated; vancomycin: fast infusions can cause severe non-IgE–mediated reactions

It should be noted that local anesthetics rarely cause systemic allergic reactions or anaphylaxis. Nevertheless, local anesthetic "allergy" is commonly reported by patients, often hindering minor surgical or dental procedures. Drug testing and challenge can exclude such diagnosis to allow safe use of local anesthetics in the future. For urgent procedures in patients with a convincing history of anaphylaxis to conventional local anesthetics, it is possible to use diphenhydramine as a local anesthetic instead, even though it may be less effective and shorter lasting than, eg, lidocaine.[23]

Radiocontrast Media

Conventional high-osmolality radiocontrast media (RCM) may cause anaphylaxis in about 1% of patients. One in 1000 patients may experience severe anaphylaxis. Death from RCM-induced anaphylaxis occurs in about 1 in 75,000 patients.[24] The newer low-osmolality contrast media are less likely to induce anaphylaxis, reducing the rate of RCM associated anaphylaxis by about 80%. A patient with previous anaphylaxis to RCM has an about 20% to 40% risk of experiencing anaphylaxis again upon reexposure. Premedicating may significantly reduce this risk. There are a number of different pretreatment regimens, most of which use antihistamines and systemic corticosteroids as listed in Table 9–8.[7]

Exercise-Induced Anaphylaxis

An uncommon reason for anaphylaxis is vigorous physical exertion. Typically, symptoms start during exercise, with feelings of unusual warmth, pruritus with possible urticaria, flushing, and fatigue. Exercise-induced reactions can progress to lower and upper airway obstruction and collapse. Death may occur more commonly than reported because death during exercise is usually associated with other etiologies such as primary cardiac causes. The pathophysiologic mechanism of exercise induced anaphylaxis has yet to be elucidated. In the majority of these cases, one or more contributory factors are required to make allergic symptoms appear in addition to the exercise. Typically, these patients do not experience anaphylaxis with exercise alone or when exposed to the co-triggers alone, but only if both exercise and contributory factor(s) coincide. Most commonly, exercise-induced anaphylaxis occurs only sporadically in any given patient (whenever coexposed to the co-trigger), rendering a self-diagnosis by the patient very difficult. By unknowingly reexposing themselves to the same co-triggers, many patients may experience more than one episode of exercise anaphylaxis before the diagnosis is finally established. Examples of co-triggers are food ingestion (a specific food or any food), nonsteroidal anti-inflammatory drugs (NSAIDs), alcohol, or high pollen counts in pollen-allergic patients.[7] Exposure to the contributing factor typically occurs before exercise and less commonly during or after exercise. For example, NSAIDs may have been taken up to 24 hours prior to exercise, or the offending food may have been ingested within 6 hours prior to exercise. Among specific foods involved, wheat, other grains, nuts, and seafood have been reported most commonly, and IgE sensitization can often be confirmed by skin testing over time.

Table 9–8. Pretreatment Regimen for Patients at Risk for Radiocontrast Media–Induced Anaphylaxis

Medication, Dose, Route	Time Until Procedure
Prednisone 50 mg orally	13 hours
Prednisone 50 mg orally	7 hours
Prednisone 50 mg orally	1 hour
Diphenhydramine 50 mg orally	1 hour

> Exercise-induced anaphylaxis is rare. In most cases, exposure to a second trigger is required (eg, specific food ingestion such as wheat up to 6 hours prior to exercise or a medication, eg, NSAIDs).

Idiopathic and Unusual Causes of Anaphylaxis

When no clear trigger of anaphylaxis can be identified, patients are diagnosed as having idiopathic anaphylaxis. While up to 30% of anaphylaxis cases were thought to be idiopathic in the past, better diagnostic tools and enhanced awareness have allowed identifying more unusual causes of anaphylaxis that may previously been labeled as idiopathic. Some unusual triggers include allergenic spices and herbs, hidden food ingredients, or mislabeled food containing known allergens. Other allergenic exposures have been found due to contamination. For example, nutritional bee pollen supplements may be contaminated with pollen, or flour may be contaminated with storage mites, triggering anaphylaxis in mite-sensitized patients.[25–27] Another interesting recent discovery is hypersensitivity to the oligosaccharide alpha-galactose (alpha-gal), a carbohydrate antigen in mammalian meat (eg, beef, pork, or lamb). In contrast to usual, immediate-type food allergies that mostly affect children, patients sensitized to alpha-gal are mostly adults and may experience anaphylaxis only 3 to 6 hours after meat ingestion.[28] It has been speculated that many of these patients may have originally been sensitized by exposure to alpha-gal containing tick saliva by frequent tick bites, because alpha-gal allergy is significantly more prevalent in areas where tick bites are common.[28,29] Idiopathic anaphylaxis remains as a diagnosis of exclusion after all possible causes have been carefully taken into consideration.

> Idiopathic anaphylaxis is a diagnosis of exclusion.

CONTRIBUTORY FACTORS FOR ANAPHYLAXIS

Risk Factors for Severe Anaphylaxis

Certain factors are known to be associated with more severe courses of anaphylaxis (Table 9–9). For example, a history of previous anaphylaxis renders a patient more susceptible to having a severe reaction again when reexposed to the same allergen. In addition, asthma has not only been associated with a higher risk of experiencing anaphylaxis but also with more severe courses of anaphylaxis, particularly if the asthma is poorly controlled.[30–32] Other chronic lung diseases (COPD, interstitial lung disease) and cardiovascular disease (eg, coronary heart disease) have been associated with an increased risk of fatal anaphylaxis.[33,34] Potentially underlying conditions, such as mast cell disorders (eg, mast cell activation syndrome or systemic mastocytosis) can lower the threshold of severe allergic reactions for a patient. In addition, the amount of allergen that the patient may have ingested (food/drug) or has been injected (immunotherapy or anesthetics) also plays a role in how severe an allergic reaction may be in a sensitized individual. Whenever such factors are known in a given patient, the threshold of initiating anaphylaxis treatment, including epinephrine injection, should be very low. In some cases, such as accidental reexposure to an allergen that had caused severe anaphylaxis in the past, anaphylaxis treatment may be initiated even without waiting until all anaphylaxis criteria are fulfilled.[10]

Table 9–9. Risk Factors for Severe Anaphylaxis and "Amplifiers" of Allergic Reactions

Risk Factors for Severe Anaphylaxis
• Accidental reexposure to allergen that has caused anaphylaxis in recent past
• High-dose allergen exposure
• Asthma, particularly if poorly controlled
• Other chronic lung diseases (eg, chronic obstructive pulmonary disease, interstitial lung disease)
• Cardiovascular disease
• Concomitant usage of certain antihypertensive medication (beta-receptor antagonists, alpha adrenergic receptor antagonists, ACE inhibitors)
• Mast cell disorder (systemic mastocytosis or mast cell activation syndrome)
• Increased half-life of anaphylaxis mediators (eg, decreased degradation of PAF due to intrinsically low levels of PAF-acetylhydrolase)
Potential Amplifiers of Allergic Reactions
• Mast cell disorders
• Exercise
• Infections (viral, bacterial)
• Fever
• Emotional stress
• Lack of sleep
• Premenstrual period

Note. ACE = Angiotensin-converting enzyme; *PAF* = platelet-activating factor.

Certain antihypertensive medications have been associated with a more severe or fatal course of anaphylaxis (beta-receptor antagonists, Angiotensin-converting enzyme (ACE) inhibitors, and alpha-adrenergic blockers) and with reduced response to epinephrine during anaphylaxis treatment.[35–38] The explanation for this is that because of inhibition by these medications, endogenous or exogenous epinephrine and other compensatory mechanisms cannot fully exert their effects. For example, if a patient on beta-receptor antagonists requires epinephrine during anaphylaxis, epinephrine may not exert its effects on beta-receptors, and its effect on bronchodilation and vasoconstriction may be significantly reduced. Similarly, ACE inhibitors antagonize the metabolism of bradykinin and substance P, two potent vasodilators that play an important role during anaphylaxis.[39,40] If these intrinsic vasodilators are abundantly secreted during anaphylaxis and not sufficiently removed from the circulation because of inhibition of ACE, epinephrine may not be able to sufficiently compensate for their effects (ie, epinephrine may not be sufficiently effective in antagonizing hypotension and vascular leakage).[41]

If none of the above risk factors for severe anaphylaxis apply in a given patient, other inherent abnormalities of the patient's immune response have to be considered. For example, abnormally slow degradation of inflammatory mediators may play a role in some individuals (eg, platelet activation factor, PAF, or substrates of ACE). However, laboratory testing for these conditions is currently performed only in research settings.[42–44]

"Amplifiers" of Systemic Allergic Reactions

Apart from the above-mentioned risk factors for severe anaphylaxis, there are a number of factors that may "amplify" an allergic reaction (ie, increase their clinical manifestations). For instance, patients may have no or only a mild allergic reaction to an allergen when in their usual state of health, but may experience overt systemic reactions or anaphylaxis when certain cofactors come into play. Such cofactors include vigorous physical exertion, concomitant viral or bacterial infections, fever, lack of sleep, the premenstrual period, and emotional stress (see Table 9–9).[45,46] Other intrinsic or extrinsic nonimmunologic mast cell activators (see Table 9–5) can also act as amplifiers during an allergic reaction.

LABORATORY TESTS

As previously mentioned, the clinical picture of anaphylaxis can sometimes be confused with other differential diagnoses. Unfortunately, there is currently no immediate, real-time test available to confirm the diagnosis. However, it is possible to confirm the diagnosis of anaphylaxis retrospectively by measuring mediators that are released form mast cells during anaphylaxis (Table 9–10).

> No laboratory test is currently available to confirm the diagnosis of anaphylaxis in real time, while it is occurring. Nevertheless, blood samples obtained shortly after the onset of anaphylaxis can be sent for serum tryptase levels that can retrospectively confirm the diagnosis in unclear cases.

Serum or Plasma Tryptase

Tryptase is produced by mast cells (and in small amounts also by basophils). The mature forms of tryptase (mature beta-tryptase) are stored in mast cell granules together with histamine and released into plasma and tissue upon activation of mast cells during anaphylaxis. An elevated blood tryptase level is highly specific for mast cell activation and degranulation. It is therefore useful in distinguishing anaphylaxis from other differential diagnoses (eg, severe asthma, septic or cardiogenic shock, vasovagal syncope, or carcinoid syndrome). Total serum tryptase can be commercially measured by standardized methods. Baseline levels (ie, in absence of anaphylaxis) range between 1 and 11 ng/mL with small variations between laboratories. To detect elevated tryptase levels, the blood sample should be obtained within 30 minutes to 2 hours after onset of anaphylaxis. Tryptase levels may be elevated over 100 ng/mL during anaphylaxis and correlate relatively well with the drop in blood pressure. Levels typically return to baseline after 4 to 6 hours (with a half-life of about 2 hours).[47,48]

One major limitation in the use of tryptase levels is food-induced anaphylaxis. For unclear reasons, tryptase levels are rarely elevated in food-induced anaphylaxis, as opposed to drug-induced or stinging insect–induced anaphylaxis.

In the absence of anaphylaxis, plasma tryptase consists mainly of immature forms of tryptase (alpha and beta–protryptases). Elevated baseline tryptase levels may be a sign of spontaneous mast cell activation. In rare cases, baseline tryptase levels may be abnormally elevated, indicating an abnormal activation or number of mast cells. Therefore, if tryptase levels are elevated at baseline or do not return to baseline more than 24 hours after resolution of the anaphylactic event, the patient should be

Table 9–10. Laboratory Tests in Anaphylaxis and Mast Cell Disorders

Test	When to Obtain the Sample	Advantages	Limitations/Comments
Total tryptase (plasma or serum)	• 30–120 minutes after onset of anaphylaxis • At baseline when mast cell activation syndrome suspected	• Highly specific • Widely commercially available	• Often not elevated in food-induced anaphylaxis • Levels return to normal typically within 4–6 hours • Baseline tryptase levels should be obtained to rule out mast cell disorders >24 hours after resolution of anaphylaxis
Mature tryptase (plasma or serum)	• Baseline	• More specific for mast cell disorders then total tryptase	• Limited availability
Histamine (plasma)	• 5–20 minutes after onset of anaphylaxis		• Short half-life make it impractical • False-positive results by clotting or basophil breakage due to blood drawing technique
Histamine metabolites in urine (24-hour urine collection)	• Urine collection to be started as soon as possible after onset of anaphylaxis • Consider at baseline in suspected mast cell activation syndrome	• May distinguish an aspirin-responsive subset of patients with mast cell activation syndrome	• Rarely this may be the only elevated marker in patients with mast cell activation syndrome (with normal tryptase and 11-beta PGF2)
11-beta prostaglandin F2-alpha (11-beta PGF2, 24 hour urine collection)	• Urine collection to be started as soon as possible after onset of anaphylaxis • Consider at baseline in suspected mast cell activation syndrome	• May distinguish an aspirin-responsive subset of patients with mast cell activation syndrome	• This may be the only elevated marker in some patients with mast cell activation syndrome (with normal tryptase and urine-histamine metabolites)

referred to an allergist or hematologist for evaluation of possible systemic mastocytosis or mast cell activation disorder.

Rarely, baseline tryptase levels may also be increased because of other medical conditions (acute myelocytic leukemia, hypereosinophilic syndrome, myelodysplastic syndromes, or end-stage renal disease).[7,49,50]

Histamine and Its Metabolites

Mast cells (and basophils) produce and store large amounts of histamine, a biogenic monoamine with a very short plasma half-life (1 to 2 minutes). After degranulation of mast cells and basophils in anaphylaxis, histamine is released into the surrounding tissue and plasma. Plasma histamine levels peak within minutes and typically return to baseline within 15 to 30 minutes. Because of its fleeting nature, measurement of serum histamine is less useful for confirming a diagnosis of anaphylaxis.[51] In addition, histamine may be falsely elevated in blood samples (eg, by nonspecific histamine release from basophils during clotting or cell lysis when blood is aspired through narrow needles under vacuum).[52]

Histamine metabolites degrade less rapidly and may start to appear in the urine 30 to 60 minutes after onset of anaphylaxis. To measure these, urine should be collected for 24 hours as soon as possible after onset of anaphylaxis. Similar to tryptase, histamine and its metabolites may also be elevated at baseline in patients with systemic mastocytosis. Rarely, only histamine, but not tryptase levels may be elevated in anaphylaxis, or vice versa.[53,54]

Prostaglandins and Leukotrienes

Apart from histamine and tryptase, mast cells produce a large number of other inflammatory mediators, some of which are stored in the mast cell granules and some newly synthesized after mast cell activation. Prostaglandin D2 (PGD2) is one of the main cyclooxygenase products in mast cells but is also produced by other cells that play key roles in anaphylaxis such as eosinophils and T cells.[55–58] PGD2 is thought to play an important role in mediating symptoms of anaphylaxis. Like histamine, it is rapidly metabolized in plasma but its main metabolite, 11-beta PGF2-alpha, can be measured in urine.[48]

Leukotriene C4 (LTC4) is another inflammatory mediator produced by mast cells. Similar to PGD2, it is rapidly cleared from the circulation, and its final metabolite, LTE2, can be measured in urine. However, its sensitivity and specificity have not been well studied in anaphylaxis, so its clinical use is limited at this time.

TREATMENT OF ANAPHYLAXIS

It is important to remember that the most common cause of fatal anaphylaxis is cardiovascular and/or respiratory failure (severe bronchospasm/laryngeal edema). In addition, it has been estimated that up to 35% of the intravascular volume may shift to the extravascular tissue during severe anaphylaxis, potentially causing a fatal "empty heart syndrome."[59] Immediate epinephrine injection and proper positioning can largely prevent such catastrophic outcomes, both in clinical and out-of-hospital environments. Immediate treatment is indicated when the abovementioned diagnostic criteria of anaphylaxis are fulfilled, or if anaphylaxis is reasonably expected in a patient who starts displaying allergic symptoms (eg, after reexposure to an allergen that has previously caused anaphylaxis).

> Immediate epinephrine injection and proper positioning can largely prevent catastrophic outcomes of anaphylaxis.

In severe anaphylaxis, symptoms typically develop rapidly, often allowing a diagnosis just by looking at the patient (acute skin rash/urticaria, swelling or flushing, trouble breathing) and may further be supported by the history (e.g., exposure to known or potential allergen within past 30 min.). Anaphylaxis treatment should be initiated without any delay (ie, epinephrine injection and positioning). In the clinical setting, the provider should not wait until an assistant brings a blood pressure machine or pulse oximeter, as all this can unnecessarily delay treatment. Vital signs can be obtained once epinephrine and oxygen supplementation have been provided and the patient has been properly positioned. In case of hypotension, intravenous fluid replacement must be promptly initiated (Table 9–11). Oxygen supplementation, nebulizer treatment, and other supportive medicines should then be given as soon as possible, or simultaneously if staffing allows.

However, many times anaphylaxis symptoms develop slowly and physicians as well as patients are hesitant to inject epinephrine. As a general rule, when the risk of anaphylaxis is high (eg, if reexposed to a food allergen that had previously caused anaphylaxis), epinephrine should be given even if the diagnostic criteria for anaphylaxis are not yet fulfilled. In all other cases, where allergic symptoms develop (eg, urticaria) but do not yet fulfill anaphylaxis criteria, high doses of oral antihistamines should be given immediately, and the patient must be closely observed for any worsening signs or symptoms. In the clinic setting, such patients should be placed in an area where uninterrupted observation by trained staff for at least 30 to 60 minutes can be provided.

Table 9–11 shows a treatment scheme adapted from the most recent published practice parameter guidelines set forth by an expert panel representing the 3 largest professional allergy specialty organizations,

Table 9-11. Treatment of Anaphylaxis in Children and Adults

1. **Epinephrine (adrenaline) 1:1000 solution (= 1 mg/mL).** Repeat every 5–10 minutes if necessary.

   >12 years and adults: 0.2–0.5 mL IM anterolateral thigh (standard dose = 0.3 mL)

   >6 months and <12 years: 0.01 mg/kg

   <6 months: 0.05 mL IM

2. **Positioning: Keep patient as much reclined as tolerated, particularly if signs of cardiovascular depression; elevate legs if possible**

3. **Oxygen supplementation, beta-agonist (albuterol) and ipratropium bromide inhalation**

4. **IV access, intravenous fluids (normal saline) if still hypotensive* after epinephrine**

   Remember: 35% of the intravascular volume can be shifted to the extravascular space within the first 10 minutes of anaphylaxis

   **Low systolic BP for is defined as:*
   - *Age 1 month up to 1 year: <70 mm Hg*
   - *1 to 10 years: < (70 mm Hg + (2 × age))*
   - *>10 years and adults: <90 mm Hg or >30% drop from individual's usual baseline*

5. **If patient is on beta-blocker and inappropriately responding to epinephrine: Glucagon**

   Adults: Initial: 1–5 mg IV; followed by an infusion of 5–15 mcg/minute; (May be given IM or SC if no intravenous access). Titrate the infusion rate to achieve an adequate clinical response

   Children: Initial: 20–30 mcg/kg IV (maximum: 1 mg); followed by an infusion of 5–15 mcg/min. Titrate the infusion rate to achieve an adequate clinical response

6. **Antihistamines**

   Adults: H1-receptor antagonist (diphenhydramine = Benadryl 50 mg orally or 25–50 mg IV) and H2-receptor antagonist (eg, famotidine = Pepcid 20 mg IV—infuse slowly)

   Children (2 to 12 years): H1-receptor antagonist (diphenhydramine = Benadryl 1–1.25 mg/kg IV) and H2-receptor antagonist (famotidine = Pepcid 0.25–0.5 mg/kg IV—infuse slowly)

7. **Corticosteroids: do not help acutely but can prevent prolonged anaphylaxis; important in status asthmaticus**

   Adults: Prednisone 40–80 mg orally

   Children: Prednisone or prednisolone 1–2 mg/kg orally

If severe or prolonged hypotension, severe bronchospasm, or laryngeal edema:

- **Secure airway. Intubate if necessary.**
- **Epinephrine IV infusion (Caution! May cause cardiovascular complications)**

  Adults: Infuse between 1 and 10 ug/min. Prepare solution: Dilute epinephrine 1 mg (=1 mL vial of 1:1000, 1 mg/mL) in 250 mL of D5W or normal saline (resulting in a concentration of epinephrine 4 ug/mL), start infusion at 1 ug/min (15 drops/min or 15 mL/hour) and titrate as needed to a maximum of 10 ug/min (150 drops/min or 150 mL/h).

  Children: Infuse E at 0.1 ug/kg/min. Prepare solution: 0.6 × body weight (in kg) = mg diluted to total 100 mL saline; then 1 mL/h delivers 0.1 ug/kg/min

For status asthmaticus:

- **Magnesium sulfate ($MgSO_4$), IV—infuse over 15–20 minutes**

  Adults: 2 g magnesium sulfate as a single dose

  Children: 25–75 mg magnesium sulfate/kg/dose (maximum dose: 2 g) as a single dose

Note. I.V. = intravenous, *I.M.* = intramuscular, *SC* = subcutaneous.

the American Academy and American College of Asthma, Allergy and Immunology, as well as the Joint Council of Asthma, Allergy, and Immunology.[7] A properly stocked anaphylaxis treatment box (Figure 9–2 and Table 9–12) with a copy of the treatment plan should be readily available at all times in any clinical setting where anaphylaxis may possibly occur (allergy testing, allergy immunotherapy, drug or food challenges and desensitizations, and surgeries). Due to its rare occurrence, physicians are rarely skilled and comfortable in handling anaphylactic emergencies. Therefore, it is very useful to conduct regular mock trainings for physicians and assistant staff.

It should be noted that even though H1-receptor antagonists and corticosteroids may theoretically help to prevent prolonged or biphasic reactions, to date studies about their utility in preventing such complications are inconclusive.[7]

Apart from the above-presented treatment schemes for anaphylaxis, anecdotal reports of successfully using epinephrine hypodermal injections for the treatment of uvular swelling in the setting of anaphylaxis exist.[60] Similarly, there are reports of improving respiratory symptoms with epinephrine inhalation in anaphylaxis. The use of racemic epinephrine through nebulizer inhalation may theoretically be considered as an adjunct in the treatment of anaphylaxis when there is upper airway edema (not requiring intubation). However, this may not replace injectable epinephrine because penetration into the tissue may be insufficient, and plasma concentrations are far lower than what can be reached by one

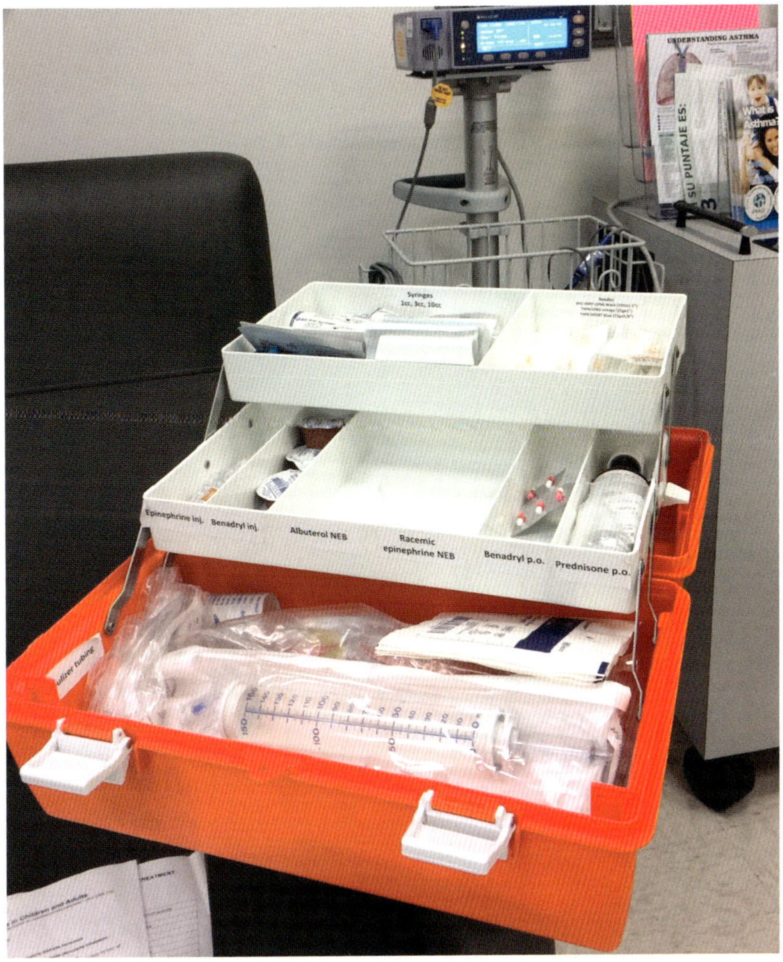

Figure 9–2. Anaphylaxis treatment box.

Table 9–12. Content Checklist for an "Anaphylaxis Emergency Treatment Box"

1. Medication			
Name	***Form***	***Dose Per Unit***	***Minimum Quantity***
☐ Benadryl	Tablets or capsules	25 mg	20
☐ Benadryl	IV solution	50 mg/mL	4
☐ Epinephrine	Injectable 1:1000	1:1000 (1 mg/mL)	5
☐ Prednisone	Tablets	20 mg	10
☐ Albuterol	Vial for nebulizer	0.083%, 3 mL	5
☐ Ipratropium bromide	Vial for nebulizer	0.5 mg	5
☐ Glucagon	Injectable, vial		1
☐ Sodium chloride 0.9%	IV solution	1000 mL	2
☐ Magnesium sulfate	IV solution		1
2. Equipment			
☐ Tubing, mouthpieces, and face masks for nebulizer treatment and oxygen delivery			
☐ Nasal cannula			
☐ Syringes 1 mL, 5 mL, 10 mL			
☐ Needles for subcutaneous and intramuscular injections in different sizes			
☐ Angiocath sets and tubing for IV infusion			
☐ Alcohol pads, gauze, medicinal tape			

Note. Note that IV H2-receptor antagonists are not listed as they usually require refrigeration for storage. In addition to the listed contents, medication and equipment for vasopressor infusion may be considered (eg, dopamine).

epinephrine injection.[7] Therefore, epinephrine inhalation is not part of the general recommendations in treating anaphylaxis.

Self-Treatment of Anaphylaxis

Patients at risk of accidental exposure to a known allergen or history of idiopathic anaphylaxis must be familiarized with a treatment plan of anaphylaxis and trained in using an epinephrine autoinjector (Figure 9–3). In addition, family members or other persons who spend much time in the vicinity of the patients should be able to initiate anaphylaxis treatment and inject epinephrine (eg, babysitters, school nurses, and even teachers). Apart from health-care providers, some professional websites provide useful guidance and education for patients and relatives, including simplified anaphylaxis treatment plans that can be carried along with the epinephrine autoinjector and oral antihistamines (http://www.foodallergy.org).

Common Barriers to Initiate Anaphylaxis Treatment

It has been shown that epinephrine has not only been insufficiently prescribed to patients at risk, but is also greatly underused by patients and parents who carry autoinjectors.[61] In addition, it is not only patients who feel hesitant to self-inject epinephrine: even medical providers frequently withhold epinephrine injections, despite clinical indications that require its use.[62]

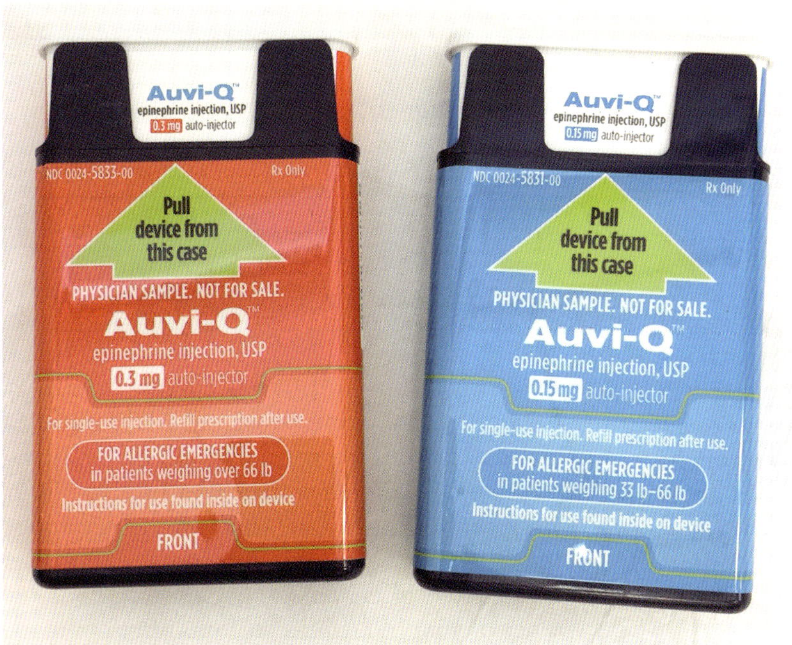

A

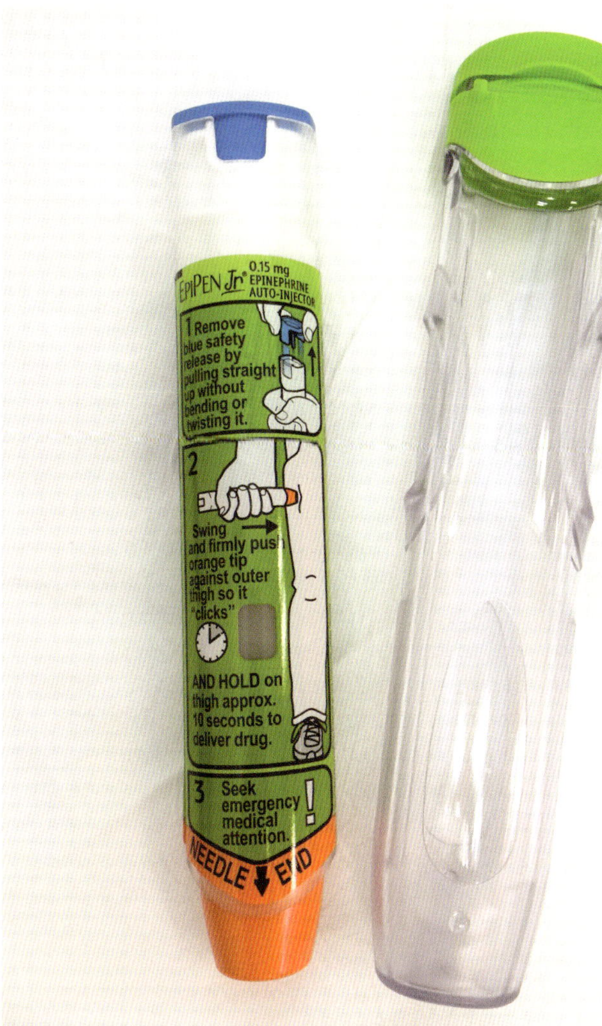

B

Figure 9-3. Examples of epinephrine autoinjectors. **A.** The "talking" Auvi-Q device (Red: contains one dose of 0.3 mg for children and adults ≥30 kg; Blue: pediatric, contains one dose of 0.15 mg for children up to 30 kg). After removal of the plastic protector (*green arrow*), the Auvi-Q device starts giving audio-instructions on how to use it. **B.** Epipen. The picture shows the "Epipen junior" containing one pediatric dose of 0.15 mg. For usage, it has to be removed from the case (shown next to the Epipen) and unlocked (remove blue plastic cap from the top). The orange tip has then to be pressed firmly onto the frontolateral thigh for 10 seconds. After use, the orange plastic tip automatically slides over the used needle for protection from needle injuries. The "adult" version of the Epipen (not shown) contains 0.3 mg and has a yellow instead of green label. Its use is otherwise identical. The needles are thin and measure approximately 12 mm in length for the pediatric versions (junior) and 15 to 16 mm for the "adult" versions.

> Epinephrine autoinjectors need to be prescribed to all patients at risk for anaphylaxis.

Hesitance due to fear of needle injection, pain, and side effects are ubiquitous barriers among providers, patients, and parents. Most autoinjectors come with practice devices, and any patient who is prescribed an autoinjector must be shown how to use it in the office (see Figure 9–3). Having to read instructions for the first time during an anaphylaxis attack is not a good idea. Patients need to be reassured that they do not have to press any button to trigger the injection, that the injection will not hurt significantly (pressure from the outer case blocks most of the needle stick pain), that the drug should not be used after its expiration date (usually 1 year), that the medicine cannot get overheated (eg, do not leave the injector in the glove compartment of a car) and finally, that they should seek further medical care (eg, emergency department) if the reaction was serious enough to warrant use of the autoinjector. To overcome fear from the injection, some providers include real-life epinephrine autoinjection when training their patients how and when to use epinephrine autoinjectors. For parents and patients, other psychologic methods such as exchanging experiences may also help. Blogs may be accessed through websites (eg, http://www.allergickid.com/2013/10/overcoming-my-fear-of-epi-pen.html).

Adverse Effects of Epinephrine Injections

Common side effects of epinephrine include palpitations, tachycardia, sweating, and headaches and should be explained to the patient during the first time that epinephrine is prescribed. Rare and potentially severe side effects include arrhythmias and symptomatic hypertension, stroke, or heart attack. Cardiovascular complications may occur in up to 10% of patients receiving intravenous bolus injections of epinephrine. The intravenous route has also been associated with a much higher incidence of erroneous epinephrine overdosage.[63] In contrast, hypertension and transient cardiac ischemia only occur in approximately 1% of patients receiving intramuscular (IM) epinephrine, and life-threatening adverse events are rare. Nevertheless, the benefits of epinephrine treatment in anaphylaxis almost always outweigh the potential risks.[7]

> Severe side effects (ie, severe cardiovascular complications) from epinephrine injections in the doses used for anaphylaxis are rare.

For patients, an additional barrier occurs at times when they misunderstand the instructions to seek medical attention after using the epinephrine autoinjector, thinking that they may not use it at all if they cannot go to a nearby emergency room after injection. However, this recommendation has been established to ensure proper observations for recurrence of anaphylactic symptoms after epinephrine levels decrease in plasma (plasma half-life 2 to 3 minutes) or biphasic reactions. It is very important to clearly explain to patients this rationale behind seeking medical advice after using epinephrine. The patient should understand that even if he or she cannot, or does not want to come to the hospital after epinephrine use, it is still better to use epinephrine and not to go the hospital, rather than not use epinephrine at all.

Occasionally, patients decline IM injections (eg, because of previously experienced side effects) or the correct needle for intramuscular injection is not available (eg, for obese patients).[64] In such cases, it is advisable to inject epinephrine subcutaneously, rather than delay or withhold epinephrine injection. Epinephrine reaches the highest peak plasma concentration when injected intramuscularly in the anterolateral thigh compared to subcutaneous injections or IM injections in the upper arm (deltoid muscle).[65] Nevertheless, the subcutaneous route may well be effective in many cases, even though it has not been systematically studied in anaphylaxis.[66] Again, the most common and worst mistake in treating anaphylaxis is to delay the epinephrine injection.

New, promising research is underway examining sublingual preparations of epinephrine for anaphylaxis. However, clinical efficacy studies have yet to be conducted with these preparations.[67]

Avoidance of Allergen Reexposure

It is intuitive that if the cause of anaphylaxis is known, patients should be instructed to strictly avoid reexposure. If the patient is allergic to a common food allergen (ie, peanut, milk, egg, wheat, soy, shellfish, tree nuts), they can often rely on food labeling, at least in the United States where labeling of common food allergens has recently become legally mandated. This becomes more difficult if the allergenic food is an unusual allergen or food additive that is not required to be listed on the label. Similarly, restaurant or delicatessen food may be a source of food allergens by cross-contamination through shared cooking tools (eg, food prepared with the same utensils or cookware). Cross-reactive food may also cause problems, such as different types of fish or shellfish in seafood allergic patients, or cross-reactive medications in drug-allergic patients.

MAST CELL DISORDERS

Mast cell disorders are rare diseases in which there are either too many mast cells, or they are overactive, or both. Systemic mast cell disorders affect mostly adults who typically present with recurrent systemic allergic reactions and anaphylaxis, often without an obvious trigger. In general, patients with systemic mast cell disorders have a decreased threshold of anaphylaxis, both to allergenic triggers and contributory factors of anaphylaxis (see Table 9–5). Anaphylaxis symptoms that occur during acute episodes are indistinguishable from anaphylaxis in otherwise healthy patients (see Table 9–1). However, patients with systemic mast cell disorders may also feel chronically fatigued and experience neuropsychiatric changes (depression, attention deficit, irritability).[68,69] Chronic mast cell mediator release can also cause osteopenia as well as gastritis and gastroduodenal ulcers.[70]

There are also cutaneous forms of mastocytosis, where mast cells proliferate and aggregate in the skin. Urticaria pigmentosa is its most common skin presentation (Figure 9–4). The diagnosis is confirmed by skin biopsy. Cutaneous mastocytosis can occur in up to 80% of patients with systemic mastocytosis and may be an important hint to establish the diagnosis, particularly in adults. Cutaneous mastocytosis without systemic involvement also exists and is almost exclusively prevalent in children whose mastocytic skin lesions start in early infancy.[71] Isolated cutaneous mastocytosis typically has a benign

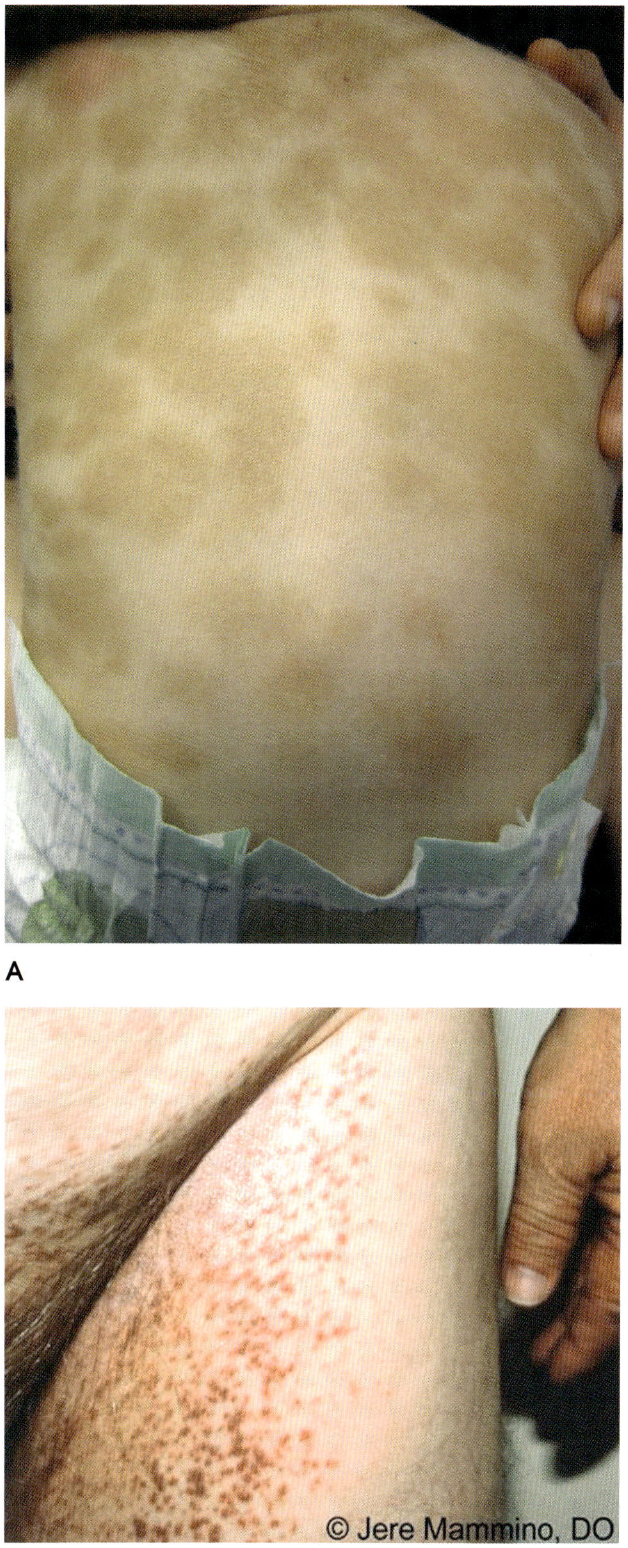

A

B

Figure 9–4. Urticaria pigmentosa in an infant (**A**) and an adult (**B**). (A. Reprinted with a Creative Commons License from James Heilman, MD. B. Reprinted with permission from Jere Mammino, DO.)

course and resolves spontaneously by adolescence. However, if the skin lesions appear after the age of 2 years, systemic mastocytosis almost always coexists.[50,68,71]

Mast cell disorders are not inherited, even though rare familial forms have been reported.[72]

Classification of Systemic Mast Cell Disorders

Different classifications of mast cell disorders exist. Based on their pathogenesis, mast cell disorders can be classified into those caused by an identifiable defect of the mast cell (primary mast cell disorder) and those in which no primary cause can be identified (idiopathic).

Systemic Mastocytosis

Systemic mastocytosis is the best characterized primary mast cell disorder. In 95% of patients, the underlying mast cell defect consists of a point mutation in the KIT gene that encodes the transmembrane receptor "c-kit" on mast cells. C-kit is the receptor for stem cell factor (SCF), which is critical for mast cell proliferation, differentiation, and survival (Figure 9–5). While SCF is also a growth factor for many other hematopoietic cells, these other cells typically lose their c-kit receptors relatively early in their development in contrast to mast cells that retain the c-kit receptor. The point mutation most commonly associated with mastocytosis is D816V, which causes a constitutive gain in c-kit function, (ie, activation without binding of SCF) (see Figure 9–5). The diagnostic criteria for systemic mastocytosis are outlined in Table 9–13.

The clinical behavior and prognosis are highly variable and range from indolent forms (relatively benign course) to aggressive systemic mastocytosis, mast cell leukemia, and other malignant hematologic disorders.[58] Very rare are malignant solid mast cell tumors (eg, in skin or bone).

Mast Cell Activation Syndrome

Mast cell activation syndromes can be primary, which are termed *monoclonal mast cell activation syn-*

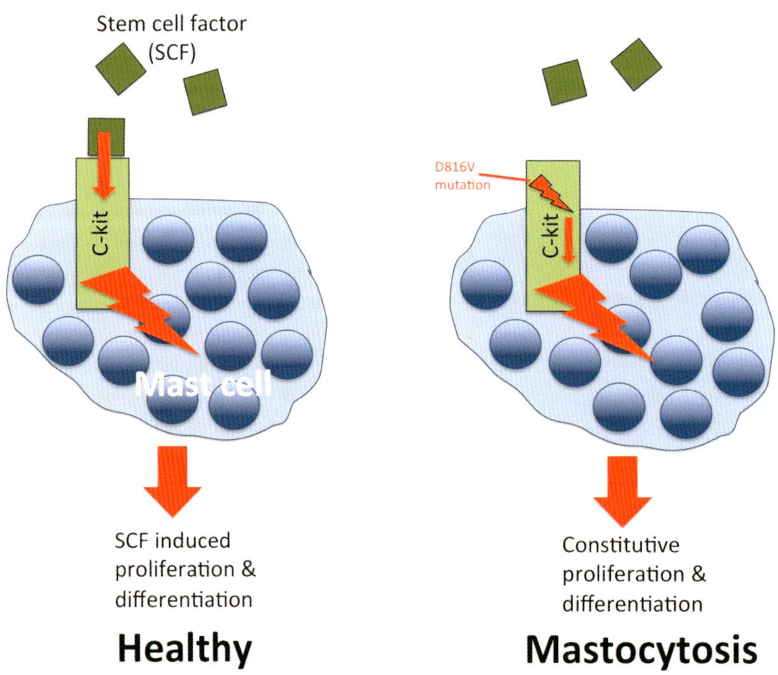

Figure 9–5. Mast cell activation through c-kit in healthy individuals (*left*) and in mastocytosis patients with the c-kit mutation (*right*).

Table 9-13. Summary of World Health Organization's (WHO) Diagnostic Criteria for Systemic Mastocytosis

Major Criterion
Multifocal, dense infiltrates of mast cells (≥15 mast cells in aggregates) detected in marrow and/or other extracutaneous organ(s)
Minor Criteria
1. >25% of mast cells in infiltrates are immature or atypical
2. Point mutation at codon 816 of *KIT*
3. Expression of abnormal mast cell marker(s) (CD25, CD2)
4. Total tryptase persistently >20 ng/mL in absence of associated clonal myeloid disease

Note. The diagnosis can be established if either the major criterion plus 1 minor criterion is fulfilled, or if 3 minor criteria are fulfilled.

Table 9-14. Suggested Diagnostic Criteria of Mast Cell Activation Syndrome (Primary or Idiopathic)

Episodic symptoms consistent with mast cell mediator release affecting ≥2 organ systems, eg
Skin: urticaria, angioedema, flushing
Gastrointestinal: nausea, vomiting, diarrhea, abdominal cramping
Cardiovascular: hypotensive syncope or near syncope, tachycardia
Respiratory: wheezing
Naso-ocular: conjunctival injection, pruritus, nasal stuffiness
Positive laboratory test:
Elevated serum tryptase, 24-hour urine histamine metabolites, or 11-beta-prostaglandin F2 at baseline
For primary (monoclonal) mast cell activation syndrome proof of mast cell defect (c-kit mutation or CD25/CD2 expression on mast cells)

drome. When no primary mast cell defect is identifiable, it is either idiopathic (unclear cause) or secondary. The term *secondary* refers to any situation in which mast cells are more activated than usual, and therefore encompasses a wide variety of conditions that have already been discussed elsewhere, including IgE-mediated allergies, nonimmunologic mast cell activation, and autoimmune urticaria.[73]

In mast cell activation syndromes, no mast cell infiltrates can be found in bone marrow or other organs. Cutaneous mastocytosis is absent. Nevertheless, mast cell abnormalities may be present (eg, c-kit mutation, CD25/CD2 expression) in some patients. Although strict criteria have not been established for mast cell activation syndromes, the diagnostic criteria listed in Table 9–14 summarizes those used in the recent literature.[73–75]

Treatment of Mastocytosis and Mast Cell Activation Syndromes

All patients with suspected mastocytosis or mast cell activation syndrome should be evaluated by an allergist and/or hematologist. Cytoreductive therapies may be necessary in aggressive or leukemic forms. Symptomatic treatment with high-dose antihistamines (H1 and H2 receptor antagonists), leukotriene antagonists, and mast cell stabilizers can significantly improve symptoms.[76] Some patients may respond to aspirin treatment, particularly if urine prostaglandin levels are elevated.[75] Aspirin blocks the production of prostaglandin D2 and may therefore reduce symptoms associated with PGD2 (eg, flushing, hypotension, bronchospasm). However, because patients with mast cell disorders may also be more susceptible to the nonimmunologic histamine and leukotriene-releasing effects of NSAIDs, graded aspirin challenge under clinical supervision should be considered.[77]

Masitinib, a tyrosine kinase inhibitor (inhibiting c-kit) has been found effective in the treatment of neuropsychiatric symptoms in mastocytosis patients.[69] Doxepin, a tricyclic antidepressant and potent antihistamine, as well as other antidepressants may also be helpful. Gastrointestinal symptoms can be treated with oral cromolyn, H2-receptor antagonists, and proton pump inhibitors. Osteopenia or osteoporosis may require bisphosphonates if vitamin D and calcium supplements are insufficient to prevent progression.

Treatment of Patients With Mast Cell Disorders and Coexisting Allergies

As mentioned above, patients with mast cell disorders are more susceptible to developing severe allergic symptoms or anaphylaxis to any nonimmunologic or immunologic trigger, including IgE-mediated allergies. While drug treatment of allergic disorders largely overlaps with the treatment of mast cell disorders, allergy immunotherapy may present a particularly high risk for anaphylaxis in patients with mast cell disorders. Immunotherapy to environmental allergens may therefore be contraindicated, even though this has not been systematically studied. Venom immunotherapy should be considered in venom-allergic patients with mast cell disorders, when the risk of experiencing severe anaphylaxis with a hymenoptera sting is higher than experiencing anaphylaxis due to venom immunotherapy.[78] The presence of a mast cell disorder is considered to be an indication for long-term continuation of venom immunotherapy since these patients are at a high risk for fatal anaphylaxis after an insect sting.

REFERENCES

1. Moneret-Vautrin DA, Morisset M, Flabbee J, Beaudouin E, Kanny G. Epidemiology of life-threatening and lethal anaphylaxis: a review. *Allergy.* Apr 2005;60(4):443–451.
2. Brown AF, McKinnon D, Chu K. Emergency department anaphylaxis: a review of 142 patients in a single year. *J Allergy Clin Immunol.* Nov 2001;108(5):861–866.
3. Lieberman P, Camargo CA, Jr, Bohlke K, et al. Epidemiology of anaphylaxis: findings of the American College of Allergy, Asthma and Immunology Epidemiology of Anaphylaxis Working Group. *Ann Allergy Asthma Immunol.* Nov 2006;97(5):596–602.
4. Decker WW, Campbell RL, Manivannan V, et al. The etiology and incidence of anaphylaxis in Rochester, Minnesota: a report from the Rochester Epidemiology Project. *J Allergy Clin Immunol.* Dec 2008;122(6):1161–1165.
5. Lin RY, Anderson AS, Shah SN, Nurruzzaman F. Increasing anaphylaxis hospitalizations in the first 2 decades of life: New York State, 1990–2006. *Ann Allergy Asthma Immunol.* Oct 2008;101(4):387–393.
6. Wood RA, Camargo CA, Jr, Lieberman P, et al. Anaphylaxis in America: the prevalence and characteristics of anaphylaxis in the United States. *J Allergy Clin Immunol.* Feb 2014;133(2):461–467.
7. Lieberman P, Nicklas RA, Oppenheimer J, et al. The diagnosis and management of anaphylaxis practice parameter: 2010 update. *J Allergy Clin Immunol.* Sep 2010; 126(3):477–480, e471–442.
8. Sampson HA, Munoz-Furlong A, Campbell RL, et al. Second symposium on the definition and management of anaphylaxis: summary report—Second National Institute of Allergy and Infectious Disease/Food Allergy and Anaphylaxis Network symposium. *J Allergy Clin Immunol.* Feb 2006;117(2):391–397.
9. Campbell RL, Hagan JB, Manivannan V, et al. Evaluation of national institute of allergy and infectious diseases/food allergy and anaphylaxis network criteria for the diagnosis of anaphylaxis in emergency department patients. *J Allergy Clin Immunol.* Mar 2012;129(3):748–752.
10. Sampson HA, Munoz-Furlong A, Bock SA, et al. Symposium on the definition and management of anaphylaxis: summary report. *J Allergy Clin Immunol.* Mar 2005; 115(3):584–591.
11. Sampson HA, Mendelson L, Rosen JP. Fatal and near-fatal anaphylactic reactions to food in children and adolescents. *N Engl J Med.* Aug 6 1992;327(6):380–384.
12. Simons FECC. Anaphylaxis: rapid recognition and treatment. *UpToDate (online).* 2014; http://www.uptodate.com/contents/anaphylaxis-rapid-recognition-and-treatment?source=machineLearning&search=anaphylaxis&selectedTitle=1%7E150&sectionRank=2&anchor=H2 - H2. Accessed February 20, 2015.
13. Simons FE, Simons KJ. Histamine and H1-antihistamines: celebrating a century of progress. *J Allergy Clin Immunol.* Dec 2011;128(6):1139–1150, e1134.
14. Khodoun MV, Strait R, Armstrong L, Yanase N, Finkelman FD. Identification of markers that distinguish IgE-from IgG-mediated anaphylaxis. *Proc Natl Acad Sci USA.* Jul 26 2011;108(30):12413–12418.
15. Weiss ME, Nyhan D, Peng ZK, et al. Association of protamine IgE and IgG antibodies with life-threatening reactions to intravenous protamine. *N Engl J Med.* Apr 6 1989; 320(14):886–892.
16. Johansson SG, Bieber T, Dahl R, et al. Revised nomenclature for allergy for global use: report of the Nomenclature Review Committee of the World Allergy Organization, October 2003. *J Allergy Clin Immunol.* May 2004;113(5):832–836.
17. Jerschow E, Lin RY, Scaperotti MM, McGinn AP. Fatal anaphylaxis in the United States, 1999–2010: temporal patterns and demographic associations. *J Allergy Clin Immunol.* Dec 2014;134(6):1318–1328, e1317.
18. Kasera R, Singh BP, Lavasa S, Prasad KN, Sahoo RC, Singh AB. Kidney bean: a major sensitizer among legumes in asthma and rhinitis patients from India. *PloS One.* 2011;6(11):e27193.
19. Asero R, Antonicelli L, Arena A, et al. Causes of food-induced anaphylaxis in Italian adults: a multi-centre study. *Int Arch Allergy Immunol.* 2009;150(3):271–277.
20. Evans MO, 2nd, Coop CA. Novel treatment of allergic fungal sinusitis using omalizumab. *Allergy Rhinol.* Jan 2014;5(3):172–174.
21. Collins J, Devos G, Hudes G, Rosenstreich D. Allergic bronchopulmonary aspergillosis treated successfully for one year with omalizumab. *J Asthma Allergy.* 2012;5:65–70.
22. Alenius H, Kurup V, Kelly K, Palosuo T, Turjanmaa K, Fink J. Latex allergy: frequent occurrence of IgE antibodies to a cluster of 11 latex proteins in patients with spina bifida and histories of anaphylaxis. *J Lab Clin Med.* May 1994;123(5):712–720.

23. Bartfield JM, Jandreau SW, Raccio-Robak N. Randomized trial of diphenhydramine vs benzyl alcohol with epinephrine as an alternative to lidocaine local anesthesia. *Ann Emerg Med.* Dec 1998;32(6):650–654.
24. Katayama H, Yamaguchi K, Kozuka T, Takashima T, Seez P, Matsuura K. Adverse reactions to ionic and nonionic contrast media. A report from the Japanese Committee on the Safety of Contrast Media. *Radiology.* Jun 1990; 175(3):621–628.
25. Greenberger PA, Flais MJ. Bee pollen-induced anaphylactic reaction in an unknowingly sensitized subject. *Ann Allergy Asthma Immunol.* Feb 2001;86(2):239–242.
26. Sanchez-Borges M, Suarez-Chacon R, Capriles-Hulett A, Caballero-Fonseca F. An update on oral anaphylaxis from mite ingestion. *Ann Allergy Asthma Immunol.* Feb 2005; 94(2):216–220; quiz 220–212, 306.
27. Puglisi G, Frieri M. Update on hidden food allergens and food labeling. *Allergy Asthma Proc.* Nov–Dec 2007;28(6): 634–639.
28. Commins SP, Platts-Mills TA. Anaphylaxis syndromes related to a new mammalian cross-reactive carbohydrate determinant. *J Allergy Clin Immunol.* Oct 2009;124(4): 652–657.
29. Gonzalez-Quintela A, Dam Laursen AS, Vidal C, Skaaby T, Gude F, Linneberg A. IgE antibodies to alpha-gal in the general adult population: relationship with tick bites, atopy, and cat ownership. *Clin Exp Allergy.* Aug 2014; 44(8):1061–1068.
30. Gonzalez-Perez A, Aponte Z, Vidaurre CF, Rodriguez LA. Anaphylaxis epidemiology in patients with and patients without asthma: a United Kingdom database review. *J Allergy Clin Immunol.* May 2010;125(5):1098–1104, e1091.
31. Iribarren C, Tolstykh IV, Miller MK, Eisner MD. Asthma and the prospective risk of anaphylactic shock and other allergy diagnoses in a large integrated health care delivery system. *Ann Allergy Asthma Immunol.* May 2010; 104(5):371–377.
32. Pumphrey RS. Lessons for management of anaphylaxis from a study of fatal reactions. *Clin Exp Allergy.* Aug 2000; 30(8):1144–1150.
33. Greenberger PA, Rotskoff BD, Lifschultz B. Fatal anaphylaxis: postmortem findings and associated comorbid diseases. *Ann Allergy Asthma Immunol.* Mar 2007;98(3):252–257.
34. Mulla ZD, Simons FE. Concomitant chronic pulmonary diseases and their association with hospital outcomes in patients with anaphylaxis and other allergic conditions: a cohort study. *BMJ Open.* 2013;3(7).
35. Triggiani M, Patella V, Staiano RI, Granata F, Marone G. Allergy and the cardiovascular system. *Clin Exp Immunol.* Sep 2008;153(suppl 1):7–11.
36. Watson A. Alpha adrenergic blockers and adrenaline. A mysterious collapse. *Aust Fam Physician.* Aug 1998; 27(8):714–715.
37. Rueff F, Przybilla B, Bilo MB, et al. Predictors of severe systemic anaphylactic reactions in patients with Hymenoptera venom allergy: importance of baseline serum tryptase-a study of the European Academy of Allergology and Clinical Immunology Interest Group on Insect Venom Hypersensitivity. *J Allergy Clin Immunol.* Nov 2009;124(5):1047–1054.
38. Nassiri M, Babina M, Dolle S, Edenharter G, Rueff F, Worm M. Ramipril and metoprolol intake aggravate human and murine anaphylaxis: evidence for direct mast cell priming. *J Allergy Clin Immunol.* Feb 2015;135(2):491–499.
39. Kaplan AP, Joseph K. Pathogenic mechanisms of bradykinin mediated diseases: dysregulation of an innate inflammatory pathway. *Adv Immunol.* 2014;121:41–89.
40. Byrd JB, Touzin K, Sile S, et al. Dipeptidyl peptidase IV in angiotensin-converting enzyme inhibitor associated angioedema. *Hypertension.* Jan 2008;51(1):141–147.
41. Mueller UR. Cardiovascular disease and anaphylaxis. *Curr Opin Allergy Clin Immunol.* Aug 2007;7(4):337–341.
42. Vadas P, Gold M, Perelman B, et al. Platelet-activating factor, PAF acetylhydrolase, and severe anaphylaxis. *N Engl J Med.* Jan 3 2008;358(1):28–35.
43. Summers CW, Pumphrey RS, Woods CN, McDowell G, Pemberton PW, Arkwright PD. Factors predicting anaphylaxis to peanuts and tree nuts in patients referred to a specialist center. *J Allergy Clin Immunol.* Mar 2008;121(3): 632–638, e632.
44. Pravettoni V, Piantanida M, Primavesi L, Forti S, Pastorello EA. Basal platelet-activating factor acetylhydrolase: prognostic marker of severe Hymenoptera venom anaphylaxis. *J Allergy Clin Immunol.* Apr 2014;133(4):1218–1220.
45. Simons FE, Ardusso LR, Bilo MB, et al. World Allergy Organization anaphylaxis guidelines: summary. *J Allergy Clin Immunol.* Mar 2011;127(3):587–593, e581–522.
46. Anagnostou K, Clark A, King Y, Islam S, Deighton J, Ewan P. Efficacy and safety of high-dose peanut oral immunotherapy with factors predicting outcome. *Clin Exp Allergy.* Sep 2011;41(9):1273–1281.
47. Schwartz LB, Yunginger JW, Miller J, Bokhari R, Dull D. Time course of appearance and disappearance of human mast cell tryptase in the circulation after anaphylaxis. *J Clin Invest.* May 1989;83(5):1551–1555.
48. van der Linden PW, Hack CE, Poortman J, Vivie-Kipp YC, Struyvenberg A, van der Zwan JK. Insect-sting challenge in 138 patients: relation between clinical severity of anaphylaxis and mast cell activation. *J Allergy Clin Immunol.* Jul 1992;90(1):110–118.
49. Lindner PS, Pardanani B, Angadi C, Frieri M. Acute nonlymphocytic leukemia in systemic mastocytosis with biclonal gammopathy. *J Allergy Clin Immunol.* Sep 1992; 90(3, pt 1):410–412.
50. Frieri M, Claus M, Martinez S, Annunziato D, Kosuri S, Lin J. Fever, hemorrhagic bullae and gastritis in a 20-month-old male. *Ann Allergy.* Sep 1989;63(3):179–183.
51. Halmerbauer G, Hauk P, Forster J, Urbanek R, Kaufmehl K, Koller DY. In vivo histamine release during the first minutes after deliberate sting challenges correlates with the severity of allergic symptoms. *Pediatr Allergy Immunol.* Feb 1999;10(1):53–57.
52. Schwartz LB. Laboratory tests to support the clinical diagnosis of anaphylaxis. *UpToDate (online).* 2014; http://www.uptodate.com/contents/laboratory-tests-to-support-the-clinical-diagnosis-of-anaphylaxis?source=search_

result&search=laboratory+tests+anaphylaxis&selectedTitle=1%7E150. Accessed June 3, 2015.
53. Lin RY, Schwartz LB, Curry A, et al. Histamine and tryptase levels in patients with acute allergic reactions: an emergency department-based study. *J Allergy Clin Immunol.* Jul 2000;106(1, pt 1):65–71.
54. Laroche D, Vergnaud MC, Sillard B, Soufarapis H, Bricard H. Biochemical markers of anaphylactoid reactions to drugs. Comparison of plasma histamine and tryptase. *Anesthesiology.* Dec 1991;75(6):945–949.
55. Tanaka K, Ogawa K, Sugamura K, Nakamura M, Takano S, Nagata K. Cutting edge: differential production of prostaglandin D2 by human helper T cell subsets. *J Immunol.* Mar 1 2000;164(5):2277–2280.
56. Luna-Gomes T, Magalhaes KG, Mesquita-Santos FP, et al. Eosinophils as a novel cell source of prostaglandin D2: autocrine role in allergic inflammation. *J Immunol.* Dec 15 2011;187(12):6518–6526.
57. Celestin J, Frieri M. Eosinophilic disorders in various diseases. *Curr Allergy Asthma Rep.* Feb 2012;12(1):18–24.
58. Frieri M, Linn N, Schweitzer M, Angadi C, Pardanani B. Lymphadenopathic mastocytosis with eosinophilia and biclonal gammopathy. *J Allergy Clin Immunol.* Jul 1990; 86(1):126–132.
59. Fisher MM. Clinical observations on the pathophysiology and treatment of anaphylactic cardiovascular collapse. *Anaesth Intensive Care.* Feb 1986;14(1):17–21.
60. Peltz S, Bateman HE, Reyes R, Oppenheimer J, Bielory L. Hypodermic epinephrine spray and uvular angioedema revisited. *J Allergy Clin Immunol.* Feb 1996;97(2):717–718.
61. Campbell RL, Luke A, Weaver AL, et al. Prescriptions for self-injectable epinephrine and follow-up referral in emergency department patients presenting with anaphylaxis. *Ann Allergy Asthma Immunol.* Dec 2008;101(6):631–636.
62. Ross MP, Ferguson M, Street D, Klontz K, Schroeder T, Luccioli S. Analysis of food-allergic and anaphylactic events in the National Electronic Injury Surveillance System. *J Allergy Clin Immunol.* Jan 2008;121(1):166–171.
63. Campbell RL, Bellolio MF, Knutson BD, et al. Epinephrine in anaphylaxis: higher risk of cardiovascular complications and overdose after administration of intravenous bolus epinephrine compared with intramuscular epinephrine. *J Allergy Clin Immunol.* Jan–Feb 2015;3(1):76–80.
64. Johnstone J, Hobbins S, Parekh D, O'Hickey S. Excess subcutaneous tissue may preclude intramuscular delivery when using epinephrine autoinjectors in patients with anaphylaxis. *Allergy.* Jun 2015;70(6):703–706.
65. Simons FE, Gu X, Simons KJ. Epinephrine absorption in adults: intramuscular vs subcutaneous injection. *J Allergy Clin Immunol.* Nov 2001;108(5):871–873.
66. Chowdhury BA, Meyer RJ. Intramuscular vs subcutaneous injection of epinephrine in the treatment of anaphylaxis. *J Allergy Clin Immunol.* Apr 2002;109(4):720; author reply 720–721.
67. Rawas-Qalaji M, Rachid O, Mendez BA, Losada A, Simons FE, Simons KJ. Adrenaline (epinephrine) microcrystal sublingual tablet formulation: enhanced absorption in a preclinical model. *J Pharm Pharmacol.* Jan 2015; 67(1):20–25.
68. Akin C, Metcalfe DD. Systemic mastocytosis. *Annu Rev Med.* 2004;55:419–432.
69. Moura DS, Sultan S, Georgin-Lavialle S, et al. Depression in patients with mastocytosis: prevalence, features and effects of masitinib therapy. *PloS One.* 2011;6(10):e26375.
70. Doyle LA, Sepehr GJ, Hamilton MJ, Akin C, Castells MC, Hornick JL. A clinicopathologic study of 24 cases of systemic mastocytosis involving the gastrointestinal tract and assessment of mucosal mast cell density in irritable bowel syndrome and asymptomatic patients. *Am J Surg Pathol.* Jun 2014;38(6):832–843.
71. Frieri M, Quershi M. Pediatric mastocytosis: a review of the literature. *Pediatr Allergy Immunol Pulmonol.* Dec 1 2013;26(4):175–180.
72. Longley BJ, Jr, Metcalfe DD, Tharp M, et al. Activating and dominant inactivating c-KIT catalytic domain mutations in distinct clinical forms of human mastocytosis. *Proc Natl Acad Sci USA.* Feb 16 1999;96(4):1609–1614.
73. Frieri M, Patel R, Celestin J. Mast cell activation syndrome: a review. *Curr Allergy Asthma Rep.* Feb 2013;13(1):27–32.
74. Akin C, Valent P, Metcalfe DD. Mast cell activation syndrome: proposed diagnostic criteria. *J Allergy Clin Immunol.* Dec 2010;126(6):1099–1104, e1094.
75. Ravi A, Butterfield J, Weiler CR. Mast cell activation syndrome: improved identification by combined determinations of serum tryptase and 24-hour urine 11beta-prostaglandin2alpha. *J Allergy Clin Immunol.* Nov–Dec 2014;2(6):775–778.
76. Hamilton MJ, Hornick JL, Akin C, Castells MC, Greenberger NJ. Mast cell activation syndrome: a newly recognized disorder with systemic clinical manifestations. *J Allergy Clin Immunol.* Jul 2011;128(1):147–152, e142.
77. Steinke JW, Negri J, Liu L, Payne SC, Borish L. Aspirin activation of eosinophils and mast cells: implications in the pathogenesis of aspirin-exacerbated respiratory disease. *J Immunol.* Jul 1 2014;193(1):41–47.
78. Castells MC, Akin C. Treatment and prognosis of systemic mastocytosis. *UpToDate (online).* 2014; http://www.uptodate.com/contents/treatment-and-prognosis-of-systemic-mastocytosis?source=see_link&anchor=H10-H10. Accessed February 19, 2015.

10

Allergic Skin Diseases

Luz Fonacier, Melanie Chong, Ryan Steele, and Marcella R. Aquino

INTRODUCTION

As the largest organ of the human body, the skin is involved in many diseases that may be encountered by ear, nose, and throat (ENT) physicians. In atopic dermatitis, especially during infancy, the dermatitis primarily involves the face, scalp, and extensor surface of the extremities. Irritant and allergic contact dermatitis of the head and neck is common, and the North American Contact Dermatitis Group Patch test results for 2009 through 2010 lists the face and eyelids as the third and fourth most frequent body site involved in dermatitis referred for patch testing. Drug eruptions can affect not only the skin but also the mucous membranes. The ENT physician may encounter these manifestations either as the primary or secondary diagnosis and should therefore learn to recognize and manage them.

ATOPIC DERMATITIS

Atopic dermatitis (AD) affects approximately 20% of the population in developing countries[1] and up to 18% of children and 2% of adults in the United States alone. There is also a significant economic burden associated with AD, with $3.8 billion spent on health care expenditures annually in the United States.[2] The atopic march is a concept in allergy used to describe the natural progression of allergic disease from AD to food allergy, asthma, and allergic rhinitis. This progression is believed to begin with AD, often occurring in infancy, with other allergic disorders developing throughout childhood. AD is a chronic inflammatory disease defined by pruritic skin lesions, often beginning before the age of 5 years.[3] It commonly affects the face, scalp, and flexor regions in children with the affected body distribution changing with age. By adulthood, only 60% of affected individuals have had a resolution of their AD,[4] and it remains a lifelong disease burden for many patients.

Pathophysiology

Epidermal Barrier Dysfunction

Our understanding of the underlying mechanisms of AD has evolved from an emphasis on the adaptive immune response and the Th1-Th2 balance as an inciting event to a focus on epithelial barrier dysfunction as the primary event in disease pathogenesis. Breakdown of the skin barrier can lead to subsequent immunodysregulation and IgE-mediated disease that all play a role in progression of AD.

The epidermis serves to restrict water loss from the body and to prevent the entrance of pathogens. In order to form this barrier, the keratinocytes that make up the epithelium replace their plasma membranes with a cornified envelope. This insoluble layer helps to regulate the essential barrier functions of the epidermis, and its failure plays a critical role in the pathogenesis of AD. Individuals with AD have increased transepidermal water loss as a consequence of multiple abnormalities including reduced lipids such as sphingosine and ceramide[1] and, in some, dysfunctional filaggrin causing abnormal keratinization of the cornified envelope. Filaggrin is a protein that binds to keratin fibers in epithelial cells, becoming integrated into the lipid envelope; it is critical to water retention in the skin and maintenance of pH via its amino acid breakdown products.[5] Individuals with mutations in the filaggrin gene (*FLG*) have an earlier disease onset of AD, increased disease severity, and are at higher risk for allergic sensitization. Increased transepidermal water loss can be seen in both lesional and nonlesional skin in AD patients.[1]

> Breakdown of the skin barrier leads to water loss and dermatitis flare, which can be worsened by infectious agents such as bacteria or yeasts, and allergens.

Immunodysregulation

Multiple immunohistological and immunoregulatory abnormalities can be seen in the skin of AD patients. The keratinocytes present in AD have abnormal responses to environmental triggers, favoring the production of cytokines and chemokines of a Th2 profile (atopic) in acute lesions and subsequent promotion of Th1 responses leading to chronic inflammatory lesions. The Th2 responses of acute lesions are promoted from specific allergenic triggers through antigen-presenting dendritic cells, and superantigens—antigens from bacterial colonization leading to nonspecific activation of T-cell receptors. In acute AD there is an increase in cytokines including IL-4 and IL-13, while chronic lesions are characterized by increased IL-12 and IFN-γ (a Th1 cytokine). In addition to changes in the cytokine profile of AD patients, keratinocytes in the skin overexpress thymic stromal lymphopoietin (TSLP). TSLP has effects on multiple cell types including T cells, eosinophils, and mast cells; it functions by promoting an allergic Th2 response. Antigens that are processed by Langerhans cells in the skin of AD patients interact with naïve T cells in regional lymph nodes and promote Th2 responses, leading to the production of IgE.[1]

IgE-Mediated Disease

IgE-mediated allergies may also be a trigger for disease flare in patients with AD, notably food and environmental triggers. There is an early association between food allergy and the appearance of AD, with a prevalence of IgE-mediated food allergy of 35% among children with AD.[6] For patients with confirmed allergies to specific foods (such as egg, milk, peanut, and fish allergens),[5] avoidance of these foods can result in clinical improvement but not resolution of their AD symptoms. For patients with environmental allergies such as dust mites, environmental control measures that lower allergen loads have led to symptomatic improvement.[5]

> Atopic dermatitis is a pruritic chronic inflammatory skin condition marked by epidermal barrier dysfunction and immunologic abnormalities.

Head and Neck AD

The diagnosis of AD is based on a thorough history and clinical exam. Although supporting laboratory evaluations such as increased serum IgE, peripheral eosinophilia, and skin biopsy may aid in diagnosis of AD or its associated comorbid atopic conditions, they are usually not required for presumed diagnosis and treatment. Care must be taken, however, in distinguishing AD of the head and neck from other causes of regional dermatitis including photodermatoses and contact dermatitis, discussed later in the chapter.

Airborne Pattern Atopic Dermatitis

Airborne pattern AD closely resembles the distribution of photodermatitis; however, its occurrence tends to peak with the appearance of seasonal environmental allergens. For those individuals sensitized to perennial allergens such as dust mites, disease flares may occur at any time. Certain environmental allergens are protease enzymes and act on the epidermal barrier, causing activation of the protease-activated receptor-2 (PAR-2). Activation of PAR-2 directly mediates pruritus and also causes keratinocytes to release inflammatory cytokines. Identified proteins that activate this pathway are found in many allergenic substances, including dust mite, cockroach, and the pollens of ragweed, birch, cedar, juniper, and cypress trees.[7,8] The airborne pattern variant of AD described here is generally not responsive to antihistamines and immunotherapy. In these patients, allergen avoidance measures should be emphasized.

Role of Microbials in Atopic Dermatitis

Staphylococcus Aureus

It is estimated that *S. aureus* may be cultured from more than 90% of skin lesions in AD, as opposed to 5% of healthy controls.[5] The proteases of this species help to degrade the epidermal barrier, and recurrent staphylococcal pustulosis can add to the disease burden of AD. *S. aureus* may also exert noninfectious damage to the skin in AD. Studies have shown that *S. aureus* acts as a superantigen and thus may play a role in increasing inflammation in AD.[9] In addition to the possible superantigen mediated effects of some of its toxins, *S. aureus* exotoxin δ-toxin has potent mast-cell degranulating activity.[10]

Malassezia

In patients with AD of the head and neck that do not respond to traditional therapies such as topical steroids and moisturizers, consideration must be given to colonization with *Malassezia* yeasts.[11] *Malassezia* species on the skin of AD patients can exacerbate underlying disease, with the forehead, eyelids, and neck being the most commonly affected areas.[2] Patients with AD of the head and neck have also been shown to react more frequently to *Malassezia* on skin prick testing and have elevated levels of *Malassezia* specific-IgE compared to patients with AD without head and neck involvement.[2] Increases in *Malassezia* populations correlate with increases of sebum production in adolescence, although sensitization can occur well into adulthood and lead to a new onset of AD on the face, neck, and upper chest, where counts of the yeast are the highest.[2] Studies examining the mechanisms underlying sensitization of patients with AD of the head and neck to *Malassezia* have demonstrated that it is an MHC-restricted immune response causing worsening of AD. [2]

HSV and Molluscum Contagiosum

Patients with AD are also more susceptible to viral infections, including herpes simplex virus (HSV) and molluscum contagiosum. HSV infections may manifest as generalized eruptions known as eczema herpeticum, and complications such as corneal involvement may necessitate emergency care. Viral culture and polymerase chain reaction (PCR) from recently unroofed vesicles may aid in the diagnosis of these cases. Molluscum contagiosum may require treatment or coverage of lesions due to the contagious nature of the disease, although most cases will spontaneously resolve.[5]

Treatment

Effective treatment of AD of the head and neck requires consideration of both the disease mechanisms and the anatomic location of the lesions being treated (Figure 10–1). Understanding that dysfunction of the epidermal barrier is responsible for initial disease pathogenesis in AD, its restoration and decreasing transepidermal water loss can significantly alleviate symptoms and restore barrier function. Bathing will help to restore water

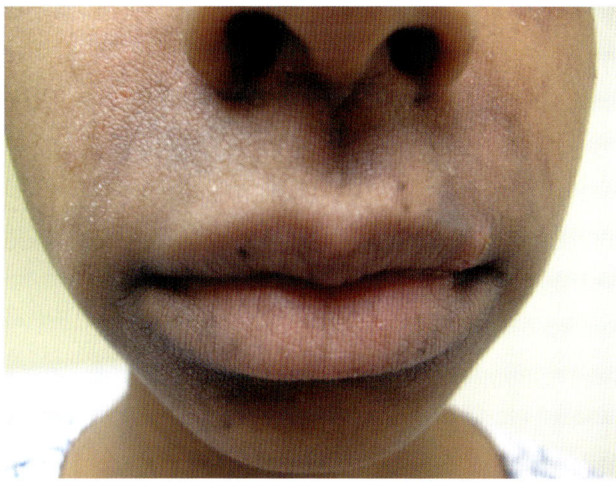

Figure 10–1. Atopic dermatitis of the face.

content, and should be done for 10 to 15 minutes with a wet washcloth or towel covering the face and neck. This may need to be repeated several times a day depending on disease severity. Once hydrated, the skin should be patted dry of excess water, and moisturizer immediately applied in order to prevent evaporation.

Adequate moisturization may decrease the need for topical pharmacoactive treatments. When considering moisturizing agents, oils, lotions, creams, and ointments are available. Those with preservatives and fragrances may be irritating to the skin of AD patients, and/or cause sensitization via allergic contact dermatitis (ACD). Lotions and creams have higher water content and are practical choices for application to highly visible areas such as the head and neck. Due to their higher water content, lotions may have a drying effect secondary to evaporation. Petroleum jelly is inexpensive but generally cosmetically less appealing for head and neck application. It does not act as a moisturizer but as a sealant after hydration of the skin. Ointments are generally more accepted if applied at night. There are also non-FDA-regulated prescription products classified as medical devices that are marketed for pruritic dermatoses and aim to restore lipid content and hydration to the skin in AD (EpiCeram, MimyX, Eletone, Atopiclair).[5]

> Therapy is aimed at restoration of the epidermal barrier, possible treatment of microbiologic agents contributing to disease, and control of allergen exposure.

Topical corticosteroids, while the mainstay of treatment in AD, should be used with caution in head and neck dermatitis. They are effective for the short-term management of mild to moderate AD[3]; however, their use on the face and neck may be problematic as these areas are susceptible to associated adverse events including telangiectasia, skin atrophy, rosacea, and perioral dermatitis.[12] Nonsteroidal alternatives exist in the form of the calcineurin inhibitors, tacrolimus[5] and pimecrolimus.[3] These are well-tolerated alternatives that may be used in head and neck dermatitis. Studies with pimecrolimus in children with mild to moderate facial AD have shown improvement in dermatitis severity and pruritus.[3] Despite the FDA black box warning for the calcineurin inhibitors, and some provider hesitancy in prescribing them, a joint task force concluded the risk-benefit ratios of these agents are similar to conventional therapies for chronic relapsing AD.[5] Side effects include transient burning or stinging at the site of application.

> Although topical corticosteroids are a mainstay of treatment in atopic dermatitis, their prolonged use in head and neck dermatitis can be problematic. The use of moisturizing agents and topical calcineurin inhibitors such as tacrolimus and pimecrolimus can be effective long-term disease management strategies.

Bacterial, viral, and fungal infections can all contribute to a worsening of AD symptoms, and treatment of these infections may improve therapy outcomes. *S. aureus* should be treated when there is an active systemic or overlying local infection. The treatment of *S. aureus* as a colonizing organism in uninfected AD patients is more controversial, and long-term oral antibiotic therapy should be avoided.[13] For systemic infections, first- and second-generation cephalosporins given for a 7 to 10 day duration is usually effective (eg, cephalexin, cefadroxil, cefdinir). Methicillin-resistant *Staphylococcus aureus* (MRSA) may be treated with clindamycin, doxycycline, minocyline, or trimethoprim/sulfamethoxazole. Topical mupirocin applied 3 times a day for the same duration is also effective for localized infections. Neomycin should be avoided if possible, as this is a common skin sensitizer that causes contact dermatitis.

> Antimicrobial therapy may be an adjunctive treatment modality in active bacterial infections or recalcitrant head and neck dermatitis with evidence of yeast colonization.

For patients with eczema herpeticum, systemic antiviral therapy with either acyclovir or valacyclovir may be necessary. Recurrent cases may require long-term suppression. Cases of molluscum contagiosum on the head and neck may be treated with curettage, or cryotherapy. Patients with recalcitrant head and neck AD lesions colonized with *Malassezia* may benefit from an empiric, 1 to 2 month daily treatment course of itraconazole or ketoconazole followed by long-term weekly treatment.[2]

CONTACT DERMATITIS

Contact dermatitis (CD) of head and neck is not uncommon and could be due to an irritant or an allergen (allergic contact to dermatitis-ACD). This problem can be caused by a single agent, by simultaneous exposure to multiple agents, or have an additive, synergistic, or antagonistic effect. An example would be titanium dioxide in facial cosmetics that adsorbs gold released from a hand that has touched jewelry or eyeglass frames and facilitates the development of facial and eyelid dermatitis (Table 10–1).

It is not unusual for patients to have both an ACD superimposed on an irritant contact dermatitis (ICD) because an exposure to an irritant may enhance penetration of the allergen and upregulation of pro-inflammatory cytokines.[14] There are a few important clinical differences between ACD and ICD. ICD is due to nonimmunologic, direct tissue damage of the skin and may manifest as burning, stinging, and soreness (more than itching) of erythematous, edematous skin usually with sharply demarcated borders. ACD is more common in the genetically predisposed and previously sensitized atopic individual and is a type IV delayed hypersensitivity response. Itching is prominent, and the rash manifests as erythema, edema, vesicles, papules, and/or lichenification.

> Contact dermatitis can manifest as a non-immunologic (irritant contact dermatitis) and/or an immunologic (allergic contact dermatitis) dermatologic reaction.

Clinical Manifestations

Face

Allergic CD of the face may be generalized or primarily affect periorbital, perioral, or specific regions such as the forehead (Figure 10–2).

Sensitizers in commercial facial products are commonly found in cosmetics that come in almost daily and direct contact with the skin. However, facial ACD can also occur due to ectopic transfer of allergens to the face by the hands from other regions of the body. Airborne aeroallergens (eg, tree, weed pollens) may also cause an eczematous dermatitis of the exposed areas such as the face and neck, especially during their specific pollinating seasons.[15]

> Allergic contact dermatitis of the face can be due to products applied directly on the skin, ectopic transfer of allergens to the face by the hands from other regions of the body, or even airborne aeroallergens.

Eyelid. Allergic CD is the most common cause of isolated periorbital and eyelid dermatitis.[16] Other causes include ICD, AD, seborrheic dermatitis, and blepharitis. The most common sources of causative allergens are found in cosmetic products (eg, facial cream, eye shadow) and ophthalmic therapeutics. The most common sensitizers are fragrance mix, Balsam of Peru, thimerosal, neomycin sulfate, and nickel.[16,17] "Ectopic dermatitis" from nail polish can manifest on the eyelids and the neck and is usually due to toluene-sulfonamide formaldehyde resin in the nail polish (Figure 10–3).

Lip. Eczematous lip dermatitis (cheilitis) is an acute or chronic inflammation of the lips manifesting as itching, burning, redness, and edema with fissuring. Irritant CD is the most common cause of cheilitis, especially in children. Chemical irritants include saliva, lip cosmetics, or other oral products and physical irritants including cold exposure, low humidity, dryness, or wind. Other causes of cheilitis are ACD and AD. Allergic contact cheilitis (ACC) is more common in women[18] and often involves the lip vermillion and its border and extends to contiguous skin presenting with concomitant perioral dermatitis. The oral mucosa is typically spared. Fragrance mix, Balsam of Peru, and nickel are the most common positive allergens on patch testing.[18] Sources of fragrances include oral hygiene products (eg, toothpastes, mouthwashes, flavorings, compounds used for dental impressions), cosmetics, and lip products (eg, lipsticks, glosses, lip balms). Lip products were

Table 10-1. Common Allergens Involved in Contact Dermatitis of the Head and Neck

Contact Allergen	Common Exposures
Nickel sulfate	Jewelry
Wool alcohols (lanolin)	Cosmetics, skin-care products (creams, lotions, ointments), soaps and cleansers, facial masks, sunscreen, hair-care products (shampoos, hair sprays), over-the-counter and prescription medications for skin
Neomycin sulfate	Topical antibiotics
Potassium dichromate	Dental cement, pigments in inks and paints, cosmetics
Caine mix	Topical anesthetics
Fragrance mix	Fragrances
Colophony	Cosmetics, sunscreens, adhesives
Paraben mix	Preservatives in topical formulations, cosmetics
Balsam of Peru	Cosmetics, fragrances , dental hygiene products, topical medications
Ethylenediamine dihydrochloride	Topical medications, piperazine-related antihistamines, aminophylline, hydroxyzine hydrochloride
Cobalt dichloride	Jewelry, paints, cobalt-based pigments
Carba mix	Rubber products, shampoos, disinfectants
Black rubber mix	Hair dye, rubber products
Methylchloroisothiazolinone (MCI), methylisothiazolinone (MI)	Cosmetics, skin-care products (creams, lotions, moisturizers), soaps and cleansers, wipes, hair-care products (conditioners, shampoos, coloring agents)
Quaternium-15	Cosmetics, skin-care products
Methyldibromo glutaronitrile	Skin-care products, shampoos
p-Phenylenediamine	Hair dyes, cosmetics, black henna tattoo
Formaldehyde	Cosmetics
Thimerosal	Preservative in contact lens solutions, cosmetics
Thiuram	Rubber products, adhesives
Diazolidinyl urea	Hair-care products, skin-care products, cosmetics
Quinoline mix	Paste bandages, prescription and nonprescription topical antibiotics and antifungal creams, skin-care products
Tixocortol-21-pivalate	Related topical corticosteroids
Gold sodium thiosulfate	Gold or gold-plated jewelry, dental restorations
Imidazolidinyl urea	Soaps and cleansers, hair-care products, cosmetics, skin-care products
Budesonide	Topical corticosteroids, intranasal corticosteroid spray, inhaled corticosteroids
Hydrocortizone-17-butyrate	Topical corticosteroids
Mercaptobenzothiazole	Rubber products, nitrile or neoprene (rubber bands, earphones and headphones, masks)
Bacitracin	Topical antibiotics, bandaids, ophthalmic and otic solutions

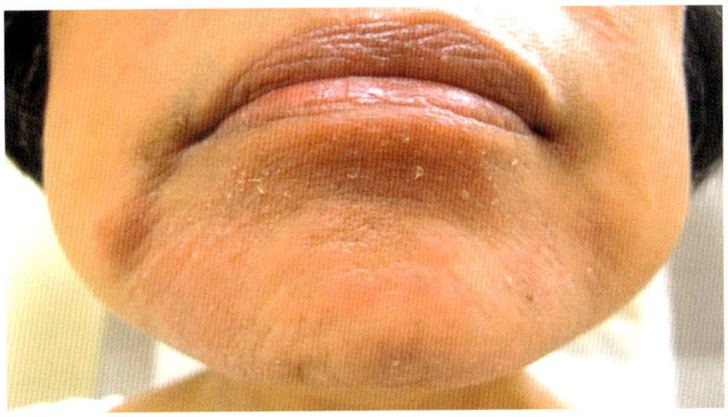

Figure 10-2. Perioral and facial dermatitis due to allergic contact dermatitis.

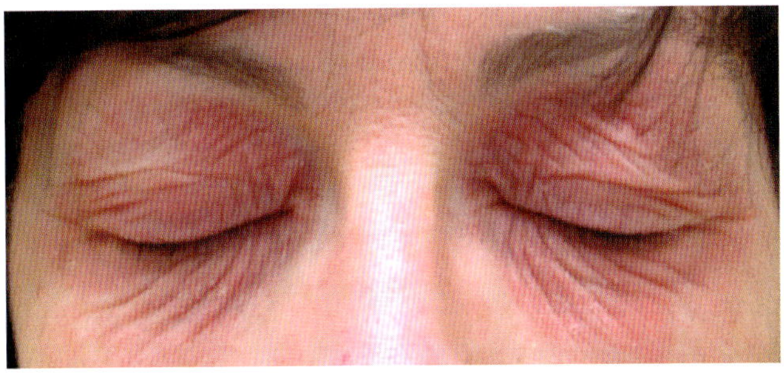

Figure 10-3. Eyelid dermatitis.

the most common sources of allergens for ACC in females, and toothpastes were the most common in males. The flavoring chemicals such as spearmint, menthol, peppermint, carvone, cinnamal, and anethole are common relevant allergens in toothpaste. In lip balm, propolis, lanolin, coconut oil, almond oil, peppermint oil, and vitamin E are potential sensitizers. Topical medications (eg, neomycin, budesonide, tetracaine) have also been reported as causes of ACC. Ectopic transfer of allergen must also be considered in ACC, such as ectopic transfer of nickel by the hands or from direct contact from other sources such as kissing their partners or children.

Oral Mucosa

Although often suspected, ACD is not a common cause of chronic oral mucosal inflammatory conditions such as burning mouth syndrome, lichenoid tissue reactions, stomatitis, gingivitis, orofacial granulomatosis, or recurrent aphthous stomatitis. In a large study of 331 patients presenting with oral symptoms, patch testing to a comprehensive panel of flavorings, preservatives, acrylates, medications, and metals showed the most frequent positive reactions to potassium dicyanoaurate, nickel, gold sodium thiosulfate, fragrance mix, Balsam of Peru, beryllium, cobalt, and acrylate.[19] However, based on available clinical data, there is insufficient evidence to confirm a causative role or relevance of the positive patch test to the aforementioned oral syndromes.[19] Irritant CD from chemical and traumatic injury during dental treatment may be the most common causes of contact reactions involving mucous membranes.

Head and Neck

Females are twice as likely as males to have ACD due to cosmetics involving the head and neck.[20] However, nickel remains the most common contact sensitizer and is more frequent in women than men likely due to greater exposure to nickel in jewelry. Common sensitizers in hair products include paraphenylenediamine (hair dye), glyceryl thioglycolate (permanent wave solutions), cocamidopropyl betaine (surfactant in shampoo), fragrances, methylchloroisothiazolinone/methylisothiazolinone, quaternium-15, imidazolidinyl urea (preservatives) and other ingredients such as propylene glycol, vitamin E, paraben, benzophenones, iodopropynyl butylcarbamate, and methyldibromoglutaronitrile/phenoxyethanol. Allergic CD involving the scalp is most frequently caused by sensitization to medical products, hair tints, and bleaches.

> Contact dermatitis should be considered in the differential diagnosis of a dermatitis that involves the head, neck, and oral mucosa.

Special Considerations

Nickel

Nickel is the most common allergen in positive patch test reactions. The worldwide prevalence of ACD due to nickel is estimated to be 8.6%; however, it reaches up to 17% in the female population.[21] Primary sensitization usually occurs from nonoccupational sources, with body piercing as the most common source. Investigations have demonstrated that nickel sensitization is significantly higher in individuals with pierced ears vs those with unpierced ears. More than one ear piercing may also be associated with a greater frequency of nickel sensitization.[22]

Nickel sensitization through occupational exposure commonly manifests as a chronic hand eczema. However, traces of nickel can be transferred to the face through direct contact.[23] Industrial exposure to nickel occurs from the production of stainless steel, nickel alloys and cast iron, electroplating and electroforming, alkaline batteries, coins, hair dye, and nickel-plated hand tools.[24] Recently, nickel in mobile cell phones has been implicated as a potential source of exposure, especially in individuals who present with a persistent facial dermatitis involving the preauricular and cheek area.[25]

Dental Implants

Cases of ACD due to dental implants have been reported and are thought to be due to a delayed type hypersensitivity reaction that occurs when biologic fluids contact the metal alloy. This leads to corrosion of the metal alloy and release of metal ions that interact with endogenous proteins to form metal-protein complexes that can activate T lymphocytes through several unclear mechanisms. However, a delayed-type hypersensitivity response is most frequently observed.[26] Mercury amalgam is the most frequently used material in dental practice and the most common metal to induce a contact allergy. Other metals (copper, zinc, palladium, cobalt, tin, gold) have also been implicated although less frequently. Although metal-associated CD commonly presents as an eczematous reaction overlying the site of the implant, ACD from dental implants usually presents as an oral lichenoid reaction.[27] Burning mouth syndrome (BMS) and "burning lip syndrome" (a subype of BMS) have also been associated with allergy to cobalt, nickel, mercury, gold, and bone cement components contained in dental implants.[28] Removal of the implant may lead to resolution of symptoms and failure to improve may suggest an alternative diagnosis.[29]

> Metal hypersensitivity through exposure to nickel-containing products including dental implants has been reported to cause symptoms in both the skin and oral mucosa.

Fragrance

Fragrances are the most common cause of ACD from cosmetics in the United States. They contain hundreds of different chemicals and are regularly present in cosmetics, personal care products, household products, and medicaments, either to achieve an appealing scent or to mask unpleasant odors. Labeling of products with regard to fragrance can be confusing and nonstandardized, with some manufacturers using the term *fragrance free*, yet the product contains large numbers of botanical extracts which can be sensitizing as well. Current labeling laws do not require manufacturers to label a specific fragrance as present in a product, and regulation of fragrance ingredients in cosmetics exempts fragrance formulas as "trade secrets." Therefore, some essential oils (tea tree oil, ylang-ylang oil, jasmine flower oil, peppermint oil, lavender oil, citrus oil) and "covert fragrances" that may be used as preservatives rather than for aroma (bensaldehyde, benzyl alcohol, bisabolol, citrus oil, unspecified essential oils) can also cause ACD and may not appear on labels. In toothpastes, flavoring chemicals are the most frequent relevant allergens, including mint derivatives such as spearmint, menthol, peppermint, carvone as well as cinnamal, and anethole. In lip balm, propolis produced by bees, lanolin, coconut oil, almond oil, peppermint oil, and vitamin E are potential sensitizers. It is necessary to perform patch testing to detect hypersensitivity to this group of allergens. The documentation of fragrance allergy necessitates instituting an avoidance protocol that eliminates all culprit fragranced cosmetics and personal hygiene products.

Cocoamidopropyl Betaine (CAPB)

CAPB is an amphoteric surfactant that is often found in shampoos, bath products, eye and facial cleaners, liquid detergents, surface cleaners, pet care products, and other skin and hair care products. Allergic CD to CAPB typically presents as eyelid, facial, scalp, and/or neck dermatitis. Sensitization occurs from shampoos (including baby shampoo) and other toiletry products that include liquid shower gels, roll-on deodorants, and facial cleansers. According to the North American Contact Dermatitis Group (NACD), 1.1% of patients tested had a positive reaction to CAPB.[30]

Corticosteroids

Surprisingly, topical corticosteroids are not uncommon causes of facial and perioral dermatitis. ACD to TCS affects 0.5% to 5.8% of patients suspected of ACD and should be suspected if a rash worsens, rather than improves after the topical application, or fails to respond to topical corticosteroids. In such cases, the patient should be referred to an allergist or dermatologist for evaluation and patch testing.

> Delayed-type hypersensitivity to topical corticosteroids can be challenging to identify and should be considered in a dermatitis that does not respond to treatment, or initially responds, then worsens with prolonged use of topical corticosteroids.

Topical corticosteroids are classified according to their potency and allergenicity. The potency and side effects of TCS are related to saturation of the glucocorticoid receptors in different cell types. They are classified as class 1 (superpotent) to class 7 (least potent). The allergenicity of topical corticosteroids based on 2 immune recognition sites on the molecule is classified into groups A, B, C, D-1, and D-2[31] (Table 10–2). There is considerable cross-reactivity within the groups and possible cross-reactivity between them, so avoidance of topical corticosteroids within each class is recommended once allergy to one of these drugs has been confirmed by patch testing.

Patch testing to corticosteroids is complicated by the inherent, anti-inflammatory nature of the drug itself, which results in frequent false-negative results if tested at too a high concentration or there is failure to perform delayed patch test readings. Although rare, patients sensitized to topical corticosteroids by skin contact can develop systemic contact dermatitis with administration of the corticosteroids by an oral, intravenous (IV), intramuscular (IM), or inhalation route.[32]

Vehicle and preservatives in topical preparations of corticosteroids[33,34] are common causes of ACD and must also be tested. Vehicle ingredients that are well-known allergens are propylene glycol (most common), sorbitan sesquioleate (second most common), formaldehyde-releasing preservatives, parabens, methylchloroisothiazolinone/methylisothiazolinone, and lanolin. Lanolin is used as the base of many topical medications including topical corticosteroids and moisturizers.

Patch testing should therefore be performed if possible to the steroid allergy screening agents [tixocortol pivalate (group A), budesonide (group B), hydrocortisone butyrate (group D)], the patient's own topical corticosteroids, and vehicle and preservatives (propylene glycol, sorbitan sesquioleate, formaldehyde, imidazolidinylurea, diazolidinylurea, paraben mix, fragrance mix, lanolin, MCI/MI). If patch testing is not available and ACD to topical corticosteroids is suspected, use of a class C steroid with a vehicle with no "common" allergens is suggested. (Examples include Topicort ointment [desoximetasone 0.25% ointment] and Topicort gel [desoximetasone 0.05% gel]). Another option is the use of a nonsteroidal medication such as tacrolimus ointment (0.1%, 0.03%).

Diagnosis and Differential Diagnosis

An essential part of the diagnosis of ACD is a detailed history of occupational exposures and daily activities. However, only 10% to 20% of contact allergens can be accurately predicted in this way even by experienced physicians.[35] Another challenging aspect of diagnosis includes the extensive list of cutaneous conditions that can mimic ACD including AD, seborrheic dermatitis, impetigo, psoriasis, dermatophytosis, lichen simplex chronicus, prurigo nodularis, nummular eczema, and polymorphous light eruption. Systemic diseases such as Wiskott-Aldrich syndrome, X-linked agammaglobulinemia, hyper IgE syndrome, acrodermatitis enteropathica, connective tissue diseases, mycosis fungoides, as well as systemic drug reactions should also be considered in the differential diagnosis of ACD involving the head and neck.[36]

Table 10-2. Structural Groups of Corticosteroids: Cross-Reactivity Based on 2 Immune Recognition Sites—C 6/9 and C16/17 Substitutions

Topical Corticosteroids	Systemic Corticosteroids
Group A: Hydrocortisone and tixocortol pivalate: has C17 or C21 short-chain ester	
Cloprednol	Cortisone acetate
Dichlorisone acetate	Hydrocortisone-21-acetate
Fludrocortisone acetate	Methylprednisolone acetate (Depo Medrol)
Fluorometholone (FML Ophthalmic Ointment)	
Fluprednisolone acetate	Prednisone
Hydrocortisone (Egocort, Cortaid)	Prednisolone acetate
Hydrocortisone-2-sodium	
Medrysone	
Meprednisone	
Methylprednisolone acetate	
Prednisone sodium phosphate	
Prednisolone acetate (Pred Forte eye drops)	
Tixocortol	
Group B: Acetonides: has C16 C17 cis-ketal or –diol additions	
Amcinonide	Triamcinolone
Budesonide (Pulmicort, Butacort, and Entocort)	Triamcinolone benetonide
Desonide	Triamcinolone diacetate
Fluocinolone acetonide (Synalar)	Triamcinolone hexacetonide
Fluocinonide (Metosyn)	
Flumoxonide	
Flunisolide (Aerospan)	
Halcinonide (Halog)	
Triamcinolone acetonide (Aristocort)	
Group C: Nonesterified betamethasone: has C16 methyl group	
Betamethasone sodium phosphate	Betamethasone
Desoximetasone (Topicort)	Dexamethasone acetate
Dexamethasone-sodium phosphate	Paramethasone acetate
Diflucortolone (pivalate, valerate)	
Flumethasone	
Fluocortin butyl	
Fluocortolone (hexanoate, pivalate, caproate) (Ultraproct)	
Fluprednidene acetate	
Halometasone	

Table 10-2. *continued*

Topical Corticosteroids	Systemic Corticosteroids
Group D1: has C16 methyl group and halogenated B ring	
Alclometasone dipropionate (Aclovate)	Beclomethasone dipropionate
Betamethasone 17 valerate (Betnovate, Beta)	Betamethasone dipropionate
Betamethasone dipropionate (Diprosone)	
Clobetasol propionate (Dermol, Dermovate)	
Clobetasone 17 butyrate (Eumovate)	
Diflorasone diacetate (ApexiCon)	
Fluticasone propionate (Cutivate)	
Halobetasol (Ultravate)	
Mometasone furoate (Elocon)	
Group D2: labile esters without C16 methyl or B ring halogen substitution	
Hydrocortisone aceponate	
Hydrocortisone 17-butyrate (Locoid)	
Hydrocortisone-17-valerate	
Prednicarbate (Dermatop)	
Methylprednisolone aceponate	

Patch testing is the gold standard for the diagnosis of ACD. The T.R.U.E. Test system is preloaded with 35 common allergens and a negative control; however, the use of a larger system such as the North American Contact Dermatitis series which ranges from 65 to 70 allergens may pick up relevant allergens that may be missed by the T.R.U.E. Test alone. The chambers are applied onto the back and held in place with hypoallergenic tape for 48 hours. Although simple to perform, patch test interpretation requires expertise. Oral corticosteroids and/or immunosuppressants can suppress patch test results, but there are no supporting data that guide the duration of steroid reduction or withdrawal prior to performing patch testing. If necessary, patch testing should be performed while on the lowest possible dose of the immunosuppressant medication. Topical corticosteroids and immunosuppressants at the site of patch testing should be avoided 5 to 7 days prior to testing as the anti-inflammatory effects of these agents can diminish a positive result[36] (Figures 10–4 and 10–5).

> Patch testing is the gold standard tool to diagnose contact dermatitis.

The repeat open application test can also be performed to identify contact allergens and is best suited for the evaluation of leave-on products (ie, cosmetics). It is especially useful for eyelid dermatitis as eyelid skin may be more reactive than skin in other areas, such as the back. The test involves the repeated application of the product to the antecubital fossa or back of the ear twice daily for up to 1 to 2 weeks to observe for the development of dermatitis. Skin biopsy may also be helpful to differentiate ACD from morphologically similar cutaneous conditions.[36]

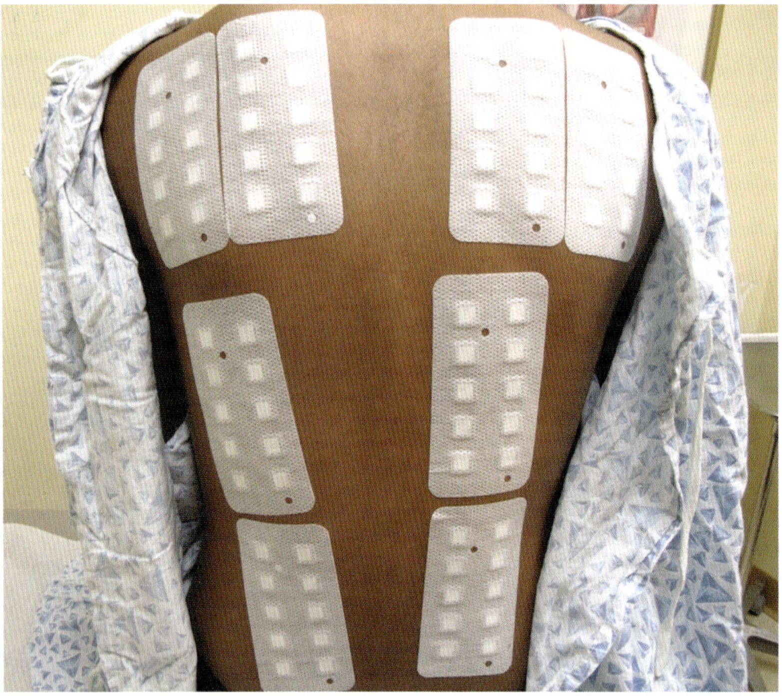

Figure 10-4. Patch tests applied onto the patient's back.

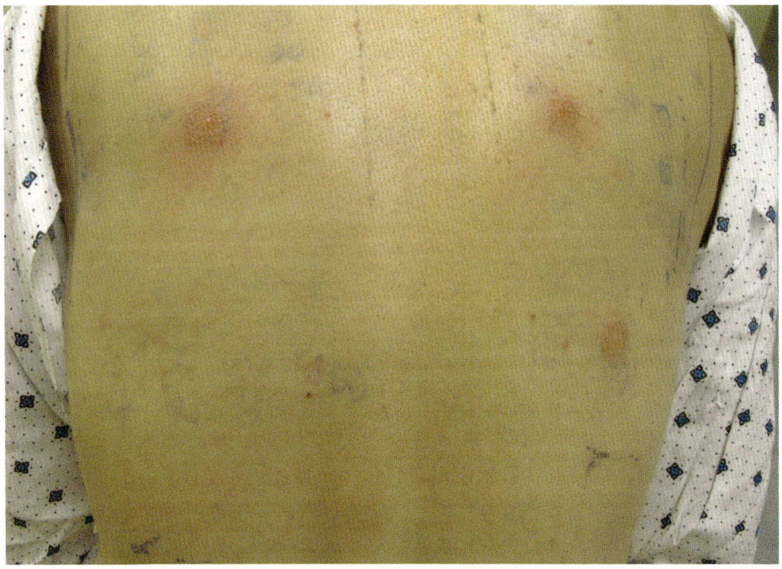

Figure 10-5. Erythematous papules representing positive results after removal of patch tests.

Treatment

Identification and avoidance of the offending agent is the key to successful ACD therapy. It is important to give the patients not only a list of ingredients to which they are reacting but also a list of alternative products that they can safely use. Two databases are available in the United States that can provide a list of products that are free of the suspected allergens: Contact Allergen Management Program, CAMP (http://www.contactderm.org) and Mayo Clinic's *Contact Allergen Replacement Database*, CARD (http://www.SkinSAFEapp.com). Metal testing kits are also available to detect the presence of nickel (Nickel Spot Test) and cobalt (Cobalt Spot Test) in common consumer products and are helpful for an individual with these specific metal allergies.

In circumstances where avoidance is not possible, topical corticosteroids are first-line agents. When the dermatitis involves areas of thin skin, such as the face, ointments and fluorinated corticosteroids should be avoided. Lower-potency topical corticosteroids are best suited in this area and should be used sparingly to avoid skin thinning and atrophy. Systemic corticosteroids are reserved for dermatitis involving >20% of the body. Adjunctive medications in acute ACD include cold compresses and calamine lotion for temporary symptom relief. Hydration of the skin with emollients, moisturizers, and/or barrier creams may also be helpful to reduce exposure to the irritant or allergic contact allergen. Although commonly prescribed, the use of antihistamines is generally not effective to relieve pruritus in ACD. Topical and/or systemic antibiotics (against staphylococcus or ß-hemolytic streptococcus) are warranted if lesions of ACD become secondarily infected.[36]

Successful treatment for ACD that is refractory to topical corticosteroids has been reported with certain immunomodulatory agents (ie, azathioprine, cyclosporine, thalidomide) and UVA/UVB light therapy.[37,38] Although successful in AD, the role of topical T-cell selective inhibitors of inflammatory cytokines (ie, tacrolimus) in ACD has not been established.[36] Contact dermatitis can be a lifelong condition, so early diagnosis and proper management to prevent complications (ie, infection) are crucial. Surveys on the quality of life of patients with persistent contact dermatitis show severe impairment, especially in those with dermatitis involving the face.[39]

DRUG ALLERGY

Gell and Coombs Classification of Drug Eruptions

Drug eruptions have been classified according to Gell and Coombs system of hypersensitivity based on particular cell involvement. Some reactions are immediate in nature (type 1) whereas others are delayed (types 2 through 4). Type 1–mediated reactions are due to development of drug-specific IgE antibodies which upon encountering an allergen cause mast cell and basophil degranulation. Symptoms may include urticaria, angioedema, hypotension, pruritus, emesis, diarrhea, bronchospasm, and anaphylaxis.[40] Type 2 reactions are mediated by drug-specific IgG or IgM antibodies directed at drug hapten-coated cells; these cytoxic drug reactions usually affect the hematopoietic system presenting with hemolytic anemia, thrombocytopenia, neutropenia, or granulocytopenia.[40,41] Type 3–mediated reactions occur from tissue deposition (skin, kidney) of drug-antibody complexes and complement activation.[40] Patients may present with serum sickness, vasculitis, or glomerulonephritis.[41] Type 4 reactions are the most commonly encountered; these delayed reactions can be furthered divided into 4 subtypes—IVa (monocytes), IVb (eosinophils), IVc (CD4 or $CD8^+$ T cells), and IVd (neutrophils)—based on cellular involvement and clinical presentation.[42] Phenotypically, rashes vary from maculopapular eruptions to eczematous, pustular, or bullous lesions. (This is reviewed in more detail in Chapter 2).

Immunologic Mechanisms of Drug Allergy

Immunologic drug hypersensitivity reactions are hypothesized to occur via a few different mechanisms. Small-sized molecules that would not be typically immunogenic may become so by binding with larger proteins (hapten hypothesis); penicillin binding to albumin is a classic example.[41] With the prohapten hypothesis, the agent becomes immunogenic only after metabolism; this reactive intermediate agent then binds with proteins (eg, sulfamethoxazole). The pharmacologic interaction with immune receptors (p-I concept) proposes that drugs directly interact with immune receptors and elicit a response.[41] (Reviewed in more detail in Chapter 8.)

Many drug reactions occur in the head and neck and cause abnormalities in the skin, mucosa, or conjunctiva. Their manifestations can be variable and can include urticaria, eczema, pigmentation, folliculitis, and ulcerations.

> Immunologic drug reactions can be due to either immediate or delayed hypersensitivity.

Drug-Associated Mucosal Diseases

Erythema Multiforme

Erythema multiforme (EM) is an acute mucocutaneous immune-mediated disease; the exact prevalence is not known but is believed to be less than 1%.[43] It is seen most commonly in adults but also occurs in children. Lesions are target shaped and occur on arms and trunk in a symmetrical distribution; ulcerative oral, genital, or ocular lesions can occur concurrently.[44] There has been debate whether EM is part of the spectrum of cutaneous disorders including Stevens-Johnson syndrome (SJS) and toxic epidermal necrolysis (TEN). However, most authorities identify EM as a separate disorder.[44] EM is mostly attributed to infectious etiologies with the vast majority of cases due to herpes simplex virus (HSV). Other infectious agents include *Mycoplasma pneumoniae*, EBV, CMV, adenovirus, *Corynebacterium*, *Salmonella* and *Streptococcus pneumoniae*.[43,45] Other causes of EM include medication-induced (NSAIDs, antiepileptics, antibiotics, allopurinol), malignancy (leukemia, lymphoma), autoimmunity (sarcoidosis, lupus), radiation, and immunization (hepatitis B, smallpox).[43,45]

Prodromal symptoms may be present in patients with mucosal involvement a week or more before the onset of disease.[43] Classically, skin lesions present with a central dusky area which is surrounded by dark red zone followed by a lighter zone with another erythematous zone at the periphery. However, varying types of papular lesions may be seen that display poorly defined borders.[46] Mucosal involvement is estimated to occur in 25% to 50% of patients,[43] although a prevalence of up to 70% has been reported[45]; it usually occurs at the same time as the rash, but also can proceed or follow rash onset.[47]

EM tends to be a self-limited disease. However, recurrent EM (frequent episodes) and persistent EM (continuous disease) have been reported. Resolution of EM usually occurs over 1 to 2 weeks.[43] Typically, disease onset and resolution will occur within a 1-month period., although disease courses in which mucosal involvement is present, may take longer.[43] Cutaneous lesions heal without scarring but a postinflammatory hypopigmentation or hyperpigmentation may be seen transiently[45]; ocular involvement can lead to keratitis, conjunctival scarring, uveitis, or visual impairment.[48]

The diagnosis of EM is made clinically. If EM is suspected, patients should be evaluated for HSV (PCR, viral culture, serology) as it is the most common cause of disease.[47] If respiratory symptoms are present, consider *Mycoplasma pneumoniae*. Also obtain history of new medication use.

Treatment of EM depends on disease severity and progression. If a medication is suspected, promptly discontinue its use. Mild cases can be treated with topical corticosteroids and oral antihistamines for itch.[47] For EM caused by active herpes infection, treat with antiviral therapy, and consider antibiotics for patients with EM due to *Mycoplasma*.[47] In patients with oral involvement, treatment options include topical corticosteroid gels, antiseptic washes, and anesthetics.[47] With severe oral involvement that is limiting oral intake, causing pain, or causing difficultly with speaking, patients may require systemic corticosteroids at a dose of 40 to 60 mg daily tapered over to 2 to 4 weeks.[45] Consultation with ophthalmology is recommended for patients with ocular involvement.

> Erythema multiforme is an acute mucocutaneous disease with typical target-shaped cutaneous lesions primarily caused by infections, in particular herpes simplex virus.

Stevens-Johnson Syndrome (SJS) and Toxic Epidermal Necrolysis (TEN)

Stevens-Johnson syndrome is a severe cutaneous adverse reaction with erythematous skin, epidermal detachment, and involvement of mucous membranes.[49] Patients will display hemorrhagic lesions on mucous membranes including eyes, lips, mouth, vulva, penis, urethra, anus, and/or trachea[49] (Figures 10–6 and 10–7).

SJS is believed to exist along a spectrum with TEN based on skin involvement. In SJS less than 10% body surface area is involved; in SJS/TEN overlap syndrome there is 10% to 30% body surface area involvement, and in TEN there is more than 30% body surface area involvement.[46] These skin diseases cause a great deal of morbidity and can have a mortality rate of up to 30%.[50]

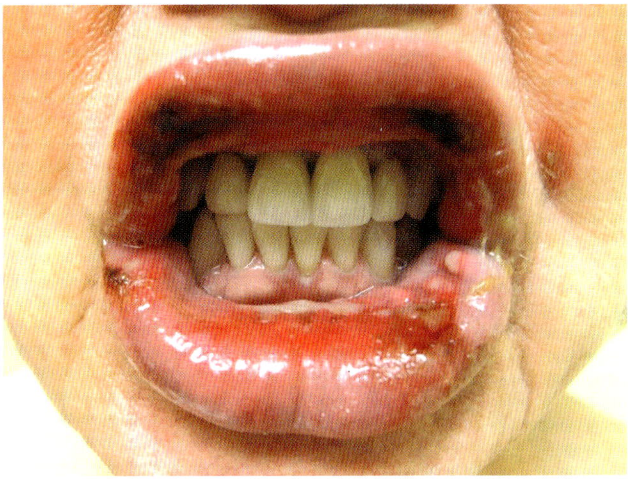

Figure 10-6. Oral mucositis in SJS.

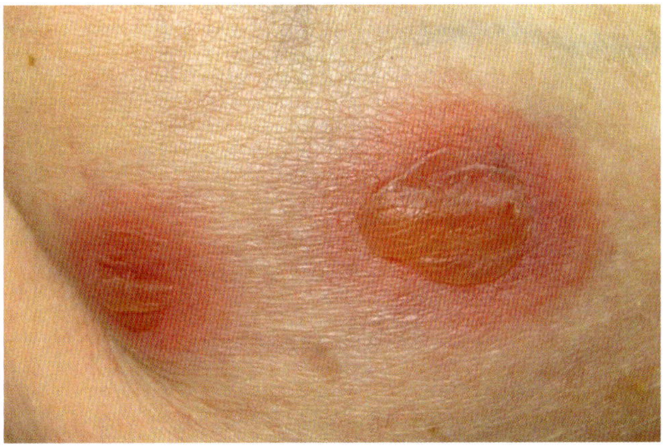

Figure 10-7. Blisters in SJS.

The etiology of TEN is due to epidermal necrosis; however, its exact mechanism is not fully understood; cells including CD8$^+$T cells and natural killer (NK) cells and the tumoricidal and bactericidal molecule granulysin (found in the cytoplasmic granules of CD8+ and NK cells)[51] are found in SJS and may contribute to disease.[49] As opposed to EM, drug hypersensitivity is the most likely cause of disease in SJS and TEN; however, infections with mycoplasma, influenza, and cytomegalovirus (CMV) have also been reported as causes of SJS and TEN.[51] Medications highly implicated in SJS/TEN are oxicam-NSAIDs, allopurinol, anti-epileptics (carbamazepine, lamotrigine, phenytoin, phenobarbital), nevirapine, and antimicrobials (sulfonamide antibiotics).[50] Drugs that have been started within the previous 4 weeks of symptom onset are the most likely agents.[50] Genetic factors also likely play a role; in Han Chinese patients who develop SJS with carbamazepine, a strong association has been found with the HLA-B*1502 haplotype.[52] Another strong association has been seen in Chinese patients who develop SJS/TEN due to allopurinol and who have the HLA-B*5801 haplotype.[53]

Identifying and discontinuing any suspected agents and correct diagnosis are the first steps in therapy. Other therapeutic measures are supportive and may aid in preventing long-term complications. Patients with extensive skin involvement/detachment are best cared for in intensive care units at specialized institutions (burn units).[49] Due to the extensive skin involvement, water is lost rapidly, and skin thermoregulatory mechanisms are compromised. Room temperature should be increased to 30°C to 32°C (86°F–90°F) and fluids need to be replaced.[49] Nutritionally, patients require caloric replacement (1500 calories over the first 24 hours with 500 calorie increments daily).[49] It is essential to monitor for infection and prompt treatment with antimicrobials is needed as sepsis is one of the most frequent causes of death in these patients. Genital erosions should be treated with wet dressing and/or sitz baths in females to prevent scarring and strictures; oral and lip erosions can be treated with antiseptic mouth washes and ointments, respectively.[49] Eye care is of the utmost importance to prevent corneal scarring. Other therapies include immunomodulatory treatments with corticosteroids, replacement immunoglobulin (IVIG), and cyclosporine. Evidence mostly comes from case reports and case series and is conflicting. A recent meta-analysis of 13 studies of IVIG in patients with SJS/TEN[54] demonstrated a strong inverse relationship between IVIG dose (≥2 g/kg) and standardized mortality rate, but another meta-analysis failed to show benefit from either IVIG or corticosteroids.[55] The use of plasmapheresis, hyperbaric oxygen, and cyclophosphamide have also been reported in the literature as treatment options, but evidence is limited.[49] Mortality rates are assessed by SCORTEN (Score of Toxic Epidermal Necrolysis: severity of illness score) based on patient age, ≥10% body surface area detachment, underlying malignancy, tachycardia, serum glucose, serum bicarbonate, and BUN.[56] Long-term possible complications include hyper- or hypopigmented skin lesions, pruritus, reversible hair loss, partial or complete nail loss, impaired taste, vaginal adhesions, esophageal strictures, urethral strictures, sicca syndrome due to lacrimal duct damage, and visual loss.[49]

> Stevens-Johnson syndrome and toxic epidermal necrolysis are severe cutaneous drug eruptions primarily caused by medications and cause high morbidity and mortality. Prompt recognition of disease, discontinuation of causative agents, supportive care measures, and initiation of immunomodulatory agents are necessary for management.

Drug-Induced Oral Lichenoid Lesions

Lichenoid drug lesions have similar appearance to other causes of lichen planus in the mouth. It can present clinically with white striae, papules, plaques with erythema, or erosion of the oral mucosa with symptoms varying from burning sensation to severe pain.[57] Lesions may not appear for months to a few years after the drug has been started. Patients may also have cutaneous lichenoid lesions or present solely with oral lesions.[58] Diagnosis is often difficult as there is no specific testing that will diagnosis lichenoid drug eruptions; improvement of lesions once the drug is discontinued and recurrence if the drug is restarted, are supportive of the diagnosis.[59] Medications that have been implicated include antiretrovirals (zidovudine),[57,60] antihypertensives,[59,61] imatinib,[62-64] olanzapine, anti-epileptics,[65,66] oral hypoglycemic agents,[59] gold salts, [59] NSAIDs,[67] and penicillamine. Corticosteroid suspensions[59,66] are often used as initial therapy, but definitive treatment involves recognition of the entity and prompt withdrawal of drug.

> Lichenoid drug eruptions in the mouth resemble lichen planus and may occur months to years after a medication is started; a high index of suspicion is needed to identify these lesions.

Drug-Induced Anosmia

Loss of smell has been linked to weight loss, decreased appetite, and poor quality of life.[68] Most evidence for loss of smell due to medications comes from clinical case reports.[69] Many medications have been implicated in smell dysfunction including antimicrobials (ciprofloxacin, doxycycline, amikacin, pentamidine, terbinafine), chemotherapeutics, antithyroid agents, antidepressants, lipid-lowering agents, aspirin, zinc, and antihypertensives (enalapril, nifedipine, propranolol)[69–71] (Table 10–3). A prospective study of 87 patients[72] undergoing chemotherapy for breast and gynecologic cancers that evaluated smell before, during, and after chemotherapy found that smell decreased significantly during therapy but returned after completion of therapy; older patients had more dysfunction than younger patients, and taxene-based therapy caused the most severe dysfunction in taste and smell.

> Medications are an underrecognized cause of anosmia. Antimicrobials, antihypertensives/cardiac medications, and chemotherapeutic agents have all been linked to anosmia.

Drug-Induced Black Hairy Tongue

Black hairy tongue is a black, brown, yellow, or greenish discoloration of the tongue due to abnormally hypertrophied filiform papillae from defective desquamation.[73,74] Most patients are asymptomatic; however, taste alterations, pain, burning, halitosis, or nausea have also been noted.[74] Precipitating or aggravating factors include poor oral hygiene, medication-induced dry mouth (including medications that can cause xerostomia such as NSAIDs, antibiotics, antihypertensives, antihistamines), radiation therapy of head and neck, tobacco use, oxygenating oral mouth rinses (sodium perborate, sodium peroxide, and hydrogen peroxide), and caffeine intake (tea, coffee).[73–75] Medications that have been implicated in causing black hairy tongue include antimicrobials (erythromycin, ampicillin, ceftriaxone, doxycycline, sulfamethoxazole), lansoprazole, and antipsychotics (olanzapine)[71,73,74] (Table 10–4). The

Table 10-3. Drug-Induced Anosmia[69–71]

Antimicrobials	Amikacin Ciprofloxacin	Doxycycline Ganciclovir	Levofloxacin Pentamidine	Terbinafine
Antihypertensives	Enalapril	Nifedipine	Propranolol	
Carbonic anhydrase inhibitors	Acetazolamide	Methazolamide	Pyrazinamide	
Other	Aspirin Cocaine	Cromolyn Interferon α	Methoxsalen Minoxidil	Zinc

Table 10-4. Medication-Induced Black Hairy Tongue (Lingua Villosa Nigra)[73,74,76]

Antimicrobials	Amoxicillin Ampicillin Ceftriaxone	Clarithromcyin Doxycycline Methicillin	Minocycline Nafcillin Penicillin	Streptomycin Sulfamethoxazole Tetracycline
Benzodiazepines	Clonazepam			
Tricyclic antidepressants	Amitriptyline Amoxapine	Clomipramine Desipramine	Nortriptyline	
Other	Fluoxetine Lansoprazole	Methyldopa Nicotine	Olanzapine Phenelzine	Tranylcypromine

disease is benign and treatment options including brushing tongue, improved oral hygiene, smoking cessation, and discontinuation of suspected drug allergen are effective.[76]

> Black hairy tongue is usually an asymptomatic discolorization of the tongue from medications, dry mouth, poor dental hygiene, tobacco use, or oral mouth rinses.

REFERENCES

1. Zheng T, Yu J, Oh MH, Zhu Z. The atopic march: progression from atopic dermatitis to allergic rhinitis and asthma. *Allergy Asthma Immunol Res*. 2011;3(2):67–73.
2. Darabi K, Hostetler SG, Bechtel MA, Zirwas M. The role of *Malassezia* in atopic dermatitis affecting the head and neck of adults. *J Am Acad of Dermatol*. 2009;60(1):125–136.
3. Hoeger PH, Lee KH, Jautova J, et al. The treatment of facial atopic dermatitis in children who are intolerant of, or dependent on, topical corticosteroids: a randomized, controlled clinical trial. *Br J Dermatol*. 2009;160(2):415–422.
4. Spergel JM. From atopic dermatitis to asthma: the atopic march. *Ann Allergy Asthma Immunol*. 2010;105(2):99–106; quiz 7–9, 17.
5. Boguniewicz M AM, Fonacier L. Atopic dermatitis and contact dermatitis. In: Adelman DC, Casale TB, Corren J, eds. *Manual of Allergy and Immunology*. 5th ed. Philadelphia, PA: Lippincott Wiliams & Wilkins; 2012:215–227.
6. Eigenmann PA, Sicherer SH, Borkowski TA, Cohen BA, Sampson HA. Prevalence of IgE-mediated food allergy among children with atopic dermatitis. *Pediatrics*. 1998; 101(3):E8.
7. Gunawan H, Takai T, Ikeda S, Okumura K, Ogawa H. Protease activity of allergenic pollen of cedar, cypress, juniper, birch and ragweed. *Allergol Int*. 2008;57(1):83–91.
8. Jeong SK, Kim HJ, Youm JK, et al. Mite and cockroach allergens activate protease-activated receptor 2 and delay epidermal permeability barrier recovery. *J Invest Dermatol*. 2008;128(8):1930–1939.
9. Cardona ID, Cho SH, Leung DY. Role of bacterial superantigens in atopic dermatitis: implications for future therapeutic strategies. *Am J Clin Dermatol*. 2006;7(5):273–279.

10. Nakamura Y, Oscherwitz J, Cease KB, et al. Staphylococcus delta-toxin induces allergic skin disease by activating mast cells. *Nature*. 2013;503(7476):397–401.
11. Sugita T, Suto H, Unno T, et al. Molecular analysis of *Malassezia* microflora on the skin of atopic dermatitis patients and healthy subjects. *J Clin Microbiol*. 2001;39(10): 3486–3490.
12. Hengge UR, Ruzicka T, Schwartz RA, Cork MJ. Adverse effects of topical glucocorticosteroids. *J Am Acad of Dermatol*. 2006;54(1):1–15; quiz 6–8.
13. Bath-Hextall FJ, Birnie AJ, Ravenscroft JC, Williams HC. Interventions to reduce *Staphylococcus aureus* in the management of atopic eczema: an updated Cochrane review. *Br J Dermatol*. 2010;163(1):12–26.
14. Pedersen LK, Johansen JD, Held E, Agner T. Augmentation of skin response by exposure to a combination of allergens and irritants—a review. *Contact Dermatitis*. 2004;50(5):265–273.
15. Gordon LA. Compositae dermatitis. *Australas J Dermatol*. 1999;40(3):123–128; quiz 9–30.
16. Feser A, Plaza T, Vogelgsang L, Mahler V. Periorbital dermatitis—a recalcitrant disease: causes and differential diagnoses. *Br J Dermatol*. 2008;159(4):858–863.
17. Temesvari E, Ponyai G, Nemeth I, Hidvegi B, Sas A, Karpati S. Periocular dermatitis: a report of 401 patients. *J Eur Acad Dermatol Venereol*. 2009;23(2):124–128.
18. Zug KA, Kornik R, Belsito DV, et al. Patch-testing North American lip dermatitis patients: data from the North American Contact Dermatitis Group, 2001 to 2004. *Dermatitis*. 2008;19(4):202–208.
19. Torgerson RR, Davis MD, Bruce AJ, Farmer SA, Rogers RS, 3rd. Contact allergy in oral disease. *J Am Acad of Dermatol*. 2007;57(2):315–321.
20. Warshaw EM, Buchholz HJ, Belsito DV, et al. Allergic patch test reactions associated with cosmetics: retrospective analysis of cross-sectional data from the North American Contact Dermatitis Group, 2001–2004. *J Am Acad of Dermatol*. 2009;60(1):23–38.
21. Thyssen JP, Linneberg A, Menne T, Johansen JD. The epidemiology of contact allergy in the general population—prevalence and main findings. *Contact Dermatitis*. 2007;57(5):287–299.
22. Dotterud LK, Falk ES. Metal allergy in north Norwegian schoolchildren and its relationship with ear piercing and atopy. *Contact Dermatitis*. 1994;31(5):308–313.
23. Meding B. Differences between the sexes with regard to work-related skin disease. *Contact Dermatitis*. 2000;43(2): 65–71.
24. Torres F, das Gracas M, Melo M, Tosti A. Management of contact dermatitis due to nickel allergy: an update. *Clin Cosmet Investig Dermatol*. 2009;2:39–48.
25. Aquino M, Mucci T, Chong M, Lorton MD, Fonacier L. Mobile phones: potential sources of nickel and cobalt exposure for metal allergic patients. *Pediatr Allergy Immunol Pulmonol*. 2013;26(4):181–186.
26. Hallab N, Merritt K, Jacobs JJ. Metal sensitivity in patients with orthopaedic implants. *J Bone Joint Surg Am*. 2001; 83A(3):428–436.
27. Basko-Plluska JL, Thyssen JP, Schalock PC. Cutaneous and systemic hypersensitivity reactions to metallic implants. *Dermatitis*. 2011;22(2):65–79.
28. Dutree-Meulenberg RO, Kozel MM, van Joost T. Burning mouth syndrome: a possible etiologic role for local contact hypersensitivity. *J Am Acad of Dermatol*. 1992;26(6):935–940.
29. Mallo Perez L, Diaz Donado C. Intraoral contact allergy to materials used in dental practice. A critical review. *Med Oral*. 2003;8(5):334–347.
30. Fransway AF, Zug KA, Belsito DV, et al. North American Contact Dermatitis Group patch test results for 2007–2008. *Dermatitis*. 2013;24(1):10–21.
31. Wilkinson SM. Corticosteroid cross-reactions: an alternative view. *Contact Dermatitis*. 2000;42(2):59–63.
32. Jacob SE, Zapolanski T. Systemic contact dermatitis. *Dermatitis*. 2008;19(1):9–15.
33. Ferguson AD, Emerson RM, English JS. Cross-reactivity patterns to budesonide. *Contact Dermatitis*. 2002; 47(6):337–340.
34. Lepoittevin JP, Drieghe J, Dooms-Goossens A. Studies in patients with corticosteroid contact allergy. Understanding cross-reactivity among different steroids. *Arch Dermatol*. 1995;131(1):31–37.
35. Wilkinson JD SS. *Contact Dermatitis Textbook of Dermatology*. 6th ed. Oxford, UK: Blackwell Science Ltd.; 1998.
36. American Academy of Allergy A, Immunology, American College of Allergy A, Immunology. Contact dermatitis: a practice parameter. *Ann Allergy Asthma Immunol*. 2006;97(3, suppl 2):S1–S38.
37. Cohen DE, Heidary N. Treatment of irritant and allergic contact dermatitis. *Dermatol Ther*. 2004;17(4):334–340.
38. Li LY, Cruz PD, Jr. Allergic contact dermatitis: pathophysiology applied to future therapy. *Dermatol Ther*. 2004; 17(3):219–223.
39. Kadyk DL, McCarter K, Achen F, Belsito DV. Quality of life in patients with allergic contact dermatitis. *J Am Acad of Dermatol*. 2003;49(6):1037–1048.
40. Riedl MA, Casillas AM. Adverse drug reactions: types and treatment options. *Am Fam Physician*. 2003;68(9): 1781–1790.
41. Khan DA. Drug allergy. In: Adelman DC, Casale TB, Corren J, eds. *Manual of Allergy and Immunology*. 5th ed. Philadelphia, PA: Lippincott Williams & Wilkins; 2012: 292–324.
42. Pichler WJ. Delayed drug hypersensitivity reactions. *Ann Intern Med*. 2003;139(8):683–693.
43. Huff JC, Weston WL, Tonnesen MG. Erythema multiforme: a critical review of characteristics, diagnostic criteria, and causes. *J Am Acad of Dermatol*. 1983;8(6):763–775.
44. Assier H, Bastuji-Garin S, Revuz J, Roujeau JC. Erythema multiforme with mucous membrane involvement and Stevens-Johnson syndrome are clinically different disorders with distinct causes. *Arch Dermatol*. 1995;131(5): 539–543.
45. Samim F, Auluck A, Zed C, Williams PM. Erythema multiforme: a review of epidemiology, pathogenesis, clinical features, and treatment. *Dent Clin North Am*. 2013;57(4): 583–596.

46. Bastuji-Garin S, Rzany B, Stern RS, Shear NH, Naldi L, Roujeau JC. Clinical classification of cases of toxic epidermal necrolysis, Stevens-Johnson syndrome, and erythema multiforme. *Arch Dermatol*. 1993;129(1):92–96.
47. Sokumbi O, Wetter DA. Clinical features, diagnosis, and treatment of erythema multiforme: a review for the practicing dermatologist. *Int J Dermatol*. 2012;51(8):889–902.
48. Huff JC. Erythema multiforme. *Dermatol Clin*. 1985;3(1): 141–152.
49. Mockenhaupt M. Stevens-Johnson syndrome and toxic epidermal necrolysis: clinical patterns, diagnostic considerations, etiology, and therapeutic management. *Semin Cutan Med Surg*. 2014;33(1):10–16.
50. Mockenhaupt M, Viboud C, Dunant A, et al. Stevens-Johnson syndrome and toxic epidermal necrolysis: assessment of medication risks with emphasis on recently marketed drugs. The EuroSCAR-study. *J Invest Dermatol*. 2008;128(1):35–44.
51. Schwartz RA, McDonough PH, Lee BW. Toxic epidermal necrolysis: Part I. Introduction, history, classification, clinical features, systemic manifestations, etiology, and immunopathogenesis. *J Am Acad of Dermatol*. 2013;69(2):173 e1–13; quiz 85–86.
52. Chung WH, Hung SI, Hong HS, et al. Medical genetics: a marker for Stevens-Johnson syndrome. *Nature*. 2004; 428(6982):486.
53. Hung SI, Chung WH, Liou LB, et al. HLA-B*5801 allele as a genetic marker for severe cutaneous adverse reactions caused by allopurinol. *Proc Natl Acad Sci USA*. 2005; 102(11):4134–4139.
54. Barron SJ, Del Vecchio MT, Aronoff SC. Intravenous immunoglobulin in the treatment of Stevens-Johnson syndrome and toxic epidermal necrolysis: a meta-analysis with meta-regression of observational studies. *Int J Dermatol*. 2015;54(1):108–115.
55. Roujeau JC, Bastuji-Garin S. Systematic review of treatments for Stevens-Johnson syndrome and toxic epidermal necrolysis using the SCORTEN score as a tool for evaluating mortality. *Ther Adv Drug Saf*. 2011;2(3):87–94.
56. Bastuji-Garin S, Fouchard N, Bertocchi M, Roujeau JC, Revuz J, Wolkenstein P. SCORTEN: a severity-of-illness score for toxic epidermal necrolysis. *J Invest Dermatol*. 2000;115(2):149–153.
57. Arirachakaran P, Hanvanich M, Kuysakorn P, Thongprasom K. Antiretroviral drug-associated oral lichenoid reaction in HIV patient: a case report. *Int J Dent*. 2010; 2010:291072.
58. Korstanje MJ. Drug-induced mouth disorders. *Clin Exp Dermatol*. 1995;20(1):10–18.
59. Kaomongkolgit R. Oral lichenoid drug reaction associated with antihypertensive and hypoglycemic drugs. *J Drugs Dermatol*. 2010;9(1):73–75.
60. Ficarra G, Flaitz CM, Gaglioti D, et al. White lichenoid lesions of the buccal mucosa in patients with HIV infection. *Oral Surg Oral Med Oral Pathol*. 1993;76(4):460–466.
61. Fessa C, Lim P, Kossard S, Richards S, Penas PF. Lichen planus-like drug eruptions due to beta-blockers: a case report and literature review. *Am J Clin Dermatol*. 2012; 13(6):417–421.
62. Brazzelli V, Muzio F, Manna G, et al. Photoinduced dermatitis and oral lichenoid reaction in a chronic myeloid leukemia patient treated with imatinib mesylate. *Photodermatol Photoimmunol Photomed*. 2012;28(1):2–5.
63. Gomez Fernandez C, Sendagorta Cudos E, Casado Verrier B, Feito Rodriguez M, Suarez Aguado J, Vidaurrazaga Diaz de Arcaya C. Oral lichenoid eruption associated with imatinib treatment. *Eur J Dermatol*. 2010; 20(1):127–128.
64. Sendagorta E, Herranz P, Feito M, et al. Lichenoid drug eruption related to imatinib: report of a new case and review of the literature. *Clin Exp Dermatol*. 2009;34(7): e315–316.
65. Artico G, Bruno IS, Seo J, Hirota SK, Acay R, Migliari DA. Lichenoid reaction to carbamazepine in the oral mucosa: case report. *An Bras Dermatol*. 2011;86(4, suppl 1):S152–S155.
66. Woo V, Bonks J, Borukhova L, Zegarelli D. Oral lichenoid drug eruption: a report of a pediatric case and review of the literature. *Pediatr Dermatol*. 2009;26(4):458–464.
67. Bagan JV, Thongprasom K, Scully C. Adverse oral reactions associated with the COX-2 inhibitor rofecoxib. *Oral Dis*. 2004;10(6):401–403.
68. Hummel T, Nordin S. Olfactory disorders and their consequences for quality of life. *Acta Otolaryngol*. 2005; 125(2):116–121.
69. Doty RL, Bromley SM. Effects of drugs on olfaction and taste. *Otolaryngol Clin North Am*. 2004;37(6):1229–1254.
70. Malaty J, Malaty IA. Smell and taste disorders in primary care. *Am Fam Physician*. 2013;88(12):852–859.
71. Litt JZ. *Litt's Drug Eruptions & Reactions Manual*. 19th ed. Boca Raton, FL. CRC Press, 2013.
72. Steinbach S, Hummel T, Bohner C, et al. Qualitative and quantitative assessment of taste and smell changes in patients undergoing chemotherapy for breast cancer or gynecologic malignancies. *J Clinical Oncol*. 2009; 27(11):1899–1905.
73. Thompson DF, Kessler TL. Drug-induced black hairy tongue. *Pharmacotherapy*. 2010;30(6):585–593.
74. Vano-Galvan S, Jaen P. Black hairy tongue. *Cleve Clin J Med*. 2008;75(12):847–848.
75. Lawoyin D, Brown RS. Drug-induced black hairy tongue: diagnosis and management challenges. *Dent Today*. 2008; 27(1):60, 2–3; quiz 93, 58.
76. Sarti GM, Haddy RI, Schaffer D, Kihm J. Black hairy tongue. *Am Fam Physician*. 1990;41(6):1751–1755.

11

Food Allergy and Food-Related Disorders

Antonella Cianferoni, Laura M. Gober, and Jonathan M. Spergel

OVERVIEW OF FOOD ALLERGY

Adverse food reactions are any type of abnormal clinical response associated with food ingestion ranging from food intolerance to food-related anaphylaxis.[1,2] Food intolerances are by far the most common type of adverse reactions to food, are often not reproducible, and are dose dependent. They are defined as an adverse physiologic response to a food, and may be due to the intrinsic characteristics of the food (ie, toxic contaminant, pharmacologic active component) or of the patient (ie, metabolic disorders, idiosyncratic responses, or psychological disorder). Food allergy is a reproducible and abnormal immunologic response to a food.[1–5] Based on the immunological mechanism involved, food allergies may be further subdivided into categories of (1) immunoglobulin E (IgE) mediated; (2) cell mediated, when cellular components of the immune system are responsible for the food allergy. These primarily involve the gastrointestinal (GI) tract; or (3) mixed IgE/cell mediated, when both IgE and immune cells are involved in the reaction[1–5] (Figure 11–1).

Patient's perceived IgE-mediated food allergy prevalence is approximately 25%; however, the actual prevalence confirmed by food challenges is only between 2% and 8%. IgE-mediated food allergy is most common in children under 3 years of age (6% to 8%) and decreases with age, affecting 2% to 4% of adults.[6–8] Recent studies report a significant increase in the prevalence of food allergy and food-induced anaphylaxis,[9–11] with a doubling in peanut allergy prevalence in children in the United States and England in the last decade.[12,13] Given the short time in which this increase occurred, environmental factors (ie, introduction of food later in the infant diet, methods of food preparation, and increased use of antacids) are more likely to be involved than genetic factors.[14–16] The latest estimates are that the incidence of fatal food allergies is 1 in 800000 per year in children and 1 in 4 million for adults, with a total of about 200 fatalities per year. In addition, serious reactions due to foods are reported to be between 0.5 and 16 cases per 100000 person-years.[17–20]

FOOD-INDUCED ANAPHYLAXIS

Food-induced anaphylaxis (FIA) is a serious systemic allergic reaction that may cause death rapidly in an otherwise healthy individual (Table 11–1).[21] In children, FIA presents in up to 40% of cases with GI symptoms, such as nausea, abdominal pain, vomiting, and less commonly, diarrhea.[22] Such symptoms may be the only ones that occur after food ingestion, or other organs may be involved, making them part of an anaphylactic reaction.[23,24] Mouth itch, throat pain, and throat tightness are also frequent symptoms and may either be an early sign of anaphylaxis (see Table 11–1) or could be mild and self-limited. The latter group of symptoms may also be due to oral allergy syndrome, a reaction caused by cross-reactivity between certain foods (typically raw fruit and vegetable) and pollens.[23,24]

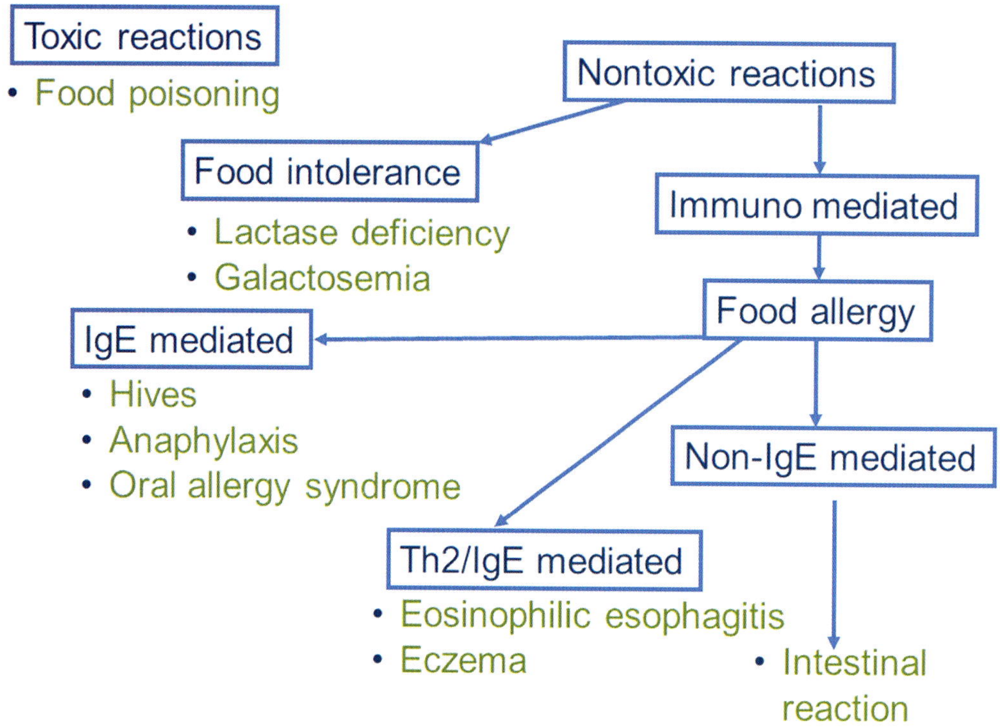

Figure 11-1. Classification of adverse reactions to foods. Adapted from Cianferoni A, Spergel JM. Food allergy: review, classification and diagnosis. *Allergol Int.* 2009;58(4):457–466.

Table 11-1. Symptoms of Anaphylaxis

Clinical Criteria for the Diagnosis of Anaphylaxis	
Anaphylaxis is possible when any one of the following three criteria are fulfilled:	1. Acute onset of an illness with involvement of skin, mucosal tissue, or both and at least one of the following: a. Respiratory compromise b. Reduced blood pressure 2. Two or more of the following that occur rapidly after exposure to a likely allergen for that patient (minutes to 2 hours): a. Involvement of the skin or mucosal tissue (eg, generalized hives; itch or flushing; swollen lips, tongue-uvula; rhinorrhea; conjunctivitis) b. Respiratory compromise (eg, dyspnea, bronchospasm, stridor, hypoxia) c. Cardiovascular compromise (eg, dizziness, hypotension, collapse) d. Persistent gastrointestinal symptoms (eg, crampy abdominal pain, vomiting) 3. Hypotension after exposure to known allergen for that patient (minutes to 2 hours): Hypotension for children is defined as systolic blood pressure <70 mm Hg from 1 month to 1 year (<70 mm Hg + (2 · age)) from 1 to 10 years, and <90 mm Hg from 11 to 17 years.

Source: Adapted from Sampson HA, Munoz-Furlong A, Campbell RL, et al. Second symposium on the definition and management of anaphylaxis: summary report—second National Institute of Allergy and Infectious Disease/Food Allergy and Anaphylaxis Network symposium. *Ann Emerg Med.* 2006;47(4):373–380.

Virtually every type of food can be a cause of FIA (Table 11–2).[25–33] Most commonly implicated foods throughout the world include peanuts, tree nuts, milk, egg, sesame seeds, fish, and shellfish.[17,20,34–37] Peanuts and tree nuts are disproportionately represented in severe and fatal outcomes, and in emergency department visits for food anaphylaxis particularly in the United States, Germany, Australia, and the United Kingdom.[37–45] Milk is the third most common food responsible for fatal or near-fatal food-induced anaphylactic reactions (8% to 15% cases)[46–48] and globally is one of the most common causes of anaphylaxis in young children.[22,42,49,50]

Most infants with IgE-mediated cow's milk or hen egg allergies develop clinical tolerance by the third year of life, but about 10% to 25% of infants with IgE-mediated cow's milk allergy retain their sensitivity, and about 50% develop sensitivity to other foods.[19,46,51] Shellfish, peanut, sesame seed, and tree nut allergies are more persistent, with chance of becoming tolerant only about 20% for peanut and sesame seeds, and only about 10% for tree nuts.[52–55]

Pathogenesis

FIA is a typical IgE-mediated allergic reaction (ie, it is immediate, reproducible, and readily diagnosed by detection of food-specific IgE). When a specific antigen binds the IgE linked to the FcεRI, it causes

Table 11-2. Foods Causing Anaphylaxis

Confirmed Foods Causing Food-Induced Anaphylaxis			
Almond	Chicory	Lupine	Pistachio
Apple	Cinnamon	Mandarin	Poppy seed
Artichoke	Clove	Mango	Potato
Avocado	Coconut	Manioc	Pumpkin seed
Banana	Codfish	Mushroom	Quinoa
Barley	Coriander	Medlar	Rice
Beer	Corn	Melon	Royal jelly
Bell pepper	Cotton seed	Milk	Sage
Blueberry	Crab	Millet	Salmon
Brazil nut	Cucumber	Mustard	Sesame seeds
Buckwheat	Dill	Nutmeg	Shrimp
Cabbage	Egg	Oat	Soy
Camomile	Fig	Olive	Squid
Carrot	Garlic	Orange	Strawberry
Cashew	Ginger	Oyster	Tangerine seeds
Cassava	Hazelnut	Peach	Tilapia
Catfish	Honey	Peanut	Tomato
Cauliflower	Lentil	Peas	Tuna
Celery	Lettuce	Pecan	Walnut
Cherry	Linen seed	Pepper	Wheat
Chestnut	Lobster	Pine nut	Wine

Note. Foods were confirmed on PubMed to cause food-induced anaphylaxis.

receptor cross-linking and consequent release of preformed mediators (histamine, tryptase, carboxypeptidase A, proteoglycans, and some cytokines) and newly synthesized ones (leukotrienes, bradykinins, and cytokines including tumor necrosis factor [TNF]-α, and platelet-activating factor [PAF]).[3] These mediators cause the characteristic clinical features of anaphylaxis, including vasodilatation, angioedema, bronchoconstriction, and increased mucus production[56,57] (Figure 11–2).

Serum tryptase levels (a specific marker of mast cell activation) are usually increased (typically >10 ng/mL) in the first 6 hours after an anaphylactic reaction. However, up to 50% of patients with documented FIA do not exhibit increased serum tryptase levels, suggesting histamine release coming from tryptase negative cells, such as basophils.[58]

The intrinsic molecular properties of food allergens help determine whether the allergen preferentially induces allergic immune responses and their severity.[58,59] Characteristics common to "major" food allergens include being water-soluble glycoproteins, being 10 to 70 kD in size, and being relatively stable to heat, acid, and proteases.[60] (See Chapter 2 for a more detailed discussion about allergen structure and components.)

Treatment

For the treatment of food allergy–induced anaphylaxis, intramuscular injection of epinephrine is the primary, lifesaving treatment. All other treatments, including antihistamines, glucocorticoids,

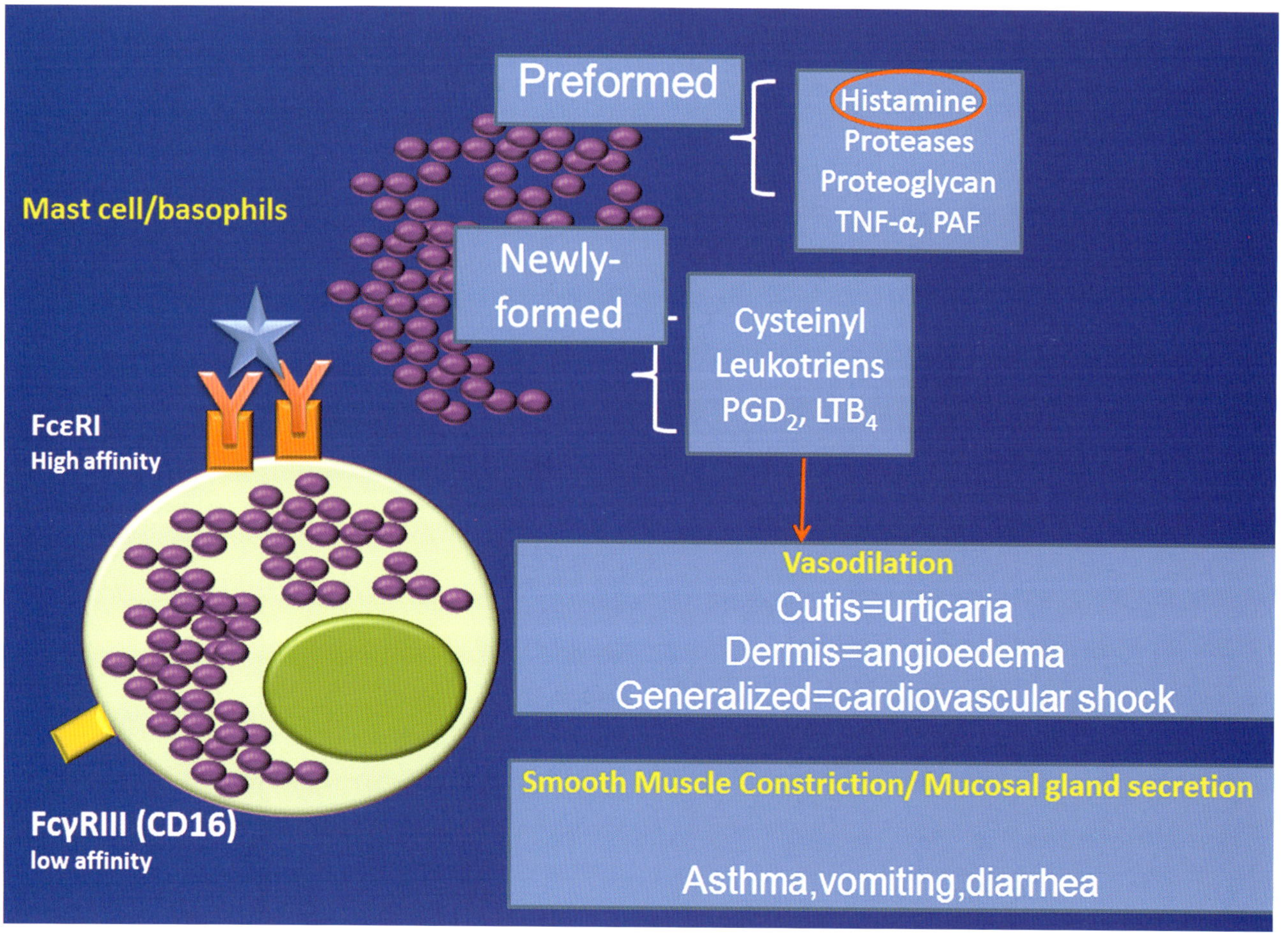

Figure 11–2. Pathogenesis of anaphylaxis. Mediators of anaphlylaxis. Allergen binds to cross-linked IgE on mast cells or basophils at the FcεRI receptor, releasing both preformed and newly formed mediators, leading to vasodilation, anaphylaxis, wheezing, and vomiting.

and β-agonists, either alone or in combination, are considered to be ancillary anaphylaxis treatments. Injected epinephrine is an agonist for the adrenergic receptors (α-1, β-1, β-2) and rapidly reverses anaphylaxis by causing bronchodilation and vasoconstriction.[4,35,46,48,57,61] The severity of a previous allergic reaction is not predictive of the severity of future allergic reactions. For that reason, the National Institutes of Health (NIH) guidelines for food allergy management encourage prescribing an epinephrine autoinjector for all patients with documented IgE-mediated food allergy.[38,48,62]

Oral Immunotherapy

One promising technique for treatment of food allergy is oral immunotherapy (OIT). Tolerance is defined as being able to eat a specific food for 1 month without a reaction, while desensitization is defined as being able to increase the amount of food ingested without experiencing multiple systemic reactions (reviewed in Vickery and Burks[63]). Overall, the reported experience is that 50% to 90% of patients have been desensitized using this technique. However, the rate of true tolerance is much lower closer to 25%.

The proposed mechanism is thought to be an induction of regulatory T cells with low-dose antigen exposure, or lymphocyte anergy or deletion with high antigen doses. Interestingly, there are a series of humoral immunologic changes induced by OIT including a rise in food-specific immunoglobulin G4 (IgG4) antibodies. In addition, a transient initial increase in serum levels of food-specific immunoglobulin E (IgE) antibodies is seen in the first 12 months of OIT, followed by a subsequent decrease.[64]

OIT protocols have been reported for cow's milk (CM), egg white, fish, apple, orange, celery, and peanut.[62,64–66] Patients are generally started on a very small daily dose and advanced very slowly over months to a maintenance dose. For milk OIT, the success rates have ranged from 60% to 90% depending on the study design. The development of true food tolerance was 10-fold higher in the treated group compared to the controls.[67]

For the treatment of egg allergy, 55% of patients passed a food challenge compared to 0% in the control group. However, only 27% maintained the desensitization when egg was discontinued for 2 months.[68] Similar success has been seen with peanut allergy with desensitization results in the 80% to 90% range. For example, in the patients who completed one clinical study, 90% were able to tolerate 3900 mg of peanut.[69] However, only 50% maintained tolerance after stopping peanut for 1 month after 4 years of peanut therapy.[70] Since many patients have multiple-food allergies, Nadeau and colleagues have tried multiple food OIT. OIT was done with 2 foods in 6 participants, 3 foods in 8, 4 foods in 5, and 5 foods in 6.[71]

There are significant limitations to this therapy. All OIT protocols are associated with significant side effects. Side effects occur 34 times more frequently in the treated patents compared to control subjects, and almost 10% of the treated patients experienced a systemic reaction requiring epinephrine. [67] Almost all patients experience some allergic symptoms during desensitization, and only 60% to 90% are able to achieve the final maximum dose. In addition, only 25% maintain tolerance after 2 years of therapy, which might increase to 50% after 4 years of therapy (seen in one study). It is not recommended for regular clinical care at the current time.

Primary Prevention of Food Allergy

The recently published LEAP study examined whether the introduction of allergy-prone infants (with severe eczema and/or egg allergy) to peanuts at an early age would reduce the subsequent development of peanut allergy.[72] Infants 4 to 11 months old were randomized to regular peanut product ingestion or complete peanut avoidance for the first 5 years of life. The study intervention demonstrated (intention to treat analysis) that there was a reduction in the rate of peanut allergy from 17.2% in the peanut avoidance group to 3.2% in the peanut consumption group, representing a greater than 80% reduction in the rate of peanut allergy. The study confirms previous observational studies and the recommendation for early food introduction.[73] There is no one perfect way to prevent food allergies. However, consistent with all current recommendations, the introduction of solid foods after age 4 to 6 months is recommended.

ORAL ALLERGY SYNDROME

Oral allergy syndrome (OAS) is a relatively common form of food allergy and occurs in patients with allergic rhinitis. The symptoms are itching and/

or mild swelling of the mouth and throat immediately following ingestion of certain uncooked fruits (including nuts) or raw vegetables. The symptoms result from allergic cross-reactivity with the pollen-related proteins in these foods. Most patients do not have systemic allergic reactions.

Oral allergy syndrome is also known as pollen-food allergy syndrome (PFAS). There is a slight difference between the 2. In OAS, the symptoms are localized to the oropharynx and in PFAS, patients have localized and systemic symptoms.[1,2] It is one of the most types of common food allergy seen in 5% to 15% of the general population depending on the country studied.[74,75] It is more common in patients with allergic rhinitis, in particular birch pollen, where it can occur up to 24% of the patients.[76] Sensitization to other pollens is also a risk factor. One study found that 20% of the grass allergic patients has OAS symptoms.[77]

Most patients have symptoms localized to the oropharynx. But, 2% to 10% will have systemic symptoms with pollen-related foods. The most common oral symptoms are pruritus, tingling, mild erythema, and minor swelling of the lips, oral mucosa, palate, and throat, sometimes accompanied by a sensation of throat swelling. Symptoms occur while or shortly after (within 5 to 10 minutes of) ingesting the fruit, nut, or vegetable. The foods tend to cross-react with individual pollens (Table 11–3). Interestingly, the symptoms classically only occur with fresh fruits or vegetables. When the food is cooked, the cross-reactive protein is denatured, eliminating the reaction.[2]

Table 11-3. Foods Inducing Oral Allergy Syndrome

Pollen	Food
Birch	Apple, peach, apricot, cherry, plum, pear, almond, hazelnut, carrot, celery, parsley, fennel, coriander, soybean, and peanut
Sycamore	Hazelnut, peach, apple, kiwi, peanut, corn, chickpea, lettuce, and green beans
Ragweed	Cantaloupe, honeydew, watermelon, zucchini, cucumber, and bananas
Mugwort	Carrot, celery, parsley, caraway, coriander, bell pepper, black pepper, garlic, mustard, and onion
Grass	Watermelon, cantaloupe, honeydew, white potato, tomato, orange, peanut, and kiwi

EOSINOPHILIC ESOPHAGITIS

Eosinophilic esophagitis (EoE) is a food allergy with symptoms related to esophageal dysfunction. The symptoms typically last hours to days suggesting a non-IgE-mediated mechanism of disease. As typically IgE-mediated symptoms occur 2 to 4 hours after ingestion, the delays of symptoms indicate a non-IgE mechanism. The symptoms of EoE vary in different age groups. Infants and toddlers present with failure to thrive, persistent gastroesophageal symptoms not responsive to PPI treatment, and feeding difficulties, such as gagging, difficulties in advancing solid food introduction, and food refusal. Young children more often exhibit gastroesophageal reflux disease (GERD) symptoms, abdominal pain, and frequent vomiting. As children age and eventually become teenagers and adults, they tend to develop signs of esophageal fibrosis such as dysphagia and food impaction[78,79] (Figure 11–3).

EoE Diagnosis

A careful history should be obtained to elicit the presence of the above-described symptoms, especially dysphagia and related coping mechanisms (ie, drinking a lot of fluids during meals, chewing food for a long time, or cutting food in small pieces).[80–84] Because of the high rate of atopic comorbidities in EoE patients (ie, allergic rhinitis, asthma, IgE-mediated food allergy, and/or eczema), a complete allergy evaluation for food and environmental allergies is recommended.[85] Once EoE is suspected, its presence needs to be confirmed by esophageal gastroduodenal endoscopy and biopsy (EGD). The diagnosis of EoE requires a minimum of 15 eosinophils/high-power field (eos/hpf) on at least one esophageal biopsy specimen, with eosinophilia limited to the esophagus, after ruling out GERD.[86] Multiple biopsies (4 or more) of both the proximal and dis-

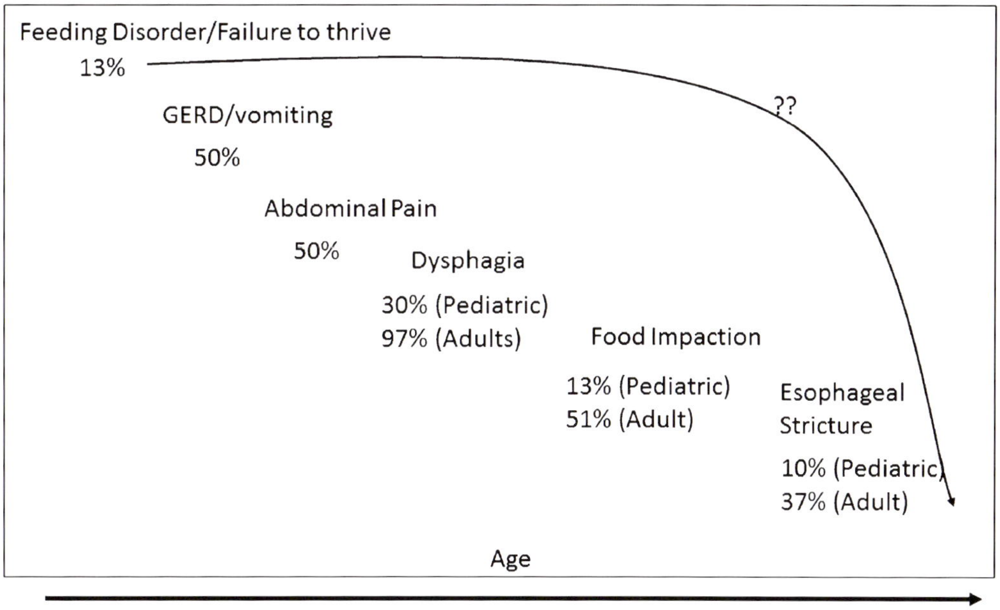

Figure 11–3. Natural history of eosinophilic esophagitis. A proposed natural history of eosinophilic esophagitis based on progression of symptoms and esophageal dysfunction. The percentage of patients presenting with each symptom is represented. Adapted from Spergel JM, Brown-Whitehorn TF, Beausoleil JM, Shuker M, Verma R, Liacouras, CA. 14 years of eosinophilic esophagitis: clinical features and prognosis. *J Pediatr Gastroenterol Nutr.* 2009 Jan;48(1):30–36.

tal esophagus should be collected during diagnostic and follow-up endoscopic procedures, as the disease is often patchy[86,87] (Table 11–4).

EoE Histology and Etiology

EGD macroscopically can show mucosal fragility, furrowing, white mucosal plaques, esophageal trachealization, esophageal narrowing, stricture, and mucosal tearing, or can be totally normal. Therefore, biopsies should be collected not only from macroscopically abnormal esophagus, but also from normal appearing areas. Microscopically, in addition to esophageal eosinophilia, the biopsies can show superficial layering, eosinophilic microabscesses, extracellular eosinophil granules, basal cell hyperplasia, dilated intercellular spaces, and lamina propria fibrosis.[86,87]

Esophageal fibrosis and esophageal strictures are known complications of EoE. Endoscopic stricture dilation is a common procedure performed in adults with EoE to provide short-term symptomatic relief.[88] Fortunately, this complication is extremely rare in pediatric patients, and mechanical dilations are rarely if ever performed in children.[80,89] Based on symptom progression from those of esophageal dysfunction observed in young children to fibrotic changes typical of older children and adults, it appears that EoE is a progressive disease.[80] In over 562 patients followed for 1 to 14 years (average 3.2 years), only 11 patients who were only allergic to either milk, egg, or grains and were treated with an elimination diet, had a true remission, and were able to reintroduce those foods without experiencing an exacerbation. Given the chronic nature of the disease, it is believed that therapy should be initiated in every diagnosed patient and for most, lifelong therapy will be required.[80]

In most patients, foods have been identified as the trigger of EoE.[80,89–91] In a cohort of 315 pediatric patients, the most common food allergen, proven to be causing EoE by biopsies taken after diet and after reintroduction of the foods, are milk, followed by

Table 11–4. Diagnostic Criteria for Eosinophilic Esophagitis

Esophagogastroduodenoscopy with biopsy after 8 to 12 weeks PPI monotherapy (20 to 40 mg twice a day in adults and 1 mg/kg twice a day in children) for 8 to 12 weeks) or if PH meter negative	
Typical endoscopy findings:	• Typically thickening, furrowing, white plaques, concentric rings, and stricture • 20% to 30% of patients may have an endoscopically normal esophagus
Biopsy:	• Multiple biopsy specimens, at least 4 to 5 from distinct esophageal levels (proximal, middle, and distal) • Pathology—Eosinophils 15 per high-power field at 400× light microscopy only in esophagus • Typically accompanied by basal zone hyperplasia

Source: Adapted from Liacouras CA, Furuta GT, Hirano I, et al. Eosinophilic esophagitis: updated consensus recommendations for children and adults. *J Allergy Clin Immunol.* 2011;128(1):3–20, e26; quiz 21–22.

wheat, egg, beef, soy, and chicken.[92] In adults, milk, egg, and wheat are the most common EoE allergens.[93] These same foods have been found to be related to EoE in multiple studies in different countries.[94]

Identification of the trigger food in EoE is challenging for a number of reasons:

1. Standard allergy tests (skin tests or serum IgE) have a very low positive predictive value (PPV) for determining the foods that are causing the esophageal inflammation.[80,95]
2. The introduction of skin test–negative foods (ie, milk or wheat) into the diet can induce clinical disease.[89,92]
3. Unlike IgE-mediated reactions, the development of EoE symptoms after a food introduction does not occur within 2 hours but can be delayed for days or months.[89–93]
4. There are reports of children who outgrew IgE-mediated food allergy, or had successfully undergone an oral desensitization treatment for food allergy, who later developed EoE from the same food, suggesting that the pathogenesis of EoE is different than the IgE-mediated pathogenesis of food allergy.[96]

EoE Pathogenesis

It is felt that the eosinophilic inflammation in EoE is due to esophageal epithelial cell-derived thymic stromal lymphopoietin (TSLP) that induces typical Th2 inflammation[97,98] and is strongly influenced by a genetic predisposition.[97–100] Esophageal biopsies and blood samples of patients with active EoE show increased expression of Th2 cytokines and chemokines (interleukin [IL]-5, IL-4, IL-13, IL-15, TSLP, and eotaxin 3). In addition, cells involved in allergic inflammation: T cells, mast cells, basophils, invariant natural killer T cells (iNKTs), and esophageal epithelial cells are present[100–102] (Table 11–5). Although eosinophils are pathognomonic of EoE inflammation in the absence of GERD, they are not essential for the pathogenesis of EoE and are most likely a consequence of the local Th2 inflammation. Evidence for this comes from clinical trials with anti-IL-5 that show that patients can remain symptomatic even when the treatment depletes eosinophils from the esophagus.[103,104] This only partial reduction of esophageal inflammation and symptom reduction in these anti-IL5 trials suggests that, as in all atopic diseases, Th2 cytokines have redundant functions, so that eliminating a single cytokine is not sufficient to control EoE.[105,106]

Additional evidence for a role for TSLP in EoE is the fact that it induces the development of a unique basophil subpopulation, which secretes pro-Th2 cytokines (IL-4, IL-6, CCL3, CCL4, and CCL12) independently from IgE stimulation.[107,108] Genetic confirmation for the role of TSLP comes from the demonstration that SNPs on the TSLP gene, which are associated with its dysregulated expression, have

Table 11-5. Cytokine and Chemokine Expression in Human Eosinophilic Esophagitis (EoE)

Publication	Cytokine/Chemokine Finding
Cytokines	Increased TSLP
	Increased TGF-b
	Increased expression of IL-5
	TNF-α was increased in epithelial cells
	Eosinophils express "activation" markers: 60% express IL-13 and IL-4
	41% of intestinal eosinophils express IL-13 at baseline, circulating eosinophils do not express IL-4 or IL-13
Leukotrienes	No increase in cysLT
Chemokines	50-fold increase in eotaxin-3 in biopsy
	Increased RANTES
Adhesion expression	Phospho-Smad2/3, VCAM

Source: Adapted from Merves J, Muir A, Modayur Chandramouleeswaran P, et al. Eosinophilic esophagitis. *Ann Allergy Asthma Immunol.* 2014;112(5):397–403.

been linked to EoE as well as other atopic diseases such as eczema, asthma, and allergic rhinitis.[109]

Another epithelial factor, eotaxin-3/CCL-26 is a potent eosinophil and mast cell chemoattractant that plays a major role in EoE pathogenesis. Interestingly its gene is overexpressed in EoE subjects, both in esophageal biopsies and peripheral blood, and a gain-of-function polymorphism in the eotaxin-3 gene is associated with an increased risk of EoE in children.[99] It has also been demonstrated that esophageal epithelial cells can secrete the chemokine RANTES (CCL5)[110] which may play a role in the migration and activation of IL-13 producing iNKT cells in EoE. An additional inflammatory pathway in EoE may involve human esophageal epithelial cells that express toll-like receptors[111,112] and produce pro-inflammatory cytokines and chemokines in response to both pathogen-associated molecular patterns (PAMPs) and danger-associated molecular patterns (DAMPs).[111]

Another genetic marker for EoE is an SNP (rs77569859 G/A) located in proximity to the calpain 14 (*CAPN14*) gene on chromosome 2p23 that has been associated with an increased risk for developing this disease. *CAPN14* is specifically expressed in the esophagus and is upregulated in patients with active disease and after exposure of epithelial cells to IL-13.[113,114] The exact role of *CAPN14* in esophageal epithelial cells and EoE remains unknown.

EoE Treatment

Dietary Management

For the treatment of EoE, there are 2 basic approaches: diet and medication. Diet removes the cause of EoE, but sometimes the quality of life is poor as multiple foods need to be removed. Three different approaches exists for diet: targeted elimination diets, six food elimination diet (SFED), or elemental formulas[80,89,90,93] (Table 11–6).

An elemental diet is the most effective diet treatment for EoE with histological and clinical resolution in greater than 95% of pediatric and adult patients after 6 weeks of this therapy.[80,89,115] However, elemental diets are very difficult to establish, often require nasogastric or gastric tube feeding to achieve caloric goals, have poor palatability, and are difficult to sustain long term.[86,115] Hence, elimination diets based on removal of the 6 most common food allergens[88] (SFED) or of the foods positive to skin

Table 11-6. Diet Options in Eosinophilic Esophagitis

History not accurate	Reactions may be delayed several days Reactions may persist several days More than one food can cause reaction
Elemental formula	Remove all foods and use only elemental formula; success rate greater than 90%
Empiric diet	Remove the most common foods (milk, egg, soy, nut, peanut, fish); success rate 50% to 70%
Allergen testing directed diet	Prick skin test, atopy patch test (PPV (75% to 87%; 92% for milk), NPV 87% to 100%, milk low 40%) Most commonly identified foods: milk, egg, soy, peanuts, beef, chicken, wheat, corn, peas, and potato Success rates: 50% to 70%

Source: Adapted from Greenhawt M, Aceves SS, Spergel JM, Rothenberg ME. The management of eosinophilic esophagitis. *J Allergy Clin Immunol Pract.* 2013;1(4):332–340; quiz 341–332.

prick tests (SPTs) and atopy patch tests (APTs) (targeted elimination diets) have been tried with a similar rates of improvement.[116,117] SFED showed similar effectiveness both in children and adults with symptom scores decreased in 74% to 94% of patients.[90,93]

Approximately two-thirds of children with EoE have positive skin tests to at least one food allergen, but their positive predictive value (PPV) is poor especially for key foods such as milk and wheat.[80,118] To increase the PPV of skin testing in predicting the foods that trigger EoE, food allergy patch tests (APTs) have been used.[80,118] In a study of 361 children with biopsy specimen-diagnosed EoE and a relevant food allergy trigger, and who had eliminated foods based on SPT and APT, it was found that 77%, had biopsy-proven improvement. In general, targeted elimination diets are based on skin testing plus milk elimination (since milk skin tests are usually negative, this food is involved in EoE pathogenesis in up to 70% of cases).[93] The major advantage of a targeted elimination diet based on SPT/APT requires that fewer foods be removed compared to a SFED. However, both methods are acceptable options.[92]

Medication

Some patients prefer medications to diet therapy. Swallowed inhaled corticosteroids such as swallowed fluticasone or budesonide have low bioavailability, less potential for systemic side effects and are considered "topical." They are very effective (although not as effective as oral corticosteroids) and induce EoE remission in up to 80% of patients. Aerosolized fluticasone propionate is administered from a metered dose inhaler (110 mcg × 2 puffs twice daily for children more than 8 years of age, and 220 mcg × 2 puffs twice daily for children year more than 8 years of age) without a spacer.[119–122] Budesonide is delivered as slurry, which is made by mixing each 1 mg Pulmicort Respule (liquid budesonide intended for nebulized administration),[123,124] with 10 g (10 packets) of sucralose (Splenda) or a teaspoon of applesauce or honey to create a volume of approximately 8 mL.[123,124] The dose of swallowed budesonide in children under the age of 10 years is typically 1 mg/day and 2 mg/day in those who are older than 10 years of age. After administration of topical steroids, no food or drink is allowed for 30 minutes. Aerosolized corticosteroids may be difficult for young children to ingest, as they are often bitter to taste and require twice daily administration.

Although both of these topical steroids are used in clinical practice, one study that compared the effectiveness of nebulized vs viscous topical corticosteroid in EoE showed that viscous budesonide results in a significantly higher esophageal exposure to the steroid and to a consequent greater reduction in esophageal eosinophil infiltration.[125] Moreover, topical budesonide but not fluticasone is able to reverse esophageal fibrosis.[126,127] While topical steroids are effective for treatment, clinical and histological features of EoE return upon discontinuation.[128] Topical steroids have been shown to be safe in limited studies that have analyzed their effect in the short term. The only major side effect has been oral and/or esophageal candidiasis in up to 10% of patients. It has been also shown that fluticasone 220 mcg twice a day may induce a mild inhibition of morning serum cortical level.[86,123] However, there are no studies on the side effects of long-term use of topical steroids because no study longer than 1 year has been conducted on bone health and children's growth. From experience with topical steroid use in asthma, it is known that moderate or high doses of topical steroids, similar to those used to treat EoE, are associated with significant growth reduction in children.[129,130] Moreover, there are many unanswered question related to chronic topical steroid use. In particular, there is no consensus about dosage, formulation, frequency, or how to obtain a remission using only minimal doses of steroids. In addition, further research needs to be performed with regard to steroid resistance, the effect of corticosteroids on esophageal fibrosis, the need to treat to histological normalcy, quality-of-life issues, growth, and the consequences of prolonged use (eg, adrenal suppression).[86]

Esophageal Dilation

Esophageal fibrosis and esophageal strictures are known complications of EoE. Endoscopic stricture dilation is a common procedure performed in adults with EoE to provide short-term symptomatic relief. However it should be used only in an emergency situation or only if patients have failed dietary and medical therapy. It is important to remember that esophageal mucosal fragility is a known feature of EoE,[86] and stricture dilation in EoE is associated with increased risk of complications including pain, bleeding, and esophageal perforation.[86,131]

EOSINOPHILIC GASTROENTERITIS

Eosinophilic gastroenteritis (EG) is a chronic illness thought to affect approximately 0.02% to 0.03% of the population.[132] Most commonly it affects adults, but EG has also been described in children. There are shared similarities between EG and eosinophilic esophagitis (EoE) which include tissue eosinophilic inflammation, peripheral eosinophilia, coexisting allergic diseases (eg, allergic rhinitis and/or asthma), and sensitization to multiple food allergens. Also, EG, like EoE, is more prevalent in males. Despite many similarities to other eosinophilic gastrointestinal disorders (EGID) like EoE, EG varies greatly in clinical presentation. This clinical variation occurs due to different segments of the gastrointestinal tract being affected as well as the degree of eosinophilic inflammation in the tissues.

Clinical Presentation and Histopathology

The clinical manifestations of EG depend largely on the area of the gastrointestinal tract affected by eosinophilic inflammation. Patients with gastric involvement will present with nausea, vomiting, and early satiety. Duodenal involvement characteristically presents with malabsorption and protein-losing enteropathy. Both gastric or duodenal involvement can present with abdominal pain and bloating. It is not uncommon for patients to have simultaneous duodenal and gastric involvement. Since the jejunem and ileum are not routinely biopsied during an endoscopy, the incidence of EG in these segments is unknown. Diarrhea and constipation can also be presenting symptoms.[133] Presentation also varies depending on tissue layers affected and degree of eosinophilic inflammation. EG can be further divided into subtypes based on depth of eosinophilic infiltration.[134,135] The subtypes are based on dominant involvement of different areas: mucosa, muscularis propria, and serosa. The prevalence of these subtypes is unknown and difficult to ascertain from reports in the medical literature. The surgical literature mainly cites muscularis involvement with reports of obstruction requiring surgical intervention while the nonsurgical medical literature mainly reports patients with mucosal involvement. Subserosal involvement is associated with eosinophilic ascites. It is unclear if these subtypes represent a spectrum of the same disease or different disease entities. EG can present with other manifestations, such as gastric ulcers that do not respond to PPI.[136,137] Hepatobiliary tree involvement can occur and may present as pancreatitis or eosinophilic cholangitis.[138,139] Eosinophilic strictures occur in only 5% to 10% which is quite different from EoE where there is a higher incidence of strictures.[136] When strictures occur, patients can present with acute bowel obstruction with nausea, vomiting, cramping, and abdominal bloating.[140] There is also a degree of functional obstruction due to tissue edema and decreased gastrointestinal motility.

Pathogenesis

EG may also be food-allergen driven because select patients improve with diet.[137] It is also a Th2- mediated disease since peripheral blood mononuclear cells from EG patients have increased IL-5 expression.[141] The CD4$^+$ T cell responses between EG, IgE-mediated peanut allergy, and healthy controls are different. EG was associated with an IL-5$^+$, IL-13$^+$ T cell response to foods, while those with peanut allergy showed an IL-5$^-$, IL-13$^+$ Th2 response.[142] Further study of these IL-5$^+$ Th2 cells has demonstrated that they are highly differentiated and require multiple repeat challenges by a food allergen in vivo to express the Th2 cytokines.[143]

Diagnosis

Eosinophilic gastroenteritis is diagnosed when clinical symptoms suggestive of EG are corroborated by a positive biopsy showing eosinophilic inflammation. Biopsies should be obtained from 5 to 6 sites per affected segment (eg, duodenum), and the gross appearance of the biopsies and tissue and may be normal on endoscopy, both features similar to EoE. Eosinophils in ascites fluid can also be diagnostic of EG. Other etiologies for gastrointestinal eosinophilia need to be excluded. The number of eosinophils considered pathogenic is still unclear in EG. The number proposed for diagnosis is 30 eos/hpf in the stomach and 50 eos/hpf in the duodenum.[144,145] The presence of eosinophils in particular tissue layers such as epithelial eosinophils, intraglandular eosinophils, or eosinophils in the muscularis propria layer make the diagnosis of EG more likely, as do pseudopolyps.[146] Pseudopolyps are composed of dense collagen deposits with overlying epithelium, which differ from true polyps which have hyperplastic glandular or epithelial components. Gastric pseudopolyps are the most common presentation of EG occurring in up to 25% of EG patients. Small bowel pseudopolyps have been observed but are much less frequent.[147] Patients with EG may also have esophageal eosinophilia with one pediatric study reporting 12% of EoE patients also having elevated gastric eosinophils (>10 eos/hpf). Another study of adult EG patients observed up to 25% of patients with concurrent esophageal eosinophilia (≥15 eos/hpf).[147] The patients with gastric eosinophils were clinically indistinguishable from those without gastric eosinophilia.[148] Peripheral eosinophilia is present in the majority of patients with EG and can be quite high with absolute eosinophil count into the thousands, but peripheral eosinophilia is not a diagnostic criteria.[134,149]

Patients with an absolute blood eosinophil count (AEC) greater than or equal to 1500 eosinophils/mm^2 should be screened for hypereosinophilic syndrome (HES). HES can present with gastrointestinal symptoms, but the distinction is that in eosinophilic gastrointestinal disorders (EGIDs), the eosinophilia is restricted to the gastrointestinal tract alone. Clinical history should include a careful drug and travel history to rule out secondary causes of eosinophilia. Stool should be sent for ova and parasite screening and serology for *Strongyloides stercoralis* should be obtained. For patients where there is a concern for HES, additional studies can be sent such as TCR clonality studies (T cell clonality in lymphocytic HES), FIP1-like 1/platelet-derived growth factor receptor α fusion gene studies (commonly seen in myeloid HES), and cardiac echocardiogram (to rule out the endomycocardial fibrosis that is seen in HES with cardiac involvement).[147] The diagnosis of eosinophilic granulomatosis with polyangiitis (EGPA or Churg-Strauss syndrome) should be considered in patients with significant lung disease or presence of nasal polyps. These patients can present with dysphagia, anorexia, vomiting, abdominal pain, and bloody diarrhea. Chest x-ray may be helpful in diagnosis with migratory infiltrates common in EGPA. Serum antinuclear cytoplasmic antibodies also may be useful.

Treatment

Diet

Eosinophilic gastroenteritis is a chronic disease with remission being the treatment goal. Due to the effectiveness of dietary management for the treatment of EoE, dietary therapy has been tested in EG and may be effective for a subpopulation. One pediatric case series of 6 patients with protein-losing enteropathy due to EG showed improvement within 4 weeks on an elemental diet.[137] Similarly, an adult case series of 9 patients with EG using the 6 food elimination diet (SFED; no milk, soy, eggs, wheat, fish/shellfish, peanut/tree nuts) showed that diet could reduce clinical symptoms. In the adult case series, 2 patients were placed on an elemental diet and both responded within 4 weeks while only 4 of the 7 patients treated with the elimination diet showed resolution of eosinophilia in the GI tract and blood.[150]

Corticosteroids

Elemental diets can be difficult to implement and have poor patient adherence. Most patients are therefore treated initially with systemic steroids, which are very effective in inducing remissions. Doses of 0.5 to 1 mg/kg/day given once daily in the morning will typically lead to remission within 2 to 14 days. Once symptoms are controlled, steroids should be tapered over at least 2 weeks. The goal is to use the smallest dose possible to maintain remission and to avoid systemic steroid side effects. Due to the risk of side effects, the use of topical or swallowed steroids is recommended once remission is achieved. Swallowed budesonide is well studied in EG and has low oral bioavailability.[151,152] For EG a different preparation is used than the swallowed viscous budesonide used to treat EoE. Entocort is a widely available, commercial formulation of budesonide that produces controlled release of drug in the ileum with very minimal gastric delivery. These capsules are taken once daily at bedtime on an empty stomach using a patient-prepared solution. Patients are instructed to open the Entocort capsule, crush the contents into a powder, and dissolve it in 15 to 30 mL of water and juice. Patients with suspected predominantly ileal disease can use the intact Entocort capsules for optimal ileal activity. The starting dose for swallowed budesonide is typically 9 mg once daily. Once a patient has been off systemic steroids for a few months, the budesonide dose can be tapered slowly over a few months to achieve a desired dosing range of 3 to 6 mg/day for long-term use in maintaining remission. Swallowed fluticasone has been used in EoE patients successfully, and in such a study, it was shown to also decrease gastric eosinophils.[148] Fluticasone is commercially available as an asthma inhaler, which can be used for this disease although it is unclear how much drug reaches more distal segments of the gastrointestinal tract.

Biological Agents and Other Medications

Due to the presence of IL-5^{+} Th2-driven inflammation, monoclonal anti-IL-5, reslizumab, has been used to treat EG in an open-label clinical trial of 4 patients and is very effective in decreasing peripheral eosinophilia.[153] Reslizumab showed only moderate improvement in tissue eosinophilia. Another promising drug that has not yet been tested in EG is a monoclonal antibody targeting the IL-5 receptor, benralizumab which has been used in clinical trials to treat eosinophilic asthma.[154] Another monoclonal antibody (anti-IgE), omalizumab, was not effective in treating tissue eosinophilia in EG similar to its negative results in EoE.[155]

Other allergy drugs have been trialed in EG with varying results. Montelukast has been used for treatment of EG and EoE. A retrospective case series of EoE and EGID pediatric patients showed improvement in clinical symptoms, while other reports have shown no benefit and no effect on sustaining remission of EG.[115,156] Sodium cromolyn has also been used to treat EG with some case reports showing disease improvement and other showing no effect in treating EGID.[115,157,158] There have been 2 case reports on the use of suplatast, an anti-Th2 drug that inhibits Th2 cytokine expression, and successful treatment was shown, but this drug is not commercially available in the United States and requires further study to demonstrate effectiveness in EG.[159,160]

> Eosinophilic gastroenteritis is a chronic illness characterized by eosinophilic inflammation in the stomach and small bowel. Currently treatment relies heavily on systemic and topical steroids.

EOSINOPHILIC COLITIS

Introduction

Eosinophilic colitis (EC) is a chronic inflammatory disorder associated with eosinophilic infiltration and inflammation into a segment of the gastrointestinal tract the colon. EC occurs in a higher frequency in atopic individuals like other eosinophilic gastrointestinal disorders (EGID). Eosinophilic colitis is seen in young infants within the spectrum of food protein–induced enterocolitis.[161] EC can also occur in older children and adults, although it is the least frequent form of EGID even when colitis is present along with inflammation in other segments of the gastrointestinal system.[162,163]

Clinical Presentation

Like eosinophilic gastroenteritis (EG), EC can be subdivided into 3 subtypes depending on the dominantly involved tissue layer: mucosa, muscularis propria, and serosa. The clinical presentation of EC varies widely depending on the subtype and the degree of inflammation present.[164] The mucosa-predominant variant presents with protein-losing enteropathy, malabsorption, and diarrhea.[165] Muscularis-predominant disease with transmural inflammation leads to symptoms of intestinal obstruction and has been associated with volvulus, intussusception, and even intestinal perforation.[166,167] Disease involving the serosa presents with eosinophilic ascites, which can be diagnosed by the high% of eosinophils in the fluid.[168] All of these subtypes can have more severe presentations compared to other forms of EGID, and often require hospitalization for acute management.

Diagnosis

The diagnosis of EC relies on clinical symptoms characteristic of the disease and a positive biopsy or ascites fluid analysis demonstrating eosinophilia with no secondary cause for eosinophilia. Peripheral eosinophilia is quite common but is not necessary for the diagnosis of EC. Unlike EoE, there is no consensus on the degree of tissue eosinophils needed to diagnosis EC, but a suggested diagnostic cutoff of 20 eosinophils per high-power field (hpf) or greater has been used. Part of the obstacle is that the normal range of eosinophils in the colon varies depending on location, with a normal range of less than 10 eosinophils/hpf in the rectum compared to greater than 30 eosinophils/hpf in the cecum. This also emphasizes the importance of choosing biopsy locations during diagnostic endoscopy and obtaining multiple biopsies from each site. Since other diseases have been associated with gastrointestinal eosinophilia, it is important to exclude secondary causes of tissue eosinophilia in the colon before the diagnosis of EC is made. These include medications, parasitic infections, inflammatory bowel disease, and other autoimmune disorders. Drug-induced EC has been described from various medications including clozapine,[169] carbamazepine,[170] rifampicin,[171] nonsteroidal anti-inflammatory drugs,[172,173] tacrolimus,[174] and gold.[175] Inflammatory bowel disease, in particular Crohn disease, has been linked to severe eosinophilic inflammation in the colon.[176] Eosinophilia in the colon has also been observed in certain autoimmune connective tissue diseases such as scleroderma, polymyositis, and dermatomyositis.[165,177] EC has also been observed following bone marrow transplantation.[178]

Pathogenesis

The pathogenesis of EC is not well defined. Most infantile EC is food driven as are other forms of food protein–induced enterocolitis, with cow's milk and soy protein being the main causative foods. The degree of sensitivity can vary, with reports of EC occurring in breastfed infants and infants on casein hydrolysate formulas. Further supporting a role for food allergens in the development of EC is the finding that mast cells have been noted to accumulate in the colon interstitium.[179] Furthermore, similar to other eosinophilic GI disorders, Th2-driven inflammation is thought to be involved with IL-5 and eotaxin considered to be potentially important in EC pathogenesis.

Treatment

Currently, the mainstay of treatment for EC is systemic steroids. The majority of cases will respond within 2 weeks of treatment with a slow taper over weeks suggested after remission is reached. Relapse is frequent so recurrent systemic steroid courses are required in most patients. Due to the concern for long-term steroid dependence, swallowed steroids have been used to maintain remission. Swallowed budesonide has been effective in case reports in treating right colon disease, but further studies need to be done to corroborate this effect and to define whether it is effective therapy for left-sided colonic disease.[151] The need for steroid-sparing agents has led to the use of many other drugs in isolated case reports. The antihistamine, ketotifen, an H1 antagonist, decreased symptoms as well as tissue eosinophilia.[180,181] Anti-IL-5 (mepolizumab) has been used with some success.[182] Another monoclonal antibody (anti-IgE), omalizumab, has been tried with reported success.[145] For the infantile form, dietary elimination works without the need for further medications or the use of corticosteroids.

> Eosinophilic colitis is a rare entity. The more common form of EC seen in infants is food driven and treated successfully with food elimination, but for older children and adults the current mainstay of treatment is systemic corticosteroids with limited use of topical corticosteroids, especially for more distal disease.

FOOD PROTEIN–INDUCED ENTEROCOLITIS

Food protein–induced enterocolitis (FPIES) is a non-IgE–mediated food allergy which characteristically presents with delayed-onset vomiting with or without diarrhea typically occurring 2 to 6 hours postingestion of the causative food.[183] The delayed presentation in FPIES is a stark contrast to IgE-mediated food allergies which present within minutes of ingestion.[23] FPIES typically presents in the first 6 to 9 months of life[184] or at the time when solid foods are first introduced. Once patients are on elimination diets, symptoms on reexposure can be as acute or even more severe as the initial presentation.

Clinical Presentation

Food protein–induced enterocolitis is a rare disease with a reported prevalence of 0.34%.[185] Like IgE-mediated food allergies and other atopic disorders such as asthma and allergic rhinitis, FPIES is on the rise with multiple studies demonstrating a 2-fold to 3-fold increase in cases in the past 2 decades.[162,186] This disease mainly occurs in infants and toddlers with the majority of patients outgrowing symptoms by 5 years of age. A recent study documented that many patients outgrow their reactions much sooner, with 35% no longer having reactions to causative foods by age 2 years and 70% by age 3 years.[187] There have been reported cases of adolescents still reactive to causative foods, but these are quite rare. FPIES presents with delayed-onset vomiting with or without diarrhea approximately 2 hours postingestion of the causative food. An estimated 20% of patients will have a more severe presentation with pallor, dehydration, lethargy, and shock.[164] Infants presenting with FPIES to cow's milk or soy who ingest one of these formulas on a daily basis may present less dramatically with chronic vomiting, diarrhea, failure to thrive, and bloody stools. Interestingly, after a period of avoidance, these children may develop repetitive vomiting and even shock after reexposure to milk or soy. Since solids are usually not ingested every day, the presentation of FPIES from solid foods may be more dramatic, lacking the chronicity of symptoms seen with FPIES to milk or soy. Breastfed infants typically do not have acute symptoms to a food until they are fed food directly. Due to the severity of presentation in some cases of FPIES, patients may be misdiagnosed with sepsis or meningitis; thus, FPIES should be considered in the differential diagnosis of an afebrile child with suspected sepsis, especially if all cultures are negative. If prolonged, chronic diarrhea can eventually develop mucous and blood in the stool.

In the past, milk and soy were usually linked to the majority of FPIES cases. Recent studies have corroborated that milk and soy are the most likely but that many other foods should be considered as culprits. Physicians should be aware that grains, vegetables, and meats, in particular poultry, can be causative foods, especially in exclusively breastfed infants starting solids.[183] One study of the largest reported cohort of FPIES patients (n = 462) presenting to a pediatric allergy clinic showed that the most common foods involved were milk (67%), soy (41%), rice (19%), oat (16%), and egg (11%).[185] In this cohort, 43% of patients with FPIES to milk also reacted to soy, which is comparable to prior published data on cross-reactivity between milk and soy, and 42% of those with FPIES to a grain also reacted to 2 or more grains. Rice is the most common grain culprit in FPIES reactions and is one of the first solid foods to be introduced in the United States. This study also showed that age of presentation varied depending on causative food. Patients with FPIES to milk and soy presented on average at 7 months of age compared counterparts who presented with FPIES to solids on average at 12 months of age. Although less common, FPIES has been identified to a wide variety of foods including meats, peanuts, tree nuts, fruits, and vegetables (Figure 11–4). Since some children may have FPIES to more than one food, it is important to identify which foods are safest to identify at home vs which should be done in a controlled setting.

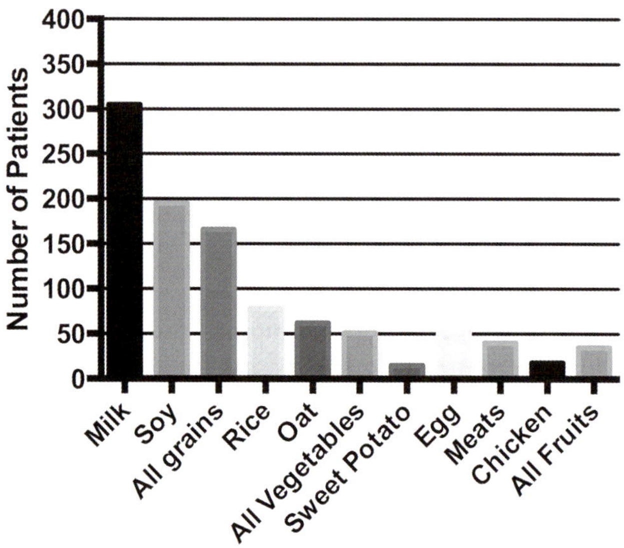

Figure 11–4. Foods that cause food protein induced enterocolitis (FPIES) reactions. Foods were identified as causing symptoms 2 to 4 hours after exposure. The *y*-axis indicates the number of individual patients with a reaction to a single food or a group of foods.

Pathogenesis

The mechanism for FPIES is thought to be non-IgE mediated since the onset of symptoms is delayed by hours. It is hypothesized that there is a breakdown in oral tolerance during a key time in infancy during which these foods are introduced. Gastrointestinal tracts of infants have immature intestinal barriers, decreased proteolytic enzyme activity in the gut, and higher gastric pH.[188] This may be why many children outgrow food reactions by 2 to 3 years of age after reaching gut maturity.[189] Surprisingly, breastfeeding has not been shown to be protective, with the same rates of FPIES as formula-fed infants.[187] The delayed onset of symptoms is also consistent with a cell-mediated immunologic response. Intestinal biopsies of FPIES patients show decreased expression of transforming growth factor–β (TGF-β)[188] which is important in B cell class switching for IgA production and plays a role in epithelial barrier function. More recently, tumor necrosis factor α (TNF-α) has been implicated as playing a role in FPIES patients presenting with hypotension or fever.[190] T cells of patients with active cow's milk allergy produce more TNF-α, when exposed in vitro to cow's milk after a short-term milk-free diet, compared to children without cow's milk allergy (including a portion of children who have outgrown their cow's milk allergy).[191] Food allergy skin testing is typically negative to causative foods in FPIES and is not useful in diagnosis. Specific serum food IgE levels are also not helpful since these tend to correlate with an immediate onset reaction to a food. Patients may have elevation in peripheral blood polymorphonuclear leukocyte count and if a severe reaction occurs, may have acidemia. Methemoglobinemia has been described postreaction and is thought to result from an increase in nitrates in the intestine. Although endoscopy is not part of the recommended workup for FPIES, some patients may have this procedure done, and biopsies may reveal crypt abscesses, mild villous injury in the small intestine, and diffuse inflammation in the colon.

Diagnosis

The diagnosis of FPIES relies heavily on history of maternal and child's diet. As noted above, food allergy skin prick or blood testing is not useful in the disorder. Atopy patch testing has been used in identifying causative foods in FPIES in the past, but several studies have shown it is not as helpful in diagnosis as was previously thought, with up to 45% false negative rate reported in one study.[187,192] The gold standard for diagnosis of FPIES is a physician-observed oral food challenge, preferably in a hospital setting. Unfortunately, there are currently no laboratory tests available for the diagnosis of FPIES. The lack of testing for FPIES may also lead to delayed diagnosis. One study found that most patients were diagnosed after 2 reactions although some patients in the cohort were not diagnosed until the fifth reaction despite a high rate of severe reactions including shock.[183]

Treatment

Currently, the only treatment options are the avoidance of causative foods as well as dietary exclusion of other foods not yet introduced that have a high likelihood of cross-reactivity (eg, other grains). Some children with cow's milk allergy will tolerate a casein hydrolysate formula, but some require an elemental formula. In children presenting with FPIES prior to starting solid food, the introduction of solids should be delayed until 6 to 7 months of age. When it is likely that a child has outgrown this disease, foods should be introduced one at a time, and initially as a hospital-based food challenge. Some patients at risk for more severe reactions may warrant having an IV in place prior to the start of the challenge. When patients react, it is important to push IV fluids aggressively as patients can quickly develop dehydration and shock. One issue with FPIES challenges is that when children react, it may take hours until resolution of nausea and vomiting. If they are unable to maintain hydration on their own with oral intake, they require admission for observation and continued hydration. In recent years, ondansetron (Zofran) given orally or intramuscularly (IM), has been helpful in shortening the recovery time and severity of presentation when administered during a failed FPIES challenge. Ondansetron is a selective serotonin 5-HT3 receptor antagonist approved for the treatment of nausea and vomiting in oncology patients treated with chemotherapy or radiation although it has become popular in recent years in ER patients with acute gastroenteritis. It is thought to work by inhibiting serotonin receptors on the vagal nerve responsible for eliciting the vomiting reflex. Case reports have demonstrated that when used after a positive challenge, patients had resolution of vomiting and nausea within 30 minutes of administration.[193] Another benefit is that it can be administered intravenously. Ondansetron has minimal side effects and does not cause sedation but has been associated with QT prolongation, so it should be avoided in certain patients such as those with prolonged QT syndrome.

> Food protein–induced enterocolitis is a delayed reaction to a food that is most common in early childhood. It can be managed quite successfully by food avoidance, and most children will outgrow these reactions during school-age years. If done in the appropriate setting, foods can be safely added using a challenge protocol when it is deemed appropriate for each child.

FOOD PROTEIN-INDUCED PROCTOCOLITIS

Food protein-induced proctocolitis has symptoms limited to colon and rectum and presents with mucus or blood in the stool. Interestingly, about 50% of infant cases occur in breastfed infants.[194,195] The typical clinical case is a healthy infant who has mucus or blood in the stool. The infant may be fussy but is growing well.[196] Food protocolitis typically presents around 2 to 8 weeks of age and resolves around 1 year of age. There is one case series of similar findings in older children (2 to 14 years of age) that resolve with milk elimination.[197] The most common causative foods are cow's milk (65%), egg (19%), corn (6%), and soy (3%).[194,195]

The mechanism is unknown but is thought to be non-IgE mediated based on the poor predictive values of IgE testing and the delayed nature of symptom onset. The diagnosis is based on clinical criteria (symptom presentation and resolution of symptoms upon withdrawal of the presumed food antigen). Food allergy skin prick testing and blood allergy testing are not recommended. Biopsies are only recommended when symptoms do not resolve after removal of milk, soy, and egg. Colonoscopies show mild colitis with patchy erythema and loss of vascularity.[198] In patients with food protein–induced proctocolitis, mucosal changes are frequently confined to the rectum, although they may rarely extend further up the colon. Biopsies typically reveal high numbers of eosinophils (including eosinophilic abscesses) in the lamina propria and muscularis mucosa as well as lymphoid nodular hyperplasia.[199]

CELIAC DISEASE

Celiac disease or gluten sensitivity is caused by an immune reaction to gluten, a common protein constituent of wheat, barley, and rye. It is not a typical IgE-mediated food allergy since the immune reaction to gluten induces inflammation of the small intestine characterized by villous atrophy and lymphocyte infiltrate. The diagnosis of celiac disease is based on biopsy and serologic studies. IgA antibodies to a protein component of gluten (gliadin), to intestinal connective tissue (endomysium), and the target intestinal autoantigen, tissue transglutaminase, are pathognomonic for celiac disease.[200,201]

Tissue transglutaminase (TTG) is a ubiquitous intracellular enzyme that is released by endothelial cells and fibroblasts in response to mechanical injury. TTG cross-links glutamine-rich proteins such as gluten proteins from wheat. TTG also deamidates glutamine residues in gluten to glutamic acid increasing their binding to HLA-DQ2 and DQ8, which potentiates their capacity to stimulate T-cells leading to autoimmune inflammation.[202]

The disorder is common, occurring in 0.5% to 1% of the general population in most countries.[203] It is increased in certain genetic subpopulations (those with the HLA locus DR3-DQ2 and/or DR4-DQ8) and is associated with other diseases including type 1 diabetes and autoimmune thyroid disease.

The symptoms vary from classic gastrointestinal symptoms to those more typical of autoimmunity. Children can present with a large constellation of symptoms including abdominal pain, constipation, and diarrhea. The villous atrophy leads to malsabsorption and subsequent failure to thrive, osteopenia, anemia, and fatigue. Celiac disease is associated with neuropathies, arthritis, kidney disease, tooth enamel defects, infertility, and increased hepatic transamines.[204] The treatment is strict avoidance of gluten.

CONCLUSION

The symptoms and severity of food allergy reactions vary based on the pathogenetic mechanism and location of disease. Food allergies can be severe and life threatening (food allergy–induced anaphylaxis) or mild with limited symptoms (food protein–induced proctocolitis). The diagnosis of food allergy is based both on history and diagnostic testing. The gold standard is a food challenge, where the food is administered and the symptoms are monitored. However, for patients with delayed food reactions (ie, eosinophilic esophagitis or other eosinophilic gastrointestinal diseases), a biopsy of the affected tissue after an extended period of time on the food might be needed to confirm the diagnosis. Whenever possible, the primary treatment of all types of food allergy is avoidance. New research is examining ways to desensitize or induce food tolerance, but the research is still investigational.

REFERENCES

1. Sampson HA. Food allergy. Part 1: immunopathogenesis and clinical disorders. *J Allergy Clin Immunol.* 1999;103(5, pt 1):717–728.
2. Boyce JA, Assa'ad A, Burks AW, et al. Guidelines for the diagnosis and management of food allergy in the United States: report of the NIAID-sponsored expert panel. *J Allergy Clin Immunol.* 2010 Dec;126(6, suppl):S1–58.
3. Sampson HA. Food allergy. Part 2: diagnosis and management. *J Allergy Clin Immunol.* 1999;103(6):981–989.
4. Nowak-Wegrzyn A, Sampson HA. Adverse reactions to foods. *Med Clin North Am.* 2006;90(1):97–127.

5. Lee LA, Burks AW. Food allergies: prevalence, molecular characterization, and treatment/prevention strategies. *Annu Rev Nutr.* 2006;26:539–565.
6. Venter C, Pereira B, Voigt K, et al. Prevalence and cumulative incidence of food hypersensitivity in the first 3 years of life. *Allergy.* 2008;63(3):354–359.
7. Sicherer SH, Munoz-Furlong A, Sampson HA. Prevalence of seafood allergy in the United States determined by a random telephone survey. *J Allergy Clin Immunol.* 2004;114(1):159–165.
8. Pereira B, Venter C, Grundy J, Clayton CB, Arshad SH, Dean T. Prevalence of sensitization to food allergens, reported adverse reaction to foods, food avoidance, and food hypersensitivity among teenagers. *J Allergy Clin Immunol.* 2005;116(4):884–892.
9. Sheikh A, Hippisley-Cox J, Newton J, Fenty J. Trends in national incidence, lifetime prevalence and adrenaline prescribing for anaphylaxis in England. *J R Soc Med.* 2008;101(3):139–143.
10. Sheikh A, Alves B. Hospital admissions for acute anaphylaxis: time trend study. *BMJ.* 2000;320(7247):1441.
11. Poulos LM, Waters AM, Correll PK, Loblay RH, Marks GB. Trends in hospitalizations for anaphylaxis, angioedema, and urticaria in Australia, 1993–1994 to 2004–2005. *J Allergy Clin Immunol.* 2007;120(4):878–884.
12. Sicherer SH, Sampson HA. Peanut allergy: emerging concepts and approaches for an apparent epidemic. *J Allergy Clin Immunol.* 2007;120(3):491–503; quiz 504–495.
13. Grundy J, Matthews S, Bateman B, Dean T, Arshad SH. Rising prevalence of allergy to peanut in children: data from 2 sequential cohorts. *J Allergy Clin Immunol.* 2002;110(5):784–789.
14. Schaub B, Lauener R, von Mutius E. The many faces of the hygiene hypothesis. *J Allergy Clin Immunol.* 2006;117(5):969–977; quiz 978.
15. Du Toit C, Katz Y, Sasieni P, et al. Early consumption of peanuts in infancy is associated with a low prevalence of peanut allergy. *J Allergy Clin Immunol.* 2008;122(5):984–991.
16. Bach JF. The effect of infections on susceptibility to autoimmune and allergic diseases. *N Engl J Med.* 2002;347(12):911–920.
17. Decker WW, Campbell RL, Manivannan V, et al. The etiology and incidence of anaphylaxis in Rochester, Minnesota: a report from the Rochester Epidemiology Project. *J Allergy Clin Immunol.* 2008;122(6):1161–1165.
18. Bohlke K, Davis RL, DeStefano F, Marcy SM, Braun MM, Thompson RS. Epidemiology of anaphylaxis among children and adolescents enrolled in a health maintenance organization. *J Allergy Clin Immunol.* 2004;113(3):536–542.
19. Yocum MW, Butterfield JH, Klein JS, Volcheck GW, Schroeder DR, Silverstein MD. Epidemiology of anaphylaxis in Olmsted County: a population-based study. *J Allergy Clin Immunol.* 1999;104(2, pt 1):452–456.
20. Mullins RJ. Anaphylaxis: risk factors for recurrence. *Clin Exp Allergy* 2003;33(8):1033–1040.
21. Sampson HA, Munoz-Furlong A, Campbell RL, et al. Second symposium on the definition and management of anaphylaxis: summary report—second National Institute of Allergy and Infectious Disease/Food Allergy and Anaphylaxis Network symposium. *Ann Emerg Med.* 2006;47(4):373–380.
22. Novembre E, Cianferoni A, Bernardini R, et al. Anaphylaxis in children: clinical and allergologic features. *Pediatrics.* 1998;101(4):E8.
23. Cianferoni A, Spergel JM. Food allergy: review, classification and diagnosis. *Allergol Int.* 2009;58(4):457–466.
24. Cianferoni A, Muraro A. Food-induced anaphylaxis. *Immunol Allergy Clin North Am.* 2012;32(1):165–195.
25. Monreal P, Botey J, Pena M, Marin A, Eseverri JL. Mustard allergy. Two anaphylactic reactions to ingestion of mustard sauce. *Ann Allergy.* 1992;69(4):317–320.
26. Gloor M, Kagi M, Wuthrich B. [Poppyseed anaphylaxis]. *Schweiz Med Wochenschr.* 1995;125(30):1434–1437.
27. Dechamp C, Bessot JC, Pauli G, Deviller P. First report of anaphylactic reaction after fig (*Ficus carica*) ingestion. *Allergy.* 1995;50(6):514–516.
28. Subiza J, Subiza JL, Hinojosa M, et al. Anaphylactic reaction after the ingestion of chamomile tea: a study of cross-reactivity with other composite pollens. *J Allergy Clin Immunol.* 1989;84(3):353–358.
29. Miell J, Papouchado M, Marshall AJ. Anaphylactic reaction after eating a mango. *BMJ.* 1988;297(6664):1639–1640.
30. Savonius B, Kanerva L. Anaphylaxis caused by banana. *Allergy.* 1993;48(3):215–216.
31. Bock SA. Anaphylaxis to coriander: a sleuthing story. *J Allergy Clin Immunol.* 1993;91(6):1232–1233.
32. Blaiss MS, McCants ML, Lehrer SB. Anaphylaxis to cabbage: detection of allergens. *Ann Allergy.* 1987;58(4):248–250.
33. Parker JL, Yunginger JW, Swedlund HA. Anaphylaxis after ingestion of millet seeds. *J Allergy Clin Immunol.* 1981;67(1):78–80.
34. Sampson HA, Munoz-Furlong A, Bock SA, et al. Symposium on the definition and management of anaphylaxis: summary report. *J Allergy Clin Immunol.* 2005;115(3):584–591.
35. Muraro A, Roberts G, Clark A, et al. The management of anaphylaxis in childhood: position paper of the European Academy of Allergology and Clinical Immunology. *Allergy.* 2007;62(8):857–871.
36. Neugut AI, Ghatak AT, Miller RL. Anaphylaxis in the United States: an investigation into its epidemiology. *Arch Inter Med.* 2001;161(1):15–21.
37. Clark S, Camargo CA, Jr. Epidemiology of anaphylaxis. *Immunol Allergy Clin North Am.* 2007;27(2):145–163, v.
38. Bock SA. The incidence of severe adverse reactions to food in Colorado. *J Allergy Clin Immunol.* 1992;90(4, pt 1):683–685.
39. Iribarren C, Tolstykh IV, Miller MK, Eisner MD. Asthma and the prospective risk of anaphylactic shock and other allergy diagnoses in a large integrated health care delivery system. *Ann Asthma Allergy Immunol.* 2010;104(5):371–377.

40. Hompes S, Kohli A, Nemat K, et al. Provoking allergens and treatment of anaphylaxis in children and adolescents—data from the anaphylaxis registry of German-speaking countries. *Pediatr Allergy Immunol.* 2011;22(6):568–574.
41. Liew WK, Williamson E, Tang ML. Anaphylaxis fatalities and admissions in Australia. *J Allergy Clin Immunol.* 2009;123(2):434–442.
42. Rudders SA, Banerji A, Clark S, Camargo CA, Jr. Age-related differences in the clinical presentation of food-induced anaphylaxis. *J Pediatrics* 2011;158(2):326–328.
43. Crespo JF, James JM, Fernandez-Rodriguez C, Rodriguez J. Food allergy: nuts and tree nuts. *Br J Nutrit.* 2006;96(suppl 2):S95–S102.
44. Summers CW, Pumphrey RS, Woods CN, McDowell G, Pemberton PW, Arkwright PD. Factors predicting anaphylaxis to peanuts and tree nuts in patients referred to a specialist center. *J Allergy Clin Immunol.* 2008;121(3):632–638, e632.
45. Lack G, Fox D, Northstone K, Golding J. Factors associated with the development of peanut allergy in childhood. *New Engl J Med.* 2003;348(11):977–985.
46. Bock SA, Munoz-Furlong A, Sampson HA. Fatalities due to anaphylactic reactions to foods. *J Allergy Clin Immunol.* 2001;107(1):191–193.
47. Bock SA, Munoz-Furlong A, Sampson HA. Further fatalities caused by anaphylactic reactions to food, 2001–2006. *J Allergy Clin Immunol.* 2007;119(4):1016–1018.
48. Pumphrey RS, Gowland MH. Further fatal allergic reactions to food in the United Kingdom, 1999–2006. *J Allergy Clin Immunol.* 2007;119(4):1018–1019.
49. Hoffer V, Scheuerman O, Marcus N, et al. Anaphylaxis in Israel: experience with 92 hospitalized children. *Pediatr Allergy Immunol.* 2011;22(2):172–177.
50. Silva R, Gomes E, Cunha L, Falcao H. Anaphylaxis in children: a nine years retrospective study (2001–2009). *Allergol Immunopathol (Madr).* 2012 Jan-Feb;40(1):31–36.
51. Host A, Halken S, Jacobsen HP, Christensen AE, Herskind AM, Plesner K. Clinical course of cow's milk protein allergy/intolerance and atopic diseases in childhood. *Pediatr Allergy Immunol.* 2002;13(suppl 15):23–28.
52. Skolnick HS, Conover-Walker MK, Koerner CB, Sampson HA, Burks W, Wood RA. The natural history of peanut allergy. *J Allergy Clin Immunol.* 2001;107(2):367–374.
53. Fleischer DM, Conover-Walker MK, Matsui EC, Wood RA. The natural history of tree nut allergy. *J Allergy Clin Immunol.* 2005;116(5):1087–1093.
54. Fleischer DM, Conover-Walker MK, Christie L, Burks AW, Wood RA. The natural progression of peanut allergy: resolution and the possibility of recurrence. *J Allergy Clin Immunol.* 2003;112(1):183–189.
55. Agne PS, Bidat E, Agne PS, Rance F, Paty E. Sesame seed allergy in children. *Eur Ann Allergy Clin Immunol.* 2004;36(8):300–305.
56. Stone SF, Cotterell C, Isbister GK, Holdgate A, Brown SG. Elevated serum cytokines during human anaphylaxis: identification of potential mediators of acute allergic reactions. *J Allergy Clin Immunol.* 2009;124(4):786–792, e784.
57. Simons FE. Anaphylaxis. *J Allergy Clin Immunol.* 2010;125(2, suppl 2):S161–S181.
58. Arias K, Chu DK, Flader K, et al. Distinct immune effector pathways contribute to the full expression of peanut-induced anaphylactic reactions in mice. *J Allergy Clin Immunol.* 2011;127(6):1552–1561, e1551.
59. Radauer C, Breiteneder H. Evolutionary biology of plant food allergens. *J Allergy Clin Immunol.* 2007;120(3):518–525.
60. Eigenmann PA. Anaphylactic reactions to raw eggs after negative challenges with cooked eggs. *J Allergy Clin Immunol.* 2000;105(3):587–588.
61. Keet C. Recognition and management of food-induced anaphylaxis. *Pediatr Clinic North Am.* 2011;58(2):377–388, x.
62. Spergel JM, Beausoleil JL, Fiedler JM, Ginsberg J, Wagner K, Pawlowski NA. Correlation of initial food reactions to observed reactions on challenges. *Annals Allergy Asthma Immunol.* 2004;92(2):217–224.
63. Vickery BP, Burks W. Oral immunotherapy for food allergy. *Curr Opin Pediatr.* 2010;22:765.
64. Syed, A, Garcia MA, Lyu SC, et al. Peanut oral immnotherapy results in increased antigen-induced regulatory T-cell function and hypomethylation of forkhead box protein (FOXP3). *J Allergy Clin Immunol.* 2014: 133:500–510.
65. Patriarca G, Nucera E, Roncallo C, et al. Oral desensitizing treatment in food allergy: clinical and immunological results. *Aliment Pharmacol Ther.* 2003;17:459–465.
66. Morisset M, Moneret-Vautrin DA, Guenard L, et al. Oral desensitization in children with milk and egg allergies obtains recovery in a significant proportion of cases. A randomized study in 60 children with cow's milk allergy and 90 children with egg allergy. *Eur Ann Allergy Clin Immunol.* 2007;39:12–19.
67. Brozek JL, Terracciano L, Hsu J, et al. Oral immunotherapy for IgE-mediated cow's milk allergy: a systematic review and meta-analysis. *Clin Exp Allergy.* 2012;42:363–374.
68. Burks AW, Jones SM, Wood RA, et al. Oral immunotherapy for treatment of egg allergy in children. *N Engl J Med.* 2012;367(3):233–243.
69. Jones, SM, Pons L, Roberts JL, et al. Clinical efficacy and immune regulation with peanut oral immunotherapy. *J Allergy Clin Immunol.* 2009;123:292–300.
70. Vickery BP, Scurlock AM, Kulis M, et al. Sustained unresponsiveness to peanut in subjects who have completed peanut oral immunotherapy. *J Allergy Clin Immunol.* 2014;133:468–475.
71. Begin P, Dominguez T, Wilson SP, et al. Phase 1 results of safety and tolerability in a rush oral immunotherapy protocol to multiple foods using Omalizumab. *Allergy Asthma Clin Immunol.* 2014;10:7.
72. Du Toit G, Roberts G, Sayre PH, et al. Randomized trial of peanut consumption in infants at risk of peanut allergy. *N Engl J Med.* 2015;372:803–813.

73. Fleisher DM, Spergel JM, Assa'ad, AH, Pongracic JA. Primary Prevention of allergic diseases through nutritional interventions. *J Allergy Clin Immunol Pract*. 2013;1: 29–36.
74. Kleine-Tebbe J, Herold DA. Cross-reactive allergen clusters in pollen-associated food allergy. *Hautarzt*. 2003: 54:130–137.
75. Osterballe M, Mortz CG, Hansen TK, et al. The prevalence of food hypersensitivity in young adults. *Pediatr Allergy Immunol*. 2009;20:868–892.
76. Osterballe M, Hansen TK, Mortz CH, Bindslev-Jensen C. The clinical relevance of sensitization to pollen-related fruits and vegetables in unselected pollen-sensitized adults. *Allergy*. 2005:60:218–225.
77. Ricci G, Righetti F, Menna G, et al. Relationship between Bet v1 and Bet v2 specific IgE and food allergy in children with grass pollen respiratory allergy. *Mol Immunol*. 2005;42:1251–1257.
78. Spergel JM, Andrews T, Brown-Whitehorn TF, Beausoleil JL, Liacouras CA. Treatment of eosinophilic esophagitis with specific food elimination diet directed by a combination of skin prick and patch tests. *Ann Allergy Asthma Immunol*. 2005;95(4):336–343.
79. Noel RJ, Putnam PE, Rothenberg ME. Eosinophilic esophagitis. *N Engl J Med*. 2004;351(9):940–941.
80. Spergel JM, Brown-Whitehorn TF, Beausoleil JL, et al. 14 years of eosinophilic esophagitis: clinical features and prognosis. *J Pediatr Gastroenterol Nutr*. 2009;48(1):30–36.
81. Straumann A. Eosinophilic esophagitis: a bulk of mysteries. *Dig Dis*. 2013;31(1):6–9.
82. Straumann A. The natural history and complications of eosinophilic esophagitis. *Gastrointest Endosc Clin N Am*. 2008;18(1):99–118; ix.
83. Spergel JM, Shuker M. Nutritional management of eosinophilic esophagitis. *Gastrointest Endosc Clin N Am*. 2008;18(1):179–194; xi.
84. Spergel JM, Cianferoni A. Treatment of eosinophilic esophagitis. *Expert Opin Orphan Drugs*. 2013;1(4):261–272.
85. Furuta GT, Liacouras CA, Collins MH, et al. Eosinophilic esophagitis in children and adults: a systematic review and consensus recommendations for diagnosis and treatment. *Gastroenterology*. 2007;133(4):1342–1363.
86. Liacouras CA, Furuta GT, Hirano I, et al. Eosinophilic esophagitis: updated consensus recommendations for children and adults. *J Allergy Clin Immunol*. 2011;128(1): 3–20, e26; quiz 21–22.
87. Collins MH. Histopathologic features of eosinophilic esophagitis. *Gastrointest Endosc Clin N Am*. 2008;18(1): 59–71; viii–ix.
88. Schoepfer AM, Gonsalves N, Bussmann C, et al. Esophageal dilation in eosinophilic esophagitis: effectiveness, safety, and impact on the underlying inflammation. *Am J Gastroenterol*. 2010;105(5):1062–1070.
89. Kelly KJ, Lazenby AJ, Rowe PC, Yardley JH, Perman JA, Sampson HA. Eosinophilic esophagitis attributed to gastroesophageal reflux: improvement with an amino acid-based formula. *Gastroenterology*. 1995;109(5):1503–1512.
90. Kagalwalla AF, Sentongo TA, Ritz S, et al. Effect of six-food elimination diet on clinical and histologic outcomes in eosinophilic esophagitis. *Clin Gastroenterol Hepatol*. 2006;4(9):1097–1102.
91. Gonsalves N. Food allergies and eosinophilic gastrointestinal illness. *Gastroenterol Clin North Am*. 2007;36(1): 75–91, vi.
92. Spergel JM, Brown-Whitehorn TF, Cianferoni A, et al. Identification of causative foods in children with eosinophilic esophagitis treated with an elimination diet. *J Allergy Clin Immunol*. 2012;130(2):461–467, e465.
93. Gonsalves N, Yang GY, Doerfler B, Ritz S, Ditto AM, Hirano I. Elimination diet effectively treats eosinophilic esophagitis in adults; food reintroduction identifies causative factors. *Gastroenterology*. 2012;142(7):1451–1459, e1451; quiz e1414–1455.
94. Greenhawt M, Aceves SS, Spergel JM, Rothenberg ME. The management of eosinophilic esophagitis. *J Allergy Clin Immunol Pract*. 2013;1(4):332–340; quiz 341–332.
95. Assa'ad AH, Putnam PE, Collins MH, et al. Pediatric patients with eosinophilic esophagitis: an 8-year follow-up. *J Allergy Clin Immunol*. 2007;119(3):731–738.
96. Maggadottir SM, Hill DA, Ruymann K, et al. Resolution of acute IgE-mediated allergy with development of eosinophilic esophagitis triggered by the same food. *J Allergy Clin Immunol*. 2014;133(5):1487–1489, 1489, e1481.
97. Rothenberg ME, Spergel JM, Sherrill JD, et al. Common variants at 5q22 associate with pediatric eosinophilic esophagitis. *Nature Genetics*. 2010;42(4):289–291.
98. Sherrill JD, Gao PS, Stucke EM, et al. Variants of thymic stromal lymphopoietin and its receptor associate with eosinophilic esophagitis. *J Allergy Clin Immunol*. 2010; 126(1):160–165, e163.
99. Blanchard C, Wang N, Stringer KF, et al. Eotaxin-3 and a uniquely conserved gene-expression profile in eosinophilic esophagitis. *J Clin Invest*. 2006;116(2):536–547.
100. Straumann A, Kristl J, Conus S, et al. Cytokine expression in healthy and inflamed mucosa: probing the role of eosinophils in the digestive tract. *Inflamm Bowel Dis*. 2005;11(8):720–726.
101. Blanchard C, Stucke EM, Rodriguez-Jimenez B, et al. A striking local esophageal cytokine expression profile in eosinophilic esophagitis. *J Allergy Clin Immunol*. 2011;127(1):208–217, 217, e201–207.
102. Kinoshita Y, Furuta K, Ishimura N, Ishihara S. Elevated plasma cytokines in Japanese patients with eosinophilic esophagitis and gastroenteritis. *Digestion*. 2012;86(3): 238–243.
103. Straumann A, Conus S, Grzonka P, et al. Anti-interleukin-5 antibody treatment (mepolizumab) in active eosinophilic oesophagitis: a randomised, placebo-controlled, double-blind trial. *Gut*. 2010;59(1):21–30.
104. Spergel JM, Rothenberg ME, Collins MH, et al. Reslizumab in children and adolescents with eosinophilic esophagitis: results of a double-blind, randomized, placebo-controlled trial. *J Allergy Clin Immunol*. 2012; 129(2):456–463, 463, e451–453.

105. Otani IM, Anilkumar AA, Newbury RO, et al. Anti-IL-5 therapy reduces mast cell and IL-9 cell numbers in pediatric patients with eosinophilic esophagitis. *J Allergy Clin Immunol.* Jun 2013;131(6):1576-1582.
106. Assa'ad AH, Gupta SK, Collins MH, et al. An antibody against IL-5 reduces numbers of esophageal intraepithelial eosinophils in children with eosinophilic esophagitis. *Gastroenterology.* 2011;141(5):1593–1604.
107. Siracusa MC, Saenz SA, Hill DA, et al. TSLP promotes interleukin-3-independent basophil haematopoiesis and type 2 inflammation. *Nature.* 2011;477(7363):229–233.
108. Noti M, Wojno ED, Kim BS, et al. Thymic stromal lymphopoietin-elicited basophil responses promote eosinophilic esophagitis. *Nat Med.* 2013;19(8):1005–1013.
109. Soumelis V, Reche PA, Kanzler H, et al. Human epithelial cells trigger dendritic cell mediated allergic inflammation by producing TSLP. *Nat Immunol.* 2002;3(7):673–680.
110. Jyonouchi S, Smith CL, Saretta F, et al. Invariant natural killer T cells in children with eosinophilic esophagitis. *Clin Exp Allergy.* 2014 Jan;44(1):58–68.
111. Lim DM, Narasimhan S, Michaylira CZ, Wang ML. TLR3-mediated NF-{kappa}B signaling in human esophageal epithelial cells. *Am J Physiol Gastrointest Liver Physiol.* 2009;297(6):G1172–G1180.
112. Mulder DJ, Lobo D, Mak N, Justinich CJ. Expression of toll-like receptors 2 and 3 on esophageal epithelial cell lines and on eosinophils during esophagitis. *Dig Dis Sci.* 2012;57(3):630–642.
113. Kottyan LC, Davis BP, Sherrill JD, et al. Genome-wide association analysis of eosinophilic esophagitis provides insight into the tissue specificity of this allergic disease. *Nat Genet.* 2014;46(8):895–900.
114. Sleiman PM, Wang ML, Cianferoni A, et al. GWAS identifies four novel eosinophilic esophagitis loci. *Nat Commun.* 2014;5:5593.
115. Liacouras CA, Spergel JM, Ruchelli E, et al. Eosinophilic esophagitis: a 10-year experience in 381 children. *Clin Gastroenterol Hepatol.* 2005;3(12):1198–1206.
116. Spergel JM, Beausoleil JL, Mascarenhas M, Liacouras CA. The use of skin prick tests and patch tests to identify causative foods in eosinophilic esophagitis. *J Allergy Clin Immunol.* 2002;109(2):363–368.
117. Spergel JM, Brown-Whitehorn T. The use of patch testing in the diagnosis of food allergy. *Curr Allergy Asthma Rep.* 2005;5(1):86–90.
118. Spergel JM, Brown-Whitehorn T, Beausoleil JL, Shuker M, Liacouras CA. Predictive values for skin prick test and atopy patch test for eosinophilic esophagitis. *J Allergy Clin Immunol.* 2007;119(2):509–511.
119. Konikoff MR, Noel RJ, Blanchard C, et al. A randomized, double-blind, placebo-controlled trial of fluticasone propionate for pediatric eosinophilic esophagitis. *Gastroenterology.* 2006;131(5):1381–1391.
120. Noel RJ, Putnam PE, Collins MH, et al. Clinical and immunopathologic effects of swallowed fluticasone for eosinophilic esophagitis. *Clin Gastroenterol Hepatol.* 2004; 2(7):568–575.
121. Teitelbaum JE, Fox VL, Twarog FJ, et al. Eosinophilic esophagitis in children: immunopathological analysis and response to fluticasone propionate. *Gastroenterology.* 2002;122(5):1216–1225.
122. Caldwell JM, Blanchard C, Collins MH, et al. Glucocorticoid-regulated genes in eosinophilic esophagitis: a role for FKBP51. *J Allergy Clin Immunol.* 2010;125(4):879–888, e878.
123. Aceves SS, Bastian JF, Newbury RO, Dohil R. Oral viscous budesonide: a potential new therapy for eosinophilic esophagitis in children. *Am J Gastroenterol.* 2007; 102(10):2271–2279; quiz 2280.
124. Dohil R, Newbury R, Fox L, Bastian J, Aceves S. Oral viscous budesonide is effective in children with eosinophilic esophagitis in a randomized, placebo-controlled trial. *Gastroenterology.* 2010;139(2):418–429.
125. Dellon ES, Sheikh A, Speck O, et al. Viscous topical is more effective than nebulized steroid therapy for patients with eosinophilic esophagitis. *Gastroenterology.* 2012;143(2):321–324 e321.
126. Aceves SS, Newbury RO, Chen D, et al. Resolution of remodeling in eosinophilic esophagitis correlates with epithelial response to topical corticosteroids. *Allergy.* 2010;65(1):109–116.
127. Lucendo AJ, Arias A, De Rezende LC, et al. Subepithelial collagen deposition, profibrogenic cytokine gene expression, and changes after prolonged fluticasone propionate treatment in adult eosinophilic esophagitis: a prospective study. *J Allergy Clin Immunol.* 2011;128(5):1037–1046.
128. Liacouras CA, Furuta GT, Hirano I, et al. Eosinophilic esophagitis: updated consensus recommendations for children and adults. *J Allergy Clin Immunol.* 2011; 128(1):3–20, e26; quiz 21–22.
129. Kelly HW, Sternberg AL, Lescher R, et al. Effect of inhaled glucocorticoids in childhood on adult height. *N Engl J Med.* 2012;367(10):904–912.
130. Turpeinen M, Pelkonen AS, Nikander K, et al. Bone mineral density in children treated with daily or periodical inhaled budesonide: the Helsinki Early Intervention Childhood Asthma study. *Pediatr Res.* 2010;68(2): 169–173.
131. Dellon ES, Gonsalves N, Hirano I, et al. ACG clinical guideline: evidenced based approach to the diagnosis and management of esophageal eosinophilia and eosinophilic esophagitis (EoE). *Am J Gastroenterol.* 2013;108(5): 679–692; quiz 693.
132. Spergel JM, Book WM, Mays E, et al. Variation in prevalence, diagnostic criteria, and initial management options for eosinophilic gastrointestinal diseases in the United States. *J Pediatr Gastroenterol Nutr.* 2011;52(3): 300–306.
133. Khan F, Chaudhry MA, Nusrat S, Qureshi N, Ali T. Constipation—another manifestation of eosinophilic gastroenteritis. *J Okla State Med Assoc.* 2012;105(4–5):134, 136.
134. Talley NJ, Shorter RG, Phillips SF, Zinsmeister AR. Eosinophilic gastroenteritis: a clinicopathological study

of patients with disease of the mucosa, muscle layer, and subserosal tissues. *Gut.* 1990;31(1):54–58.
135. Chang JY, Choung RS, Lee RM, et al. A shift in the clinical spectrum of eosinophilic gastroenteritis toward the mucosal disease type. *Clin Gastroenterol Hepatol.* 2010; 8(8):669–675; quiz e688.
136. Kristopaitis T, Neghme C, Yong SL, Chejfec G, Aranha G, Keshavarzian A. Giant antral ulcer: a rare presentation of eosinophilic gastroenteritis—case report and review of the literature. *Am J Gastroenterol.* 1997;92(7): 1205–1208.
137. Chehade M, Magid MS, Mofidi S, Nowak-Wegrzyn A, Sampson HA, Sicherer SH. Allergic eosinophilic gastroenteritis with protein-losing enteropathy: intestinal pathology, clinical course, and long-term follow-up. *J Pediatr Gastroenterol Nutr.* 2006;42(5):516–521.
138. Lyngbaek S, Adamsen S, Aru A, Bergenfeldt M. Recurrent acute pancreatitis due to eosinophilic gastroenteritis. Case report and literature review. *JOP.* 2006;7(2): 211–217.
139. Schoonbroodt D, Horsmans Y, Laka A, Geubel AP, Hoang P. Eosinophilic gastroenteritis presenting with colitis and cholangitis. *Dig Dis Sci.* 1995;40(2):308–314.
140. Yun MY, Cho YU, Park IS, et al. Eosinophilic gastroenteritis presenting as small bowel obstruction: a case report and review of the literature. *World J Gastroenterol.* 2007;13(11):1758–1760.
141. Jaffe JS, James SP, Mullins GE, Braun-Elwert L, Lubensky I, Metcalfe DD. Evidence for an abnormal profile of interleukin-4 (IL-4), IL-5, and gamma-interferon (gamma-IFN) in peripheral blood T cells from patients with allergic eosinophilic gastroenteritis. *J Clin Immunol.* 1994;14(5):299–309.
142. Prussin C, Lee J, Foster B. Eosinophilic gastrointestinal disease and peanut allergy are alternatively associated with IL-5+ and IL-5(−) T(H)2 responses. *J Allergy Clin Immunol.* 2009;124(6):1326–1332, e1326.
143. Upadhyaya B, Yin Y, Hill BJ, Douek DC, Prussin C. Hierarchical IL-5 expression defines a subpopulation of highly differentiated human Th2 cells. *J Immunol.* 2011; 187(6):3111–3120.
144. Lwin T, Melton SD, Genta RM. Eosinophilic gastritis: histopathological characterization and quantification of the normal gastric eosinophil content. *Mod Pathol.* 2011; 24(4):556–563.
145. DeBrosse CW, Case JW, Putnam PE, Collins MH, Rothenberg ME. Quantity and distribution of eosinophils in the gastrointestinal tract of children. *Pediatr Dev Pathol.* 2006;9(3):210–218.
146. Jimenez-Rivera C, Ngan B, Jackson R, Ahmed N. Gastric pseudopolyps in eosinophilic gastroenteritis. *J Pediatr Gastroenterol Nutr.* 2005;40(1):83–86.
147. Prussin C. Eosinophilic gastroenteritis and related eosinophilic disorders. *Gastroenterol Clin North Am.* 2014;43(2):317–327.
148. Ammoury RF, Rosenman MB, Roettcher D, Gupta SK. Incidental gastric eosinophils in patients with eosinophilic esophagitis: do they matter? *J Pediatr Gastroenterol Nutr.* 2010;51(6):723–726.
149. Zhang L, Duan L, Ding S, et al. Eosinophilic gastroenteritis: clinical manifestations and morphological characteristics, a retrospective study of 42 patients. *Scand J Gastroenterol.* 2011;46(9):1074–1080.
150. Gonsalves N, Doerfler B, Yang G, Hiro I. A prospective clinical trial of six food elimination diet or elemental diet in the treatment of adults with eosinophilic gastroenteritis. *Gastroenterology.* 2009;2009(136):A20.
151. Tan AC, Kruimel JW, Naber TH. Eosinophilic gastroenteritis treated with non-enteric-coated budesonide tablets. *Eur J Gastroenterol Hepatol.* 2001;13(4):425–427.
152. Siewert E, Lammert F, Koppitz P, Schmidt T, Matern S. Eosinophilic gastroenteritis with severe protein-losing enteropathy: successful treatment with budesonide. *Dig Liver Dis.* 2006;38(1):55–59.
153. Kim YJ, Prussin C, Martin B, et al. Rebound eosinophilia after treatment of hypereosinophilic syndrome and eosinophilic gastroenteritis with monoclonal anti-IL-5 antibody SCH55700. *J Allergy Clin Immunol.* 2004;114(6):1449–1455.
154. Laviolette M, Gossage DL, Gauvreau G, et al. Effects of benralizumab on airway eosinophils in asthmatic patients with sputum eosinophilia. *J Allergy Clin Immunol.* 2013;132(5):1086–1096, e1085.
155. Foroughi S, Foster B, Kim N, et al. Anti-IgE treatment of eosinophil-associated gastrointestinal disorders. *J Allergy Clin Immun.* 2007;120(3):594–601.
156. Daikh BE, Ryan CK, Schwartz RH. Montelukast reduces peripheral blood eosinophilia but not tissue eosinophilia or symptoms in a patient with eosinophilic gastroenteritis and esophageal stricture. *Annals Allergy Asthma Immunol.* 2003;90(1):23–27.
157. Van Dellen RG, Lewis JC. Oral administration of cromolyn in a patient with protein-losing enteropathy, food allergy, and eosinophilic gastroenteritis. *Mayo Clin Proc.* 1994;69(5):441–444.
158. Perez-Millan A, Martin-Lorente JL, Lopez-Morante A, Yuguero L, Saez-Royuela F. Subserosal eosinophilic gastroenteritis treated efficaciously with sodium cromoglycate. *Dig Dis Sci.* 1997;42(2):342–344.
159. Shirai T, Hashimoto D, Suzuki K, et al. Successful treatment of eosinophilic gastroenteritis with suplatast tosilate. *J Allergy Clin Immunol.* 2001;107(5):924–925.
160. Ishido K, Tanabe S, Higuchi K, et al. Eosinophilic gastroenteritis associated with giant folds. *Dig Endosc.* 2010; 22(4):312–315.
161. Nowak-Wegrzyn A, Muraro A. Food protein-induced enterocolitis syndrome. *Curr Opin Allergy Clin Immunol.* 2009;9(4):371–377.
162. Mehr S, Kakakios A, Frith K, Kemp AS. Food protein-induced enterocolitis syndrome: 16-year experience. *Pediatrics.* 2009;123(3):e459–464.
163. Guajardo J, Plotnick L, Fende J, Collins M, Putnam P, Rothenberg M. Eosinophil-associated gastrointestinal disorders: a World-Wide-Web based registry. *J Pediatrics.* 2002;141(4):576–581.

164. Klein NC, Hargrove RL, Sleisenger MH, Jeffries GH. Eosinophilic gastroenteritis. *Medicine (Baltimore).* 1970; 49(4):299–319.
165. Clouse RE, Alpers DH, Hockenbery DM, DeSchryver-Kecskemeti K. Pericrypt eosinophilic enterocolitis and chronic diarrhea. *Gastroenterology.* 1992;103(1):168–176.
166. Shin WG, Park CH, Lee YS, et al. Eosinophilic enteritis presenting as intussusception in adult. *Korean J Intern Med.* 2007;22(1):13–17.
167. Box JC, Tucker J, Watne AL, Lucas G. Eosinophilic colitis presenting as a left-sided colocolonic intussusception with secondary large bowel obstruction: an uncommon entity with a rare presentation. *Am Surg.* 1997;63(8): 741–743.
168. Ong GY, Hsu CC, Changchien CS, Lu SN, Huang SC. Eosinophilic gastroenteritis involving the distal small intestine and proximal colon. *Chang Gung Med J.* 2002; 25(1):56–61.
169. Friedberg JW, Frankenburg FR, Burk J, Johnson W. Clozapine-caused eosinophilic colitis. *Ann Clin Psychiatry.* 1995;7(2):97–98.
170. Anttila VJ, Valtonen M. Carbamazepine-induced eosinophilic colitis. *Epilepsia.* 1992;33(1):119–121.
171. Lange P, Oun H, Fuller S, Turney JH. Eosinophilic colitis due to rifampicin. *Lancet.* 1994;344(8932):1296–1297.
172. Bridges AJ, Marshall JB, Diaz-Arias AA. Acute eosinophilic colitis and hypersensitivity reaction associated with naproxen therapy. *Am J Med.* 1990;89(4):526–527.
173. Jimenez-Saenz M, Gonzalez-Campora R, Linares-Santiago E, Herrerias-Gutierrez JM. Bleeding colonic ulcer and eosinophilic colitis: a rare complication of nonsteroidal anti-inflammatory drugs. *J Clin Gastroenterol.* 2006; 40(1):84–85.
174. Saeed SA, Integlia MJ, Pleskow RG, et al. Tacrolimus-associated eosinophilic gastroenterocolitis in pediatric liver transplant recipients: role of potential food allergies in pathogenesis. *Pediatr Transplant.* 2006;10(6):730–735.
175. Chisholm JC, Jr., Martin HI. Eosinophilic gastroenteritis with rectal involvement: case report and a review of literature. *J Natl Med Assoc.* 1981;73(8):749–753.
176. Rubio CA. A method for the detection of eosinophilic granulocytes in colonoscopic biopsies from IBD patients. *Pathol Res Pract.* 2003;199(3):145–150.
177. Barbie DA, Mangi AA, Lauwers GY. Eosinophilic gastroenteritis associated with systemic lupus erythematosus. *J Clin Gastroenterol.* 2004;38(10):883–886.
178. Ashida T, Shimada T, Kawanishi K, Miyatake J, Kanamaru A. Eosinophilic colitis in a patient with acute myeloid leukemia after allogeneic bone marrow transplantation. *Int J Hematol.* 2003;78(1):76–78.
179. Inamura H, Kashiwase Y, Morioka J, Suzuki K, Igarashi Y, Kurosawa M. Accumulation of mast cells in the interstitium of eosinophilic colitis. *Allergol Immunopathol.* 2006;34(5):228–230.
180. Suzuki J, Kawasaki Y, Nozawa R, et al. Oral disodium cromoglycate and ketotifen for a patient with eosinophilic gastroenteritis, food allergy and protein-losing enteropathy. *Asian Pac J Allergy Immunol.* 2003;21(3): 193–197.
181. Melamed I, Feanny SJ, Sherman PM, Roifman CM. Benefit of ketotifen in patients with eosinophilic gastroenteritis. *Am J Med.* 1991;90(3):310–314.
182. Stein ML, Collins MH, Villanueva JM, et al. Anti-IL-5 (mepolizumab) therapy for eosinophilic esophagitis. *J Allergy Clin Immunol.* 2006;118(6):1312–1319.
183. Nowak-Wegrzyn A, Sampson HA, Wood RA, Sicherer SH. Food protein-induced enterocolitis syndrome caused by solid food proteins. *Pediatrics.* 2003;111(4, pt 1): 829–835.
184. Powell GK. Food protein-induced enterocolitis of infancy: differential diagnosis and management. *Compr Ther.* 1986;12(2):28–37.
185. Katz Y, Goldberg MR, Rajuan N, Cohen A, Leshno M. The prevalence and natural course of food protein-induced enterocolitis syndrome to cow's milk: a large-scale, prospective population-based study. *J Allergy Clin Immunol.* 2011;127(3):647–653 e641–643.
186. Sopo SM, Giorgio V, Dello Iacono I, Novembre E, Mori F, Onesimo R. A multicentre retrospective study of 66 Italian children with food protein-induced enterocolitis syndrome: different management for different phenotypes. *Clin Exp Allergy.* 2012;42(8):1257–1265.
187. Ruffner MA, Ruymann K, Barni S, Cianferoni A, Brown-Whitehorn T, Spergel JM. Food protein-induced enterocolitis syndrome: insights from review of a large referral population. *J Allergy Clin Immunol Pract.* 2013; 1(4):343–349.
188. DeMeo MT, Mutlu EA, Keshavarzian A, Tobin MC. Intestinal permeation and gastrointestinal disease. *J Clin Gastroenterol.* 2002;34(4):385–396.
189. Sampson HA, Scanlon SM. Natural history of food hypersensitivity in children with atopic dermatitis. *J Pediatrics.* 1989;115(1):23–27.
190. Chung HL, Hwang JB, Park JJ, Kim SG. Expression of transforming growth factor beta1, transforming growth factor type I and II receptors, and TNF-alpha in the mucosa of the small intestine in infants with food protein-induced enterocolitis syndrome. *J Allergy Clin Immunol.* 2002;109(1):150–154.
191. Benlounes N, Candalh C, Matarazzo P, Dupont C, Heyman M. The time-course of milk antigen-induced TNF-alpha secretion differs according to the clinical symptoms in children with cow's milk allergy. *J Allergy Clin Immunol.* 1999;104(4, pt 1):863–869.
192. Jarvinen KM, Nowak-Wegrzyn A. Food protein-induced enterocolitis syndrome (FPIES): current management strategies and review of the literature. *J Allergy Clin Immunol Pract.* 2013;1(4):317–322.
193. Holbrook T, Keet CA, Frischmeyer-Guerrerio PA, Wood RA. Use of ondansetron for food protein-induced enterocolitis syndrome. *J Allergy Clin Immunol.* 2013;132(5): 1219–1220.
194. Lake AM. Allergic bowel disease. *Adolesc Med Clin.* 2004; 15(1):105–117, ix–x.

195. Lake AM. Food-induced eosinophilic proctocolitis. *J Pediatr Gastroenterol Nutr.* 2000;30(suppl):S58–S60.
196. Pittschieler K. Cow's milk protein-induced colitis in the breast-fed infant. *J Pediatr Gastroenterol Nutr.* 1990; 10(4):548–549.
197. Ravelli A, Villanacci V, Chiappa S, Bolognini S, Manenti S, Fuoti M. Dietary protein-induced proctocolitis in childhood. *Am J Gastroenterol.* 2008;103(10):2605–2612.
198. Arvola T, Ruuska T, Keranen J, Hyoty H, Salminen S, Isolauri E. Rectal bleeding in infancy: clinical, allergological, and microbiological examination. *Pediatrics.* 2006;117(4):e760–768.
199. Winter HS, Antonioli DA, Fukagawa N, Marcial M, Goldman H. Allergy-related proctocolitis in infants: diagnostic usefulness of rectal biopsy. *Mod Pathol.* 1990;3(1):5–10.
200. Hill ID. What are the sensitivity and specificity of serologic tests for celiac disease? Do sensitivity and specificity vary in different populations? *Gastroenterology.* 2005;128(4, suppl 1):S25–S32.
201. Pittschieler K, Ladinser B. Coeliac disease: screened by a new strategy. *Acta Paediatr Suppl.* 1996;412:42–45.
202. Molberg O, McAdam SN, Korner R, et al. Tissue transglutaminase selectively modifies gliadin peptides that are recognized by gut-derived T cells in celiac disease. *Nat Med.* 1998;4(6):713–717.
203. Hill ID, Dirks MH, Liptak GS, et al. Guideline for the diagnosis and treatment of celiac disease in children: recommendations of the North American Society for Pediatric Gastroenterology, Hepatology and Nutrition. *J Pediatr Gastroenterol Nutr.* 2005;40(1):1–19.
204. Schuppan D, Dieterich W. Pathogenesis, epidemiology, and clinical manifestations of celiac disease in adults. *UpToDate.* 2014. http://www.uptodate.com/home/index.html. Accessed February 1, 2015.

12

Environmental and Occupational Allergies

Kristin Schmidlin and Jonathan A. Bernstein

INTRODUCTION

Airborne allergens encountered in the environmental and occupational setting are a major cause of allergic disease, including rhinitis and asthma. Environmental allergens can be divided into indoor domestic allergens, which include arthropod, mammalian, and fungal allergens, and outdoor allergens, such as pollens and molds. Allergens encountered in the workplace can elicit rhinitis symptoms either through allergic sensitization secondary to an immune-mediated response, or based on a non-immune-mediated, irritant response. There are countless exposures in the workplace that may be sensitizing or irritating agents, including but not limited to pesticides, cleaning products, and paint fumes.

The prevalence of allergic sensitization is increasing worldwide, both in developed and developing countries, and this has become a global public health issue in the recent years.[1] For example, in the United States alone, the percentage of people aged 6 years and older with at least one sensitization to inhalant allergens has reached nearly 50%, based on the results from the National Health and Nutrition Examination Survey (NHANES) 2005–2006.[2] The reasons behind this growing prevalence of allergic sensitization are not well elucidated, but it is thought to be a multifactorial process, and in part related to "westernization" of the world.[3]

Environmental and occupational allergies are significant causes of morbidity resulting in increased medical costs, reduced work productivity, and lost school days in patients suffering from these diseases.[4] Although allergic rhinitis (AR) is typically considered a benign disease, it is known to significantly affect patients' quality of life adversely, and has been associated with conditions such as headaches, cognitive impairment, fatigue, and sleep disturbances.[4] Medical costs related to allergic diseases are substantial and significantly contribute to the economic burden of health care on society. It is estimated that the cost of AR, including loss of productivity, in the United States in 2002 totaled $11.58 billion.[5] Additionally, the cost of asthma in the United States is estimated to be $14 billion annually.[6]

This chapter discusses the different classifications of environmental and occupational allergies, including environmental and occupational causes of respiratory health problems. Additionally, the epidemiology, underlying mechanisms causing disease, and the genetic and environmental determinants associated with these conditions are reviewed. The final part of this chapter focuses on the diagnosis, assessment, management, and prevention of environmental and occupational allergies.

> Allergic sensitization is an increasing issue worldwide and can be due to exposures encountered in the outdoor or indoor environment, including the workplace.

DEFINITIONS AND CLASSIFICATION

There are numerous allergens that cause environmental and occupational allergies. AR is the most common manifestation of atopic disease and is due to immunoglobulin E (IgE)-mediated inflammation of the nasal mucosa.[7] It is characterized by one or more of the following symptoms: nasal congestion, anterior or posterior rhinorrhea, sneezing, and nasal itching.[8] Additionally, people with environmental and occupational allergies can experience ocular, ear, throat, and respiratory symptoms, either in combination with rhinitis or each other, or as separate disease processes.

Environmental and occupational allergies can be divided into different classifications based on the type of aeroallergen sensitization or on the temporal relationship of symptoms to triggers, either in relation to seasonal exposures or location-specific exposures. Classically, AR has been categorized as either seasonal or perennial allergic rhinitis based on the type of aeroallergen sensitization involved.[9] More recently, an international working group released the Allergic Rhinitis and Its Impact on Asthma (ARIA) guidelines that proposed replacing the terms *seasonal* and *perennial* allergic rhinitis with the terms *intermittent* (symptoms that are present less than 4 days a week or for less than 4 weeks) and *persistent* (more than 4 days a week and for more than 4 weeks) allergic rhinitis.[10] The ARIA guidelines indicate that seasonal and perennial may not be the best descriptors for allergic disease for several reasons, including the fact that some pollens and molds can be both seasonal and perennial allergens based on geographic location.[4,11] For the purposes of this book chapter, the terms *seasonal* and *perennial* AR will continue to be used since the classification system proposed in the ARIA guidelines has not yet been uniformly agreed upon.

Allergic Rhinitis

Outdoor environmental aeroallergens, including tree pollen, grass pollen, weed pollen, and fungal spores are responsible for the symptoms of seasonal allergic rhinitis (SAR). By definition, SAR occurs during the season of active pollination of the inciting allergens; symptoms occur secondary to release of bioactive mediators after IgE specific to the pollen antigen cross-links high-affinity IgE receptors (FcεRI) on mast cells and basophils. In general, in most of the United States, trees pollinate in the spring, grass pollinates from late spring to early summer, and weeds pollinate from late summer and early fall. However, these pollination seasons can be longer and vary between different geographic regions and climate conditions.[12]

Flowering trees (also known as angiosperms) are typically more allergenic than seed-bearing trees (also known as gymnosperms).[13] Tree pollens range from 20 to 50 μm in size while weed pollens typically range in size from 10 to 20 μm and grass pollen averages around 50 μm in size.

Perennial allergic rhinitis (PAR) is characterized by year-round symptoms of rhinitis, with symptoms that occur during at least 9 months out of the year.[14] Symptoms are caused by an IgE-mediated immune response to perennial allergens. The aeroallergens implicated in PAR are primarily from indoor and domestic environments, and include house-dust mites, cockroaches, pets, rodents, and indoor mold spores.

House-dust mites are microscopic arachnids that feed on human and animal dander (shed skin). They are found in bedding, upholstery, carpeting, and products with woven or stuffed material, including stuffed animals.[13] House-dust mites thrive in warm, humid environments because they directly absorb water from the air and require anywhere from 55% to 75% humidity to survive, depending on the ambient temperature.[3] The 2 main species associated with PAR are *Dermatophagoides farinae* and *Dermatophagoides pteronyssinus*. Their main allergens, Der f 1 and Der p 1, are primarily contained in the mite's gut and fecal particles that range in size from 10 to 20 μm. Given that these allergens frequently attach to larger airborne particles, they tend to settle quickly from the air onto surfaces such as bedding and flooring.[15]

Cockroaches are another source of indoor allergen contributing to PAR symptoms. The two main species encountered in the United States are *Blatella germanica* (German cockroach) and *Periplaneta americana* (American cockroach); Oriental cockroach (*Blatta orientalis*) can also be found in regions of the United States but less information is available regarding sensitization prevalence. Cockroaches feed on discarded human food items and are attracted to densely populated areas, including multifamily homes and apartment complexes. The major allergens implicated in causing allergic symptoms are Bla g 1, Bla g 2, and Per a 1, which are isolated from the body, feces, saliva, and secretions of the cockroach. Similar to house-dust mites, cockroach allergens tend to be contained in larger particles (10–40 μm), and are therefore found in settled dust rather than suspended in ambient air. Cockroach sensitization is extremely prevalent in individuals living in the inner city, and it is estimated that nearly 40% of urban children are sensitized to cockroach allergens.[16] Cockroach sensitization has also been shown to play an essential role in asthma severity and has been associated with increased asthma morbidity among asthmatic children with evidence of elevated cockroach antigen levels in their homes.[17]

Mammalian pets are a major source of indoor allergens that can lead to PAR. It is estimated that at least two-thirds of the US population has at least one pet dog or cat and many homes have multiple animals. The primary dog allergen is Fel d 1, while Can f 1 is the major cat allergen that cause allergic disease. Both allergens are isolated from the animals' saliva, dander, and hair and in contrast to mite and roach allergens, are relatively small in size (<10 μm), enabling them to remain dispersed in ambient air.[18,19] The Fel d 1 is very stable and can take several months to degrade once the primary source of allergen has been removed from the home. Additionally, it can be detected in dust samples taken from homes without cats, indicating that the allergen can be passively transferred on shoes and clothing to other environments leading to symptoms in non-cat–owning but sensitized subjects.[19,20]

Rodents, including mice and rats, are important sources of allergens contributing to PAR, especially among inner-city populations. The main mouse allergens are Mus m 1 and Mus m 2, which are found in mouse urine, dander, and hair follicles. Mouse urine is easily aerosolized and because it is also contained in a small particle (<10 μm), it can remain suspended in the ambient air for long periods of time.[21]

Mold species can be both seasonal and perennial allergens depending on climate and geographic location. Outdoor mold spores typically peak in mid-summer and disappear after the first frost in regions with cold winter seasons. Mold spores are smaller than pollen grains, ranging anywhere from 2 to 50 μm in size. The small particle size of fungal spores allows them to be deposited throughout the respiratory tract, from the upper airways all the way down to the small alveoli of the lungs, resulting in significant upper and lower respiratory symptoms.[22] The most common indoor molds implicated in allergic sensitization include *Aspergillus* and *Penicillium*. *Alternaria* is a common outdoor mold that can also be found indoors especially if windows are left open. Fungal spores thrive in moist, humid environments, and therefore it is not surprising that they are often found in damp basements or in homes with water damage. (See Chapter 2 for additional discussion of allergen structure and components.)

Occupational Rhinitis

Occupational rhinitis (OR) falls into the category of "work-related rhinitis" (WRR) along with work-exacerbated rhinitis (WER). OR is defined as "an inflammatory disease of the nose, characterized by intermittent or persistent symptoms of nasal congestion, sneezing, rhinorrhea, and itching, and/or variable nasal airflow limitation with or without hypersecretion due to causes and conditions attributable to a particular work environment and not related to stimuli encountered outside the workplace."[23] OR commonly coexists with occupational asthma (OA), and it is thought that for a given suspected causal agent, the development of OR may precede the development of OA.[24] OR can be further divided into allergic and nonallergic categories.

Allergic OR is caused by an immunologically mediated hypersensitivity reaction that occurs after a latency period. IgE-mediated immune reactions typically occur with high-molecular-weight (HMW) agents, although some low-molecular-weight (LMW) agents such as trimellitic anhydride (TMA) and platinum salts have also been implicated as sensitizing agents.[25] There are also non-IgE, immune-mediated reactions that can occur when LMW agents act as haptens, but this mechanism has not been fully characterized to date.[23] IgE-mediated sensitization to protein allergens in the workplace, including flour, laboratory animals, animal products, and other substances, has also been implicated in the development of allergic OR.[4,26]

Nonallergic OR, or irritant-induced OR, is a non-immune–mediated response that is caused by irritant exposures and does not require a latency period before symptoms develop. Irritant exposures that can lead to OR include grain dust constituents, flour dust, fuel oil ash, volatile organic compounds, fumes, vapors, and ozone, all of which can elicit neutrophilic inflammation of the nasal mucosa.[4,27] Symptoms of nonallergic OR may be present only during exposure to irritants at work, or they can be persistent both inside and outside the workplace.[23] The term *corrosive rhinitis* has been used to describe a severe form of irritant-induced OR and is characterized by permanent inflammation of the nasal mucosa after exposure to high concentrations of corrosive chemicals.[28]

Another disorder that falls into the nonallergic OR spectrum is reactive upper airways dysfunction syndrome (RUDS), which can occur when an individual is exposed to high concentrations of irritant compounds leading to transient or persistent symptoms of rhinitis and is analogous to RADS (reactive airways dysfunction syndrome) in the lower respiratory tract.[29] RUDS (also referred to as irritant-induced rhinitis) can occur after a single chemical exposure or after multiple exposures to high concentrations of compounds, such as chlorine, smoke, or certain air pollutants.[30] Due to lack of knowledge on the natural history and pathogenesis of RUDS, this condition remains poorly defined but should be considered when the clinical history is consistent with an acute toxic exposure leading to rhinitis symptoms.

Work-exacerbated rhinitis (WER) is another type of WRR and is defined as "pre-existing or concurrent allergic or non-allergic rhinitis that is worsened by workplace exposures."[28] WER is not caused by the work environment, as is the case with OR, but instead, symptoms are aggravated by conditions at work, including exposures to irritant agents, physical factors such as cold temperatures, strong odors, and second-hand smoke exposure.[23] IgE-mediated sensitization to occupational agents is typically not detected in cases of WER; therefore, this condition is thought to be a type of nonallergic work-related rhinitis.[23]

Occupational Asthma

Occupational asthma (OA) includes work-related asthma (WRA) and work-exacerbated asthma (WEA). OA is defined as "a disease with variable airflow limitations and/or hyperresponsiveness and/or inflammation due to causes and conditions attributable to a particular occupational environment and not to stimuli encountered outside the workplace."[31] OA can be further classified into sensitizer-induced and nonsensitizing, irritant-induced OA, depending on the mechanism through which disease is elicited.[32]

Sensitizer-induced OA is characterized by a latency period, typically of 1 to 3 years, during which time workers are exposed to either HMW or LMW agents and become sensitized.[33] Once the workers develop allergen-specific IgE, with continued exposure they are at increased risk of developing rhinitis and asthma. However, many LMW chemicals act as irritants and elicit respiratory symptoms through less well-defined, non-IgE-mediated mechanisms. Frequently, occupational rhinitis (OR) precedes the development of asthma. For those LMW agents that elicit specific IgE-responses (ie, trimellitic anhydride), they act as haptens requiring conjugation with endogenous proteins to elicit a specific immune response.[34] Examples of HMW agents are plant or animal proteins (>1000 kD) and include cereals and grains, natural rubber latex, insects, enzymes, and laboratory animal allergens.[34] LMW agents (<1000 kD) that elicit specific immune responses include hexamethylene diisocyanate, trimellitic acid anhydrides, and platinum metallic salts.[35]

Irritant-induced OA is caused by exposure to chemicals and irritant agents encountered in the workplace, in the absence of sensitization. Typically, irritant-induced OA is characterized by the absence of a latency period, and asthma symptoms develop within 24 hours after exposure to a high concentration of the irritating chemical. This is a severe form of irritant-induced OA referred to as reactive airways dysfunction syndrome (RADS).[36] Clinical criteria for the diagnosis of RADS includes a documented absence of preceding respiratory complaints and the onset of symptoms after a single, specific high-exposure incident or accident involving an irritating gas, smoke, fume, or vapor that results in airway hyperresponsiveness and asthma symptoms (cough, wheezing, and dyspnea) within 24 hours, and that persist for at least 3 months. Pulmonary function tests may or may not show airflow obstruction, but methacholine challenge testing is usually positive, and other types of pulmonary disease must be ruled out.[36]

Work-exacerbated asthma (WEA) is another form of work-related asthma defined as the worsening of asthma symptoms attributable to workplace exposures. WEA occurs in patients with preexisting asthma not caused by exposure to, but aggravated by workplace conditions.[37] The different classifications of rhinitis and asthma symptoms related to occupational exposures are shown in Figure 12–1.

> AR can be divided into SAR and PAR based on the type of aeroallergen sensitization involved. OR often precedes OA. Allergic OR and OA can occur after sensitization to HMW and LMW agents. Irritant-induced OA and OR are also termed RUDS and RADS, respectively.

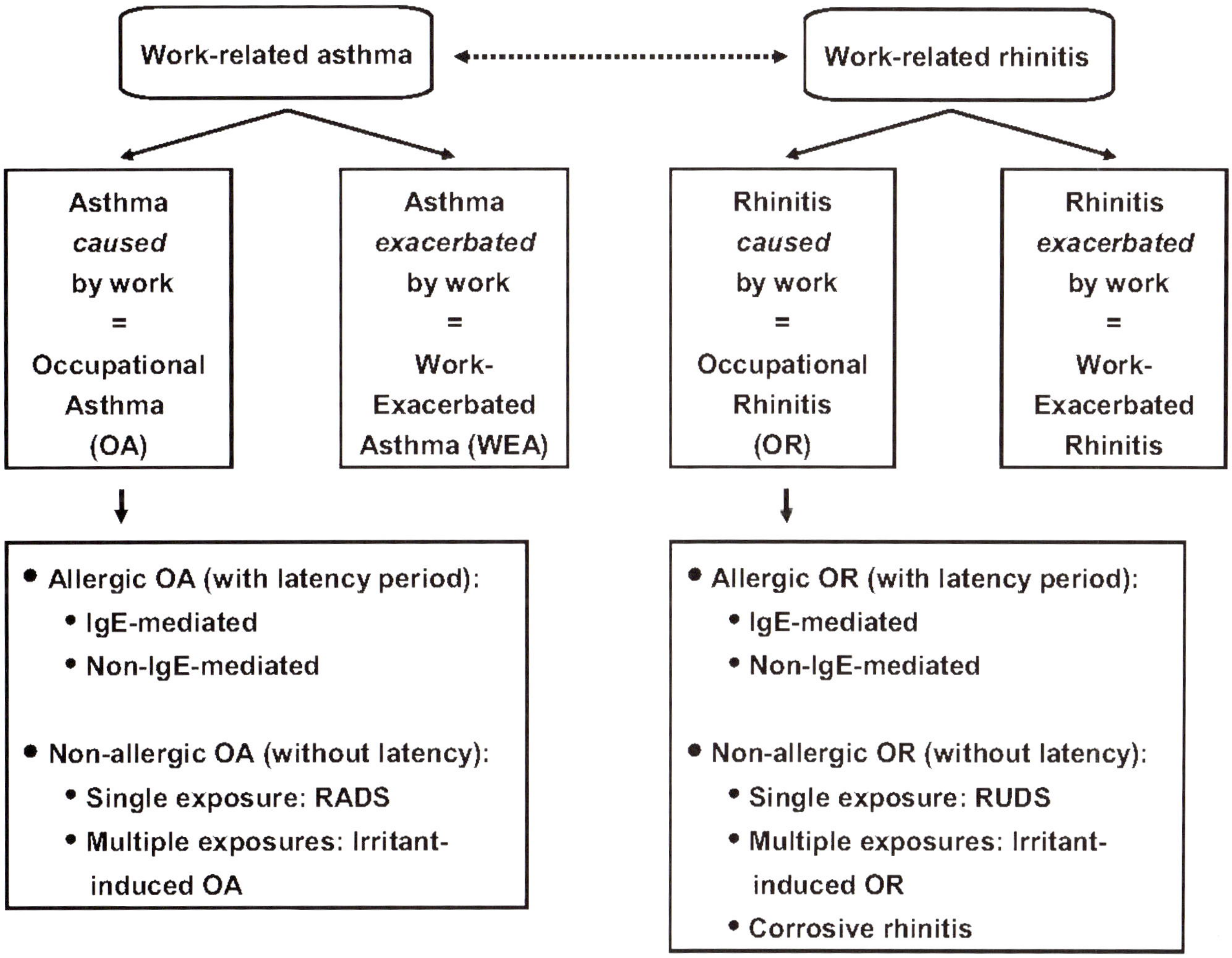

Figure 12–1. Classification of work-related upper and lower respiratory symptoms. Reprinted with a Creative Commons License from BioMed Central Ltd. Moscato G, Vandenplas O, Van Wijk RG, et al. EAACI position paper on occupational rhinitis. *Respir Res.* 2009;10(1):16.

EPIDEMIOLOGY

Allergic Rhinitis

Allergic rhinitis is a common, chronic health condition affecting up to 60 million people in the United States.[38] The prevalence of AR is estimated to range from as low as 9% to as high as 42%[39] and affects 10% to 30% of adults and up to 40% of children.[4] It is important to note that estimates of allergic rhinitis prevalence are largely based on questions referring to SAR, so the exact prevalence of AR may actually be underestimated. AR is more prevalent in individuals who are nonwhite, live in more polluted urban areas, and have a family history of allergies and atopy.[4] Additionally, AR is more common in boys than in girls during childhood, but the sex ratio becomes more equalized in adulthood, and may even be more prevalent in adult women.[4] AR tends to develop in the first few decades of life, with around 80% of cases developing before 20 years of age.[4] The prevalence of SAR appears to be increasing and is estimated to affect around 10% to 20% of the general population and accounts for 20% of all allergic rhinitis cases.[14,40] PAR comprises 40% of all cases of allergic rhinitis.[14] The prevalence of SAR is higher in children, while the prevalence of PAR is higher in adults.[41]

Occupational Rhinitis and Work-Exacerbated Rhinitis

The prevalence and incidence of OR is less well studied than allergic rhinitis and OA. However, a recent review looking at the epidemiology of OR demonstrated that the prevalence rates of OR vary depending on the types of workplace exposure.[42] When exposed to HMW agents, the prevalence rate of OR ranges from 2% to 87%.[42] Additionally, in workforces exposed to LMW agents, the prevalence of OR ranges from 3% to 48%.[42] It should be noted that prevalence data of OR depend on the methods used to diagnose the disease; therefore, the frequency of OR may actually be overestimated or underestimated depending on the diagnostic criteria (eg, patient-reported symptoms only, compared to symptoms with evidence of specific IgE antibodies). Up to 92% of patients with OA also report OR.[43] There appears to be a temporal relationship of OR with OA induced by HMW agents as rhinitis symptoms precede lower respiratory symptoms in 20% to 78% of affected individuals.[43] The prevalence of work-exacerbated rhinitis is not known, but it appears to be high based on epidemiologic surveys of work-related nasal symptoms, where there is no evidence of IgE sensitization in symptomatic patients.[23]

Risk factors for developing OR include the level of exposure, atopy, and possibly smoke exposure. There is a dose-response gradient between the level of exposure and IgE-mediated sensitization for various HMW agents, including laboratory animals, wheat, flour, and insects.[44–47] Additionally, the presence of atopy has been associated with an increased risk of IgE-mediated sensitization to various HMW agents.[42] Conversely, studies have not consistently demonstrated an association between atopy and OR secondary to LMW agents.[42]

Occupational Asthma and Work-Exacerbated Asthma

The prevalence and incidence of OA are not well defined, as there are differing definitions and diagnostic criteria used to define this disease. Additionally, the development of disease depends on numerous variables, including the type of exposure, duration of exposure, geographic location, and varying environmental conditions. However, it is estimated that up to 15% to 25% of all new adult-onset asthma diagnoses begin in the workplace.[48] It is important to note that using population-based studies and surveillance data to determine the prevalence of disease may actually underestimate OA as individuals who develop symptoms may leave the workplace without reporting the disease referred to as the "healthy worker effect" leading to "survivor bias." Based on a large prospective study, the incidence of OA appears to be 250 to 300 cases per million people per year.[49] It is estimated that irritant-induced asthma accounts for 15% to 22% of all OA cases.[50] Risk factors for developing OA include a history of a large acute inhalational event (consistent with a history of RADS), high levels of exposure to sensitizing agents, and exposure to HMW agents.[51] Occupations with the highest risk of OA include printing, woodworking, construction, metal work, nursing, agriculture and forestry, industrial cleaning, plastic work, and electrical processing.[52] It is estimated that approximately 15% to 20% of all adult-onset asthmatic patients have WEA.[53] Risk factors for developing WEA include increased age, exposure to airborne dust, temperature fluctuations, poor indoor air quality, physically demanding work, and working with chemicals and fumes.[53]

> AR affects up to 42% of the population. The prevalence of OR is dependent on the type workplace exposure but can be as high as 87% with HMW agents and 48% with LMW agents. Up to 25% of all adult-onset asthma diagnoses begin in the workplace.

MECHANISMS

Allergic Rhinitis

The mechanism for seasonal and perennial allergic rhinitis is a type 1 hypersensitivity immune response resulting in the production of specific IgE antibody to environmental allergens and involves type 2 helper (TH2) T lymphocytes. Exposure to aeroallergens over time results in sensitization, which occurs when antigen is processed by antigen-presenting cells in the nasal mucosa and then presented by major histocompatibility complex (MHC) class II molecules to $CD4^+$ T cells in regional lymph nodes. This interaction, along with costimulatory signals, results in T cells differentiating into TH2 cells. The cytokines produced by TH2 cells (IL-3, IL-4, IL-13, IL-5, GM-CSF) promote B-cell isotype switching resulting in aeroallergen-specific IgE production, mast call proliferation and infiltration into the nasal mucosa, and eosinophilic infiltration into nasal mucosa and epithelium.[4]

An early and late-phase response may be involved in the development of nasal symptoms and inflammation. The early, immediate response to allergen exposure occurs within 5 to 30 minutes secondary to IgE-mediated mast cell activation resulting in the typical nasal symptoms of allergic rhinitis (rhinorrhea, nasal congestion, and sneezing). Mast cell activation results in the release of pre-formed mediators, including histamine, tryptase, chymase, kininogenase, heparin, and other enzymes and newly formed mediators such as prostaglandin D2 and cysteinyl leukotrienes (CysLTs) synthesized by not only mast cells but also by eosinophils, basophils, and macrophages.[54–56] Release of these mediators results in mucus hypersecretion, increased vascular permeability, and vasodilation, leading to rhinorrhea, nasal obstruction, and mucosal hypertrophy.[57] Sensory nerves are also stimulated and convey sensations of nasal itch and congestion, which lead to sneezing.[4] The late-phase response occurs in 60% to 70% of individuals, which is characterized by eosinophil, basophil, and TH2 cell infiltration into the nasal mucosa.[58] This response typically occurs 4 to 8 hours after allergen exposure and is likely to be enhanced by the mediators and cytokines released during the immediate allergic response. Mediators of the late phase reaction include leukotrienes, histamine, and IL-5; histamine increases without a change in tryptase level, indicating that the source of these late phase response mediators may be basophils rather than a secondary degranulation of resident mast cells.[59] It is thought that eosinophil products, such as major basic protein and hypohalides, damage the nasal epithelium, which results in a chronic inflammatory response and leads to tissue damage.[60]

Occupational Rhinitis and Work-Exacerbated Rhinitis

The mechanism leading to symptoms in OR is also IgE mediated for HMW agents and some LMW agents. After a latency period and repeat exposure to the offending agent, symptoms of rhinitis develop through mast cell activation and release of inflammatory bioactive mediators. Non-IgE-mediated OR develops for many LMW agents, including isocyanates, persulfate salts, and wood dusts.[23] The mechanisms involved in the development of nonallergic OR, including irritant-induced OR, RUDS, and corrosive OR, are currently not well defined but may involve neurogenic pathways that lead to increased parasympathetic responses. It has been demonstrated that a number of chemical irritants, and mechanical or thermal stimuli, can activate transient response potential (TRP) ion channels leading to activation of nociceptive nerves and release of neuropeptides like substance P and calcitonin gene-related peptides (CGRP) that can cause mast cell activation.[61] The mechanisms involved in the development of work-exacerbated rhinitis have not been thoroughly investigated at this time but likely involve neurogenic mechanisms as well.[23]

Occupational Asthma and Work-Exacerbated Asthma

Mechanisms involved in the development of OA appear to be similar to those involved in non-OA.[62] An IgE-dependent mechanism associated with HMW and some LMW sensitizing agents has been implicated in many cases of OA.[62] The ensuing inflammatory responses leading to an early and late airway response result in airway infiltration of inflammatory cells, especially eosinophils, activation of lymphocytes, and airway remodeling secondary to collagen deposition in the subbasement membrane.[63]

> AR and some cases of allergic OR and OA are due to a type I hypersensitivity reaction in which specific IgE antibody to allergens are produced leading to sensitization.

GENETICS

Allergic Rhinitis

The development of AR depends on both genetic and environmental factors. Studies of disease prevalence among monozygotic and dizygotic twins show a 45% to 60% concordance rate in the development of AR among monozygotic twins and a 25% concordance rate in dizygotic twins, the latter of which approaches the prevalence rate in the general population.[58] The genes involved in the development of AR have been less studied compared to other allergic diseases such as asthma and atopic dermatitis. However, there have been a few genome-wide association studies (GWAS) and single nucleotide polymorphisms (SNPs) studies in patients with allergic rhinitis. Several studies have identified a connection between AR and regions of chromosomes 2, 3, 4, and 9.[64] Additionally, studies of SNPs have linked polymorphisms of certain transcription factors, cytokines, and their receptors, including GATA3, IL-13, IL-18, and IL-4 genes, to AR.[58,65] Another study demonstrated that a specific polymorphism involving the inducible T-cell tyrosine kinase (ITK) in $CD4^+$ T-cells is a risk factor for SAR.[66] Finally, a study involving Egyptian atopic individuals showed an association between an interferon-gamma gene polymorphism and atopic disease.[67] Of note, the results of these studies need to be interpreted cautiously due to their small sample sizes, differing inclusion criteria, and lack of reproducibility with other studies, and therefore are not generalizable to all populations.

Occupational Rhinitis and Work-Exacerbated Rhinitis

There is a paucity of studies regarding the genes involved in the development of OR and WER. More research is therefore required to identify potential genetic associations for these occupational conditions.

Occupational Asthma and Work-Exacerbated Asthma

Genetic associations have been identified in patients with OA. An association between the major histocompatibility complex (MHC) genes on chromosome 6p that encode HLA class II molecules and OA has been established.[52] One study involving patients with OA induced by rat lipocalin allergens demonstrated that 40% of patients express an HLA-DRβ1*07 phenotype.[68] There is also an association between individuals sensitized to ammonium hexachloroplatinate (ACP) and the HLA-DR3 phenotype, particularly among cases with low exposures to ACP.[69] Associations between HLA phenotype and sensitization to complex platinum salts and diisocyanates have also been described.[52] The HLA class II alleles HLA-DQA1*0104 and HLA-DQB1*0503 are significantly increased in workers with diisocyanate asthma.[70] Another gene that is potentially implicated in OA is glutathione S-transferase (GST), which is critical in protecting cells from oxidative stress products; certain GST polymorphisms are protective against isocyanate-induced OA.[71] Furthermore, workers with *N*-acetyltransferase slow acetylator genotypes are at increased risk for toluene diisocyanate (TDI)–induced asthma.[72] More recently, polymorphisms of IL-4RA, CD14, IL-13, and TNFA genes have been associated with development of isocyanate-induced OA.[70,73] There have not been any genetic studies involving WEA to date, but given its increased recognition as a variant of OA, future studies are warranted.

> The development of allergies depends on genetic and environmental factors. Polymorphisms of certain transcription factors, cytokines, and cytokine receptors have been identified in patients with AR. Specific HLA phenotypes have also been implicated in the development of OA.

ENVIRONMENTAL AND OCCUPATIONAL CAUSES OF RESPIRATORY HEALTH PROBLEMS

Sensitizing agents that are implicated in OR and OA can be divided into HMW compounds and LMW compounds based on their molecular weights. HMW compounds act as complete antigens to induce an immunologic response, whereas, LMW agents likely act as haptens to elicit an immune response.[23] Of the approximately 400 known causes of OA, most are HMW protein sensitizers.[74] Fewer than 30 reactive chemicals or LMW agents have been proven to cause OA.[74] Specific agents known to cause OR and/or OA are listed in Table 12–1. The most common HMW agents involved in OR and OA include cereals and flour, laboratory animals, shellfish allergen, natural rubber latex, plant- and animal-derived enzymes,

Table 12-1. Agents That Cause Occupational Rhinitis and Occupational Asthma

	Agent	Occupation at Risk of Exposure
High-molecular-weight agents	Baking flour	Bakers
	Cereals	Bakers, harbor workers
	Animal allergens	Laboratory workers, veterinary workers, farmers
	Insect antigens	Farmers, beekeepers
	Proteolytic enzymes	Detergent manufacturers
	Natural rubber latex	Health-care workers, latex glove manufacturers
Low-molecular-weight agents	Anhydrides	Plastic manufacturers, epoxy resin workers
	Metals	Welders, refinery workers
	Diisocyantes	Plastic and spray paint manufacturers
	Platinum salts	Refinery workers
	Cleaning agents	Custodians, domestic cleaners
	Wood dusts	Carpenters, wood workers
	Pesticides	Farmers
	Reactive dyes	Hairdressers, food industry workers, textile workers

insects and mites, and grain dust.[35,42] The most commonly implicated LMW chemicals in the development of disease include acid anhydrides, metals, diisocyanates, cleaning agents, wood dust, drugs, and chemicals.[35,42] Nonsensitizing agents capable of causing RADS and WEA are listed in Table 12–2.

> HMW agents typically lead to allergic sensitization through an IgE-mediated immune response, whereas LMW agents induce disease through non-IgE–dependent mechanisms.

DIFFERENTIAL DIAGNOSIS

The differential diagnosis of AR and OR is broad and includes nonallergic rhinitis, mixed rhinitis, WER, drug-induced rhinitis, nasal polyposis, and cerebral spinal fluid (CSF) rhinorrhea. Nonallergic rhinitis is defined as periodic or year-round symptoms of rhinitis that are not the result of an IgE-mediated immunologic response. Nonallergic rhinitis includes vasomotor rhinitis, infectious rhinitis, and nonallergic rhinitis with eosinophilia (NARES). Individuals with vasomotor rhinitis can experience rhinorrhea related to cholinergic glandular secretory activity or nasal congestion due to nociceptive neurons that have heightened sensitivity to innocuous stimuli.[4] Typical triggers for vasomotor rhinitis include temperature or barometric changes, tobacco smoke, dust, strong odors, and perfumes. Infectious rhinitis, either secondary to viral infection or acute or chronic bacterial rhinosinusitis, can often be mistaken for AR; however, time course and diagnostic studies can help distinguish between the two diseases. Patients with NARES have perennial rhinitis symptoms and the presence of nasal eosinophils on nasal smear but do not demonstrate the positive skin testing or specific IgE antibodies typically seen with AR. Additional findings on nasal mucosal biopsies of patients with NARES include mast cells with bound IgE and elevated tryptase, which is also seen in patients with AR.[75] Mixed rhinitis is diagnosed in individuals who have chronic rhinitis with evidence of IgE-mediated responses and symptoms due to both allergic and nonallergic triggers.[38] Drug-induced rhinitis can result in nasal congestion with or without rhinorrhea. Medications most commonly implicated in drug-induced rhinitis include ACE inhibitors,[76] β-blockers,[4] α-receptor antagonists,[77] and phosphodiesterase-5-selective inhibitors.[78] Nasal polyposis can be seen in up to 10% to 15% of patients with allergic rhinitis and must be excluded in patients presenting with nasal obstruction and

Table 12–2. Common Causes of Irritant-Induced Upper and Lower Respiratory Symptoms

Agent	Occupation at Risk of Exposure
Cleaning agents (bleach, chlorine, ammonia)	Custodians and domestic cleaners
Cooking vapors	Food preparation workers
Glutaraldehyde, formaldehyde	Health-care workers
Solvent vapors, paint fumes	Printers and painters
Diesel exhaust	Truck drivers and miners
Asphalt vapors	Roofers and pavers
Wood dust	Carpenters and woodworkers
Smoke	Firefighters
Sulfur dioxide	Refinery workers and power plant workers
Chemical vapors, volatile vapors	Laboratory workers and scientists

Source: Adapted from Shusterman D. Occupational irritant and allergic rhinitis. *Curr Allergy Asthma Rep.* 2014;14(4):425.

anosmia.[79] CSF rhinorrhea, which is clear rhinorrhea resulting from a CSF leak that may occur after head trauma or surgery, is also included in the differential for allergic rhinitis.[80]

The differential diagnosis of OA and WEA includes preexisting asthma and allergic asthma due to non-work–related allergens or exposures. However, preexisting asthma does not preclude the diagnosis of OA.[81] Additionally, WEA must be distinguished from OA. Other diseases that mimic asthma symptoms need to be ruled out when considering a diagnosis of OA or WEA. This includes chronic obstructive lung disease (COPD), vocal cord dysfunction (VCD), gastroesophageal reflux disease (GERD), bronchiolitis obliterans, and eosinophilic bronchitis. In patients with VCD, the vocal cords adduct inappropriately, usually during inspiration, which can lead to airway obstruction, wheezing (inspiratory), and stridor.[82] It can be difficult to distinguish VCD from OA as VCD can also occur after an irritant exposure.[83] Additionally, a spectrum of clinical responses beside asthma can occur after irritant exposures, including an enhanced cough reflex[84] and increased awareness of irritants,[85] and must be excluded when diagnosing OA or WEA. The term *sensory hyperreactivity* has been used to describe patients with upper airway symptoms triggered by irritating chemicals and exhibit increased capsaicin-induced cough sensitivity, but no airway hyper-responsiveness.[86] It is crucial to accurately diagnose OA as it can lead to health impairment, loss of work, and worsening socioeconomic status.[87]

> AR and OR must be distinguished from other types of rhinitis, including nonallergic rhinitis. OA and WEA must be differentiated from preexisting asthma and other mimickers of asthma.

DIAGNOSTIC APPROACH AND ASSESSMENT

Allergic Rhinitis

The evaluation of AR begins with a complete history, which should include the following components: specific symptoms, their onset, duration, severity and frequency, seasonality, relationship to allergen exposure, response to medications, presence of coexisting conditions such as atopic dermatitis, sinusitis, and asthma, family history of allergic conditions, social history for active or passive smoke exposure, and environmental assessment for outdoor exposures as well as indoor exposures in and out of the workplace.[4,38] For example, a history of symptoms related to pollen or animal exposure may have a high positive predictive value when diagnosing AR.[88] In addition, quality of life should be assessed during the initial evaluation as chronic conditions such as AR have been demonstrated to cause significant health and economic burdens. The physical examination should include any organ systems potentially affected by rhinitis including the nose, ears, eyes, throat, lymphatics, lungs, and skin, which may help diagnose coexisting conditions such as otitis, eustachian tube dysfunction, conjunctivitis, asthma, and atopic dermatitis. Nasal findings that support the diagnosis of AR but are not pathognomonic include mucosal pallor, edema, or hyperemia.[4] Symmetrical, asymptomatic blue-gray discolorations of the periorbital skin, known as allergic shiners, which is secondary to venous stasis, are associated with nasal congestion, and present in up to 60% of atopic individuals.[89]

While history and physical exam support the diagnosis of AR, it is confirmed by the presence of specific IgE antibody to aeroallergens measured by by either skin testing or in vitro testing that correlates with exposure. Skin prick testing (SPT) is the preferred method to diagnose AR and identify specific allergens for avoidance measures and/or therapeutic options for immunotherapy, as it is more sensitive than serum-specific IgE tests.[4] In studies using positive nasal provocation challenges as a standard, the sensitivity and specificity of SPT ranges from 85% to 87% and 79% to 86%, respectively.[90,91] The sensitivity of specific IgE immunoassays compared with SPT is estimated to be around 70% to 75%.[92] There are certain circumstances where in vitro assay is preferred to skin testing, such as in patients with chronic urticaria or other related skin conditions such as dermatographism, or patients on chronic medications capable of suppressing the skin test response which cannot be discontinued.

Occupational Rhinitis and Work-Exacerbated Rhinitis

The diagnosis of OR requires both evidence of rhinitis symptoms and demonstration that the symptoms are related to the workplace. The different steps involved in the diagnosis of OR include clinical history, nasal examination, immunological tests if applicable, and nasal provocation tests.[23] It is crucial to confirm the diagnosis objectively because misdiagnosis can have detrimental effects both financially and socially as it can impact employment.[23] Additionally, given the fact that OA frequently coexists with OR, patients presenting with possible OR should also be screened for lower airway involvement with spirometry regardless of the presence or absence of lower respiratory symptoms. Since there has been great variability on diagnostic testing for OR, a consensus diagnostic algorithm has been developed (Figure 12–2). The diagnosis of WER relies mainly on history and lack of

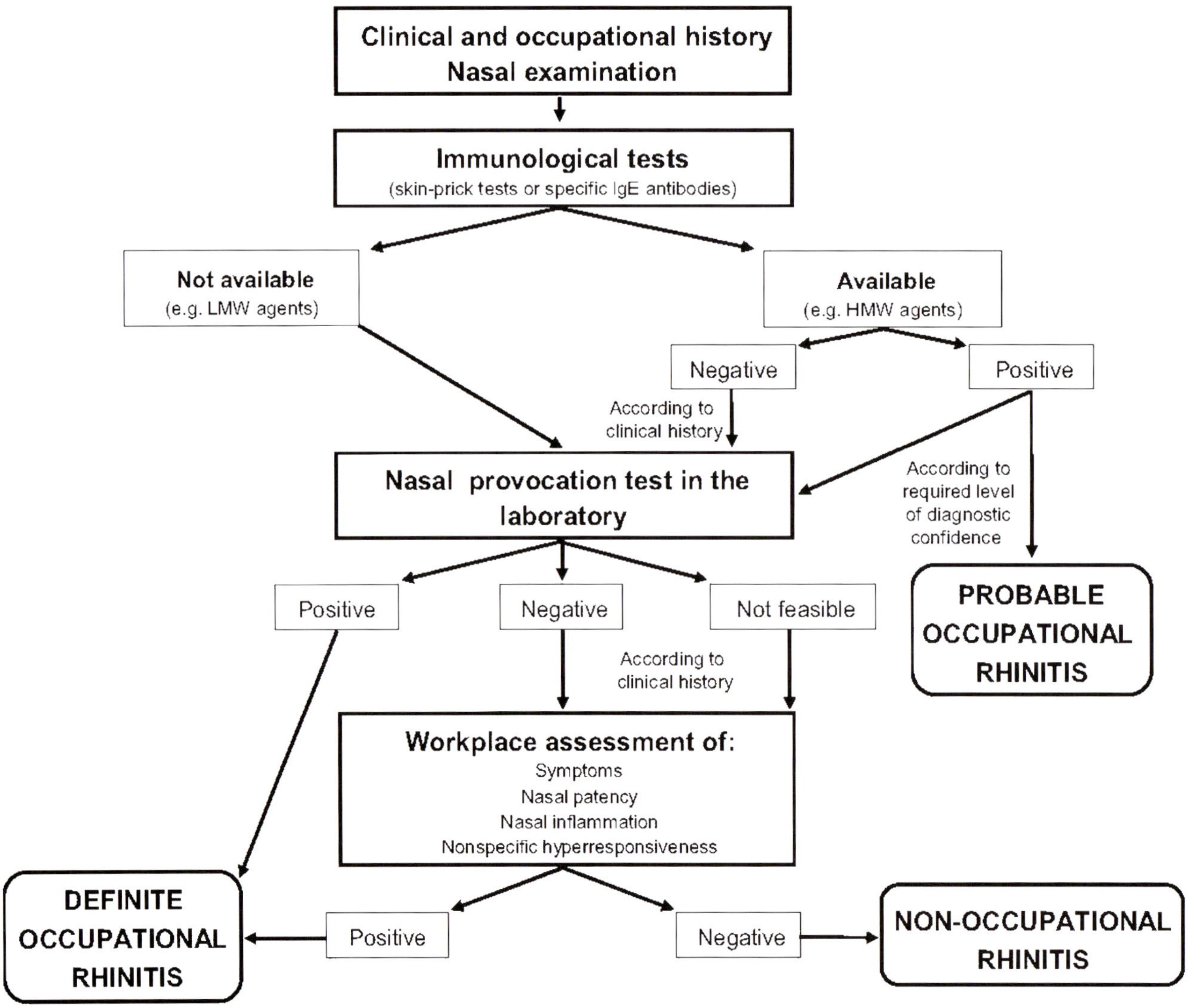

Figure 12–2. Diagnostic approach to occupational rhinitis. Reprinted with a Creative Commons License from BioMed Central Ltd. Moscato G, Vandenplas O, Van Wijk RG, et al. EAACI position paper on occupational rhinitis. *Respir Res.* 2009;10(1):16.

evidence of specific sensitization to workplace agents to distinguish it from OR.

The evaluation of OR begins with a detailed medical and occupational history. Components of the history include the following: description of the patient's current job responsibilities, any possible exposures to sensitizing agents or noxious chemicals, work processes in adjacent work areas, recent changes in work policies or materials, and workplace hygiene conditions.[23] It is critical to investigate the timing of nasal symptoms in relation to occupational exposure, as IgE-mediated allergic OR requires a latency period during which time the worker becomes sensitized. Improvement of symptoms when patients are away from work during vacation or sick leave is supportive of OR, but it should be noted that symptom onset can occur immediately while at work or as a delayed nasal response with symptoms not appearing until later in the evening at home.[93] Any measures used in the workplace to reduce or control noxious exposures, such as respiratory protection equipment or industrial hygiene strategies and their effectiveness, should also be assessed.[93] Symptoms of allergic OR are similar to AR, including rhinorrhea, nasal itching, sneezing, and nasal congestion. Symptoms experienced with nonallergic OR include nasal discomfort, rhinorrhea, nasal congestion, postnasal drainage, sinus headache, and occasionally, epistaxis.[94] Conjunctival symptoms are more likely to occur with allergic OR compared to nonallergic OR.[43]

In addition to a thorough clinical history, nasal examination similar to AR is essential to rule out other nasal pathologies such as nasal polyps, chronic rhinosinusitis, and structural abnormalities.[23] The presence of sepal perforation or ulceration may indicate exposure to corrosive substances.[95] Direct visualization of the nose by anterior rhinoscopy or endoscopy can be viewed as a subjective assessment as it does not allow quantitative assessment of nasal changes. More objective measures, such as peak nasal inspiratory flow (PNIF), rhinomanometry, and acoustic rhinometry can be used to assess nasal patency; however, these techniques require special equipment and may not always be practical for routine use.[23] Assessing for nasal inflammation may also be helpful in the diagnosis of OR. Evidence of neutrophils and eosinophils indicate the presence of Th1- and Th2-mediated inflammation, respectively. Methods used to sample nasal secretions include blown nasal secretions, microsuction techniques, nasal lavage, nasal smears, and more invasive techniques, including nasal scrapings and nasal biopsy.[23,93] Typically, nasal secretions are collected at the time of nasal provocation tests or exposure at the workplace so subjects serve as their own controls.

In cases of allergic OR where HMW agents are implicated, SPT and/or serum-specific IgE antibodies can be used to determine the presence of IgE-mediated sensitization. The sensitivity and specificity of immunological tests compared to nasal provocation tests are unknown, but it appears that their specificity may be lower than their sensitivity because positive results also occur in exposed, asymptomatic individuals.[96] The negative predictive value of SPT is high, so a negative test result makes the diagnosis of OR unlikely, provided that the appropriate allergens have been tested.[23] Some HMW agents and a few LMW agents, such as platinum salts, reactive dyes, and acid anhydrides, are available for skin prick testing. However, the use of immunological tests for this class of disorders is limited due to the lack of commercial availability of standardized extracts for many occupational agents.[23] If a patient has a suggestive clinical history in the setting of positive immunological test to a well-standardized extract, then the diagnosis of OR is very likely.[23]

The gold standard for confirming the diagnosis of OR is the nasal provocation test (NPT) using objective methods to assess nasal response.[97] NPT can be performed in the laboratory under controlled conditions (laboratory-based nasal challenge test or LNCT) or at work under natural conditions. NPT are primarily preformed to establish a connection between rhinitis symptoms and exposure at work. Despite the fact that LNCT are considered useful in the diagnosis of OR, there are limitations due to the fact that various criteria have been used for defining a positive response, but there is lack of validated comparison between NPTs using these different criteria.[98] There are established guidelines regarding the methodology of NPT, which are beyond the discussion in this chapter.[99] However, if a NPT is positive, a definitive diagnosis of OR can be established. If NPT is negative but the history is highly suggestive for OR, then further evaluation of work-related changes in nasal symptoms, nasal patency, and nasal inflammation in the workplace is recommended. In addition, assessment in the workplace may suffice for diagnosis when LNPT is not feasible.[23]

Occupational Asthma and Work-Exacerbated Asthma

Occupational asthma should be considered in all patients with adult-onset asthma. Patients must first meet the diagnostic criteria for asthma, with either reversible airflow limitation or evidence of airway hyperresponsiveness diagnosed by bronchial provocation (ie, methacholine challenge), before a diagnosis of OA can be considered. After asthma is confirmed, then the relationship between asthma and the workplace must be assessed. Diagnostic criteria for diagnosing OA are shown in Table 12–3. Diagnostic criteria for OA have been proposed by the American College of Chest Physicians and include the following: a diagnosis of asthma, onset of symptoms after entering the workplace, an association between symptoms of asthma and work, and one or more of the following: (1) workplace exposure to an agent or process known to give rise to OA, (2) significant work-related changes in FEV_1 or peak expiratory flow (PEF) rate, (3) significant work-related changes in nonspecific airway responsiveness, (4) positive response to specific inhalation challenge tests with an agent to which the patient is exposed at work, or (5) onset of asthma symptoms with a clear association to an irritant agent in the workplace.[82] There are no specific diagnostic criteria for WEA; the diagnosis relies mainly on the history of asthma symptoms worsening related to workplace conditions, which can manifest as asthma exacerbations, loss of asthma control due to change in frequency and severity of asthma symptoms, or need for increased asthma medications.[100]

Table 12–3. Diagnostic Criteria for OA

A confirmed diagnosis of asthma
Onset of symptoms after entering the workplace
An association between symptoms of asthma and work
One or more of the following:
Workplace exposure to an agent or process known to give rise to OA
Significant work-related changes in FEV_1 or peak expiratory flow (PEF) rate
Significant work-related changes in nonspecific airway responsiveness
Positive response to specific inhalation challenge tests with an agent to which the patient is exposed at work
Onset of asthma with a clear association with a symptomatic exposure to an irritant agent in the workplace

Source: Adapted from Tarlo SM, Balmes J, Balkissoon R, et al. Diagnosis and management of work-related asthma: American College of Chest Physicians consensus statement. *Chest.* 2008;134(3, suppl):1S–41S.

Once asthma has been confirmed, an employment history should be obtained and include the following components: past and current employment and start dates, work hours and schedule, description of work responsibilities, potential exposure to sensitizing or irritating agents work processes in adjacent areas, impairment of work due to symptoms, relationship of symptoms experienced before, during, or after work to a specific exposure in the workplace, duration of symptoms after leaving work, and improvement of symptoms when away from workplace. Typically patients with OA experience the onset of symptoms while at work and resolution or improvement shortly after shift is completed and during weekends and holidays. However, airway responses to LMW chemicals are more commonly isolated to late responses, and in these circumstances workers can present with evening symptoms after leaving work, and improvement may require several days away from exposure.[82] Another key component that facilitates the occupational history are material safety data sheets (MSDSs) which often provide essential information about the specific chemicals and substances used in the workplace and related standardized threshold limit values (TLVs), and permissible exposure levels (PELs).[81] In addition to the employment history, it is important to inquire about additional symptoms, including upper respiratory symptoms and rhinitis, because as already discussed, OR commonly precedes or coexists with OA. The general allergic history is also important to obtain, as atopic individuals are more likely to experience work-related asthma symptoms than nonatopic individuals, especially after exposure to HMW agents.[101]

Although a detailed history can support the diagnosis of OA, it cannot be used alone in the diagnosis due to its low positive predictive value.[102] Additional evaluation for OA includes documentation of symptomatic, functional, and inflammatory changes in response to exposure to occupational agents, which can be done via PEF monitoring, methacholine inhalation challenge, and specific inhalation challenge (SIC) testing, and immunologic testing using skin prick testing or serologic specific IgE testing when available.[32] SIC involves exposing an individual to a suspected sensitizing agent at increasing doses to cause a fall in expiratory flow volumes, an increase in airway responsiveness, and/or an increase in inflammatory biomarkers.[103] HMW agents typically elicit immediate airway responses manifesting as a decline in the forced expiratory capacity in 1 second (FEV_1) of 20% or greater within 1 hour of exposure or as a dual response, where the initial decline improves and is then followed by a secondary decline in FEV_1 several hours after the initial exposure.[104] LMW agents tend to produce immediate, late, and dual responses equally.[104] Although SIC is used as a reference standard for comparison with other diagnostic tests, it is not widely available in the United States because it requires specialized facilities to implement. Specific bronchoprovocation testing may have false-positive and false-negative results, and has generally been considered only if other test results are inconclusive or cannot be performed.[82] When the offending agent cannot be identified or a SIC is not available but is needed to confirm the diagnosis of OA, then an inhalation challenge with spirometry monitoring may be undertaken in the workplace before and after the patient's natural exposure.[82]

Ideally, lung function should be evaluated and monitored in the workplace during a known exposure to a causative agent; however, this is not always logistically possible or can be met with resistance from the employer.[105] Serial PEF monitoring at work and away from work is an inexpensive and reliable method to diagnose OA. When performed properly, compared to SIC, PEF measurements have around 64% sensitivity and 77% specificity.[106] Workers should record PEF readings 4 times daily while at work[107] and on days away from work for at least 4 weeks, including at least 2 weeks at work and 2 weeks away from work.[108] The use of data loggers can prevent fabrications of measurements, and the use of computerized peak flow meters that record effort, reproducibility, and time of readings may help prevent noncompliance issues.[82] A 20% variability in PEF rates at work compared to being away from the workplace supports the diagnosis of OA. Another method used to diagnose OA is serial measures of airway responsiveness using methacholine or histamine challenge at and away from the workplace. A provocation concentration causing a 20% fall in FEV_1 (PC_{20}) that increases more than 3-fold after a few weeks away from work, when measured within 8 weeks of the test at work, is considered significant; a 2-fold increase is considered to be of possible significance.[109] If portable spirometry is available, then measuring FEV_1 cross-shift may also be helpful in the diagnosis of OA.[82]

The use of immunologic testing with skin testing or in vitro testing may have a role in the assessment of sensitizer-induced OA. Cases of OA caused by HMW proteins and some LMW agents are associated with production of specific IgE antibodies. The SPT detects tissue-bound IgE antibodies and is highly sensitive and specific for identifying a specific IgE antibody response to protein allergens.[110] An immunologic response to a specific agent helps phenotype different forms of OA and along with an appropriate history in a worker with confirmed asthma supports this diagnosis, but is usually not diagnostic by itself.[105] One limitation of immunologic testing for OA is the lack of standardized skin test reagents and immunoassays. Test extracts and immunoassays for most HMW proteins implicated in OA are not commercially available, and those that are available often lack standardization with regard to allergenic potency.[82] However, when using validated occupational protein allergens, such as natural rubber latex, cat and dog allergen, or venom from stinging insects, a negative SPT response, which has a high negative predictive value (NPV), can exclude sensitizer-induced OA with a high degree of accuracy.[111]

The diagnosis of irritant-induced OA or RADS is frequently retrospective and relies more on a detailed history along with the objective evidence of asthma. Workers with RADS typically do not manifest the types of airway response patterns seen with

OA induced by HMW and LMW agents.[105] Diagnostic criteria for RADS and irritant-induced asthma are summarized in Table 12–4.

The diagnosis of WEA is made by confirming the diagnosis of asthma and associating the worsening of symptoms with triggers or exposures, such as cold air, dust fumes, low-level irritant chemicals, or exercise in the workplace.[109] Common allergens such as dust mites, cat dander, or fungal spores may be present above background levels in some work environments and can trigger worsening of asthma symptoms in patients with atopic asthma.[82] Aeroallergen SPT can support the diagnosis of WEA in susceptible atopic individuals. Immunologic testing is not helpful in identifying WEA due to nonallergic work triggers and therefore is not indicated for the detection of irritant-induced asthma or RADS.[82]

> History and physical exam are important in diagnosing environmental and occupational allergies. The presence of specific IgE antibody to aeroallergens and occupational allergens that correlates with symptoms upon exposure are important diagnostic tests for AR and OR, respectively. OA is confirmed by documenting an association between symptoms of asthma and a workplace exposure, in association with supportive immunologic and provocation testing when applicable.

Table 12–4. Diagnostic Criteria for RADS

New-onset respiratory symptoms
Onset of symptoms occurs after a single, specific exposure
Exposure to a high concentration of a known irritating substance
Symptoms develop within 24 hours of exposure
Symptoms persist for 3 months or more
Evidence of airway obstruction or hyperresponsiveness
Other pulmonary diseases have been excluded

Source: Adapted from Brooks SM, Weiss MA, Bernstein IL. Reactive airways dysfunction syndrome (RADS). Persistent asthma syndrome after high level irritant exposures. *Chest.* 1985;88(3):376–384.

MANAGEMENT

Allergic Rhinitis

Interventions for allergic rhinitis include decreasing exposure to environmental allergens and pharmacologic therapies including medications and/or allergen immunotherapy.[22] Even though the pollen allergens involved in SAR cannot be easily avoided due to their ubiquitous presence in the environment, individuals can at least limit their time outdoors during peak pollen seasons. Additionally, pollen levels can be reduced indoors by closing windows and using air conditioning throughout the pollen seasons. Exposure to perennial allergens, including house dust mite and domestic animals, can more easily be avoided provided multiple environmental interventions are implemented in the home. For example, controlling the humidity level and using air conditioning in the home can control the level of house dust mite and mold exposure. In addition, encasing mattresses, box springs, and pillows in zippered, allergen-proof covers is effective at reducing dust mite allergen levels in the bed.[112] High-efficiency particulate air (HEPA) filters may be useful in decreasing exposure to allergens that are small enough to stay suspended in ambient air for several hours, such as pet, rodent, and fungal allergens.[22] Ideally, in pet-allergic patients, it is best to remove pets from the home, but when this is not possible, keeping them out of the affected individual's bedroom is helpful in reducing the total allergen burden.

Pharmacotherapy of AR includes oral or topical antihistamines and intranasal corticosteroids. Oral H_1 antihistamines are considered first-line therapy for the treatment of mild-to-moderate allergic rhinitis, especially in patients with intermittent symptoms of sneezing, itching, and rhinorrhea, but are not as effective in treating nasal congestion.[113] The nonsedating, second-generation oral antihistamines, such as cetirizine, fexofenadine, and loratadine, are preferred over first-generation antihistamines, such as diphenhydramine, chlorpheniramine, and hydroxyzine, since these latter medications can cross the blood-brain barrier causing sedation and impaired performance, cognitive, and psychomotor skills.[114] Second-generation antihistamines still provide effective relief of symptoms but have a higher selectivity for peripheral H1 receptors due to their hydrophilic nature, and thus are relatively free of sedating side effects.[115] Intranasal antihistamines are also considered first-line therapy for mild-to-moderate allergic rhinitis[113] and may be more effective in treating nasal congestion compared to oral antihistamines.[116] Intranasal corticosteroids are considered first-line therapy for more moderate-to-severe chronic allergic rhinitis symptoms.[117] Intranasal corticosteroids are effective in treating all major symptoms of allergic rhinitis, including rhinorrhea, sneezing, itching, and nasal congestion.[4] Adverse effects of intranasal corticosteroids include local irritation, epistaxis, and rarely septal perforation.[4] However, when used at recommended doses, they are not typically associated with systemic side effects.

Other medications used to treat allergic rhinitis include cromolyn sodium, leukotriene receptor antagonists (LTRAs), and oral decongestants. Cromolyn sodium inhibits the degranulation of sensitized mast cells, which prevents the release of mediators responsible for the immediate symptoms of allergic rhinitis and, therefore, can actually prevent allergic events instead of just alleviating symptoms once they have begun.[118] The use of cromolyn can be considered for preventive therapy before a potential or known allergen exposure[119] as the benefit lasts up to 4 to 8 hours after dosing.[120] Leukotriene receptor antagonists are another type of medication that can be used to treat allergic rhinitis as an alternative or in addition to antihistamine and intranasal corticosteroids. Studies have shown that LTRAs improve nasal symptoms and quality of life scores compared to placebo and are as efficacious as oral antihistamines.[121]

Finally, allergen immunotherapy (AIT) is an effective treatment for allergic rhinitis and is the only treatment option that has the potential to cure AR.[122] Aeroallergen immunotherapy may prevent the development of new sensitizations[123] as well as reduce the risk for the development of asthma in children with allergic rhinitis.[124] Indications for immunotherapy include severe symptoms not responsive to medications, inability to tolerate other treatment options or reluctance to take medications long term, and patients' desire to potentially modify allergic disease.[4] Immunotherapy is typically well tolerated; side effects such as injection site or local reactions are possible, and rarely, life-threatening or fatal systemic reactions can occur.[125]

Occupational Rhinitis and Work-Exacerbated Rhinitis

The management of OR involves minimizing symptoms and improving patient quality of life as well as preventing the development of OA. The primary environmental intervention needed to treat OR is avoidance of the offending agent. Unfortunately, complete avoidance measures are often not feasible, as it requires substantial changes in one's job description, which may not be possible to implement in the workplace. If complete avoidance is not possible, then some studies have found that use of personal respiratory protection may effectively decrease OR symptoms induced by certain HMW agents, including laboratory animals[126] and natural rubber latex.[127] There are no studies assessing the use or effectiveness of medications for either allergic or nonallergic OR. As a result, medications should not be considered an acceptable alternative to the elimination or reduction of workplace exposure to the offending agent.[23] However, if patients experience ongoing symptoms despite reduction of workplace exposures, the established guidelines for treating rhinitis[4] can be used to guide pharmacologic therapies for OR.[93] There have been only a few studies involving AIT and occupational respiratory diseases to date. The safety and long-term effectiveness of AIT have not been assessed, indicating that further studies to confirm the utility of AIT for OR or OA are needed.[128] Another important aspect of managing OR is to prevent development of OA. The actual risk of developing OA in patients with rhinitis is difficult to assess, so it is difficult to decide whether a worker with OR should be completely removed from the causal exposure in an attempt to prevent OA.[93] A more effective approach may be to advise the worker to limit his or her exposure to the offending agent(s); stricter avoidance measures should be implemented if there is evidence of asymptomatic, nonspecific bronchial hyperreactivity (NSBH) or more severe rhinitis symptoms of longer duration, as the risk for developing OA may be increased.[129]

Occupational Asthma and Work-Exacerbated Asthma

Once the diagnosis of OA has been confirmed, the most effective treatment option is removal from further exposure. Complete removal has been found to reduce asthma symptoms and improve lung function, including FEV_1 and NSBH, especially in cases secondary to LMW agents.[130] If avoidance is not possible without changing jobs, then recommending that a patient leave his or her current employment should be handled with sensitivity, because workers often experience anxiety and financial concerns related to lost income secondary to unemployment or having to go on worker's compensation.[131] For irritant-induced OA where there are brief and infrequent exposures, use of personal protective equipment (PPE) such as air-supplying respirators, provide a reasonable degree of protection.[132,133] Studies evaluating the natural history of OA have found that persistence of asthma correlated with the duration of exposure and symptoms prior to diagnosis.[105] Therefore, the best outcomes occur when the diagnosis is established early; the exposure is stopped; and the asthma is not yet severe.[134] Asthma symptoms and airway hyperresponsiveness persist in approximately 70% of patients with OA, even years after removal from the sensitizing agent.[32] Pharmacologic treatment of acute or chronic OA is similar to that of non-OA, which involves inhaled short-acting $beta_2$-agonists, inhaled anticholinergics, inhaled corticosteroids with or without long-acting $beta_2$-adrenergic agonist, leukotriene-modifying agents, xanthine oxidase inhibitors, and oral corticosteroids.[135] Allergen immunotherapy may play a role in the treatment of OA caused by HMW protein allergens such as laboratory or other animal proteins.[74,105]

As long as interventions have been made to prevent future accidental exposures, workers with RADS are often able to stay in their current work environment because their asthma was usually initiated by an isolated unusual, acute exposure to a high level of a respiratory irritant.[74] Individuals with irritant-induced OA may be able to continue to work when placed in a work area with better air circulation and with reduced exposures to irritants and/or use of PPE. If workers remain in their current place of employment in an environment with reduced or no exposure to the offending agent(s), it is critical to continue monitoring the patient for clinical symptoms and for changes in lung function to ensure that their condition is not deteriorating over time.[74] The treatment of WEA depends on the worker's severity of symptoms. More severe cases of WEA may require a job change, while workers with milder symptoms may be able to remain at work if exposures are minimized and asthma medication is optimized.[37]

> Treatment of AR includes reducing allergen burden and using pharmacologic therapies including oral and topical antihistamines, nasal corticosteroids, and allergen immunotherapy. The primary treatment of OR and OA is avoidance of inciting agents.

PREVENTION

Allergic Rhinitis

Although not as extensively investigated as asthma, there is some data on the prevention of allergic rhinitis. Breastfeeding for 4 to 6 months has been shown to reduce the risk of total allergy, atopic dermatitis, and positive skin tests (both food and aeroallergens) in children up to 4 years of age.[136] Early exposure to endotoxin, which is a component of the cell wall of Gram-negative bacteria, associated with pet ownership, has been reported to provide a protective effect on the development of atopic disease.[136] There also appears to be a relationship between viral infections during early childhood and development of atopic disease, where frequent infections lead to a reduction in allergic disease by shifting the immune response from Th2 to Th1 phenotype.[137]

Occupational Rhinitis and Work-Exacerbated Rhinitis

Studies indicate that the level of exposure to sensitizing agents is the most important factor for developing IgE-mediated allergic OR, so that reducing workplace exposures to sensitizing agents is usually the most effective measure to prevent OR.[23] There is no utility in screening asymptomatic individuals for OR as the positive predictive values of available susceptibility markers are too low for screening out potentially susceptible individuals.[138] Increased awareness and education regarding the risk of OR with certain workplace exposures is crucial for preventing disease.

Occupational Asthma and Work-Exacerbated Asthma

Primary prevention measures for the development of sensitizer-induced OA include reducing worker exposure to and use of known sensitizing agents.[32] Reducing exposures can be effectively accomplished by substituting sensitizing agents with nonsensitizing agents (ie, replacing latex with nitrile gloves).[32] Additionally, optimizing occupational hygiene measures to contain work processes, using robotics instead of workers in high-exposure areas, improving ventilation, and using PPE are all important strategies for creating a healthy workplace.[139] Educating workers on measures to reduce exposures as well as the importance of adhering to handling procedures implemented at the workplace is a key component in the prevention of OA.[105] Workers who develop OR should be continuously monitored due to their increased risk of developing OA. For some workplace exposures (ie, enzymes, platinum salts, acid anhydrides, and diisocyanates), the use of comprehensive medical surveillance programs has been implemented either voluntarily or based on recommendations by governmental agencies and has been found to prevent the development of sensitization to occupational agents and development of clinical disease.[82,140–144] Finally, prevention of irritant-induced OA and WEA relies on methods to control exposures, such as isolation or enclosure of the source, improved workplace ventilation, and the use of respirators when a worker has the potential to be exposed to irritating agents.[82]

Breastfeeding, exposure to endotoxin, and viral infections have been reported to be protective for developing AR. Prevention of OR and OA primarily involves reducing or preventing exposures to known sensitizing agents.

CONCLUSIONS

Allergens encountered in the environmental and occupational setting are a major cause of allergic disease, including AR, OR, and OA. The diagnosis of these conditions requires a careful history along with appropriate immunologic testing to determine allergic sensitization. Treatment should focus on avoidance measures, pharmacotherapy, and when appropriate AIT. Early recognition of these conditions and appropriate evaluation and management leads to better long-term outcomes.

REFERENCES

1. Pawankar R, Pacheco KA, Holgate ST, Lockey RF. *World Allergy Organization (WAO) White Book on Allergy.* Milwaukee, WI: World Allergy Organization; 2011.
2. Salo PM, Arbes SJ, Jr, Jaramillo R, et al. Prevalence of allergic sensitization in the United States: results from the National Health and Nutrition Examination Survey (NHANES) 2005–2006. *J Allergy Clin Immunol.* 2014; 134(2):350–359.
3. Yoo Y, Perzanowski MS. Allergic sensitization and the environment: latest update. *Curr Allergy Asthma Rep.* 2014;14(10):465.
4. Wallace DV, Dykewicz MS, Bernstein DI, et al. The diagnosis and management of rhinitis: an updated practice parameter. *J Allergy Clin Immunol.* 2008;122(2, suppl):S1–84.
5. Schoenwetter WF, Dupclay L, Jr, Appajosyula S, Botteman MF, Pashos CL. Economic impact and quality-of-life burden of allergic rhinitis. *Curr Med Res Opin.* 2004; 20(3):305–317.
6. O'Connell EJ. The burden of atopy and asthma in children. *Allergy.* 2004;59(suppl 78):7–11.
7. Howarth PH, Salagean M, Dokic D. Allergic rhinitis: not purely a histamine-related disease. *Allergy.* 2000;55 (suppl 64):7–16.
8. Naclerio RM, Pawankar R. Allergic Rhinitis. In: Lockey RF, Ledford DK, eds. *Asthma Comorbidities, Coexisting Conditions, and Differential Diagnosis.* New York, NY: Oxford University Press; 2014:231–241.
9. Dykewicz MS, Fineman S. Executive Summary of Joint Task Force Practice Parameters on Diagnosis and Management of Rhinitis. *Ann Allergy Asthma Immunol.* 1998; 81(5, pt 2):463–468.
10. Bousquet J, Van Cauwenberge P, Khaltaev N, Aria Workshop G, World Health O. Allergic rhinitis and its impact on asthma. *J Allergy Clin Immunol.* 2001;108(5, suppl):S147–S334.
11. Bauchau V, Durham SR. Epidemiological characterization of the intermittent and persistent types of allergic rhinitis. *Allergy.* 2005;60(3):350–353.
12. Weber RW. Aeroallergen botany. *Ann Allergy Asthma Immunol.* 2014;112(2):102–107.
13. Friedlander JL, Baxi S, Phipatanakul W. Asthma and allergens. In: Bernstein JA, Levy ML, eds. *Clinical Asthma Theory and Practice.* Boca Raton, FL: CRC Press; 2014:93–97.

14. Skoner DP. Allergic rhinitis: definition, epidemiology, pathophysiology, detection, and diagnosis. *J Allergy Clin Immunol.* 2001;108(1, suppl):S2–S8.
15. Diette GB, McCormack MC, Hansel NN, Breysse PN, Matsui EC. Environmental issues in managing asthma. *Respiratory Care.* 2008;53(5):602–615; discussion 608–609.
16. Diette GB, Hansel NN, Buckley TJ, et al. Home indoor pollutant exposures among inner-city children with and without asthma. *Environ Health Perspect.* 2007;115(11): 1665–1669.
17. Rosenstreich DL, Eggleston P, Kattan M, et al. The role of cockroach allergy and exposure to cockroach allergen in causing morbidity among inner-city children with asthma. *N Engl J Med.* 1997;336(19):1356–1363.
18. Perzanowski MS, Ronmark E, Platts-Mills TA, Lundback B. Effect of cat and dog ownership on sensitization and development of asthma among preteenage children. *Am J Respir Crit Care Med.* 2002;166(5):696–702.
19. Custovic A, Simpson B, Simpson A, Hallam C, Craven M, Woodcock A. Relationship between mite, cat, and dog allergens in reservoir dust and ambient air. *Allergy.* 1999;54(6):612–616.
20. D'Amato G, Liccardi G, Russo M, Barber D, D'Amato M, Carreira J. Clothing is a carrier of cat allergens. *J Allergy Clin Immunol.* 1997;99(4):577–578.
21. Ohman JL, Jr., Hagberg K, MacDonald MR, Jones RR, Jr, Paigen BJ, Kacergis JB. Distribution of airborne mouse allergen in a major mouse breeding facility. *J Allergy Clin Immunol.* 1994;94(5):810–817.
22. Peden D, Reed CE. Environmental and occupational allergies. *J Allergy Clin Immunol.* 2010;125(2, suppl 2): S150–S160.
23. Moscato G, Vandenplas O, Van Wijk RG, et al. EAACI position paper on occupational rhinitis. *Respir Res.* 2009; 10:16.
24. Ameille J, Hamelin K, Andujar P, et al. Occupational asthma and occupational rhinitis: the united airways disease model revisited. *Occup Environ Med.* 2013;70(7): 471–475.
25. Gautrin D, Desrosiers M, Castano R. Occupational rhinitis. *Curr Opin Allergy Clin Immunol.* 2006;6(2):77–84.
26. Rodier F, Gautrin D, Ghezzo H, Malo JL. Incidence of occupational rhinoconjunctivitis and risk factors in animal-health apprentices. *J Allergy Clin Immunol.* 2003; 112(6):1105–1111.
27. Christiani DC, Malo JL, Siracus A. Upper airways involvement. In: Bernstein IL, Chan-Yeung M, Malo JL, Bernstein DI, eds. *Asthma in the Workplace.* Vol 3. New York, NY: Taylor & Francis; 2006:785–796.
28. Castano R, Theriault G. Defining and classifying occupational rhinitis. *J Laryngol Otol.* 2006;120(10):812–817.
29. Meggs WJ. RADS and RUDS—the toxic induction of asthma and rhinitis. *J Toxicol.Clin Toxicol.* 1994;32(5): 487–501.
30. Banauch GI, Dhala A, Alleyne D, et al. Bronchial hyperreactivity and other inhalation lung injuries in rescue/recovery workers after the World Trade Center collapse. *Crit Care Med.* 2005;33(1, suppl):S102–S106.
31. Bernstein IL, Bernstein DI, Chan-Yeung M, Malo JL. Definition and classification of asthma in the workplace. In: Malo JL, Chan-Yeung M, Bernstein DI, eds. *Asthma in the Workplace.* Vol 4. Boca Raton, FL: CRC Press, Taylor & Francis Group; 2013:1–5.
32. Tarlo SM, Lemiere C. Occupational asthma. *N Engl J Med.* 2014;370(7):640–649.
33. Bernstein DI. Allergic reactions to workplace allergens. *JAMA.* 1997;278(22):1907–1913.
34. Malo JL, Vandenplas O. Definitions and classification of work-related asthma. *Immunol Allergy Clin North Am.* 2011;31(4):645–662, v.
35. Malo JL, Chan-Yeung M. Agents causing occupational asthma. *J Allergy Clin Immunol.* 2009;123(3):545–550.
36. Brooks SM, Weiss MA, Bernstein IL. Reactive airways dysfunction syndrome (RADS). Persistent asthma syndrome after high level irritant exposures. *Chest.* 1985; 88(3):376–384.
37. Henneberger PK. Work-exacerbated asthma. *Curr Opin Allergy Clin Immunol..* 2007;7(2):146–151.
38. Bernstein JA. Allergic and mixed rhinitis: epidemiology and natural history. *Allergy Asthma Proc.* 2010;31(5): 365–369.
39. Settipane RA, Charnock DR. Epidemiology of rhinitis: allergic and nonallergic. *Clin Allergy Immunol.* 2007;19: 23–34.
40. Smith JM. A five-year prospective survey of rural children with asthma and hay fever. *J Allergy.* 1971;47(1):23–30.
41. Jessen M, Malm L. Definition, prevalence and development of nasal obstruction. *Allergy.* 1997;52(40, suppl):3–6.
42. Siracusa A, Desrosiers M, Marabini A. Epidemiology of occupational rhinitis: prevalence, aetiology and determinants. *Clin Exp Allergy.* 2000;30(11):1519–1534.
43. Malo JL, Lemiere C, Desjardins A, Cartier A. Prevalence and intensity of rhinoconjunctivitis in subjects with occupational asthma. *European Respir J.* 1997;10(7):1513–1515.
44. Liebers V, Hoernstein M, Baur X. Humoral immune response to the insect allergen Chi t I in aquarists and fish-food factory workers. *Allergy.* 1993;48(4):236–239.
45. Hollander A, Heederik D, Doekes G. Respiratory allergy to rats: exposure-response relationships in laboratory animal workers. *Am J Respir Crit Care Med.* 1997;155(2):562–567.
46. Musk AW, Venables KM, Crook B, et al. Respiratory symptoms, lung function, and sensitisation to flour in a British bakery. *Br J Ind Med.* 1989;46(9):636–642.
47. Houba R, Heederik D, Doekes G. Wheat sensitization and work-related symptoms in the baking industry are preventable. An epidemiologic study. *Am J Respir Crit Care Med.* 1998;158(5, pt 1):1499–1503.
48. Smith AM. The epidemiology of work-related asthma. *Immunol Allergy Clin North Am.* 2011;31(4):663–675, v.
49. Kogevinas M, Zock JP, Jarvis D, et al. Exposure to substances in the workplace and new-onset asthma: an international prospective population-based study (ECRHS-II). *Lancet.* 2007;370(9584):336–341.
50. Rosenman KD, Reilly MJ, Schill DP, et al. Cleaning products and work-related asthma. *J Occup Environ Med.* 2003;45(5):556–563.

51. Matte TD, Hoffman RE, Rosenman KD, Stanbury M. Surveillance of occupational asthma under the SENSOR model. *Chest.* 1990;98(5, suppl):173S–178S.
52. Mapp CE, Boschetto P, Maestrelli P, Fabbri LM. Occupational asthma. *Am J Respir Crit Care Med.* 2005;172(3): 280–305.
53. Saarinen K, Karjalainen A, Martikainen R, et al. Prevalence of work-aggravated symptoms in clinically established asthma. *Eur Respir J.* 2003;22(2):305–309.
54. Wagenmann M, Schumacher L, Bachert C. The time course of the bilateral release of cytokines and mediators after unilateral nasal allergen challenge. *Allergy.* 2005;60(9):1132–1138.
55. Okano M, Fujiwara T, Sugata Y, et al. Presence and characterization of prostaglandin D2-related molecules in nasal mucosa of patients with allergic rhinitis. *Am J Rhinol.* 2006;20(3):342–348.
56. Peters-Golden M, Gleason MM, Togias A. Cysteinyl leukotrienes: multi-functional mediators in allergic rhinitis. *Clin Exp Allergy.* 2006;36(6):689–703.
57. Sin B, Togias A. Pathophysiology of allergic and nonallergic rhinitis. *Proc Am Thorac Soc.* 2011;8(1):106–114.
58. Broide DH. Allergic rhinitis: Pathophysiology. *Allergy Asthma Proc.* 2010;31(5):370–374.
59. Baraniuk JN. Pathogenesis of allergic rhinitis. *J Allergy Clin Immunol.* 1997;99(2):S763–S772.
60. Gelfand EW. Inflammatory mediators in allergic rhinitis. *J Allergy Clin Immunol.* 2004;114(5, suppl):S135–S138.
61. Meggs WJ. Neurogenic switching: a hypothesis for a mechanism for shifting the site of inflammation in allergy and chemical sensitivity. *Environ Health Perspectives.* 1995;103(1):54–56.
62. Maestrelli P, Yucesoy B, Park HS, Wisnewski AV. Mechanisms, genetics, and pathophysiology. In: Malo JL, Chan-Yeung M, Bernstein DI, eds. *Asthma in the Workplace.* Vol 4. Boca Raton, FL: CRC Press, Taylor & Francis Group; 2013:40–56.
63. Maestrelli P, Boschetto P, Fabbri LM, Mapp CE. Mechanisms of occupational asthma. *J Allergy Clin Immunol.* 2009;123(3):531–542; quiz 543–544.
64. Dávila I, Mullol J, Ferrer M, et al. Genetic aspects of allergic rhinitis. *J Investig Allergol Clin Immunol.* 2009; 19(suppl 1):25–31.
65. Li ZP, Yin LL, Wang H, Liu LS. Association between promoter polymorphisms of interleukin-4 gene and allergic rhinitis risk: a meta-analysis. *J Huazhong Univ Sci Technol Med Sci.* 2014;34(3):306–313.
66. Benson M, Mobini R, Barrenas F, et al. A haplotype in the inducible T-cell tyrosine kinase is a risk factor for seasonal allergic rhinitis. *Allergy.* 2009;64(9):1286–1291.
67. Hussein YM, Ahmad AS, Ibrahem MM, et al. Interferon gamma gene polymorphism as a biochemical marker in Egyptian atopic patients. *J Investig Allergol Clin Immunol.* 2009;19(4):292–298.
68. Jeal H, Draper A, Jones M, et al. HLA associations with occupational sensitization to rat lipocalin allergens: a model for other animal allergies? *J Allergy Clin Immunol.* 2003;111(4):795–799.
69. Nicholson PJ, Cullinan P, Taylor AJ, Burge PS, Boyle C. Evidence based guidelines for the prevention, identification, and management of occupational asthma. *Occup Environ Med.* 2005;62(5):290–299.
70. Bernstein DI, Wang N, Campo P, et al. Diisocyanate asthma and gene-environment interactions with IL4RA, CD-14, and IL-13 genes. *Ann Allergy Asthma Immunol.* 2006;97(6):800–806.
71. Mapp CE, Fryer AA, De Marzo N, et al. Glutathione S-transferase GSTP1 is a susceptibility gene for occupational asthma induced by isocyanates. *J Allergy Clin Immunol.* 2002;109(5):867–872.
72. Wikman H, Piirila P, Rosenberg C, et al. N-Acetyltransferase genotypes as modifiers of diisocyanate exposure-associated asthma risk. *Pharmacogenetics.* 2002;12(3): 227–233.
73. Acouetey DS, Zmirou-Navier D, Avogbe PH, et al. Genetic predictors of inflammation in the risk of occupational asthma in young apprentices. *Ann Allergy Asthma Immunol.* 2013;110(6):423–428, e425.
74. Smith AM, Bernstein DI. Management of work-related asthma. *J Allergy Clin Immunol.* 2009;123(3):551–557.
75. Powe DG, Huskisson RS, Carney AS, Jenkins D, Jones NS. Evidence for an inflammatory pathophysiology in idiopathic rhinitis. *Clin Exp Allergy.* 2001;31(6):864–872.
76. Materson BJ. Adverse effects of angiotensin-converting enzyme inhibitors in antihypertensive therapy with focus on quinapril. *Am J Cardiol.* 1992;69(10):46C–53C.
77. Plosker GL, Goa KL. Terazosin. A pharmacoeconomic evaluation of its use in benign prostatic hyperplasia. *PharmacoEconomics.* 1997;11(2):184–197.
78. Vitezic D, Pelcic JM. Erectile dysfunction: oral pharmacotherapy options. *Int J Clin Pharm Therapeutics.* 2002; 40(9):393–403.
79. Fireman P. Allergic rhinitis. In: Fireman P, Slavin R, eds. *Atlas of Allergies.* Philadelphia, PA: JB Lippincott; 1991: 9.2–9.18.
80. Dunn CJ, Alaani A, Johnson AP. Study on spontaneous cerebrospinal fluid rhinorrhoea: its aetiology and management. *J Laryngol Otol.* 2005;119(1):12–15.
81. Tan J, Bernstein JA. Occupational asthma: an overview. *Curr Allergy Asthma Rep.* 2014;14(5):431.
82. Tarlo SM, Balmes J, Balkissoon R, et al. Diagnosis and management of work-related asthma: American College of Chest Physicians Consensus Statement. *Chest.* 2008; 134(3 suppl):1S–41S.
83. Perkner JJ, Fennelly KP, Balkissoon R, et al. Irritant-associated vocal cord dysfunction. *J Occup Environ Med.* 1998;40(2):136–143.
84. Millqvist E. Cough provocation with capsaicin is an objective way to test sensory hyperreactivity in patients with asthma-like symptoms. *Allergy.* 2000;55(6):546–550.
85. Kipen HM, Hallman W, Kelly-McNeil K, Fiedler N. Measuring chemical sensitivity prevalence: a questionnaire for population studies. *Am J Public Health.* 1995; 85(4):574–577.
86. Ternesten-Hasseus E, Farbrot A, Lowhagen O, Millqvist E. Sensitivity to methacholine and capsaicin in

patients with unclear respiratory symptoms. *Allergy.* 2002;57(6):501–507.

87. Vandenplas O, Toren K, Blanc PD. Health and socioeconomic impact of work-related asthma. *Eur Respir J.* 2003;22(4):689–697.
88. Gendo K, Larson EB. Evidence-based diagnostic strategies for evaluating suspected allergic rhinitis. *Ann Intern Med.* 2004;140(4):278–289.
89. Beltrani VS, Boguneiwicz M. Atopic dermatitis. *Dermatol Online J.* 2003;9(2):1.
90. Krouse JH, Sadrazodi K, Kerswill K. Sensitivity and specificity of prick and intradermal testing in predicting response to nasal provocation with timothy grass antigen. *Otolaryngol Head Neck Surg.* 2004;131(3):215–219.
91. Gungor A, Houser SM, Aquino BF, et al. A comparison of skin endpoint titration and skin-prick testing in the diagnosis of allergic rhinitis. *Ear Nose Throat J.* 2004; 83(1):54–60.
92. Bernstein IL, Li JT, Bernstein DI, et al. Allergy diagnostic testing: an updated practice parameter. *Ann Allergy Asthma Immunol.* 2008;100(3, suppl 3):S1–148.
93. Moscato G, Dykewicz MS, Desrosiers M, Castano R. Occupational rhinitis. In: Malo JL, Chan-Yeung M, Bernstein DI, eds. *Asthma and the Workplace.* Vol 4. Boca Raton, FL: CRC Press, Taylor & Francis Group; 2013:1–8.
94. Shusterman D. Occupational irritant and allergic rhinitis. *Curr Allergy Asthma Rep.* 2014;14(4):425.
95. Castano R, Theriault G, Gautrin D. Categorizing nasal septal perforations of occupational origin as cases of corrosive rhinitis. *Am J Ind Med.* 2007;50(2):150–153.
96. Beeson MF, Dewdney JM, Edwards RG, Lee D, Orr RG. Prevalence and diagnosis of laboratory animal allergy. *Clin Allergy.* 1983;13(5):433–442.
97. Malm L, Gerth van Wijk R, Bachert C. Guidelines for nasal provocations with aspects on nasal patency, airflow, and airflow resistance. International Committee on Objective Assessment of the Nasal Airways, International Rhinologic Society. *Rhinology.* 2000;38(1):1–6.
98. Rhinitis ETFoO, Moscato G, Vandenplas O, et al. Occupational rhinitis. *Allergy.* 2008;63(8):969–980.
99. Melillo G, Bonini S, Cocco G, et al. EAACI provocation tests with allergens. Report prepared by the European Academy of Allergology and Clinical Immunology Subcommittee on provocation tests with allergens. *Allergy.* 1997;52(35, suppl):1–35.
100. Henneberger PK, Wagner GR, Lemiere C. Asthma exacerbated at work. In: Malo JL, Chan-Yeung M, Bernstein DI, eds. *Asthma in the Workplace.* Vol 4. Boca Raton, FL: CRC Press, Taylor & Francis Group; 2013:325–335.
101. Balmes J, Becklake M, Blanc P, et al. American Thoracic Society Statement: Occupational contribution to the burden of airway disease. *Am J Respir Crit Care Med.* 2003; 167(5):787–797.
102. Malo JL, Ghezzo H, L'Archeveque J, Lagier F, Perrin B, Cartier A. Is the clinical history a satisfactory means of diagnosing occupational asthma? *Am Rev Respir Dis.* 1991;143(3):528–532.
103. Chan-Yeung M, Malo JL. Occupational asthma. *N Engl J Med.*. 1995;333(2):107–112.
104. Talini D, Novelli F, Bacci E, et al. Comparison between airway responses to high versus low molecular weight compounds in occupational asthma. *J Allergy.* 2011; 2011:781470.
105. Bernstein JA. Occupational asthma. In: Bernstein JA, Levy ML, eds. *Clinical Asthma Theory and Practice.* Boca Raton, FL: CRC Press, Taylor & Francis Group; 2014.
106. Beach J, Rowe BH, Blitz S, et al. Diagnosis and management of work-related asthma: Summary. *AHRQ Evidence Report Summaries.* 2005;(129):1–8.
107. Malo JL, Cote J, Cartier A, Boulet LP, L'Archeveque J, Chan-Yeung M. How many times per day should peak expiratory flow rates be assessed when investigating occupational asthma? *Thorax.* 1993;48(12):1211–1217.
108. Burge PS. Single and serial measurements of lung function in the diagnosis of occupational asthma. *Eur J Respir Dis.* 1982;123(suppl):47–59.
109. Chan-Yeung M, Malo JL, Tarlo SM, et al. Proceedings of the first Jack Pepys Occupational Asthma Symposium. *Am J Respir Crit Care Med.* 2003;167(3):450–471.
110. Koskela H, Taivainen A, Tukiainen H, Chan HK. Inhalation challenge with bovine dander allergens: who needs it? *Chest.* 2003;124(1):383–391.
111. Merget R, Stollfuss J, Wiewrodt R, et al. Diagnostic tests in enzyme allergy. *J Allergy Clin Immunol.* 1993;92(2):264–277.
112. Sheikh A, Hurwitz B. House dust mite avoidance measures for perennial allergic rhinitis. *Cochrane Database Syst Rev.* 2001;(4)(4):CD001563.
113. Dykewicz MS, Fineman S, Skoner DP, et al. Diagnosis and management of rhinitis: complete guidelines of the Joint Task Force on Practice Parameters in Allergy, Asthma and Immunology. American Academy of Allergy, Asthma, and Immunology. *Ann Allergy Asthma Immunol.* 1998;81(5, pt 2):478–518.
114. Cimbura G, Lucas DM, Bennett RC, Warren RA, Simpson HM. Incidence and toxicological aspects of drugs detected in 484 fatally injured drivers and pedestrians in Ontario. *J Forensic Sci.* 1982;27(4):855–867.
115. McDonald K, Trick L, Boyle J. Sedation and antihistamines: an update. Review of inter-drug differences using proportional impairment ratios. *Human Psychopharmacol.* 2008;23(7):555–570.
116. Golden SJ, Craig TJ. Efficacy and safety of azelastine nasal spray for the treatment of allergic rhinitis. *J Am Osteopath Assoc.* 1999;99(7, suppl):S7–S12.
117. Pauwels R. Mode of action of corticosteroids in asthma and rhinitis. *Clin Allergy.* 1986;16(4):281–288.
118. Pelikan Z, Snoek WJ, Booij-Noord H, Orie NG, de Vries K. Protective effect of disodium cromoglycate on the allergen provocation of the nasal mucosa. *Ann Allergy.* 1970;28(11):548–553.
119. Chandra RK, Heresi G, Woodford G. Double-blind controlled crossover trial of 4% intranasal sodium cromoglycate solution in patients with seasonal allergic rhinitis. *Ann Allergy.* 1982;49(3):131–134.

120. Taylor G, Shivalkar PR. Disodium cromoglycate: laboratory studies and clinical trial in allergic rhinitis. *Clin Allergy.* 1971;1(2):189–198.
121. Wilson AM, O'Byrne PM, Parameswaran K. Leukotriene receptor antagonists for allergic rhinitis: a systematic review and meta-analysis. *Am J Med.* 2004;116(5): 338–344.
122. Durham SR, Walker SM, Varga EM, et al. Long-term clinical efficacy of grass-pollen immunotherapy. *N Engl J Med.* 1999;341(7):468–475.
123. Pajno GB, Barberio G, De Luca F, Morabito L, Parmiani S. Prevention of new sensitizations in asthmatic children monosensitized to house dust mite by specific immunotherapy. A six-year follow-up study. *Clin Exp Allergy.* 2001;31(9):1392–1397.
124. Niggemann B, Jacobsen L, Dreborg S, et al. Five-year follow-up on the PAT study: specific immunotherapy and long-term prevention of asthma in children. *Allergy.* 2006;61(7):855–859.
125. Amin HS, Liss GM, Bernstein DI. Evaluation of near-fatal reactions to allergen immunotherapy injections. *J Allergy Clin Immunol.* 2006;117(1):169–175.
126. Slovak AJ, Orr RG, Teasdale EL. Efficacy of the helmet respirator in occupational asthma due to laboratory animal allergy (LAA). *Am Ind Hygiene Assoc J.* 1985;46(8):411–415.
127. Laoprasert N, Swanson MC, Jones RT, Schroeder DR, Yunginger JW. Inhalation challenge testing of latex-sensitive health care workers and the effectiveness of laminar flow HEPA-filtered helmets in reducing rhinoconjunctival and asthmatic reactions. *J Allergy Clin Immunol.* 1998;102(6, pt 1):998–1004.
128. Sastre J, Quirce S. Immunotherapy: an option in the management of occupational asthma? *Curr Opin Allergy Clin Immunol.* 2006;6(2):96–100.
129. Boutet K, Malo JL, Ghezzo H, Gautrin D. Airway hyperresponsiveness and risk of chest symptoms in an occupational model. *Thorax.* 2007;62(3):260–264.
130. de Groene GJ, Pal TM, Beach J, et al. Workplace interventions for treatment of occupational asthma: a Cochrane systematic review. *Occup Environ Med.* 2012; 69(5):373–374.
131. Yacoub MR, Lavoie K, Lacoste G, et al. Assessment of impairment/disability due to occupational asthma through a multidimensional approach. *Eur Respir J.* 2007;29(5):889–896.
132. Martyny J, Glazer CS, Newman LS. Respiratory protection. *N Engl J Med..* 2002;347(11):824–830.
133. American Thoracic S. Guidelines for assessing and managing asthma risk at work, school, and recreation. *Am J Respir Crit Care Med.* 2004;169(7):873–881.
134. Rachiotis G, Savani R, Brant A, MacNeill SJ, Newman Taylor A, Cullinan P. Outcome of occupational asthma after cessation of exposure: a systematic review. *Thorax.* 2007;62(2):147–152.
135. National Asthma E, Prevention P. Expert Panel Report 3 (EPR-3): Guidelines for the Diagnosis and Management of Asthma-Summary Report 2007. *J Allergy Clin Immunol.* 2007;120(5, suppl):S94–S138.
136. Stanaland BE. Therapeutic measures for prevention of allergic rhinitis/asthma development. *Allergy Asthma Proc.* 2004;25(1):11–15.
137. Abramson MJ, Walters EH. The epidemic of asthma: too much allergen or not enough infection? *Med J Australia.* 2000;172(3):119–121.
138. Cullinan P, Tarlo S, Nemery B. The prevention of occupational asthma. *Eur Respir J.* 2003;22(5):853–860.
139. Tarlo SM, Liss GM, Blanc PD. How to diagnose and treat work-related asthma: key messages for clinical practice from the American college of chest physicians consensus statement. *Polskie archiwum medycyny wewnetrznej.* 2009;119(10):660–666.
140. Nicholson PJ, Newman Taylor AJ, Oliver P, Cathcart M. Current best practice for the health surveillance of enzyme workers in the soap and detergent industry. *Occup Med.* 2001;51(2):81–92.
141. Linnett PJ. Concerns for asthma at pre-placement assessment and health surveillance in platinum refining—a personal approach. *Occup Med.* 2005;55(8):595–599.
142. Merget R, Caspari C, Dierkes-Globisch A, et al. Effectiveness of a medical surveillance program for the prevention of occupational asthma caused by platinum salts: a nested case-control study. *J Allergy Clin Immunol.* 2001;107(4):707–712.
143. Bernstein JA, Ghosh D, Sublett WJ, Wells H, Levin L. Is trimellitic anhydride skin testing a sufficient screening tool for selectively identifying TMA-exposed workers with TMA-specific serum IgE antibodies? *J Occup Environ Med.* 2011;53(10):1122–1127.
144. Bernstein DI, Jolly A. Current diagnostic methods for diisocyanate induced occupational asthma. *Am J Ind Med.* 1999;36(4):459–468.

13

Rheumatic Diseases and Vasculitides

Jennifer Guttman, Irene Blanco, and Clement E. Tagoe

INTRODUCTION

The rheumatologic diseases are a group of autoimmune disorders characterized by dysregulation of the immune system. The entities that make up this large group vary widely, but most share certain prominent clinical features. These include inflammation of the skin, joints, and structures with high connective tissue content.[1]

The upper airway is bordered by the oral cavity and nares superiorly, and the mid-trachea inferiorly. The lumen of this passageway is made up of several layers of mucosa, submucosa, and serosa, and is supported by many cartilaginous and articular structures that are rich in connective tissue. As a result, a number of the rheumatologic diseases compose an important portion of the disease processes that affect the upper respiratory tract (URT). These diseases also affect other parts of the head and neck, especially the ear, as a part of both acute and chronic inflammatory processes.[2]

DISEASES WITH PROMINENT UPPER AIRWAY FINDINGS

Rheumatoid Arthritis

Epidemiology and Pathology

Rheumatoid arthritis (RA) is an inflammatory arthropathy, affecting up to 1% of the adult population, mostly women beginning in their third and fourth decades (Table 13–1). It involves the synovial diarthrodial joints, those surrounded by a synovial fluid-containing capsule, lubricating the articulating surfaces and allowing free range of mobility. It usually affects the joints symmetrically. RA affects both the articular and extra-articular joint surfaces with pressure areas impacted the most. Pathologic deformations generally begin with inflammation and proliferation of the synovial villus, deposition of fibrin, and the formation of pannus on the surfaces of the joint. It eventually leads to erosion of the underlying cartilage and infiltration of the bone, and ultimately, destruction of the joint.[3]

Though RA primarily affects the peripheral joints, it also generates many extra articular manifestations. These manifestations can include musculoskeletal abnormalities as well as vasculitis within the blood vessel walls. Furthermore, RA can lead to serositis: inflammation of the serous tissue lining the lungs, heart, and abdomen.[4]

Head and Neck Involvement

The extra-articular manifestations of RA involve multiple structures in the head and neck including relatively often, the larynx, and the ear and nose far less frequently. Joint involvement, however, leads to most of the clinically significant otolaryngologic issues that arise. RA can involve the cricoarytenoid joint (CAJ), temporomandibular joint (TMJ), and cricothyroid joint.[3]

Table 13–1. Rheumatologic Diseases and Their Estimated Prevalence

Disease	Prevalence
Rheumatoid arthritis (RA)	1% of the adult population
Granulomatosis with polyangiitis (GPA)	30 000 people in the United States
Eosinophilic granulomatosis with polyangiitis (EGPA)	10 to 15 per million people worldwide
Giant cell arteritis (GCA)	27 cases per 100 000 people aged 50 years or older
Sjögren syndrome (SjS)	3% of the population
Cogan syndrome	Rare (no epidemiologic studies)
Polyarteritis nodosa (PAN)	2 to 9 cases per million per year in Europe
Systemic lupus erythematosus (SLE)	70 to 75 cases per 100 000
Systemic sclerosis (SSc)	240 per million in the United States
Ankylosing spondylitis (AS)	1% to 2% among Caucasions
Psoriatic arthropathy (PsA)	10% to 15% of patients with psoriasis
Polymyositis	5 per million in the United States
Sarcoidosis	1% to 5% of the population

> RA is a relatively common disease that can cause arthritis of the CAJ resulting in laryngeal inflammation and consequently, airway symptoms.

Laryngeal RA: Background and Prevalence

Together, inflammation of the CAJ and the formation of rheumatoid nodules along the vocal cords compose the main contributors to the development of laryngeal RA. Laryngeal RA is a well-studied entity, first characterized by Mackenzie in 1880.[5] In general, laryngeal RA is a benign disease process. However, it can present with a variety of upper airway complaints and in rare cases, pose a life-threatening danger.[6]

The prevalence of laryngeal RA varies among different populations and by use of different diagnostic modalities. Initial studies estimated that roughly 30% of RA patients expressed complaints related to laryngeal symptoms and up to 25% of patients had some upper airway obstruction.[7] The prevalence, however, has grown to estimates of 75% with improved diagnostic techniques.[8] In fact, laryngeal involvement is the presenting complaint in almost half of RA cases.[9]

CAJ Arthritis

Anatomy. The anatomy of the CAJ helps to explain why it is vulnerable to inflammation as RA takes its course. The CAJ sits along the back wall of the larynx, sandwiched between the cricoid and arytenoid cartilages and held up by a synovial lined ligamentous capsule. As the joint moves, it pulls on the attached arytenoids thereby changing the shape and position of the vocal cords. Consequently, swelling and scarring of the CAJ affixes the cords into the surrounding tissue. If set in an adducted position, access to the trachea will be closed without a way for air to enter or exit.[10] Up to two-thirds of laryngeal complaints in RA patients are attributable to arthritis of the CAJ.[11]

Signs and Symptoms: Acute and Chronic Disease. CAJ inflammation can occur both acutely, and as part of a chronic progression. Either may result in vocal cord fixation and airway obstruction.[7] When presenting acutely, patients usually complain of a sensation of throat fullness. Hoarseness and dysphagia are other typical complaints.[12] Acute CAJ arthritis is also associated with the development of stridor and dyspnea as well as infections along the URT.[13]

Although chronic CAJ arthritis is more common, it is difficult to detect given its more subtle advancement. Nonetheless, recurrent symptoms may be noted, including husky voice and stridor. These symptoms occur with sleep, on exertion or with infection. Indeed, the mechanical airway obstruction that happens with sleep helps to explain why obstructive sleep apnea is prevalent among RA patients.[14]

In severe cases, where ankylosis of the joint has occurred, patients experience difficulty breathing. As the joint stiffens, the vocal cords lose the ability to open and close normally. They cannot protect pharyngeal contents from entering the airway, resulting in aspiration of pharyngeal contents. Both pulmonary and cardiac infections may ensue, and can result in fatality.[15]

Diagnostic Studies. Presence of CAJ arthritis does not correlate with RA severity. However, it is most commonly seen in seropositive patients with detectable rheumatoid factor (RF).[16] Computed tomography (CT) is the imaging modality of choice for noninvasive visualization. Conventional radiography may illustrate erosion of the joint with accompanying osseous destruction. However, CT can also demonstrate thickening and erosion of the CAJ joint, arytenoid subluxation and asymmetry of the glottis or the aryepiglottic folds. Magnetic resonance imaging (MRI) can identify acute inflammation if the joint needs further assessment (Table 13–2).[12]

Direct visualization is the gold standard for diagnosing CAJ arthritis. During the acute phase, the arytenoids will appear inflamed while the vocal cords may look normal or mildly edematous. In the chronic phase, manifestations of disease include thickened mucosa overlying the arytenoids and limiting their mobility, bowing of the vocal folds and narrowing of the glottis.[17] To diagnose ankylosis in advanced disease, a normal electromyogram of the vocal muscles must be combined with visualized fixation of the CAJ. This helps rule out vocal cord paresis from recurrent laryngeal nerve damage.[11]

Table 13-2. Useful Rheumatological Diagnostic Studies

Disease Entity	Diagnostic Modalities
RA: CAJ arthritis	X-ray, CT, MRI, laryngoscopy
GPA:	
active vasculitis	c-ANCA, biopsy
subglottic stenosis	PFTs, CT, MRI, laryngoscopy
sinus involvement	CT, MRI, endoscopy
EGPA	ANCA, eosinophilic count, immunoglobulin assay
GCA	Temporal artery biopsy
SjS	Anti-Ro, Anti-La; salivary gland biopsy
AIED	Audiology
RP	CT, spirometry, biopsy
Cogan syndrome	MRI, biopsy
SSc: laryngeal involvement	Laryngoscopy
PsA	Radiography
Polymyositis	Serum CK, electromyography, muscle biopsy
Sarcoidosis: upper airway involvement	Laryngoscopy, biopsy

Cricothyroid Joint and TMJ Arthritides

RA can also involve the cricothyroid joint, which works to lengthen and tense the vocal cords. As a result, dysfunction of the joint results in complaints of limited vocal range, vocal fatigue, or hoarseness.[18] In cases of TMJ involvement, more than half of longstanding RA patients complain of pain and tenderness at the site as well as restricted mouth opening. The TMJ is sensitive to cartilage loss because of its fibrocartilage composition. Joint involvement is often bilateral, and over the course of disease, the joint may become ankylosed.[19]

In severe cases of bilateral TMJ arthritis, loss of condylar height can significantly affect jaw alignment. Flexion contractures in the muscles of mastication further displace the jaw, with compensating tongue thrusting worsening the bite. These changes can result in facial deformity, altered speech, and airway obstruction, including the development of sleep apnea as a result of pharyngeal obstruction.[20] In juvenile onset RA, loss of condylar height results in retrognathia and anterior open bite. Medical providers generally treat such cases aggressively to prevent facial abnormalities and associated breathing complications.[21] Radiographic evidence of deformity, including subcortical cysts and flattening of the condylar head and articular eminence, is present in almost 70% of cases.[22]

Atlantoaxial Subluxation

Signs and Symptoms. Atlantoaxial instability is present in one-quarter of RA patients, more frequently in men and usually in those with peripheral joint involvement. Subluxation of C1-C2 is more common than complete joint dislocation.[23] Symptoms of joint instability range from neck pain and headache to vertigo and nystagmus. Erosions of the odontoid process and apophyseal joints also result in head and neck pain.[24]

Progressive erosive disease can lead to deviation of the larynx, partially obstructing the airway. Compression of the spinal cord and brainstem can occur when the transverse ligament is altered by inflammatory changes, and may lead to cord compression resulting in paresis, parasthesias, and death.[25,26] Degree of instability and appearance on radiography correlate poorly with symptomatology even when imaging shows excess separation of the odontoid from the atlas.[27] In fact, one study found that x-ray of the spine revealed subluxation in almost 40% of RA patients who lacked localizing features.[28]

Endotracheal Intubation: Issues Related to RA in the Head and Neck

In those with CAJ disease, atlantoaxial instability or other RA pathology in nearby structures (even without airway compromise), issues can arise during endotracheal intubation. Airway obstruction may occur both during intubation and following extubation. Trauma inflicted with tube manipulation results in vocal fold edema and compromise of the URT. Furthermore, sedated patients have much more difficulty maintaining their airway.

To minimize this risk, otolaryngologic evaluation is recommended in patients with any URT symptoms including hoarseness and noisy breathing. Noninvasive measures that can decrease risk are preoperative use of glucocorticoids (GC) and postoperative racemic epinephrine. In addition, fiberoptic visualization with intubation, use of local anesthetic when possible, delayed extubation until the patient is fully alert, and preanesthetic tracheotomy are employed when appropriate.[29]

> Atlantoaxial instability puts surgical patients at high risk for airway obstruction during intubation and extubation. Appropriate precautions must be taken accordingly.

Rheumatoid Nodules and Bamboo Nodes

Rheumatoid arthritis also leads to the development of rheumatoid nodules within the vocal folds, impairing their movement. They are found in both the submucosal and subcutaneous tissue. If located at the glottic level, they are usually situated in the posterior part of the vocal folds.[30] The most common resulting symptoms include hoarse voice, dysphonia, and coughing.[31]

The histology of these nodules resembles rheumatoid nodules found in other locations with fibrinoid necrosis surrounded by palisading epithelioid macrophages as well as other mononuclear cells.[32] In addition, laryngoscopy may illustrate bamboo nodes, cystic yellow collections that accumulate within the submucosa of the vocal cords. Their presence correlates with both severity of disease and presence of antibody deposits.[33]

Rheumatoid Vasculitis. Laryngeal problems also emerge from RA-associated vasculitis. Inflammation of the vessels can lead to ischemia of the recurrent laryngeal and vagus nerves causing both impaired movement and paresis of the vocal cords. This process may be accompanied by atrophy of the laryngeal muscles and with progressive narrowing of the vasa vasorum supplying the larger vessels in the area. With the widespread use of disease modifying antirheumatic drugs (DMARDs), however, the prevalence of rheumatoid vasculitis has dropped dramatically over the last 2 decades. Less than 30 cases per every 1000 RA outpatients and 15 per 1000 inpatients were reported in one study of veterans.[34]

> Other RA airway features include rheumatoid nodules and vasculitis of the larynx.

Otologic Involvement

Conductive and sensorineural hearing defects, both generally mild, can present in patients with RA. Though usually attributed to salicylate intoxication, conductive losses are likely a result of synovial inflammation triggering ossicle erosion and shortening. Increased flaccidity of the middle ears is found in almost 40% of RA patients.[35] Sensorineural hearing loss (SNHL), on the other hand, most likely emerges from vasculitis of the vessels supplying the eighth cranial nerve.[36]

Management

Glucocorticoids (GCs) are the mainstay of treatment for active RA flares, and frequently reverse upper airway obstruction associated with acute CAJ arthritis. They are given in high doses by mouth, intravenously, or injected directly into the joint. In addition, nonsteroidal anti-inflammatory drugs (NSAIDs) are effective in reducing pain and swelling. The primary goal of therapy is to prevent advancement of disease and the formation of nodules or of fibrosis with use of DMARDs.[37] DMARDs encompass both biologic agents like tumor necrosis factor alpha (TNFα) blockers as well as nonbiologics like methotrexate, sulfasalazine and hydroxychloroquine.[37] While methotrexate is one of the most commonly used DMARDs, it may paradoxically increase susceptibility to nodule development in up to 10% of patients.[38] When larger nodules develop, removal by laryngoscopy is the treatment of choice.[39]

In patients with chronic CAJ arthritis with vocal cord involvement, medical management is often insufficient, and frequently, these patients require surgical intervention. The vocal cords may be surgically lateralized either endoscopically or by an external approach. Endoscopically, the cords can be manipulated by laser cordotomy or by arytenoidectomy. Severe cervical spine disease may prevent an endoscopic approach. Though such procedures generally improve the airway obstruction, they often leave patients with permanent hoarseness and voice changes.[40,41] In patients with severe cervical spine disease compromising the airway, tracheotomy may be indicated.[42]

For TMJ arthritis, oral pain control can sometimes require supplementation with an anesthetic or steroid injection, or by use of botulin injections into the masseter and temporalis muscles. In the past, open surgery was used for more refractory cases. However, such procedures are now rarely performed because of the tendency to develop secondary degenerative disease and prolonged neuropathic pain. Moreover, open surgery is considered high risk given the neighboring trigeminal nerve, carotid artery, and jugular vein.[43] Total joint replacement is opted for in cases of collapse, severely restricted opening or unmanageable pain.[44] Long-term follow-up of joint replacement patients has demonstrated improved jaw opening, better dietary intake, and less pain complaints in these patients.[45]

> Management of laryngeal RA typically begins with immunosuppression. Many of the anatomic complications are amenable to surgical intervention.

Vasculitides

Pathology and Epidemiology

The vasculitides are a group of diseases characterized by vessel wall inflammation causing occlusion of the lumen and resulting in organ injury. Immune activation within the vessel walls leads to the formation of either granulomas or fibrinoid necrosis. Vasculitides are chiefly classified by both their histological features and the caliber of the vessels that they affect.[46]

Granulomatous Polyangiitis

Pathology, Immunobiology, and Histology. Granulomatosis with polyangiitis (GPA, formerly Wegener's granulomatosis) is a small vessel disease that primarily affects the ear, nose, and throat with involvement of these structures in up to 95% of cases. It affects approximately 30 000 people in the United States.[47] In the lungs, the disease destroys the parenchyma resulting in cavitary nodules, alveolar hemorrhages, and interstitial lung disease. It also causes pauci-immune glomerulonephritis in the kidneys, different types of skin lesions, and mononeuritis multiplex.[48]

In cases with systemic manifestations, more than 90% have positive ELISAs (enzyme linked immunosorbent assay) for c-ANCA (cytoplasmic antineutrophil cytoplasmic antibodies), with predominant specificity against proteinase 3. Although only 60% to 80% of the limited form of GPA show this pattern of immunofluorescence, it is especially useful in monitoring disease in cases of GPA persistently localized to the head and neck which occurs in less than 5% of cases.[49,50] Though ANCA positivity is strongly suggestive of a diagnosis, only evidence of vasculitis on biopsy can confirm GPA.[51] Histological examination illustrates granulomas, poorly defined collections of histiocytic cells, mostly epithelioid, surrounded by dense inflammatory infiltrates.[52]

Head and Neck Involvement

Sinus, Nasal, and Oral Features. Of the head and neck manifestations, sinonasal involvement is most common in GPA and results in sinusitis and rhinitis with complaints that range from congestion and epistaxis to sinus pain and anosmia. The maxillary sinus is the most commonly involved site. Patients develop polyps and submucosal nodularity. Eventually, chronic inflammation results in atrophy of the sinus and erosion of the nasal cartilage. Destruction of the cartilage leads to complications that include perforation of the nasal septum, saddle nose, and formation of a fistula between the nasal sinuses and the orbits or the palate. Sinus cultures in these patients are chronically positive for *Staphylococcus aureus*, the most common agent inducing superinfection and which is often only partially responsive to antibiotics.[53]

Gingivitis can be severe and may precede other features. It serves as a useful site for biopsy. Patients develop painful, shallow ulcers of the oral mucosa as well as lesions of the hard palate. They are caused by destruction of the overlying gingiva and alveolar mucosa and result in complaints of sore throat and difficulty swallowing.[54]

Otologic Features. When GPA involves the ear, serous otitis media is the most common presentation, occurring in roughly one-third of patients. Granuloma formation in the pharyngotympanic tube (eustachian tube) and nasopharynx causes obstruction, leading to the development of otitis media. Involvement can extend to the middle ear, tympanic membrane, and mastoid bone leading to chronic otitis media. Chronic middle ear effusions can eventually produce conductive hearing loss that is irreversible. Failure to drain the middle ear adequately increases susceptibility to superinfection and suppurative otitis media.[55]

In addition, SNHL can develop from inflammation of the cochlear vasculature as well as endolymph obstruction, that together result in inner ear injury.[56,57] On examination, the tympanic membrane appears concave and colorless with obscuring of the superficial vessels.[57] In association with ear symptoms, rare cases of facial nerve palsy have been reported. These likely occur as a result of granuloma formation within the temporal bone and subsequent compression of the facial and auditory nerves.[58]

Upper Airway Features. Subglottic stenosis is considered the most serious upper airway complication of GPA and occurs in up to one-fifth of cases. It initially develops from pooling of postnasal or pharyngeal mucus, or from the disassembly of a chronic inflammatory deposition within a couple of centimeters of the vocal cords.[59] Subsequent scarring and stricture formation results in a more fixed narrowing, as illustrated on tracheoscopy performed on a group of 9 GPA patients (Figure 13–1).[60]

> In GPA, granulomas form in the ears and along the entire upper airway from the nose and facial sinuses to the subglottis.

Diagnostic Studies. Pulmonary function testing is an essential tool for evaluating those with suspected GPA. Subglottic stenosis produces a fixed tracheal obstruction generating a characteristic flow volume curve, with truncation of both inspiratory and expiratory limbs. Its shape reflects the functional degree

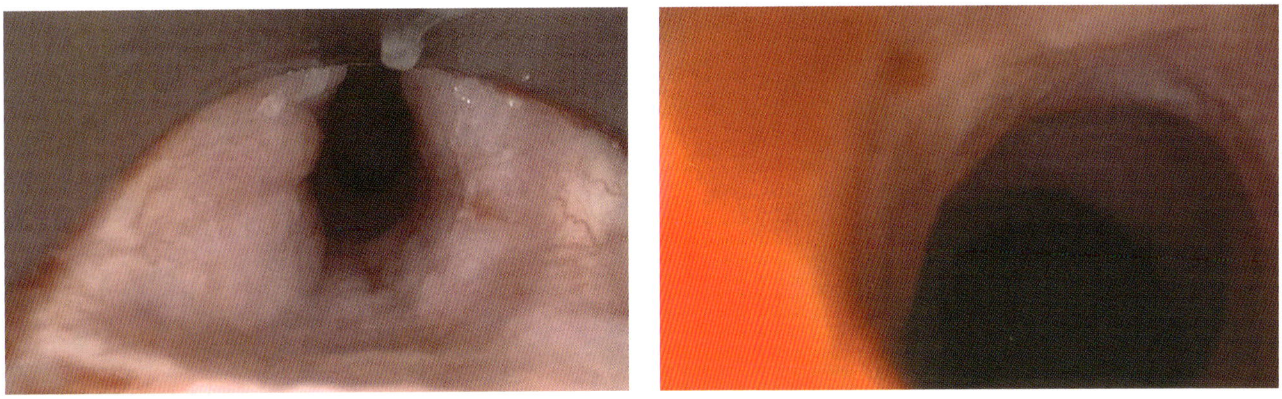

Figure 13–1. Subglottic stenosis in a patient with GPA. **A.** Pre-endoscopic balloon laryngoplasty/tracheoplasty. **B.** Postdilatation showing enlargement of airway lumen.

of obstruction rather than the anatomic size of the lesion. In fact, the flow volume curve may remain relatively intact until the lumen is reduced to less than 20% of its original area.[61]

In evaluating GPA, CT imaging of the sinuses reveals thickening of the mucosa along the nasal cavity and the paranasal sinuses, most prominently in the maxillary sinuses. Both the paranasal sinuses and the mastoid cells may appear either partially or totally opacified. During the acute phase, neither CT nor MRI can distinguish between active vasculitis and infection. However, with persistent or recurrent sinonasal involvement, characteristic findings emerge including sclerosing osteitis of the paranasal sinuses. In one-fifth of these patients, this same pattern of increased bone deposition is also seen along the mastoid cells. The nearby bone erodes with destruction of the septum and turbinates and with obliteration of the sinuses.[62] MRI is useful for actually visualizing the granulomas within the nasal cavity or paranasal sinuses.[63]

On endoscopy, the nasal and sinus mucosa look inflamed and ulcerated, and in some cases, they demonstrate a classic cobblestone appearance. Diagnosis can only be confirmed with biopsy. The nasopharynx is the most accessible site. While a specimen can show the typical granulomatous features, necrosis and superinfection may obscure the diagnostic features and necessitate repeat biopsy.[64]

Similarly, subglottic stenosis is often initially evaluated with imaging. However, CT and MRI are not sensitive enough to evaluate the extent of stenosis. Despite the risks associated, laryngoscopy is indicated to best evaluate the lesion. Active inflammation generally obscures the ability to identify granulomas or characteristic vasculitis. Nevertheless, it is helpful in excluding other causes for obstruction (Figure 13–2).[65]

Management. Vasculitic involvement of the URT requires both local and systemic immunosuppressive therapy. Local measures include topical steroids, nasal saline rinses, and surgical intervention.[66,67] Functional endoscopic sinus surgery (FESS) is a minimally invasive approach to treat sinusitis and other nasal deformities. Nonetheless, the disease process alters the anatomy and makes FESS more difficult, requiring meticulous mucosal sparing techniques and careful postoperative irrigation and debridement.[64] Nasal reconstruction with use of auricular, conchal, or costal cartilage to correct saddle nose is effective.[68] Repair of nasal septal perforation, on the other hand, is more difficult because the lesions are usually large, limiting the support of local tissue, and relapse is common. In cases where the defect is small, a silicone septal button may be inserted.[69]

Otitis media with effusion in GPA should be treated initially with irrigation. Myringotomy tube placement must be combined with systemic therapy to treat involvement of the middle ear, mastoid process, and pharyngotympanic tube.[55] The SNHL that results from ear involvement is generally irre-

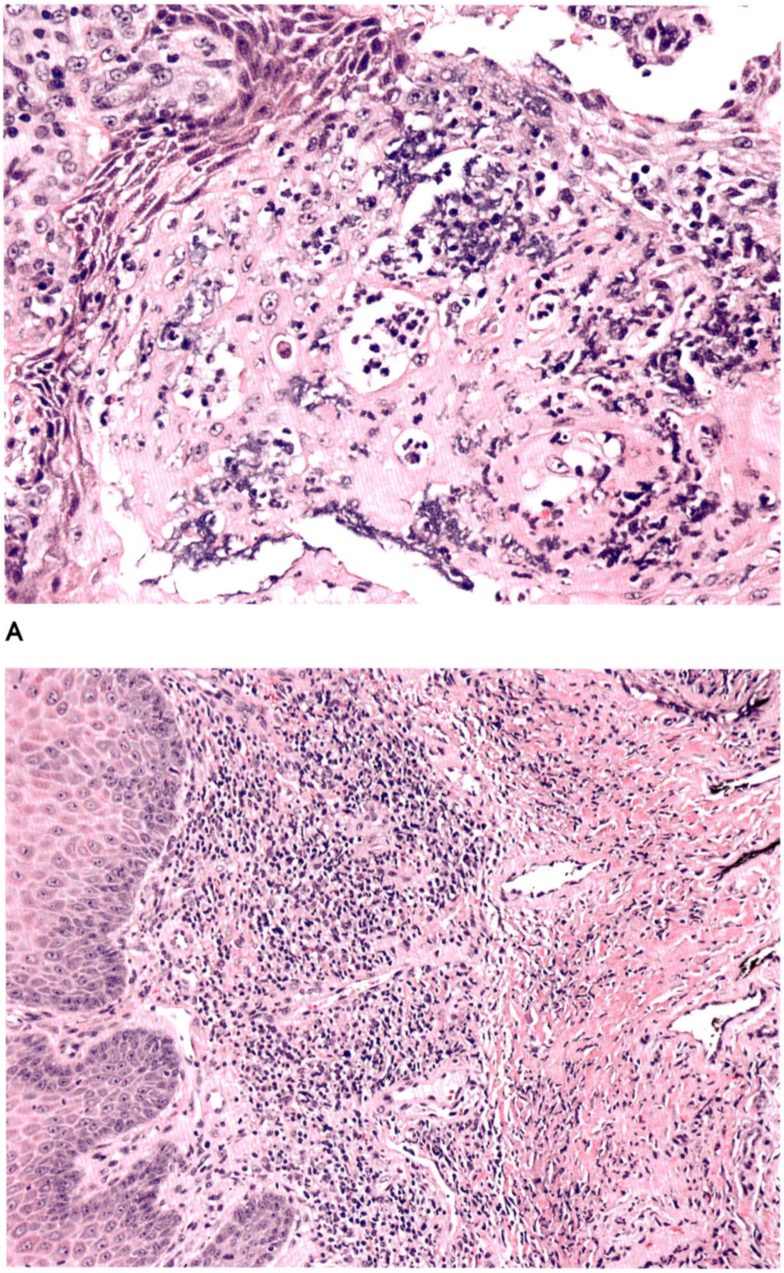

Figure 13–2. Ulcerated squamous mucosa with marked acute and chronic inflammation, microabscess formation, fibrinoid necrosis, and granulation tissue. **A.** Palatal biopsy. **B.** Gingival biopsy.

versible and treatment typically involves use of hearing aids.[70]

Subglottic stenosis requires both local management with secretion clearance and removal of the obstruction as well as adjuvant systemic GC therapy. While acute obstruction requires tracheotomy placement, different procedures have been attempted to reduce obstruction in cases of chronic subglottic stenosis. Among them, intralesional corticosteroid injection and dilatation appears to be most successful. It can often avoid the need for tracheotomy. However, repeat procedures may be required.[71,72]

Standard of care systemic therapy for the ANCA associated vasculitides such as GPA encompasses a few different options. Induction therapy generally involves the use of GCs in combination with methotrexate in the localized form, and cyclophosphamide or rituximab in systemic disease, with the addition of plasma exchange in severe cases. Use of rituximab is the favored induction regimen as a result of the RAVE trial, published in 2010, which showed that rituximab is noninferior to the highly toxic drug cyclophosphamide in inducing remission in severe ANCA associated vasculitides.[73] Maintenance therapy includes low-dose GCs plus azathioprine, methotrexate, or the second-line agent, mycophenolate mofetil.[74]

> Management of ANCA vasculitis involves an induction phase and a maintenance phase when the dose of chronic steroids is generally reduced.

Esosinophilic Granulomatosis With Polyangiitis

Eosinophilic granulomatosis with polyangiitis (also referred to as Churg-Strauss syndrome) is a much rarer small vessel vasculitis with a prevalence of about 10 to 15 per million people. It presents with a variety of otorhinolaryngological and respiratory tract manifestations and is usually accompanied by asthma. Head and neck manifestations are more prevalent in those with serology for perinuclear ANCA (p-ANCA), especially with anti-myeloperoxidase (MPO) specificity. Features of disease most commonly include sinusitis, nasal polyps, and a pseudoallergic rhinitis characterized by inflammation of the nasal airways accompanied by symptoms of rhinorrhea, itching, and nasal congestion. Other typical complaints are nasal crusting, epistaxis, and difficulty with smell.[47,75]

Unlike GPA, EGPA does not usually produce erosive lesions. Instead, polyps form and soft tissue builds up along the sinuses and orbits, and can result in compression of adjacent nerves or other nearby structures. EGPA also manifests with eosinophilic infiltration of the airway and particularly, the lungs, with corresponding symptoms of obstructed airflow. Finally, EGPA affects both the central and peripheral nervous systems and can therefore present with symptoms of vocal cord paresis.[76] Histopathology reveals granulomas both within and outside the vasculature with rich eosinophilia. Presence of ANCA, eosinophilia, and hypergammaglobulinemia help to establish the diagnosis.[77]

In EGPA, GC therapy alone can result in remission in up to 90% of cases, though in close to half, they will relapse. Cyclophosphamide or alternative immunosuppressant therapy is required in addition to GC therapy when other organs outside the head and neck are involved. Surgery may be employed to remove obstructive lesions such as compressive nasal polyps in EGPA. However, they frequently recur and require repeat intervention.[78]

> Features of EGPA include sinusitis, nonerosive nasal polyps, and rhinitis.

Giant Cell Arteritis

Giant cell arteritis (GCA) is a vasculitis of large elastic arteries which leads to aneurysm formation and stenosis, resulting in symptoms of vascular occlusion. It is most common among the elderly, with up to 27 cases per 100 000 people aged 50 years or older. GCA commonly involves the superficial temporal, vertebral, ophthalmic, and posterior ciliary arteries, and any of the extracranial arteries (Figure 13–3).[79]

Because of this extensive cranial artery disease, patients can develop a variety of head and neck manifestations. Headache is the initial complaint in almost half of cases. The other classic sign is vision changes as a result of inflammation of the ophthalmic arteries. Less frequently, patients present with pain on chewing and talking as a result of masseter ischemia causing jaw claudication. Involvement of other arteries leads to vertigo, hearing loss, and epistaxis. Oral signs of disease include glossitis and claudication of the tongue.

Early diagnosis is critical because of the reversibility of acute inflammatory changes with use of GCs. Due to the risk of high-dose steroids in the elderly population who make up the majority of GCA patients, temporal artery biopsy is indicated if there is any doubt regarding diagnosis.[80]

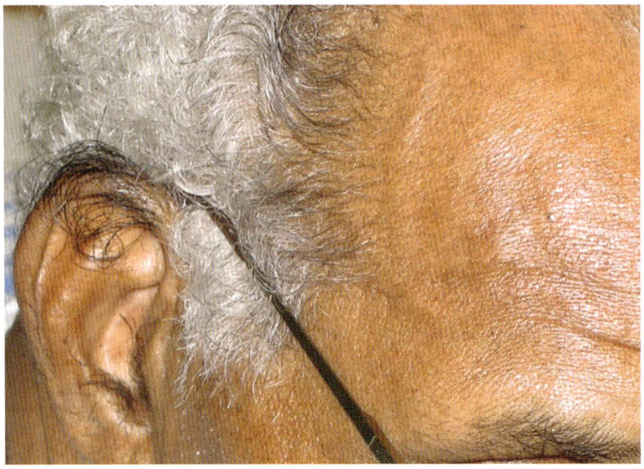

Figure 13–3. Temporal arteritis in GCA.

> GCA is a reversible cause of blindness, most commonly seen in the elderly. When suspected, patients should undergo temporal artery biopsy.

Sjögren Syndrome

Epidemiology. Sjögren syndrome (SjS) is a rheumatologic disease that primarily involves the salivary and lacrimal glands, leading to multiple ear, nose, and throat manifestations. Although Hendrik Sjogren, a Swedish ophthalmologist, reported the first case in 1933, descriptions of filamentary keratitis date back to 1882.[81,82] It is found in 3% of the population and is roughly 9 times more common in women. It most frequently presents in those between the ages of 40 and 60, and increases in prevalence with age. SjS can occur both as a primary entity or within the context of other autoimmune diseases including RA, lupus, and systemic sclerosis.[83]

Oral, Nasal, and Otologic Features. While SjS can target almost any organ in the body, mouth and eye dryness reflect the most typical features of SjS. As a result, patients develop oral ulcers, thick mucus, and fissured tongue. Patients complain of sore mouth from difficulty with chewing and swallowing and are susceptible to infection. With fungal infections, most commonly candidiasis, several oral complications may occur including pseudomembranous and erythematous mucosal lesions, atrophy of the filiform papillae, fistulae of the tongue, and angular cheilitis.[84]

SjS patients complain of decreased taste, which on exam, is linked with a reduced number of taste buds. They develop severe dental caries and periodontal disease as a result of reduced salivation.[84] Though usually mild, nasal symptoms are another feature of SjS. Epistaxis and nasal crusting are common, whereas severe dryness leading to septal perforation occurs in rare cases.[85] One-quarter of patients demonstrate symptoms localized to the ear including decreased hearing, otalgia, and tinnitus. They occur as a result of dryness of the external auditory canal, crust formation, and lymphoid mass collection along the pharyngotympanic tube.[86]

> SjS is an autoimmune disease that targets the lacrimal and salivary glands. Patients develop multiple complications as a result of the dryness and the thick mucus that result.

Upper Airway Features. Salivary gland enlargement occurs in up to 60% of cases, usually bilaterally and diffusely (termed *lymphoepithelial sialadenitis*). Massive enlargement may compromise the airway. Dryness of the airway and thick mucus adhering to the vocal folds put patients at even greater risk for respiratory difficulties. Patients often develop chronic bronchitis with production of tenacious sputum. Regular evaluation in patients with firm, palpable glands is essential because of the association of parotid gland enlargement with the development of lymphoma. Persistent enlargement may suggest either pseudolymphoma or non-Hodgkin lymphoma and indicates the need for biopsy.[87]

SjS can also involve the respiratory tract, and some patients initially present with complaints of dyspnea. Extreme dryness of the tracheobronchial mucosa (xerotrachea), may develop from decreased saliva production, causing tracheitis and putting patients at risk for bronchopneumonia. In addition, airway obstruction can occur from inflammation of the bronchus associated lymphoid tissue along the bronchial tree, especially at branch points.[88]

Diagnostic Studies. Testing for anti-Ro (SSA) and anti-La (SSB) antibodies and RF is the mainstay of initial diagnosis. Different modalities can illustrate salivary function while ultrasound, MRI, and magnetic resonance sialography demonstrate gland anatomy. For instance, with ultrasound, multiple variables can be evaluated including parenchymal homogeneity and echogenicity, size, and the appearance of the posterior glandular border. However, the use of ultrasound in standard practice remains undefined.[89,90] Biopsy of the gland shows aggregates of lymphocytes and plasma cells adjacent to the glandular ducts and replacing the acini. In 40% of cases, epimyoepithelial cell island formation can also be seen in the affected glands.[83]

In those with evidence of upper airway disease, pulmonary function testing reveals a small airway obstructive pattern suggestive of local swelling occurring at both the bronchial and bronchiolar levels. On the other hand, a restrictive pattern with low diffusion capacity may manifest as a result of a diffuse, lymphocytic interstitial pneumonitis. Chest x-ray and CT illustrate peribronchial and peribronchiolar inflammation, commonly referred to as dirty lung.[91]

Management. Treatment in SjS focuses on symptom management with measures such as oral hygiene, local lubricants, and dental fluoride. Oral muscarinic M3 receptor agonists may offer benefit to those with remaining glandular function.[92] NSAIDs are helpful in patients with tender glands. Systemic steroid therapy is reserved for those with extraglandular manifestations, especially given the increased risk for lymphoma development with use of cytotoxic drugs.[93]

> Treatment of SjS relies on the use of local hygiene and lubrication.

DISEASES WITH MARKED EAR PATHOLOGY

Autoimmune Inner Ear Disease

Definition and Epidemiology

Autoimmune inner ear disease (AIED) is an idiopathic syndrome characterized by hearing loss and frequently associated dizziness and tinnitus. While it is poorly defined, several diagnostic criteria exist, including disease restricted to the inner ear, bilateral SNHL of at least 30 decibels, and evidence of progression over a period of less than 3 months.[94,95] AIED occurs in the setting of a systemic autoimmune disease in about one-third of cases though it rarely presents as part of the initial symptomatology.[96] It accounts for less than 1% of cases of hearing impairment; however, the exact incidence remains unclear because of difficulty in diagnosis.[97]

Pathophysiology

It is well established that AIED stems from increases of both humoral and cell-mediated immune activity, but several theories exist to explain the exact mechanism. The most accepted is that there is a breakdown in immune tolerance. The inner ear is immunologically privileged, and only following some provoking event are its antigens exposed to the immune system and therefore recognized as foreign. Another explanation, the bystander theory, posits that damage to the inner ear causes the influx of immune cells which are exposed to the cochlea. These immunocytes subsequently target the endolymphatic sac leading to the death of sensory and supporting cells within the cochlea.[98–100]

> Multiple hypotheses have emerged to explain the mechanism of immune-mediated bilateral SNHL in AIED.

Diagnostic Studies and Management

Diagnostic evaluation includes audiology, nonspecific serology and inflammatory markers, and MRI to rule out a mass lesion or demyelinating disease.[101,102] Corticosteroid responsiveness, however, is the most useful way to diagnose AIED.[103] Corticosteroids are the mainstay of therapy though the level of response generally wanes with time.[104]

No prospective randomized clinical trials exist for the treatment of AIED given the rarity of this entity. However, a 4-week trial of GCs is recommended, followed by monthly audiograms to demonstrate stability. While low-dose GCs may be used for maintenance, steroid sparing therapy is favored. Available agents include cyclophosphamide, mycophenolate mofetil, and azathioprine.[95,105–107]

Biologic agents and plasmapheresis have also been used although the evidence for efficacy is anecdotal and inconclusive.[108]

Relapsing Polychondritis

Epidemiology and Pathology

Relapsing polychondritis (RP) is a rare autoimmune disorder defined by inflammation of the cartilaginous and connective tissues. Incidence has been estimated at 3.5 cases per million.[109] RP is associated with the formation of antibodies against type II collagen (anti CII) fibers and is thought to target the glycosaminoglycans and proteoglycans that make up cartilage. Affected tissues include the ears, nose, laryngotracheobronchial tree, and peripheral joints. The course of disease is highly variable, ranging from infrequent episodes to fulminant disease with significant morbidity and mortality attributable mostly to respiratory and cardiovascular involvement.[110]

Head and Neck Involvement

Otologic Features. Auricular chondritis is the most common initial symptom and eventually occurs in almost all patients. It is defined by the sudden onset of pain and swelling along the cartilage of the external ear, sparing the lobule. It usually presents bilaterally and is often accompanied by nearby lymphadenopathy. An association with ear piercing suggests that the studs used serve as an antigenic stimulus for immunocyte activation.[111]

Pharyngotympanic tube obstruction during acute inflammation can produce an otitis media that requires surgical drainage. Narrowing of the auditory canal as a result of swelling and fluid buildup may be severe enough to cause conductive hearing loss. Vasculitis of the internal auditory artery and its cochlear branches results in SNHL, which is frequently associated with symptoms of vertigo and ataxia. These attacks usually last 2 to 4 weeks. Repeated episodes, however, cause auricular cartilage destruction and lead to permanent ear deformity, such as the classic floppy pinna or cauliflower ear.[112]

Upper Airway Features. URT involvement is common with complications developing in almost half of patients. Involvement ranges in location from the nasal cartilage all the way down to the second-order bronchi. Common symptoms include cough, hoarseness, dyspnea, and neck tenderness. In cases of sudden nasal cartilage collapse, patients may develop a saddle deformity with chronic drainage and crusting.[110] Careful evaluation is essential to distinguish the etiology of the saddle nose which can also occur as part of a wide range of conditions including GPA, congenital syphilis, and leprosy, as well as a result of trauma or cocaine use.[113]

Airway obstruction occurs as a result of multiple different mechanisms. Active disease produces local swelling and can therefore compromise the airway. During later stages, a fibrous tissue mass may produce obstruction. Finally, recurrent disease leads to dissolution of the tracheobronchial cartilage with subsequent collapse of the airway.[114] In addition to these 3 primary mechanisms, thick secretions build up, and patients are at increased risk of pulmonary infection as a consequence of impaired cough, poor mucociliary clearance, atelectasis, and collapse. Airway difficulty is the chief cause of mortality in patients with RP.[115]

> Complications of the airway are common in the URT in RP. Local inflammation and subsequent scarring, cartilage collapse, and buildup of secretions extend from the nasal cartilage down to the bronchi.

Diagnostic Studies. Diagnosis can generally be made by history and physical examination alone. Nonetheless, different modalities are used for further evaluation. Disease severity is correlated with serum levels of collagen type II-specific antibodies (anti-CII), although this is not available in normal clinical practice.[116] CT scan reveals "worm eaten" cartilage with circumferential thickening. In later stages, the airway lumen will appear irregular.[117] Spirometry helps to assess the position and severity of airway involvement and to determine whether it is fixed or dynamic.[118] Biopsy specimens show loss of normal cartilage with inflammatory infiltration of the perichondrium.[119]

Management. Systemic treatment primarily involves NSAIDs, GCs, immunosuppressive agents, and dapsone with dramatic responses in many cases.

Newer studies have also shown benefit with use of plasmapheresis. Tracheotomy placement is required when the subglottic area is affected by disease.

While early tracheotomy is preferred to attempting bronchoscopy and intubation, the tracheotomy itself may cause fatal airway obstruction or tracheomalacia in rare instances. Moreover, in cases of collapse of the tracheal and bronchial rings with fixed stenoses, tracheotomy will not work to create an airway due to lack of structural support. When tracheotomy is effective, positive pressure ventilation is used to help prevent reversible airway collapse. In cases of dynamic obstruction as a product of central airway collapse, splinting of the airway with a stent may be sufficient without the need for tracheotomy placement.[120,121]

Cogan Syndrome

Epidemiology and Pathology

Cogan syndrome is a rare autoimmune disease defined by ocular and audiovestibular symptoms. Close to three-quarters of patients also have evidence of systemic disease, usually with gastrointestinal, neurological, or cardiac features, as a result of associated vasculitis. Because it is so rare, there are no epidemiologic reports of the prevalence. Nonetheless, over 100 cases have been reported in the medical literature.[122]

Both cell-mediated immunity and antibody stimulation produce the inflammation that causes Cogan syndrome. Recent studies have shown that connexin 26, a structural molecule expressed in endothelial cells of the inner ear, is one of the targeted antigens.[123] Seroepidemiological studies also support a connection between prior chlamydia infections and Cogan syndrome, especially in cases with the complications of arteriosclerosis and vasculitis. It may therefore represent the result of an infectious agent or its metabolites provoking an antibody response that cross-reacts with some of the proteins present in the audiovestibular and ocular systems.[124]

Otologic Features

Cogan syndrome is characterized by nonsyphilitic interstitial keratitis and by autoimmune inner ear disease. Inner ear manifestations include hearing loss, as well as tinnitus and vertigo. Onset of symptoms may be gradual but hearing loss is generally rapidly progressive. It can be sensorineural, conductive, or mixed, depending on the site of inflammation. Bilateral deafness eventually occurs in 70% of cases (Figure 13–4).[125]

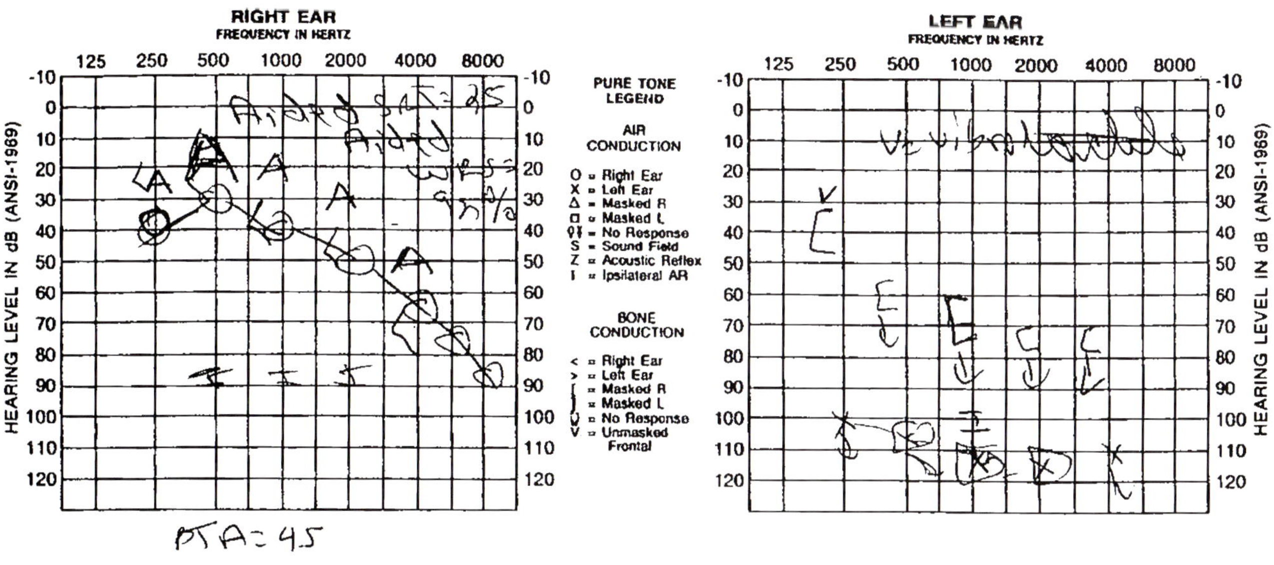

Figure 13–4. Audiology report in a patient with Cogan syndrome demonstrating moderate to severe SNHL in the right ear and profound SNHL in the left.

> Cogan syndrome is characterized by interstitial keratitis and immune-mediated inner ear disease resulting in a variety of ocular and audiovestibular symptoms.

Diagnostic Studies

Diagnosis may be difficult because of overlap with other vasculitides including Takayasu arteritis and polyarteritis nodosa. Radiographic studies are generally normal with some nonspecific findings.[126] Narrowing, calcification, and soft tissue obliteration of the vestibular labyrinth and cochlea, as seen on MRI, are highly suggestive.[127] On corneal and cochlear biopsy, histologic examination reveals both lymphocytic and plasma cell infiltration.[128]

Management

For mild symptoms of dizziness and hearing loss, local corticosteroid application is the mainstay of treatment. In more severe cases, intravenous corticosteroids result in significant improvement in hearing.[129] In long-standing cases where fibrosis and osteogenesis of the perilymphatic space have occurred, corticosteroids offer limited benefit.[130] When patients are refractory to corticosteroids, or when attempts are made to spare patients of corticosteroid use, other immunosuppressive drugs may be tried, including methotrexate, azathioprine, and TNFα blockers. In severe cases, rituximab has been shown to decrease deafness and the need for cochlear implants. However, at this time, no controlled trials exist examining the efficacy of conventional or biologic DMARDs.[131–133]

Polyarteritis Nodosa

Polyarteritis nodosa (PAN) is a necrotizing vasculitis of small and medium-sized muscular arteries affecting the systemic vasculature and usually involving the visceral circulation and sparing the pulmonary arteries. The incidence of PAN in Europe is somewhere between 2 and 9 cases per million per year.[134] Despite its tendency to affect the vasculature throughout the body, otorhinolaryngological attributes are generally limited to the ear.[135]

Sudden deafness is the presenting sign in a significant subset of PAN cases. Because otologic signs frequently follow acute otitis media, it is widely held that a viral infection serves as the antigenic stimulus for the inflammatory cascade that takes place in the ear. Involvement of the internal auditory artery causes SNHL.[136]

PAN is approached in a similar fashion to other vasculitides, with early and aggressive immunosuppressive therapy. In hepatitis B (HBV)–related cases, a short course of immunosuppressive therapy is followed by plasma exchange and antiviral therapy. One trial found that all 9 survivors of HBV treated this way achieved clinical recovery from HBV-PAN at 6 months.[137]

DISEASES WITH LESS COMMON EAR, NOSE, AND THROAT MANIFESTATIONS

Systemic Lupus Erythematosus

Epidemiology and Pathology

Systemic lupus erythematosus (SLE) is an autoimmune disease characterized by the deposition of both immune complexes and complement throughout the body causing local inflammation and tissue damage.[138] It is found 9 times more frequently in women than in men, particularly in those between the ages of 15 and 35 with an estimated prevalence of 70 to 75 per 100 000 individuals.[139,140] SLE most commonly affects the skin, kidneys, joints, blood vessels, heart, lungs, and nervous system. It can also involve the structures of the head and neck with involvement of the larynx in one-third of cases.[141]

Head and Neck Involvement

Oral and Nasal Features. Oral mucosal involvement results from deposition of inflammatory materials along both the lamina propria and the laryngeal basement membrane and is therefore associated with increased SLE activity. It leads to both nonulcerating lesions with keratotic scaling of the vermillion border and to more characteristic gray, yellow ulcers with central depression along the gingival, palatal, and buccal mucosa. Both types of lesions are generally painless. Within the submucosa, hematomas can easily develop. Most commonly, patients complain of hoarse voice and throat pain.[142]

Nasal septal perforation is another common finding, usually preceded by epistaxis and the development of foul-smelling crust.[143] Perforation occurs as a result of ischemia, as suggested by the prevalence of Raynaud's disease in these patients, as well as by immune complex deposition, enhanced blood viscosity, and frequent corticosteroid use. Generally, both the oral and nasal findings associated with SLE resolve rapidly with use of GCs.[142] Occasionally, septal perforation must be addressed with surgical closure, most effectively by the use of Silastic buttons though local ischemia often impairs the success of the underlying skin graft.[144]

Upper Airway Features. Inflammation of the larynx involves the mucosa, submucosa, and serosa and often leads to infection. Pathogens vary widely, including streptococci, mycobacteria, and candida. Biopsy of the inflamed epiglottis illustrates necrotic epithelium adjacent to a dense inflammatory infiltrate within the connective tissue.[144]

Over time, laryngeal inflammation results in scarring and stenosis, and in downstream necrotizing tracheitis. Involvement of the serosal layers of the larynx also promotes laryngitis sicca with swelling of the vocal cords and eventually, thickening and paralysis. Inflammation of the perichondrium surrounding the laryngeal cartilage and arthritis of the CAJ may also occur, causing a slight increase in the risk for respiratory difficulties.[141,145]

Vasculitis of the vasa nervorum, the vessels supplying the nerves, is felt to play an important role in producing the vocal cord palsy that is seen in patients with SLE. Moreover, vasculitis is associated with facial and trigeminal nerve dysfunction.[146] Biopsy of involved vessels shows thickened, hyalinized vessel walls with perivascular edema and lymphocytic infiltrates.[147]

Despite the low incidence of airway compromise when SLE involves the CAJ, difficulty breathing can arise from other SLE features within the URT. Inflammatory masses, composed of nonspecific inflammatory materials, collect inside the larynx. Granulomas may develop in the supraglottic area and infiltrate into the space occupied by the false vocal cords.[148] Rheumatoid nodules also form, composed of typical central zone fibrinoid necrosis with bordering mononuclear cells, in those SLE patients with overlapping RA.[149] In rare cases, these different inflammatory collections can lead to subglottic stenosis.[85,150] These lesions also promote the development of laryngeal abscesses and mediastinitis, enhancing the risk for airway compromise.[151]

SLE may also present with angioedema as a result of C1 esterase inhibitor deficiency, hypocomplementemic urticarial vasculitis syndrome, or drug therapy. Those drugs used in SLE most commonly implicated in triggering angioedema include NSAIDs and angiotensin-converting enzyme inhibitors (ACEi).[152] In almost all reported cases, symptoms of URT involvement improve with corticosteroid therapy with the exception of those presenting with pulmonary hypertension or infection. Unlike the CAJ disease that is linked with RA, in SLE, arthritis of the joint generally responds very well to treatment of the underlying disease.[145,153,154]

Otologic Features. SNHL affects greater than 20% of SLE patients. It is either unilateral or bilateral, usually affects middle and high frequencies, and is associated with high titers of antiocardiolipin antibodies. No correlation between hearing loss and disease activity has been found, likely as a result of NSAIDs and antimalarials confounding the picture. SNHL responds rapidly to aggressive GC therapy with recovery of auditory function usually within 1 month. If a patient fails treatment, cyclophosphamide may be added.[155]

> ENT manifestations of SLE include nonulcerating oral lesions, nasal septal perforation, laryngeal scarring, vasculitis, inflammatory collections along the upper airway, angioedema, and SNHL.

Systemic Sclerosis

Epidemiology and Pathology

Systemic sclerosis (SSc) is a rheumatologic disease that produces thickening and hardening of the connective tissues. Prevalence is estimated at 240 per million in the United States.[156] The accepted pathogenesis involves repeated endothelial cell injury triggering platelet aggregation and myointimal cell proliferation with subsequent deposition of collagen and elastin. While SSc primarily involves the skin, it is a systemic disease that can affect any organ, most commonly the kidneys, esophagus, heart, and lungs.[157]

Head and Neck Involvement

Facial and Oral Features. SSc frequently affects the head and neck with up to 80% of patients presenting with related complaints. Facial skin involvement is common with the progression of skin edema to tightness, telangiectasias, and calcinosis. It is associated with atrophy of the epidermis and loss of sweat glands and hair. In addition to a narrowing of the oral aperture, the oral mucosa, soft palate, and larynx become increasingly thin and rigid. As a consequence, patients often complain of difficulty opening their mouths. With disease progression, the structure of the mouth is altered, and the sclerodermatous lesions may penetrate into the underlying muscle and bone.[158]

Patients also develop xerostomia, parotitis, gingivitis, and dental problems. Plaques may form on the tongue. The tongue acquires a whitish hue and later atrophies and becomes glossy with increasing prominence of the vasculature. Tongue movement is impaired. Additionally, the periodontal membrane thickens with consequent pressure resorption. Together, these oral changes result in advanced dental disease in SSc patients.[159]

> SSc causes hardening of the facial skin and reflux producing oral strictures and laryngeal inflammation.

Upper Airway Features. Almost half of SSc patients suffer from gastroesophageal reflux disease as a consequence of lower esophageal sphincter thickening. Chronic reflux results in laryngeal inflammation and scarring, and patients complain of neck pain, dysphonia, and most commonly, dysphagia. In most cases, laryngoscopy shows interarytenoid or vestibular fold edema. Nonetheless, it must be performed with caution as both hardening of the surrounding skin and of the submental triangle makes proper alignment of the oral, pharyngeal, and laryngeal axis significantly more difficult.[160] Videoesophagoscopy is the most useful tool for careful assessment of oropharyngeal dysphagia.[161] While local treatment can be used for symptom relief, the mainstay of therapy consists of immunosuppressive therapy with or without the use of GCs.[156]

SPONDYLOARTHROPATHIES

Definition and Epidemiology

The spondyloarthropathies are a group of rheumatologic diseases with a predilection for the same body parts and with shared gene involvement. The most common entities among this group are ankylosing spondylitis, reactive arthritis, psoriatic arthritis, and enteropathic arthritis. The spondyloarthropathies most frequently affect the entheses, where tendon meets bone, the spine, and the sacroiliac joints. Together, the spondyloarthropathies affect more than 1% of US residents.[162]

Pathophysiology

The immunogenetic vulnerability that characterizes this group is associated with several genetic loci, including the HLA B27 allele. While the exact cascade leading to disease remains incompletely understood, it is well established that immunologic dysregulation leads to recruitment of macrophages and $CD4^+$ and $CD8^+$ T cells to the sites where tendons insert into bone, causing overexpression of cytokines including the proinflammatory cytokine, TNFα. As a consequence, the synovial tissue becomes inflamed and activates nearby osteoclasts. Subsequently, osteoblast activity predominates at the vertebral bodies, the periarticular bone, and the area surrounding the joints, and ultimately results in bony fusion of the joints. The spondyloarthropathies are strongly associated with certain genitourinary and gastrointestinal infections. This suggests that immune upregulation in response to bacterial antigens may persist and cause cross-reactivity with host antigens, in addition to causing a loss of tolerance to self peptides, leading to a state of chronic inflammation.[163]

Ankylosing Spondylitis

Epidemiology and Pathology

Ankylosing spondylitis (AS) is an inflammatory spondyloarthropathy characterized by infiltration of granulation tissue into the ligaments and joint capsules at the insertion sites where they meet bone. It primarily affects young men with an incidence of 1% to 2% among Caucasians.[164] Fibrocartilaginous structures are the most common targets, usually starting with the sacroiliac joints and the intervertebral discs. Proliferation of the synovium covering the articular cartilage leads to loss of the cartilage and penetration of granulation tissue into the underlying bone.[165]

Head and Neck Involvement

Over time, three-quarters of patients develop abnormal adhesions among the joints of the cervical spine resulting in what is termed *cervical ankylosis*. This puts them at high risk for fracture because of osteoporosis in the vertebral bones that develops from cytokine release.[166] Intubation must therefore proceed with caution given the restricted cervical motion. Transnasal and transoral fiberoptic intubation or retrograde intubation are generally considered safer.[167,168]

> Cervical ankylosis may develop in AS. Significant caution must be taken in intubating those patients with restricted neck motion.

AS can also involve other parts of the head and neck. The disease may affect the TMJ in almost one-quarter of AS cases. Most are asymptomatic, although signs of disease include associated chewing noises, tenderness on palpation, muscular hypertrophy, and restricted opening.[165] Cricoarytenoid arthritis can also occur, increasing the risk for vocal fold damage.[169]

Management

NSAIDs are the primary drug of choice for pain control. To prevent the progression of disease, DMARDs are used, such as sulfasalazine and anti-TNFα agents though NSAIDs have also been shown to demonstrate disease-modifying effects.[170] Physical therapy is essential in maintaining flexion in those with an anklyosed spine. Surgery may be considered in cases of severe flexion deformities. Nonetheless, neck surgery is especially risky in these patients.[171]

Psoriatic Arthropathy

Epidemiology and Pathology

Psoriasis is a papulosquamous inflammatory skin condition characterized by erythematous plaques with an overlying silvery scale.[172] Between 10% and 15% of cases are accompanied by an arthritis, termed *psoriatic arthropathy* (PsA).[173] PsA is an RF seronegative inflammatory condition in which environmental factors trigger an imbalance of T suppressor cells with subsequent lymphocyte activation and formation of immune complexes against epithelial and synovial tissues. Joint involvement is usually asymmetric and can occur almost anywhere, although most commonly affects the distal interphalangeal joints.[174]

TMJ Involvement

Up to 90% of PsA patients have findings related to TMJ dysfunction including crepitus or noise on joint movement and muscle tenderness.[175] Initially, patients with TMJ involvement complain of pain, whereas with disease progression and fibrosis formation, movement of the joint becomes limited. Severity of TMJ arthropathy is most closely associated with degree and duration of peripheral joint involvement.[176]

Diagnostic Studies

Diagnosis of PsA is often difficult because joint findings may precede skin findings. Although several criteria exist, the original diagnostic criteria of Moll and Wright are both the simplest and the most commonly used. As per their definition, PsA requires the presence of psoriasis and erosive polyarthritis along with the absence of RF serology.[177] Findings on radiography are nonspecific and include erosion and flattening of the condylar head, osteoporotic lesions, osteophytes, joint space narrowing, and subchondral sclerosis.[178] Although erosions correlate with TMJ symptoms, radiographic evidence of joint collapse may occur without signs of total occlusion.[179]

> PsA is defined by psoriasis, erosive polyarthritis, and absence of RF serology.

Management

TMJ disease within the context of PsA is generally less severe than RA-related dysfunction. However, it is managed in the same way. Oral NSAIDs and tricyclic antidepressants are employed first, while local injections may be used to reduce stiffness and more refractory pain. Joint replacement is an alternative with good long-term data in cases of total joint collapse or severe joint dysfunction.[43]

Polymyositis

Epidemiology and Pathology

Polymyositis, a form of idiopathic inflammatory myopathy (IIM), is an inflammatory muscle disease that appears either as part of a primary disease or in association with an underlying collagen vascular disease, malignancy, or infection. It is relatively uncommon, with an annual incidence in the United States estimated at 5 cases per million.[180] It is characterized by a nonsuppurative lymphocytic infiltrate that surrounds and eventually invades skeletal muscle fibers, especially along the proximal musculature. Serum creatinine kinase is elevated, and electromyography demonstrates characteristic increased fibrillations with positive sharp waves at rest and low amplitude, short duration action potentials. While the 2 studies are strongly suggestive, biopsy, revealing perimysial and endomysial mononuclear cell infiltrates, necrosis, variation in muscle fiber size, and increased connective tissue, is the most helpful in confirming the diagnosis.[181,182]

Head and Neck Involvement

Head and neck involvement is common and mostly a consequence of esophageal dysmotility and cricopharyngeal myopathy. As a result, patients complain of dysphagia and dysarthria and occasionally, have signs of aspiration.[183] Weakness of laryngeal muscles results in vocal fold flaccidity, visualized on laryngoscopy. If the posterior cricoarytenoid muscle is involved, the cords may become fixed in an adducted position causing airway obstruction.[184] In addition, the facial skin can develop either sclerodermatous changes or scaling and desquamation, especially in the related IIM, dermatomyositis. These skin changes frequently lead to a diffuse stomatitis.[159] GCs are the first line of therapy while immunosuppressive agents and intravenous immunoglobulin are reserved for refractory cases.[185]

> ENT manifestations of polymyositis include esophageal dysmotility, cricopharyngeal myopathy and vocal fold flaccidity.

SARCOIDOSIS

Epidemiology and Pathology

Sarcoidosis is an autoimmune condition formed by collections of inflammatory cells that coalesce into granulomas. They deposit in any organ, though generally, within the lung and lymph nodes. The incidence of sarcoidosis ranges from 1 to 2 cases to 35.5 cases per 10 000 people with the highest prevalence among African American females aged 20 to 40 years.[186]

Upper Airway Involvement

Although upper airway involvement is uncommon, it can occur, and in such cases, usually affects the epiglottis followed by the vestibular folds, vocal folds, and subglottis. Sarcoidosis may also affect vocal cord mobility by encroaching onto the recurrent laryngeal nerve. Patients most frequently complain of hoarseness, but they may present with obstruction because of supraglottic region involvement. Patients also present with nasal obstruction and rhinorrhea, and sometimes develop necrotizing sinus and palatal destruction, even prior to manifesting signs of systemic involvement. In untreated disease, nasal involvement can also lead to rhinophyma, a ruddy, bulbous nose caused by granulomatous infiltration (Figure 13–5).[187]

> In sarcoidosis, noncaseating granulomas may encroach the upper respiratory tract and in rare cases, lead to dysphonia or symptoms of airway obstruction.

Diagnostic Studies

On laryngoscopy, the mucosa appears pale, edematous, and diffusely enlarged. Punctate nodules and mass lesions can also be visualized. Histological examination reveals lymphocytic infiltration and patchy granulomas (Figure 13–6).[188]

Management

Studies reporting the efficacy of systemic GCs in laryngeal sarcoidosis are mixed. In cases where a well-circumscribed lesion is producing obstruction, surgical excision is the approach of choice. Though radiotherapy has been tried, it results in fibrosis and laryngeal distortion and does not appear to offer any unique benefits.[189] GCs, DMARDs, and experimental treatments including thalidomide have also been tried for skin and lung involvement.[190,191]

MISCELLANEOUS DISEASES

This chapter summarizes the primary rheumatologic diseases with features localized to the head and neck, but it is by no means exhaustive. For instance, mixed connective tissue disease shares features with lupus, SSc and polymyositis, and therefore presents with some of the same otorhinolaryngological features. Both gout and amyloidosis can lead to upper respiratory symptoms primarily through tophus buildup in the case of gout and through accumulation of proteinaceous materials along the larynx in amyloidosis (Figure 13–7). Behcet's disease is characterized by recurrent soft palate and oropharyngeal ulcers, which cause difficulty in eating, swallowing, and speaking. Unlike the oral ulcers caused by lupus, these are painful and patients sometimes present with greater than 6 at any given time.[192,193]

> Almost all rheumatologic diseases have the potential to present with features localized to the head and neck.

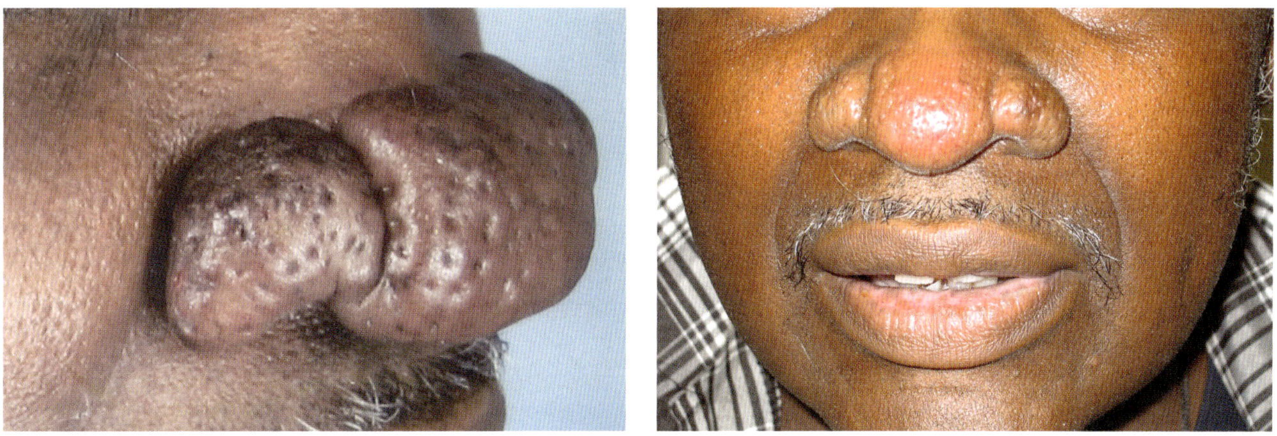

A B

Figure 13–5. Rhinophyma in sarcoidosis. **A.** Before immunosuppressive therapy. **B.** Following treatment with significant improvement in cosmetic appearance.

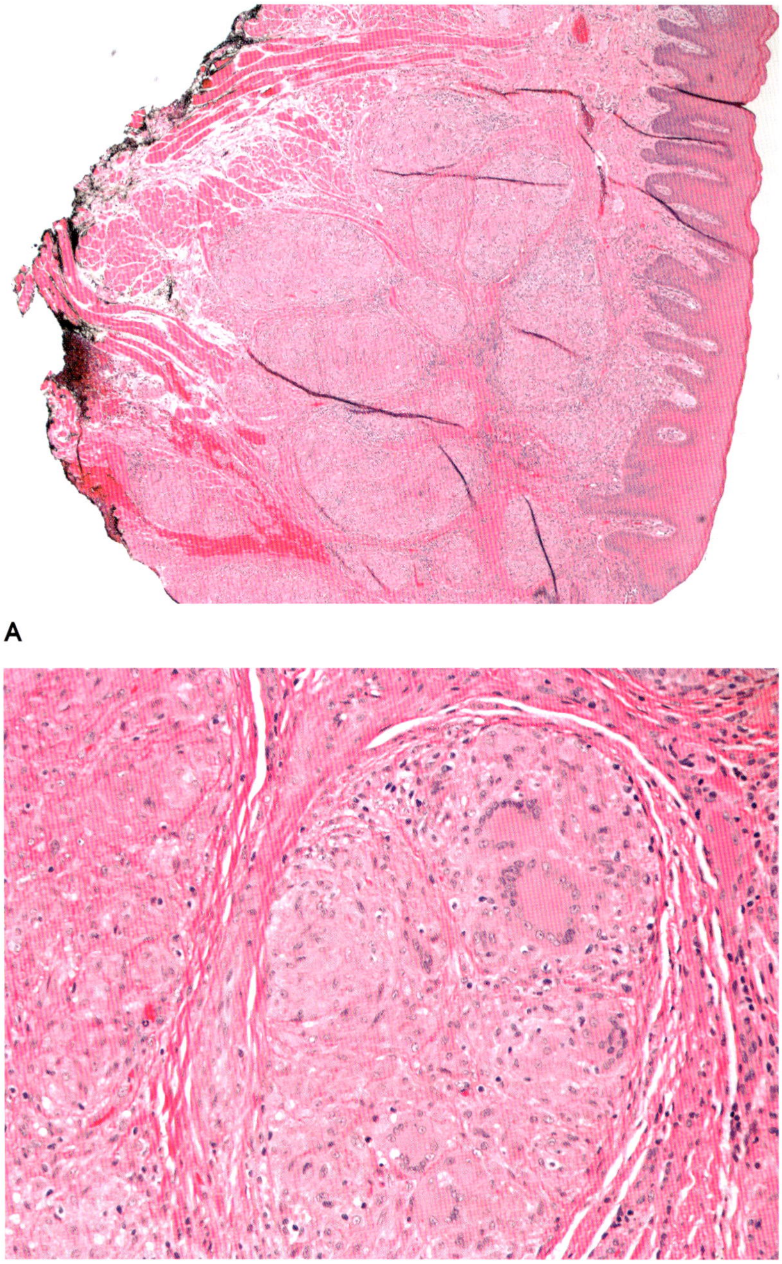

A

B

Figure 13–6. Tongue mucosa in sarcoidosis demonstrating granulomas surrounded by a lymphocytic infiltrate.

CONCLUSION

Many rheumatologic diseases present, either initially or as they take their course, by affecting otorhinolaryngological structures. These signs must be carefully evaluated and a high index of clinical suspicion for a rheumatologic process is critical for a few reasons. Firstly, complaints related to the head and neck can provide insight into a larger systemic process taking place. Secondly, if recognized early, many of these complaints are easily managed with systemic or local medical therapy or with surgical intervention. Most importantly, inflammation and

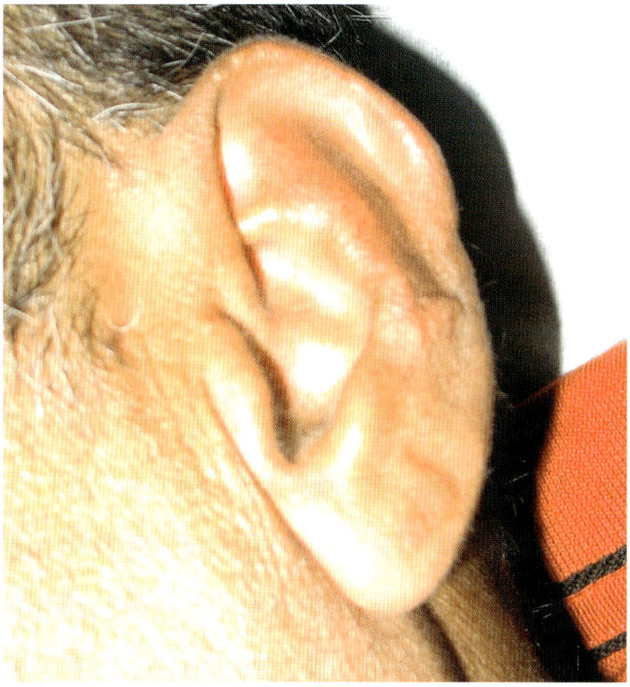

Figure 13-7. Gouty tophus of the ear.

subsequent scarring of the structures of the head and neck can lead to life-threatening complications in both the acute and more chronic settings. Therefore, a good understanding of the head and neck manifestations of rheumatologic diseases is essential for early detection and prevention of these severe end organ effects.

Acknowledgments. The authors would like to thank the following people for contributing to the figures included in this chapter: Dr. Robert Lebovics, Dr. Adam Gersten, and Dr. Elizabeth Dinces.

REFERENCES

1. Harrison TR, Anthony S. *Harrison's Principles of Internal Medicine*. 17th ed. New York, NY: McGraw-Hill Medical; 2009:885.
2. Langford CA, Van Waes C. Upper airway obstruction in the rheumatic diseases. *Rheum Dis Clin North Am*. 1997; 23(2):345–363.
3. Geterud A. Rheumatoid arthritis in the larynx. *Scand J Rheumatol*. 1991;20(3):215.
4. Prete M, Racanelli V, Digiglio L, et al. Extra-articular manifestations of rheumatoid arthritis: an update. *Autoimmun Rev*. 2011;11(2):123–131.
5. Mackenzie M. *Diseases of the Pharynx, Larynx and Trachea*. New York, NY: William Wood & Co; 1880.
6. Klipper JH, Dieppe PE. *Rheumatology*. 2nd ed. London, UK: Mosby; 1999:51.1–53.1.
7. Lofgren RH, Montgomery WW. Incidence of laryngeal involvement in rheumatoid arthritis. *N Engl J Med*. 1962; 267:193–195.
8. Hamdan AL, Sarieddine D. Laryngeal manifestations of rheumatoid arthritis. *Autoimmune Dis*. 2013;(2013). http://dx.doi.org/10.1155/2013/103081.
9. Grossman A, Martin JR, Root HS. Rheumatoid arthritis of the crico-arvtenoid joint. *Laryngoscope*. 1961;71:530–544.
10. Wang RC. Three-dimensional analysis of cricoarytenoid joint motion. *Laryngoscope*. 1998;108(4, pt 2, suppl 86): 1–17.
11. Bayar N, Kara SA, Keles I, et al. Cricoarytenoiditis in rheumatoid arthritis: radiologic and clinical study. *J Otolaryngol*. 2003;32(6):373–378.
12. Lawry GV, Pincrman ML, Hanafee WN, et al. Laryngeal involvement in rheumatoid arthritis. A clinical, laryngoscopic, and computerized tomographic study. *Arthritis Rheum*. 1984;27(8):873–882.
13. Clement F. [Stridor caused by laryngeal rheumatoid arthritis]. *Ugeskr Laeger*. 1999;161(13):1931–1932.
14. Taylor-Gjevre RM, Nair BV, Gjevre JA. Obstructive sleep apnoea in relation to rheumatic disease. *Rheumatology (Oxford)*. 2013;52(1):15–21.
15. Voulgari PV, Papazisi D, Bai M, et al. Laryngeal involvement in rheumatoid arthritis. *Rheumatol Int*. 2005;25(5): 321–325.
16. Harris ER, Grossman A, Martin JR. Cricoarytenoid joint involvement in rheumatoid arthritis: its detection and manifestation. *Arthritis Rheum*. 1973;16:553.
17. Brooker DS. Rheumatoid arthritis: otorhinolaryngological manifestations. *Clin Otolaryngol Allied Sci*. 1988; 13(3):239–246.
18. Berjawi G, Uthman I, Mahfoud L, et al. Cricothyroid joint abnormalities in patients with rheumatoid arthritis. *J Voice*. 2010;24(6):732–737.
19. Kobayashi R, et al. Ankylosis of the temporomandibular joint caused by rheumatoid arthritis: a pathological study and review. *J Oral Sci*. 2001;43(2):97–101.
20. Redlund-Johnell I. Upper airway obstruction in patients with rheumatoid arthritis and temporomandibular joint destruction. *Scand J Rheumatol*. 1988; 17(4):273–279.
21. Aliko A, Ciancaglini R, Alushi A, Tafaj A, Ruci D. Temporomandibular joint involvement in rheumatoid arthritis, systemic lupus erythematosus and systemic sclerosis. *Int J Oral Maxillofacial Surg*. 2011; 40:704–709.
22. Marbach JJ, Spiera H. Rheumatoid arthritis of the temporomandibular joints. *Ann Rheum Dis*. 1967;26(6):538–543.
23. Norton ML, Ghanma MA. Atlantoaxial instability revisited. An alert for endoscopists. *Ann Otol Rhinol Laryngol*. 1982;91(6, pt 1):567–570.
24. Harris ED. Rheumatoid arthritis: the clinical spectrum. In: Kelley W, Harris ED, Ruddy S, et al, eds. *Textbook of Rheumatology*. Philadelphia, PA: WB Saunders; 1981.

25. Keenan MA, Stiles CM, Kaufman RL. Acquired laryngeal deviation associated with cervical spine disease in erosive polyarticular arthritis. Use of the fiberoptic bronchoscope in rheumatoid disease *Anesthesiology*. 1983;58:441–449.
26. Mikulowski P, et al. Sudden death in rheumatoid arthritis with atlanto-axial dislocation. *Acta Med Scand*. 1975; 198(6):445–451.
27. Bland J. Rheumatoid subluxation of the cervical spine. *J Rheumatol*. 1990;17(2):134–137.
28. Campbell RS, Wou P, Watt I. A continuing role for preoperative cervical spine radiography in rheumatoid arthritis? *Clin Radiol*. 1995;50(3):157–159.
29. Funk D, Raymon F. Rheumatoid arthritis of the cricoarytenoid joints: an airway hazard. *Anesth Analg*. 1975; 54(6):742–745.
30. Abadir WF, Forster PM. Rheumatoid vocal cord nodules. *J Laryngol Otol*. 1974;88(5):473–478.
31. Amernik K. Glottis morphology and perceptive-acoustic characteristics of voice and speech in patients with rheumatoid arthritis. *Ann Acad Med Stetin*. 2007;53(3):55–65.
32. Kalugina Y, Petruzzelli GJ, Wojcik EM. Fine-needle aspiration of rheumatoid nodule: a case report with review of diagnostic features and difficulties. *Diagn Cytopathol*. 2003;28(6):322–324.
33. Perouse R, Coulombeau B, Cornut G, et al. Bamboo nodes: a clinical study of 19 cases. *Rev Laryngol Otol Rhinol (Bord)*. 2001;122(5):299–302.
34. Bartels C, et al. Decline in rheumatoid vasculitis prevalence among US veterans: a retrospective cross-sectional study. *Arthritis Rheum*. 2009;60(9):2553–2557.
35. Moffat DA, Ramsden RT, Rosenberg JN, et al. Otoadmittance measurements in patients with rheumatoid arthritis. *J Laryngol Otol*. 1977;91:917–927.
36. Kastanioudakis I, Skevas A, Danielidis V, et al. Inner ear involvement in rheumatoid arthritis: a prospective clinical study. *J Laryngol Otol*. 1995 Aug;109(8):713–718.
37. Singh J, Furst DE, Bharat A, et al. 2012 Update of the 2008 American College of Rheumatology recommendations for the use of disease-modifying antirheumatic drugs and biologic agents in the treatment of rheumatoid arthritis. *Arthritis Care Res*. May 2012;64(5):625–639.
38. Kerstens PJ, Boerbooms A, Jeurissen ME, et al. Accelerated nodulosis during low dose methotrexate therapy for rheumatoid arthritis. An analysis of ten cases. *J Rheumatol*. 1992;19:867–871.
39. Sorensen WT, Meller-Anderson K, Behrendt N. Rheumatoid nodules of the larynx. *J Laryngol Otol*. 1998;112: 573–574.
40. Ossoff RH, Sisson GA, Duncavage JA, et al. Endoscopic laser arytenoidectomy for the treatment of bilateral vocal cord paralysis. *Laryngoscope*. 1984;94(10):1293–1297.
41. Danino J, Goldenberg D, Joachims HZ. Submucosal arytenoidectomy: new surgical technique and review of the literature. *J Otolaryngol*. 2000;29(1):13–16.
42. Tarnowska C, et al. Fixation of the crico-arythenoid joints in rheumatoid arthritis—preliminary report. *Otolaryngol Pol*. 2004;58(4):843–849.
43. Sidebottom AJ. Current thinking in temporomandibular joint management. *Br J Oral Maxillofac Surg*. 2009; 47(2):91–94.
44. Saeed NR, McLeod NM, Hensher R. Temporomandibular joint replacement in rheumatoid-induced disease. *Br J Oral Maxillofac Surg*. 2001;39(1):71–75.
45. Mercuri LG, Edibam NR, Giobbie-Hurder A. Fourteen-year follow-up of a patient-fitted total temporomandibular joint reconstruction system. *J Oral Maxillofac Surg*. 2007;65(6):1140–1148.
46. Lane SE, Watts RA, Shepstone L, Scott DG. Primary systemic vasculitis: clinical features and mortality. *QJM*. 2005;98(2):97–111.
47. Mahr AD. Epidemiological features of Wegener's granulomatosis and microscopic polyangiitis: two diseases or one 'anti-neutrophil cytoplasm antibodies-associated vasculitis' entity? *APMIS Suppl*. 2009;(127):41–47.
48. McDonald TJ, DeRemee RA. Wegener's granulomatosis. *Laryngoscope*. 1983;93(2):220–231.
49. Carrington CB, Liebow A. Limited forms of angiitis and granulomatosis of Wegener's type. *Am J Med*. 1966;41(4): 497–527.
50. Ahmad I, Lee WC, Nagendran V, et al. Localised Wegener's granulomatosis in otolaryngology: a review of six cases. *ORL J Otorhinolaryngol Relat Spec*. 2000;62(3): 149–155.
51. Hoffman GS, Langford CA. Are there different forms of life in the antineutrophil cytoplasmic antibody universe? *Ann Intern Med*. 2005;143(9):683–685.
52. Holl-Ulrich K. Histopathology of systemic vasculitis. *Pathologe*. 2010;31(1):67–76.
53. Rasmussen N. Management of the ear, nose, and throat manifestations of Wegener granulomatosis: an otorhinolaryngologist's perspective. *Curr Opin Rheumatol*,. 2001; 13(1):3–11.
54. Wolff SM, Fauci AS, Horn RG, Dale DC. Wegener's granulomatosis. *Ann Intern Med*. 1974;81(4):513–525.
55. Takagi D, et al. Otologic manifestations of Wegener's granulomatosis. *Laryngoscope*. 2002;112(9):1684–1690.
56. Fujioka M, Okano H, Ogawa K. Front Pharmacol. Inflammatory and immune responses in the cochlea: potential therapeutic targets for sensorineural hearing loss. *Front Pharmacol*. 2014;5:287.
57. Stone JH, Francis HW. Immune-mediated inner ear disease. *Curr Opin Rheumatol*. 2000;12(1):32–40.
58. Calonius IH, Christensen CK. Hearing impairment and facial palsy as initial signs of Wegener's granulomatosis. *J Laryngol Otol*. 1980;94(6):649–657.
59. Lebovics RS, Hoffman GS, Leavitt RY, et al. The management of subglottic stenosis in patients with Wegener's granulomatosis. *Laryngoscope*. 1992;102(12, pt 1):1341–1345.
60. Schokkenbroek AA, Franssen CF, Dikkers FG. Dilatation tracheoscopy for laryngeal and tracheal stenosis in patients with Wegener's granulomatosis. *Eur Arch Otorhinolaryngol*. 2008;265(5):549–555.
61. Rosenberg DM, Weinerberger SE, Fulmer JD, et al. Functional correlates of lung involvement in Wegener's granulomatosis. Use of pulmonary function tests in staging and follow-up. *Am J Med*. 1980;69(3):387–394.

62. Lohrmann C, Uhl M, Warnartz K, et al. Sinonasal computed tomography in patients with Wegener's granulomatosis. *J Comput Assist Tomogr.* 2006;30(1):122–125.
63. Muhle C, Reinhold-Keller E, Richter C, et al. MRI of the nasal cavity, the paranasal sinuses and orbits in Wegener's granulomatosis. *Eur Radiol.* 1997;7(4):566–570.
64. Cannady SB, Batra PS, Koening C, et al. Sinonasal Wegener granulomatosis: a single-institution experience with 120 cases. *Laryngoscope.* 2009;119(4):757–761.
65. Devaney KO, Travis WD, Hoffman G, et al. Interpretation of head and neck biopsies in Wegener's granulomatosis. A pathologic study of 126 biopsies in 70 patients. *Am J Surg Pathol.* 1990;14(6):555–564.
66. Langford CA. Update on the treatment of granulomatosis with polyangiitis (Wegener's). *Curr Treat Options Cardiovasc Med.* 2012;14(2):164–176.
67. Pagnoux C, Wolter NE. Vasculitis of the upper airways. *Swiss Med Wkly.* 2012;142:w13541.
68. Congdon D, Sherrid DA, Specks U, McDonald T. Long-term follow-up of repair of external nasal deformities in patients with Wegener's granulomatosis. *Laryngoscope.* 2002;112(4):731–737.
69. Erickson VR, Hwang PH. Wegener's granulomatosis: current trends in diagnosis and management. *Curr Opin Otolaryngol Head Neck Surg.* 2007;15(3):170–176.
70. Bakthavachalam S, et al. Hearing loss in Wegener's granulomatosis. *Otol Neurotol.* 2004;25(5):833–837.
71. Wolter NE, Ooi EH, Witterick IJ. Intralesional corticosteroid injection and dilatation provides effective management of subglottic stenosis in Wegener's granulomatosis. *Laryngoscope.* 2010;120(12):2452–2455.
72. Eliachar I, Chan J, Akst L. New approaches to the management of subglottic stenosis in Wegener's granulomatosis. *Cleve Clin J Med.* 2002;69(suppl 2):SII149–51.
73. Stone JH, Peter AM, Spiera R, et al. Rituximab versus cyclophosphamide for ANCA-associated vasculitis. *N Engl J Med.* 2010;363(3):221–232.
74. Pallan L, Savage CO, Harper L. ANCA-associated vasculitis: from bench research to novel treatments. *Nat Rev Nephrol.* 2009;5(5):278–286.
75. Mohammad AJ, Jacobsson LTH, Westman KWA, et al. Incidence and survival rates in Wegener's granulomatosis, microscopic polyangiitis, Churg-Strauss syndrome and polyarteritis nodosa. *Rheumatology (Oxford).* 2009;48(12):1560–1565.
76. Kissel JT. Vasculitis of the peripheral nervous system. *Semin Neurol.* 1994;14(4):361–369.
77. Bacciu A, Bacciu S, Mercante G, et al. Ear, nose and throat manifestations of Churg-Strauss syndrome. *Acta Otolaryngol.* 2006;126(5):503–509.
78. Mahr A, Moosig F, Neurmann T, et al. Eosinophilic granulomatosis with polyangiitis (Churg-Strauss): evolutions in classification, etiopathogenesis, assessment and management. *Curr Opin Rheumatol.* 2014;26(1):16–23.
79. Goodwin JS. Progress in gerontology: polymyalgia rheumatica and temporal arteritis. *J Am Geriatr Soc.* 1992;40(5):515–525.
80. Heale, LA. Giant-cell arteritis (editorial). *Ann Intern Med.* 1978;88:710.
81. Leber T. Über die Entstehung der Netzhautablösung. Ber Versamml. *Ophthal.* Ges. Stuttg. 1882;14:165.
82. Sjogren H. *A New Conception of Keratoconjunctivitis Sicca.* Sydney: Australian Medical Publishing Co; 1943.
83. Tzioufas AG, Mitsias DI, Moutsopoulos HM. Sjögren's syndrome in rheumatology. In: Harris ED, Bidd RC, Foresteom GS, et al, eds. *Kelly's Textbook of Rheumatology.* 9th ed. Philadelphia, PA: Elsevier; 2013:1184–1185.
84. Daniels TE, Silverman S, Michalski JP, et al. The oral component of Sjögren's syndrome. *Oral Surg.* 1975;39:875–885.
85. Campbell SM, Montanaro A, Bardana EJ. Head and neck manifestations of autoimmune disease. *Am J Otolaryngol.* 1983;4(3):187–216.
86. Doig JA, Whaley K, Dick WC, et al. Otolaryngologic aspects of Sjögren's syndrome. *Br Med J.* 1971;4:460–463.
87. Kassan SS, Moutsopoulos HM. Clinical manifestations and early diagnosis of Sjögren's syndrome. *Arch Intern Med.* 2004;164(12):1275–1284.
88. Papiris SA, Tsonis IA, Moutsopoulos HM. Sjogren's syndrome. *Semin Respir Crit Care Med.* 2007;28(4):459–471.
89. Adams BK, Al Attia HM, Parkar S. Salivary gland scintigraphy in Sjögren's syndrome: are quantitative indices the answer? *Nucl Med Commun.* 2003;24(9):1011–1016.
90. Milic V, Petrovic R, Radunovic G, et al. Ultrasonography of major salivary glands could be an alternative tool to sialoscintigraphy in the American-European classification criteria for primary Sjögren's syndrome. *Rheumatology (Oxford).* 2012;51(6):1081–1085.
91. Papiris SA, Maniati M, Constantopoulos SH, et al. Lung involvement in primary Sjögren's syndrome is mainly related to the small airway disease. *Ann Rheum Dis.* 1999;58(1):61–64.
92. Vivino FB, Al-Hashimi I, Khan Z, et al. Pilocarpine tablets for the treatment of dry mouth and dry eye symptoms in patients with Sjögren's syndrome: a randomized, placebo-controlled, fixed-dose, multicenter trial. P92-01 Study Group. *Arch Intern Med.* 1999;159(2):174–181.
93. Manoussakis MN, Moutsopoulos HM. Sjogren's syndrome: current concepts. *Adv Intern Med.* 2001;47:191–217.
94. McCabe BF. Autoimmune sensorineural hearing loss. *Ann Otol Rhinol Laryngol.* 1979;88(5, pt 1):585–589.
95. Rauch SD. Clinical management of immune-mediated inner-ear disease. *Ann N Y Acad Sci,* 1997;830:203–210.
96. Amor-Dorado JC, et al. Audiovestibular manifestations in patients with limited systemic sclerosis and centromere protein-B (CENP-B) antibodies. *Medicine (Baltimore).* 2008;87(3):131–141.
97. Cai Q, Du X, Zhou B, et al. Induction of tolerance by oral administration of beta-tubulin in an animal model of autoimmune inner ear disease. *ORL.* 2009;71:135–141.
98. Adams, JC. Clinical implications of inflammatory cytokines in the cochlea: a technical note. *Otol Neurotol.* 2002;23(3):316–322.
99. Boulassel MR, Dejjouj N, Tomasi JP, Gersdorr M. Inner ear autoantibodies and their targets in patients with autoimmune inner ear diseases. *Acta Otolaryngol.* 2001;121(1):28–34.

100. Ochoa VM, Weider DJ. Development of autoimmune sensorineural hearing loss after endolymphatic sac decompression: two case reports. *Otol Neurotol.* 2003; 24(2):279–282.
101. Hirose K, Wener MH, Duckert LG. Utility of laboratory testing in autoimmune inner ear disease. *Laryngoscope.* 1999;109(11):1749–1754.
102. Ruckenstein MJ. Autoimmune inner ear disease. *Curr Opin Otolaryng Head Neck.* 2004;12:426–430.
103. Garcia Callejo FJ, Marco Algarra J, Martinez Beneyto MP, et al. Autoimmune identification of sudden hearing loss. *Acta Otolaryngol.* 2003 Jan;123(2):168–171.
104. Zeitoun H, Gray Beckman J, Arts A, et al. Corticosteroid response and supporting cell antibody in autoimmune hearing loss. *Arch Otolaryngol Head Neck Surg.* 2005; 131(8):665–672.
105. Sismanis A, Wise CM, Johnson GD. Methotrexate management of immune-mediated cochleovestibular disorders. *Otolaryngol Head Neck Surg.* 1997;116(2): 146–152.
106. Hautefort C, Loundon N, Montchilova M, et al. Mycophenolate mofetil as a treatment of steroid dependent Cogan's syndrome in childhood. *Int J Pediatr Otorhinolaryngol.* 2009;73:1477–1479.
107. Saracaydin A, Katircioglu S, Katircioglu S, Karatay MC. Azathioprine in combination with steroids in the treatment of autoimmune inner-ear disease. *J Int Med Res.* 1993;21(4):192–196.
108. Mijovic T, Zeitouni A, Colmegna I. Autoimmune sensorineural hearing loss: the otology-rheumatology interface. *Rheumatology (Oxford).* 2013;52(5):780–789.
109. Trentham DE, Le CH. Relapsing polychondritis. *Ann Intern Med,* 1998. 129(2):114–122.
110. McAdam, L.P., et al., Relapsing polychondritis: prospective study of 23 patients and a review of the literature. *Medicine (Baltimore).* 1976;55(3):193–215.
111. Serratrice J, Ené N, Granel B, et al. Severe relapsing polychondritis occurring after ear piercing. *J Rheumatol.* 2003;30(12):2716–2717.
112. Cody DT, Sones DA. Relapsing polychondritis: audiovestibular manifestations. *Laryngoscope.* 1971;81(8): 1208–1222.
113. Daniel RK, Brenner KA. Saddle nose deformity: a new classification and treatment. *Facial Plast Surg Clin North Am.* 2006;14(4):301–312, vi.
114. Mohsenifar Z, Tashkin DP, Carson SA, Bellamy PE. Pulmonary function in patients with relapsing polychondritis. *Chest.* 1982;81(6):711–717.
115. Carrión M, Girón JA, Ventura J, et al. Airway complications in relapsing polychondritis. *J Rheumatol.* 1993; 20(9):1628–1629.
116. Foidart JM, Abe S, Marting GR, et al. Antibodies to type II collagen in relapsing polychondritis. *N Engl J Med.* 1978;299(22):1203–1207.
117. Mendelson DS, Som PM, Crane R, et al. Relapsing polychondritis studied by computed tomography. *Radiology.* 1985;157(2):489–490.
118. Eng J, Sabanathan S. Airway complications in relapsing polychondritis. *Ann Thorac Surg.* 1991;51(4):686–692.
119. Kent PD, Michet CJ, Luthra HS. Relapsing polychondritis. *Curr Opin Rheumatol.* 2003;16:56–61.
120. Sarodia BD, Dasgupta A, Mehta AC. Management of airway manifestations of relapsing polychondritis: case reports and review of literature. *Chest.* 1999;116(6): 1669–1675.
121. Faul JL, Kee ST, Rizk NW. Endobronchial stenting for severe airway obstruction in relapsing polychondritis. *Chest.* 1999;116(3):825–827.
122. Cundiff J, et al. Cogan's syndrome: a cause of progressive hearing deafness. *Am J Otolaryngol.* 2006;27(1):68–70.
123. Lunardi C, et al. Autoantibodies to inner ear and endothelial antigens in Cogan's syndrome. *Lancet.* 2002;360 (9337):915–921.
124. Ikeda M, Okazaki H, Minota S. Cogan's syndrome with antineutrophil cytoplasmic autoantibody. *Ann Rheum Dis.* 2002;61(8):761–762.
125. Cheson BD. Cogan's syndrome. *Clin Adv Hematol Oncol.* 2010;8(12):833.
126. Gluth MB, et al. Cogan syndrome: a retrospective review of 60 patients throughout a half century. *Mayo Clin Proc.* 2006;81(4):483–488.
127. Casselman JW, Majoor MH, Albers FW. MR of the inner ear in patients with Cogan syndrome. *AJNR Am J Neuroradiol.* 1994;15(1):131–138.
128. St Clair EW, McCallum RM. Cogan's syndrome. *Curr Opin Rheumatol.* 1999;11(1):47–52.
129. Van Doornum S, McColl G, Walter M, et al. Prolonged prodrome, systemic vasculitis, and deafness in Cogan's syndrome. *Ann Rheum Dis.* 2001;60:69–71.
130. García Berrocal JR, Vargas JA, Vaquero M, et al. Cogan's syndrome: an oculoaudiovestibular disease. *Postgrad Med J.* 1999;75:262–264.
131. Allen NB, Cox CC, Cobo M, et al. Use of immunosuppressive agents in the treatment of severe ocular and vascular manifestations of Cogan's syndrome. *Am J Med.* 1990;88(3):296–301.
132. Touma Z, Nawwar R, Hadi U, et al. The use of TNF-alpha blockers in Cogan's syndrome. *Rheumatol Int.* 2007;27(10):995–996.
133. Orsoni JG, et al. Rituximab ameliorated severe hearing loss in Cogan's syndrome: a case report. *Orphanet J Rare Dis.* 2010;5:18.
134. Watts RA, et al. Renal vasculitis in Japan and the UK—are there differences in epidemiology and clinical phenotype? *Nephrol Dial Transplant.* 2008;23(12):3928–3931.
135. Rose GA, Spencer H. Polyarteritis nodosa. *Q J Med.* 1957;26(101):43–81.
136. Herberts G, Hillerdal O, Ranstrom S. Rhinitis, sinusitis and otitis as initial symptoms in periarteritis nodosa; Wegener's granulomatosis. *Acta Otolaryngol.* 1957;48(3):205–218.
137. Guillevin L, et al. Short-term corticosteroids then lamivudine and plasma exchanges to treat hepatitis B virus-related polyarteritis nodosa. *Arthritis Rheum.* 2004;51(3): 482–487.

138. Hahn BH. Systemic lupus erythematosus. In: Fauci AS, Braunwald E, Kasper DL, et al, eds. *Harrison's Internal Medicine*. 17th ed. New York, NY: McGraw-Hill; 2008: 2075–2082.
139. Rahman KDI. Review article: systemic lupus erythematosus. *N Engl J Med*. February 28, 2008;358(9):929–939.
140. Somers EC, et al. Population-based incidence and prevalence of systemic lupus erythematosus: the Michigan Lupus Epidemiology and Surveillance program. *Arthritis Rheumatol*. 2014;66(2):369–378.
141. Smith GA, Ward PH, Berci G. Laryngeal involvement by systemic lupus erythematosus. *Trans Sect Otolaryngol Am Acad Ophthalmol Otolaryngol*. 1977;84(1):124–128.
142. Edwards MB, Gayford JJ. Oral lupus erythematosus. Three cases demonstrating three variants. *Oral Surg Oral Med Oral Pathol*. 1971;31(3):332–342.
143. Wilkens RF, Roth GJ, Novak A, Walike JW. Perforation of nasal septum in rheumatic diseases. *Arthritis Rheum*. 1976;19:119–121.
144. Kern EB, Facer GW, McDonald TJ, et al. Closure of nasal septal perforations with a Silastic button: results in 45 patients. *ORL Digest*. 1977;39:9–17.
145. Curley JW, Byron MA, Bates GJ. Crico-arytenoid joint involvement in acute systemic lupus erythematosus. *J Laryngol Otol*. 1986;100(6):727–732.
146. Teitel AD, MacKenzie CR, Stern R, Paget SA. Laryngeal involvement in systemic lupus erythematosus. *Semin Arthritis Rheum*. 1992;22(3):203–214.
147. Minchina RA, Fastovskii Ia A, Antonova NA. Changes in the larynx in systemic lupus erythematosus and systemic scleroderma. *Zh Ushn Nos Gorl Bolezn*. 1970;30(4): 67–73.
148. Shumrick KA. Benign diseases of the hypopharynx and larynx. In: Lee JG, ed. *Textbook of Otolaryngology and Head and Neck Surgery*. New York, NY: Elsevier; 1989.
149. Schwartz IS, Grishman E. Rheumatoid nodules of the vocal cords as the initial manifestation of systemic lupus erythematosus. *JAMA*. 1980;244(24):2751–2752.
150. Smith RR, Ferguson GB. Systemic lupus erythematosus causing subglottic stenosis. *Laryngoscope*. 1976;86(5): 734–738.
151. McNellis EL, Hoang KG. Immunosuppression and systemic lupus erythematosus predisposing to laryngeal abscess. *Otolaryngol Head Neck Surg*. 1997;116(1):107–109.
152. Agah R, Bandi V, Guntupalli KK. Angioedema: the role of ACE inhibitors and factors associated with poor clinical outcome. *Intensive Care Med*. 1997;23(7):793–796.
153. Aszkenasy OM, et al. Systemic lupus erythematosus, pulmonary hypertension, and left recurrent laryngeal nerve palsy. *Ann Rheum Dis*. 1987;46(3):246–247.
154. Petri M, Katzenstein P, Hellmann D. Laryngeal infection in lupus: report of nocardiosis and review of laryngeal involvement in lupus. *J Rheumatol*. 1988;15(6):1014–1015.
155. Roverano S, et al. Asymptomatic sensorineural hearing loss in patients with systemic lupus erythematosus. *J Clin Rheumatol*. 2006;12(5):217–220.
156. Mayes MD. Scleroderma epidemiology. *Rheum Dis Clin North Am*. 2003;29(2):239–254.
157. LeRoy EC. The connective tissue in scleroderma. *Coll Relat Res*. 1981;1(3):301–308.
158. Weisman RA, Calcaterra TC. Head and neck manifestations of scleroderma. *Ann Otol Rhinol Laryngol*. 1978; 87(3, pt 1):332–339.
159. Cummings NA. The oral-mucosal manifestations of rheumatic diseases. *Rheumatology*. 1973;4:60–97.
160. Kanter GJ, Barash PG. Undiagnosed scleroderma in a patient with a difficult airway. *Yale J Biol Med*. 1998;71(1): 31–33.
161. Montesi A, Pesaresi A, Cavalli ML, et al. Oropharyngeal and esophageal function in scleroderma. *Dysphagia*. 1991;6(4):219–223.
162. Reveille JD. Epidemiology of spondyloarthritis in North America. *Am J Med Sci*. 2011;341(4):284–286.
163. Colmegna I, Cuchacovich R, Espinoza LR. HLA-B27-associated reactive arthritis: pathogenetic and clinical considerations. *Clin Microbiol Rev*. 2004;17(2):348–369.
164. Clark M, Kuman PJ, ed. *Clinical Medicine*. 7th ed. Philadelphia, PA: Saunders Elsevier; 2009.
165. Locher MC, Felder M, Sailer HF. Involvement of the temporomandibular joints in ankylosing spondylitis (Bechterew's disease). *J Craniomaxillofac Surg*. 1996;24(4): 205–213.
166. Salathe M, Johr M. Unsuspected cervical fractures: a common problem in ankylosing spondylitis. *Anesthesiology*. 1989;70(5):869–870.
167. Sinclair JR, Mason RA. Ankylosing spondylitis. The case for awake intubation. *Anaesthesia*.1984;39(1):3–11.
168. Palmer JH, Ball DR. Awake tracheal intubation with the intubating laryngeal mask in a patient with diffuse idiopathic skeletal hyperostosis. *Anaesthesia*. 2000;55(1):70–74.
169. Wojtulewski JA, Sturrock RD, Branfoot AC, Hart FD. Cricoarytenoid arthritis in ankylosing spondylitis. *Br Med J*. 1973;3(5872):145–146.
170. Haroon N, Kim TH, Inman RD. NSAIDs and radiographic progression in ankylosing spondylitis. Bagging big game with small arms? *Ann Rheum Dis*. 2012;71(10): 1593–1595.
171. Braun J, van den Berg R, Baraliakos X, et al. 2010 update of the ASAS/EULAR recommendations for the management of ankylosing spondylitis. *Ann Rheum Dis*. 2011; 70(6):896–904.
172. Gawkrodger DJ, Ardern-Jones MR. *Dermatology: An Illustrated Colour Text*. 3rd ed. Edinburg, UK: Churchill Livingstone; 2002:28.
173. Ibrahim G, Waxman R, Helliwell PS. The prevalence of psoriatic arthritis in people with psoriasis. *Arthritis Rheum*. 2009;61(10):1373–1378.
174. Gross WL, Vorwerk E, Christophers E, et al. HLA-related lymphocyte responsiveness in psoriasis. *Int Arch Allergy Appl Immunol*. 1983;70(2):151–156.
175. Kononen M. Subjective symptoms from the stomatognathic system in patients with psoriatic arthritis. *Acta Odontol Scand*. 1986;44(6):377–383.

176. Dervis E, Dervis E. The prevalence of temporomandibular disorders in patients with psoriasis with or without psoriatic arthritis. *J Oral Rehabil.* 2005;32(11): 786–793.
177. Moll JM, Wright V. Psoriatic arthritis. *Semin Arthritis Rheum.* 1973;3(1):55–78.
178. Lundberg M, Ericson S. Changes in the temporomandibular joint in psoriasis arthropathica. *Acta Derm Venereol.* 1967;47(5):354–358.
179. Kononen M. Craniomandibular disorders in psoriasis. *Community Dent Oral Epidemiol.* 1987;15(2):108–112.
180. Medsger TA, Jr, Dawson WN, Jr, Masi AT. The epidemiology of polymyositis. *Am J Med.* 1970;48(6): 715–723.
181. Wortmann RL. Inflammatory disease of muscle. In: Ruddy S, Harris ED, Sledge CB, eds. *Textbook of Rheumatology.* 6th ed. Philadelphia, PA: WB Saunders; 2001: 1273–1296.
182. Mantegazza R, Bernasconi P. Inflammatory myopathies: dermatomyositis, polymyositis and inclusion body myositis. *Madame Curie Bioscience Database.* Autstin, TX: Landes Bioscience; 2000.
183. Bohan A, Peter JB, Bowman RL, Pearson CM. Computer-assisted analysis of 153 patients with polymyositis and dermatomyositis. *Medicine (Baltimore).* 1977;56(4): 255–286.
184. Metheny JA. Dermatomyositis: a vocal and swallowing disease entity. *Laryngoscope.* 1978;88:147–161.
185. Choy EH, Isenberg DA. Treatment of dermatomyositis and polymyositis. *Rheumatology (Oxford).* 2002;41(1): 7–13.
186. Iannuzzi MC, Rybicki BA, Teirstein AS. Sarcoidosis. *N Engl J Med.* 2007;357:2153–2165.
187. Milton CM. Sarcoidosis in ENT practice. *Clin Otolaryngol Allied Sci.* 1985;10(6):351–255.
188. Devine KD. Sarcoidosis and sarcoidosis of the larynx. *Laryngoscope.* 1965;75:533–569.
189. Bower JS, Belen JE, Weg JG, Dantzker DR. Manifestations and treatment of laryngeal sarcoidosis. *Am Rev Respir Dis.* 1980;122(2):325–332.
190. Johns CJ, Michele TM. The clinical management of sarcoidosis. A 50-year experience at the Johns Hopkins Hospital. *Medicine (Baltimore).* 1999;78(2):65–111.
191. Carlesimo M, Giustini S, Rossi A, et al. Treatment of cutaneous and pulmonary sarcoidosis with thalidomide. *J Am Acad Dermatol.* 1995;32(5, pt 2):866–869.
192. Gurler A, Boyvat A, Tursen U. Clinical manifestations of Behcet's disease: an analysis of 2147 patients. *Yonsei Med J.* 1997;38(6):423–427.
193. Main DM, Chamberlain MA. Clinical differentiation of oral ulceration in Behcet's disease. *Br J Rheumatol.* 1992; 31(11):767–770.

14

Tumor Immunology

Thomas J. Ow and Missak Haigentz, Jr.

INTRODUCTION

Human malignancy and the immune system are intimately related, and immune cells appear to play a dual role in cancer development and progression. There is evidence that the immune system is constantly fighting premalignant and malignant cells and that evasion of immune surveillance is a key feature of the establishment and progression of cancer.[1] At the same time, chronic inflammation is a known risk factor for the development of several cancers, and immune cells can undergo malignant transformation leading to hematologic malignancies. Increasing knowledge of tumor immunology has led to a better understanding of carcinogenesis and of the interactions between cancer cells and the tumor microenvironment. Furthermore, understanding tumor immunology has led to novel strategies that harness the power of the immune system for cancer therapy. This chapter highlights the current understanding of the role of the immune system in cancer of the head and neck.

ROLE OF THE IMMUNE SYSTEM IN CANCER

There are two main roles that the immune system plays in human cancer—immune responses can protect against some malignancies, while in other cases the immune response can enhance the development of cancer. There is a growing understanding of both of these processes.

The Immune System in the Defense Against Cancer

The prevailing theory has been that the immune system is continuously monitoring for and destroying malignant cells, thus keeping cancers at bay. Clinical observations and epidemiology studies provide strong evidence that this is the case. Patients with AIDS secondary to human immunodeficiency virus (HIV) infection exemplify this concept, as it is clear that these patients exhibit susceptibility to both "AIDS-defining" malignancies associated with severe immunosuppression, such as Kaposi sarcoma and non-Hodgkin lymphomas, as well as an increased rate of "non-AIDS defining cancers," such as lung carcinoma.[2,3] Similarly, other patients who are immunocompromised, for instance patients requiring immunosuppression after organ transplantation, clearly have an increased rate of malignancy, particularly squamous cell cancer of the skin, lung cancer, and liver cancer.[4,5] Adding to the clinical evidence for immune protection against malignancy are studies that have demonstrated that the presence within a tumor of tumor infiltrating lymphocytes (TILs) is associated with a more favorable prognosis.[6] These include studies in esophageal cancer,[7] oral cancer,[8] and melanoma,[9] among several other tumor types. Other studies also suggest that cell type and location are important for gauging the immune response and the prognostic implications of the presence of TILs. These include studies suggesting that infiltration within the tumor is more significant,[10] as well as studies suggesting that natural killer (NK) cell infiltration,[11–14] $CD8^+$ and $CD3^+$ T cell infiltration,[6,10] and $CD8^+$/FOXP3 ratio[6] of cells are more strongly associated with improved prognosis.

In vivo laboratory models support the clinical and epidemiological evidence for tumor immune surveillance. Experimental evidence over the last several decades has provided insight into the importance of immune protection against malignancy. Largely, these experiments have been carried out using a multitude of elegant mouse models. Several studies have demonstrated that immune compromised mice appear significantly more susceptible to spontaneous as well as chemically and genetically generated cancers.[15–17] Models with several different immune defects have been studied, including loss of T cell, B cell, and NK cell function, as well as models with alterations in interferon-gamma (IFN-γ) and STAT-1 signaling.[15,17] Additionally, studies have demonstrated that aggressive tumors generated in immune-deficient mice and propagated between syngeneic immune-deficient hosts do not effectively form tumors in immune-competent, but otherwise syngeneic counterparts.[1,15–17] These models have also allowed exploration of the factors controlling these phenomena. Tumor transplant models, as well as de novo tumors in genetically engineered mouse models have been used to explore the relationship between immune cells and cancers.[16,18]

The concept of immunoediting is inherent to the current understanding of how tumors evade the immune response. Immunoediting describes the dynamic relationship between tumor cells and the immune system during the process of malignant transformation and progression.[17,19] This process is commonly broken down into 3 stages (ie, the "3 E's"): (1) elimination—the early stages of tumor cell development where tumor antigens elicit an immune response resulting in the destruction of most or all cells with malignant potential; (2) equilibrium—the stage at which an established tumor attains the ability to avoid immune destruction, but invasive and metastatic spread are kept in check by immune defenses; and (3) escape—the phase during which tumor cells gain the ability to evade the immune response and can grow, invade, and metastasize.[15,19] Interactions at the cellular and molecular levels of each of these processes have been characterized, and a brief summary of the current understanding of immunoediting follows.

The elimination phase involves both the innate and adaptive immune system, and it can be described as proceeding through four phases.[15,17] First, tumors must be recognized by the immune system, and it is thought that pro-inflammatory signals generated by malignant cells attract and activate cell components of the innate immune response, including NK cells, natural killer T (NK/T) cells, γδT cells, macrophages, and dendritic cells (DCs). This initial response leads to IFN-γ production, maturation of DCs, and signals initiating apoptosis and necrosis of tumor cells, which are then ingested by the DCs, setting the stage for the adaptive immune response. In the third phase, tumor antigens (TAs) are processed and presented to naïve $CD4^+$ T cells, which then differentiate and recruit/activate TA-specific $CD8^+$ T cells. In the fourth phase, TA-specific $CD4^+$ and $CD8^+$ T cells home toward and eliminate TA-expressing tumor cells.[15,17] The elimination phase of immunoediting is presented schematically in Figure 14–1A.

In the equilibrium phase, the tumor mass is thought to be in a constant battle with the immune forces that are active in the elimination phase. This results in constant selection pressure for tumor cells that become increasingly less immunogenic. Experimental models support this concept, as tumors generated in immune-deficient mice have been shown to be more immunogenic than tumors generated in immune-competent models.[15,20]

As tumors progress from the equilibrium phase to immune escape, tumor cells can develop several different mechanisms to evade detection and destruction. Tumor cells can simply become less antigenic. This may occur due to reduced expression of tumor antigens or a reduced availability of tumor antigens to effector cells in the tumor microenvironment, for example, due to tumor edema.[15] Cancer cells may also alter signaling pathways to evade cell death despite the presence of TAs and immune cells. For example, tumor cells may generate a cytokine milieu with factors such as IL-10, TGF-β, vascular endothelial growth factor (VEGF), and STAT3 in the tumor microenvironment, which

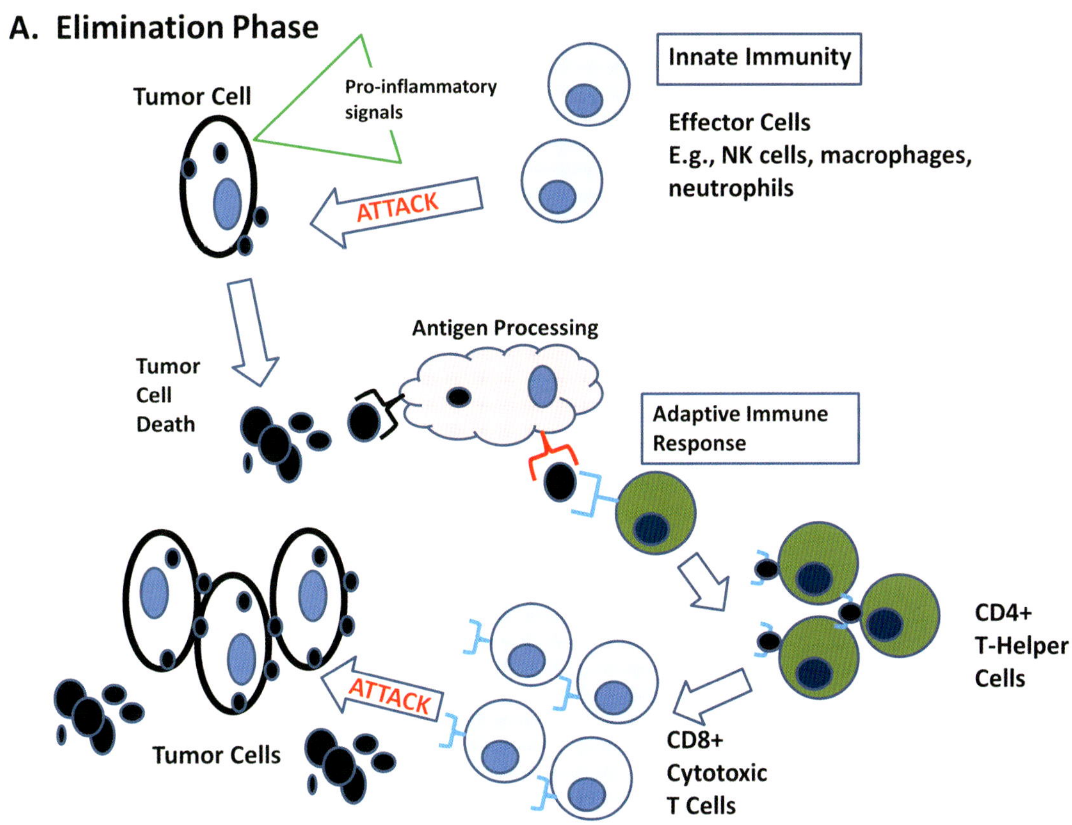

Figure 14–1. The 3 "E's" of immunoediting: **A.** Tumor immune elimination is characterized by 4 phases. Early malignant or premalignant cells are attacked and destroyed, tumor antigens are processed and presented to the adaptive immune system, tumor-specific $CD4^+$ and $CD8^+$ T cells proliferate and home to the location of the tumor, and a tumor-specific immune response results in further elimination of existing tumor cells. *continues*

can lead to suppression of immune effector cells, and/or upregulation of prosurvival signals in tumor cells, abrogating immune-mediated apoptosis.[15,19] An additional mechanism of immune escape used by tumors is to enhance the immune system's own regulatory arm. Two main immune regulatory cells are the myeloid-derived suppressor cells (MDSCs) and regulatory T cells (TRegs). MDSCs contain high levels of the enzymes arginase-1 and inducible nitric oxide synthase (iNOS)-2, which metabolize L-arginine to urea and L-citruline and nitric oxide (NO), respectively. The presence of these metabolites, particularly NO, results in inhibition of T cell function via several mechanisms. MDSCs also suppress T cells via several nonarginine–dependent mechanisms, for example, TGF-β secretion.[19] The equilibrium and escape phases of immunoediting are represented in Figures 14–1B and 14–1C.

TRegs generally function by promoting tolerance to specific "self" antigens by suppressing the induction and proliferation of effector T cells. Tumors have been shown to actively recruit TRegs in order to suppress cytotoxic T cells and avoid immune destruction.[19] This mechanism of immune evasion has recently been exploited by a new class of molecular therapeutics (immune checkpoint inhibitors) and is discussed in detail later in this chapter. Immune evasion is the most well-studied aspect of immunoediting, and a more detailed discussion of the complex mechanisms tumors utilize to survive immune destruction is beyond the scope of this chapter. The readers are directed to works by Dunn and

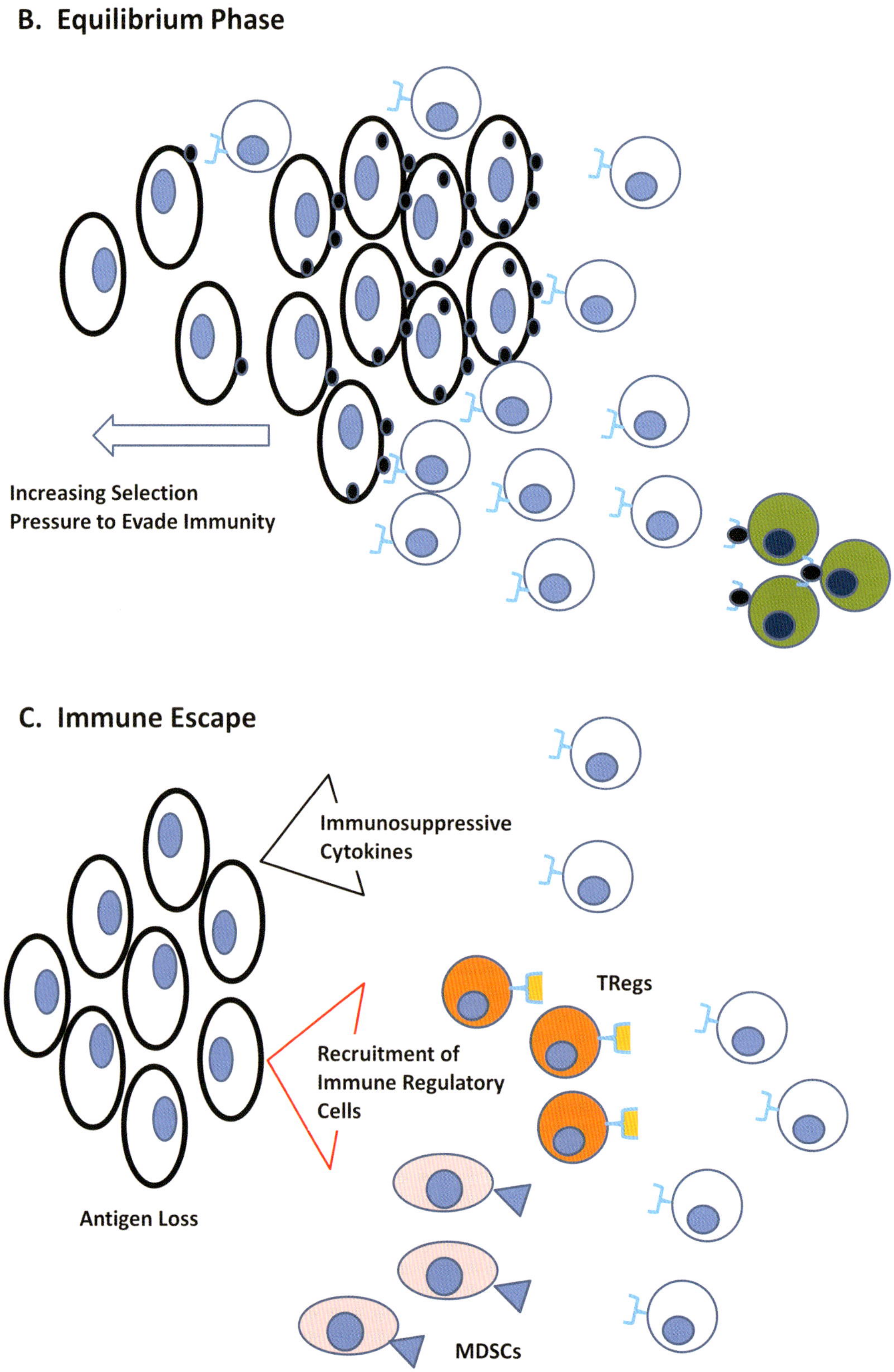

Figure 14-1. *continued* **B.** During the equilibrium phase, continuous attack of the evolving tumor results in selection pressure for tumor cells that can evade the response. **C.** Tumor cells develop multiple strategies for evading immune destruction, leading to immune escape. Tumors reduce expression of immunogenic antigens, suppressive cytokine signals suppress immune effector cells, and regulatory immune cells are recruited leading to further immune suppression. (Abbreviations: NK, natural killer; TRegs, regulatory T cells; MDSCs, myeloid derived suppressor cells.)

colleagues,[17] Kim and colleagues,[15] and Bhatia and Kumar[19] for more detailed yet concise reviews of the process of immune evasion during cancer progression.

The Immune System as Cancer Promoter

While tumors must evade immune detection to survive, it is also evident that immune cells can promote and enhance tumor progression.[1] During malignant progression, chronic or aberrant activation of immune cells can transform normal cells, and immune cells in the tumor microenvironment, especially in the setting of chronic inflammatory states, can promote the survival, invasion, and migration of tumor cells.[21] During the normal response to tissue damage, for example, after the skin is wounded, an acute inflammatory reaction is a key component of the healing process which serves to protect against infectious agents at the wound site as well as to initiate the healing process. Very shortly after tissue is damaged, complement activation and platelet degranulation provide signals to recruit inflammatory cells, namely, neutrophils and mast cells. Subsequently, macrophages migrate to the site via cytokine and chemotactic signals, and activated macrophages provide signals that lead to migration and proliferation of mesenchymal, endothelial, and epithelial components that constitute healing.[21,22] Normally, the inflammatory response to tissue damage is self-limited and subsides once the tissue is repaired. If the acute inflammatory signals are prolonged, however, this response can lead to malignant transformation and enhance invasion and metastasis. This phenomenon has led some to describe cancer as a "wound that never heals."[22,23]

There is clear clinical evidence that chronic inflammation promotes cancer. Some notable examples include the high risk of colorectal cancer in the setting of inflammatory bowel disease, *Helicobactor pylori*–induced inflammation of the stomach and risk of gastric cancer, and liver inflammation secondary to hepatitis B and C virus (HBV, HCV) infection and risk of hepatocellular carcinoma.[22,24] Additionally, though several oncogenic viruses contain oncoproteins that promote malignant transformation, such as the E6 and E7 proteins expressed by high-risk human papillomavirus (HPV), it is evident that these events coupled with a chronic inflammatory reaction promote the development of malignancy.[24] Experimental models support this concept. For example, chickens infected with Rous sarcoma virus have been shown to develop tumors at both the sites of local injection as well as at distant wounds,[25,26] and transgenic mice expressing the viral oncoprotein *v-jun* have been shown to require wounding to promote tumor development.[27]

Cells of the immune system have been shown to contribute to cancer in every phase of development and progression, promoting tumor establishment, enhancing tumor growth and proliferation, and enabling tumor invasion and metastasis. As described above, several chronic inflammatory conditions appear to predispose to the development of cancer. Inflammatory cells may produce reactive oxygen species (ROS) and reactive nitrogen intermediates (RNIs) that cause DNA damage in bystander normal cells, leading to accumulation of mutations.[21,24,28] Additionally, inflammatory cells can produce cytokines that enhance DNA damage and mutation (eg, TNF-α can increase ROS production in epithelial cells while stimulating prosurvival programs such as NF-κβ and IL-6 signaling).[21,28] Migration inhibitory factor (MIF) secreted by macrophages and T lymphocytes can suppress p53 transcriptional activity, thus leading to an increased tolerance to genotoxic stress and the capability to survive a higher mutation burden.[24] Overall, chronic inflammation can lead to tumor initiation by causing malignant transformation and by providing an environment that can enhance the survival of early malignant cells.

Interactions between established tumors and immune cells in the tumor microenvironment lead to enhanced tumor cell growth and proliferation. Immune cells can secrete IL-1, TNF, IL-6, and IL-23, supporting tumor cell survival and tumor growth.[21,28] Tumor cell cytokine signals can then lead to recruitment of specific immune cells into the tumor microenvironment, of which tumor-associated macrophages (TAMs) play an important role.[21,29] For example, as tumors outgrow their blood supply, hypoxic cells can express HIF1-α and VEGF, leading to release of VEGF and PDGF into the tumor microenvironment. This can lead to the recruitment of endothelial precursors, as well as promote migration of TAMs into the hypoxic region. TAMs can then amplify VEGF signaling and further enhance angiogenesis.[21] As tumor cells become established and begin proliferating, interactions with immune cells in the tumor microenvironment are necessary as the tumor begins to thrive.

Immune interactions also appear to play important roles in the characteristic features of malignancy —namely, invasion and metastasis. Inflammatory cells can be an important source of proteases that actively degrade the extracellular matrix at a tumor's invasive front. Myeloid cells recruited to the tumor-matrix interface have been shown to produce matrix metalloproteinases (MMP) and other factors for extracellular matrix degradation.[28] Interactions with immune cells in the microenvironment also promote and enable tumor cell metastasis. Cytokine signals such as TNF-α and NF-κβ activation can lead to upregulation of Snail and Twist, transcription factors that play a key role in tumor cell epithelial-to-mesenchymal transition (EMT).[28] Immune mediators can also generate signals for chemotaxis leading to tumor cell migration[21] as well as contribute to homing and tumor cell implantation and survival at distant metastatic sites.[28,29]

> The immune system can both prevent and promote cancer.
>
> Immunosuppression is a risk factor for the development of several cancers.
>
> Immunoediting describes the relationship between the immune system and tumor cells as cancers develop.
>
> Immunoediting consists of 3 phases: elimination, equilibrium, and escape.
>
> Several cancers are known to develop in the setting of chronic inflammation.
>
> Immune cells and cytokines can promote tumor proliferation, survival, invasion, and metastasis.
>
> Immune cells can also promote a favorable tumor microenvironment (eg, stimulate angiogenesis or contribute to the breakdown of extracellular matrix barriers).

It should be noted that the discussions above are merely a summary of the interactions between the immune system and tumor cells. The processes of immune evasion and immune support in human cancer are extremely complex, and studies over the past several decades have provided significantly more detailed accounts of these relationships than can be described within the confines of this chapter. It is important to have a basic understanding of these concepts in order to understand several key characteristics of cancers of the head and neck. Tumor immunology is particularly important in the evolving epidemiology of oropharyngeal squamous cell carcinoma and HPV infection, as well as in the consideration of exciting new immunotherapy options that have recently been developed.

THE IMMUNE SYSTEM IN HEAD AND NECK CANCERS

Cancer is associated with known deficiencies in immune surveillance, and head and neck cancers are no exception. Although mucosal head and neck squamous cell carcinomas (HNSCC) are the most common primary tumors of this region, the anatomic region is susceptible to a broad range of malignancies.

Malignancies of the Immune System (Lymphomas)

Lymphomas, primary malignancies of the immune system, often present in the head and neck region. Lymphoma is a myriad of more than 50 diseases, each with its own biology. The lymphomas are classified by their immune cell of origin (eg, B cell, T cell, NK cell) and have a widely heterogeneous aggressiveness and prognosis, ranging from chronic and quite indolent types (eg, chronic lymphocytic leukemia [CLL]) to more aggressive histological types (eg, diffuse large B cell lymphoma). Historically, the lymphomas have been broadly categorized as either Hodgkin or non-Hodgkin types, but classification of lymphomas has changed dramatically as molecular characterization based on clonal expression of cell surface markers has advanced.

Lymphoma of the head and neck most commonly involves the cervical lymph nodes, and often there is no mucosal lesion. However, involvement of lymphatic tissue in mucosal regions in the pharynx (Waldeyer ring) may masquerade as primary mucosal tumors.

The distinction of lymphoma from other malignancies of the head and neck is critical in that the disease and its treatment is systemic, primarily involving chemotherapy; rapid tumor responses are common with chemotherapy and radiotherapy. Importantly, surgery is not the primary mode of therapy for this group of malignancies and is generally reserved for excisional lymph node biopsies for diagnosis. When a diagnosis of lymphoma is suspected, a fresh surgical specimen (not formalin fixed) should be submitted for flow cytometry for immune markers to establish the exact pathological diagnosis. Consultation with a medical oncologist is imperative to help guide the staging workup and clinical management of patients.

Important types of lymphoma for the head and neck oncologist are Hodgkin lymphoma and NK cell lymphoma, because these diseases often present with head and neck symptoms. Hodgkin lymphoma, classically presenting as abnormal painless cervical lymphadenopathy in young persons (age 20s to 30s, and a second peak over age 50), is curable with aggressive chemotherapy, even in advanced stages. Extranodal NK/T cell lymphoma, nasal type (also known as "lethal midline granuloma") is a rare (more common in Asia and Central and South America) but very aggressive lymphoma associated with Epstein-Barr virus (EBV) infection that involves the nose and paranasal sinuses. NK/T cell lymphoma is also very responsive to radiotherapy or chemotherapy. The importance of including medical oncologists in the diagnosis and treatment plan of patients with suspected disease cannot be overemphasized.

Other Malignancies Associated With Immune Dysfunction

Although lymphomas are characteristically associated with immunosuppressive states (including primary disease conditions, including HIV infection and autoimmune disorders), and chronic use of immune-suppressing agents post-organ and post-bone-marrow transplantation, several other malignancies in the head and neck region can be associated with immunosuppression.

Fanconi Anemia–Associated Cancers

Fanconi anemia, an autosomal recessive or X-linked disorder affecting all races and ethnic groups, is the most common inherited form of aplastic anemia and bone marrow failure, frequently diagnosed in childhood. Multiple genes involved in normal repair of DNA interstrand cross-links have been implicated in this disorder, which also places young patients at high risk for several malignancies, particularly blood cancers (myelodysplastic syndrome and acute myeloid leukemia), as well as HNSCC and squamous cell carcinoma of the vulva. Due to deficiencies in DNA repair mechanisms, these patients are particularly susceptible to severe toxicities associated with chemotherapy and radiation. The immunologic link of Fanconi anemia–associated immunosuppression and cancer development is as yet unclear.

Cutaneous Squamous Cell Carcinomas

Skin cancers (particularly squamous cell carcinomas) are common among transplant recipients, likely associated with use of chronic immunosuppressive agents and sun exposure. Sun avoidance with particular attention to exposed head and neck sites should be strongly recommended in these patients. Consideration for a head and neck skin primary should be given to all patients presenting with a HNSCC with unknown primary site, and a thorough history from such patients should be obtained for prior skin cancer excisions.[30]

Melanoma

Cutaneous melanoma occurs with increased frequency in immunosuppressed persons, such as organ transplant recipients, and possibly in persons with HIV infection. This disease has been the prototype for the study and development of several immunomodulatory therapies (including interferon-alfa, IL-2, and now ipilimumab and pembrolizumab).

In contrast to cutaneous primaries, primary mucosal melanomas of the head and neck are rare, accounting for less than 10% of melanomas in this region.

Viral-Associated Cancers

Several viral infections are known to be oncogenic. These include Epstein-Barr virus (EBV), human papillomavirus (HPV), and the Merkel cell polyomavirus (MCV). A list of virally associated cancers affecting head and neck sites are presented in Table 14–1.

Epstein-Barr virus (EBV) infections have been associated with development of aggressive lymphomas and nasopharyngeal carcinomas. EBV infection is endemic in Southeast Asia, where the highest rates of nasopharyngeal cancers arise. The EBV infection is clonally involved in cancer; moreover, plasma EBV DNA levels (pretherapy and post-therapy) may be of prognostic value.[31] Due to their proximity to and frequent involvement of skull base structures and the sensitivity of these tumors to chemotherapy and radiation, the primary management of these tumors is frequently nonsurgical.

Merkel cell polyomavirus (MCV) is associated with Merkel cell carcinoma, a rare but aggressive skin cancer associated with severe immunodeficiency in persons with AIDS, B cell malignancies, or following organ transplantation. Indirect evidence of the role of the immune system on the development of this malignancy includes reports of spontaneous disease remissions, often following biopsy, though proof of immune stimulation following diagnostic biopsy has been lacking.[32]

A discussion of human papillomavirus (HPV) infection and head and neck cancer follows.

Table 14–1. Viral Infections Associated with Head and Neck Malignancies

Virus	Head and Neck Malignancy
Epstein-Barr virus (EBV)	Nasopharyngeal carcinoma, lymphoma
Human herpesvirus-8 (HHV-8)	Kaposi sarcoma
Human immunodeficiency virus (HIV)	Lymphoma, Kaposi sarcoma, head and neck squamous cell carcinoma
Human papillomavirus (HPV)	Head and neck squamous cell carcinoma (oropharynx)
Merkel cell polyomavirus (MCV)	Merkel cell carcinoma

Human Papillomavirus-Associated Oropharyngeal Cancers

Oncogenic human papillomavirus (HPV) infection, particularly with HPV16, has been implicated in the pathogenesis of squamous cell carcinomas of the oropharynx. Approximately 50% of tonsil cancers have been known to harbor HPV DNA.[33] Although HNSCC remains more common in older male smokers and alcohol drinkers, the incidence of oropharyngeal cancers has risen in young, never smoking males and females,[34,35] suggesting the growing importance of HPV infections. HPV-associated head and neck cancers share similar sexual risk associations with cervical cancers, namely, multiple sexual partners (specifically, high number of lifetime vaginal and oral sex partners).[36] These tumors have different biology from smoking-related head and neck cancers[37] and are associated with favorable prognosis, suggesting that HPV-associated HNSCC is a distinct clinical entity.[38,39] Tobacco smoking remains an independent risk factor for survival, with worse outcomes in patients smoking more than 10 pack-years at the time of cancer diagnosis.[40]

HPV-related cancers can be clinically detected directly by in situ hybridization for HPV DNA or indirectly by immunohistochemical evaluation of p16, a cell cycle protein often downregulated in tobacco-carcinogen–related cancers but upregulated in HPV-associated HNSCC. The use of tumor HPV-status in routine clinical decision making is currently investigational, and the treatment of HPV-associated disease is currently similar to that for HPV-unrelated cancers.[30]

Mucosal immunity is clearly involved in clearance of HPV infection, and immunodeficiency states may give rise to persistent infection leading to oncogenesis. Oral HPV infections are prevalent, though clearly not all infections develop into cancer. An estimated 7% of the US general population has evidence of oral HPV infection, and 1% of the population (approximately 3 million individuals in the United States alone) has HPV16 infection.[41] Immune system evasion of oncogenic HPV infections resulting in carcinogenesis is currently the subject of intense research efforts.

HIV-Associated Cancers

HIV-infected populations appear to be at a 3-fold increased risk of developing HNSCC, and recent epidemiological data suggest that there is an increased risk for HPV related and unrelated disease.[42] Although HPV16 is now known to be an established etiology of these malignancies and is a sexually transmitted coinfection common in persons with HIV infection, initial tumor-based studies suggest the possibility that there are additional factors in HIV-positive individuals which contribute to the excess risk.[43,44] Moderate immunosuppression may play a role in this elevated cancer risk. The etiology of HIV-associated head and neck cancers requires additional research, as does the safety and tolerability of standard multimodality therapies for this disease.

Aggressive lymphoma is prevalent and associated with advancing immunosuppression, though its incidence has declined with the development of combination antiretroviral therapies resulting in effective immune system reconstitution.[45] Persons with AIDS-associated immunosuppression also remain at risk for other viral-associated cancers affecting the head and neck, including Kaposi sarcoma (human herpes virus-8 [HHV-8] infection) and Merkel cell carcinoma (MCV infection).

> Lymphomas commonly involve the head and neck region. Fanconi anemia, which is caused by defects in DNA damage repair, is associated with several malignancies, including head and neck squamous cell carcinoma. Squamous cell carcinoma of the skin is common among patients receiving immunosuppression after organ transplant, and commonly involves head and neck sites. Malignant melanoma is common in the head and neck, and several immunotherapy approaches have been effective for this malignancy. Virus-associated malignancies are common in the head and neck region, several of which are summarized in Table 14–1.

OVERVIEW OF CANCER IMMUNOTHERAPY

Definition of Immunotherapy and Approaches

Immunotherapy is defined as any treatment that utilizes the immune system as part of the therapeutic strategy. Cancer immunotherapy therefore describes several different approaches that incorporate the immune system into prevention or treatment of cancer. These approaches can be categorized many different ways, and recent advances over the past several years have led to numerous strategies. One can divide these treatments into "active" and "passive" approaches.[46] Active cancer immunotherapy utilizes methods that expose immune cells to tumor antigens that then establish a specific immune response which is also durable due to T cell memory. Passive immunotherapy approaches are those in which antibodies or effector cells are provided to directly attack tumor cells. These approaches can be very effective but are often limited because they are transient.[46] Several other immune therapy approaches do not fit these categories or perhaps bridge both; for example, cytokine therapy can enhance the existing immune response or enable an active approach.

Modern immunotherapy can also be categorized into cell-based and antibody-based therapies. Examples of cell-based therapies include the application of vaccines developed to stimulate an immune response in vivo, or methods that involve the extraction of immune cells, such as tumor infiltrating leukocytes (TILs), dendritic cells, or NK cells, and subsequent priming of these effector cells to target antigen-bearing tumor cells prior to returning them to the host as a therapeutic agent. Antibody-based methods have rapidly advanced over the past 3 decades. Techniques such as hybridoma technology have allowed the mass production of monoclonal antibodies (MoAbs), and advances in genetics have led to the ability to synthesize both chimeric and fully humanized MoAbs that can be tailored to target specific proteins.[47] Antibodies used in cancer therapy can target tumor-specific antigens leading to destruction of the cancer cell, or they can target specific signaling molecules, resulting in inhibition or activation of signaling pathways crucial to tumor cell survival. As with the active and passive categorization, there are immunotherapy approaches that are neither cell- nor antibody-based, such as cytokine therapy, or perhaps encompass both, such as MoAbs designed as immune checkpoint inhibitors.

Cancer immunotherapy approaches are rapidly advancing, and the following sections discuss several of these strategies in more detail. A summary of these approaches is presented in Table 14–2.

Nonspecific Immune Activation

Over a century ago, it was observed that occasionally patients suffering from cancer who developed erysipelas experienced spontaneous cancer regression. William Coley, a surgical oncologist, noted this phenomenon in the late 1800s, and thus began exploring the use of bacteria to stimulate an immune response to treat malignancy. This led to the development of "Coley's Toxin," which was a mixture of killed *Streptococcus pyogenes* and *Serratia marcescens* that could be injected intravenously or directly into tumors.[48] While Coley's toxin itself has not been proven to be efficacious, the principles of this approach have led to several therapies that are actively used today. For example, interleukin-2 (IL-2) is a cytokine that acts as a signaling molecule in several aspects of the immune response. It can cause T-cell activation and differentiation, and when given systemically, can elicit a profound inflammatory and immune response. Recombinant IL-2 was studied as a therapeutic agent,[49] and it was the first cytokine that gained US Food and Drug Administration (FDA) approval for the treatment of cancer.[50] Another example is the use of bacillus Calmette-Guérin (BCG) vaccine for the treatment and prevention of early stage bladder cancer. BCG is live-attenuated *Mycobacterium bovis* which is used as a vaccine to prevent tuberculosis infection. The vaccine can generate a local immune reaction, and instillation of BCG into the urinary bladder after treatment for superficial bladder cancer has been shown to decrease cancer recurrence.[51]

A generalized immune response can be effective but is usually limited, and the systemic response is often highly toxic, as is the case with IL-2 and interferon treatment. Thus, more targeted forms of immunotherapy have been sought, and general immune enhancers, such as cytokine therapy, will perhaps be more beneficial as an adjuvant to other forms of immunotherapy.

Vaccines

A vaccine is any biological agent that is administered to a subject in order to stimulate an immune response to a specific pathogen in order to treat or prevent a disease. Vaccines for cancer treatment can be both preventive and therapeutic.

Several cancers are associated with viral infection, and therefore vaccination against oncogenic or cancer-associated viruses can be a form of cancer prevention. This has been evident in the case of vaccination against HBV. Vaccination programs against HBV in high-risk populations have been shown to be associated with decreased incidence of hepatocellular carcinoma.[52] Recently, a bivalent vaccine (Cervarix) against HPV types 16 and 18, and a quadrivalent vaccine (Gardasil) against HPV types 6, 11, 16, and 18 have been developed. HPV types 16 and 18 are associated with cervical, penile, vulvar, vaginal, anal, and oropharyngeal squamous cell cancers. It is hoped that prophylactic vaccination programs will result in decreases in the incidence of these malignancies.[53]

The concept of immune surveillance and tumor-associated antigens (TAAs) has led to attempts to develop tumor-specific vaccines for cancer therapy. Tumor vaccines can be polyvalent, derived from the antigen pool present in tumor lysates, or tumor-dendritic cell conjugates; however, processes for selecting the immunogenic antigens from these preparations on an individual basis can be arduous and costly.[54] Antigen-specific vaccines are another approach, developed from tumor-specific antigens that are commonly identified in a particular malignancy. Examples include cancer-testis antigens, which are tumor-specific antigens that are usually found only in tissues in the testes which are normally sheltered from the immune response, or overexpressed mutant proteins that are common to a malignancy.[54]

Therapeutic tumor vaccine strategies have largely been unsuccessful. This is likely due to the ability of most malignancies to evade immune detection as described earlier in this chapter. In order to improve the immune response to tumor antigens,

Table 14-2. Summary of Current Immunotherapy Approaches

Approach	Description	Examples
Nonspecific therapeutics	Agents used as cancer therapeutics by eliciting a generalized immune response	IL-2 therapy for malignant melanoma or renal cell carcinoma; Intravesicular BCG for early bladder cancer
Vaccines	Agents administered to illicit a specific immune response to a pathogen	
Preventative	Vaccines that prevent infection with oncogenic viruses, where prevention of viral infection protects against the development of cancer	HBV vaccine to prevent hepatocellular carcinoma
Therapeutic	Vaccines given that target tumor antigens directly	Tumor-associated antigens; greater success when used in combination with adoptive cell transfer methods
Cell-based therapeutics	Processes where a host's immune cells are harvested, manipulated, and returned to enhance the tumor immune response	
Adoptive T cell transfer	T cells are either enriched for TAA-specific clones (eg. TILs), activated via exposure to TAAs, or genetically altered to target TAAs (eg. CARs) and returned to the host	Adoptive T cell transfer protocols with TILs or CAR-modified T cells
Dendritic cell transfer	Dendritic cells are harvested and activated in culture with exposure to TAAs, and returned to the host	Sipuleucel-T (Provenge) for prostate cancer
Antibody therapy	MoAbs engineered to target specific antigens to treat cancer	
Elicit immune response	MoAbs target TAAs, which then elicits an immune response (eg, ADCC or CDC) resulting in tumor cell death	Rituximab targets CD20 on B cells, used to treat B cell lymphomas
Direct tumor cell killing	MoAbs target tumor cell surface receptors that lead directly to cell death (eg, via apoptosis); antibody-drug conjugates target a TAA and deliver a toxic payload	Brentuximab vedotin targets CD30 on lymphoma cells, and delivers the antimitotic agent MMAE
Functional targeting	MoAbs target a specific signaling molecule or receptor, with the goal of modifying important signaling pathways	Bevacizumab targets VEGF to inhibit VEGFR signaling important for angiogenesis; Cetuximab targets EGFR to inhibit signaling important for tumor cell proliferation and survival

continues

Table 14-2. *continued*

Approach	Description	Examples
Immune checkpoint inhibitors	Therapies that alter the immune regulatory response mechanisms that tumor cells use to evade the immune response	
CTLA-4 inhibitors	CTLA-4 is a key coregulatory receptor that results in suppression of antigen-specific $CD4^+$ T helper cells and enhances activation of TRegs	Ipilimumab targets CTLA-4 and is approved for treatment of unresectable/metastatic melanoma
PD1 pathway inhibitors	PD1 signaling reduces the immune response in peripheral tissues by generally suppressing immune effector cells and enhancing Treg response	Pembrolizumab targets the PD-1 receptor and is approved for treatment of unresectable/metastatic melanoma previously treated with ipilimumab, and when indicated, BRAF inhibition

Note. IL-2 = interleukin-2; *BCG* = Bacillus Calmette-Guérin; *HBV* = Hepatitis B virus; *TILs* = tumor infiltrating lymphocytes; *TAA* = tumor-associated antigens; *CAR* = chimeric antigen receptor; *MoAb* = monoclonal antibody; *CTLA-4* = cytotoxic T lymphocyte-associated antigen 4; *PD-1* = programmed cell death receptor 1; *EGFR* = epithelial growth factor receptor; *VEGF* = vascular endothelial growth factor; *VEGFR* = vascular endothelial growth factor receptor; *MMAE* = monomethyl auristatin E; *ADCC* = antibody-dependent cell cytotoxicity; *CDC* = complement-dependent cytotoxicity.

several adjuvants have been explored with the goal of increasing the immune reaction to tumor-specific vaccines. These include cytokines such as IL-12 and GM-CSF, oil-emulsion vehicles, and microbial derivatives administered in conjunction with the vaccine.[54] Again the efficacy of these strategies has been limited to date. To further potentiate the specific immune response to tumor antigens and harness the ability of immune cells to recognize and target malignant cells, several ex vivo cell-based therapies have been developed.

Cell-Based Therapies

In general, cell-based cancer immunotherapy involves harvesting a host's immune cells and manipulating them in order to enhance an immunologic response to a tumor prior to reintroducing them as a therapeutic. Though several immune cell types have been used in these strategies, DCs and T lymphocytes are the two most well studied. Except for Sipuleucel-T, a DC-based therapy FDA approved to treat prostate cancer, all cell-based methods are currently experimental.

Adoptive T cell transfer is a method of passive immunotherapy whereby activated T cells are transfused into the patient with the goal of attacking the patient's cancer. There are several strategies that have been developed to explore the therapeutic advantage of this concept. TILs can be extracted from the tumor mass, or peripheral T cells can be harvested and primed. In some methods, resting peripheral T cells are exposed to TAAs and activated, and activated T cells are then selected and expanded. T cells are rapidly expanded in culture using various activation and proliferation protocols, for example, by applying IL-2 and anti-CD3.[55] Extracted T cells can also be genetically manipulated to target a specific antigen prior to selection and expansion, for example, recombinant techniques can be used to generate T cells that express specific T-cell receptors (TCRs) targeting selected TAAs. Specifically, chimeric antigen receptors (CARs) have been developed to tailor T cells that can respond to any specific antigen of interest. A CAR typically grafts a single chain variable fragment (scFV) from a MoAb to the intracellular domain of the CD3-zeta costimulatory signaling protein. This "first-generation" design has since been replaced by "second-generation" and "third-generation" CARs that have additional intracellular molecules on their cytoplasmic tail that provide costimulatory signals or other modifiers that enhance activated T cell survival and response.[56] Regardless of the activation and selection techniques used, activated T cells are ultimately transfused into the patient for therapy. In several strategies, the patient is lymphodepleted prior to transfusion, and/or the T cells are given with high-dose IL-2 as an adjuvant.[57] Adoptive T cell transfer protocols are currently being studied in several malignancies. Notably, autologous TIL therapy after lymphodepletion has shown efficacy in patients with metastatic melanoma in several trials[58] and adoptive T cell transfer using CARs directed at CD19 demonstrated significant efficacy in patients with treatment-refractory acute lymphocytic leukemia.[59]

DC transfer therapy is similar to adoptive T cell transfer, in that dendritic cells can be harvested from peripheral blood and activated in culture. DCs can be activated in the presence of a specific TAA or through culture with tumor cell lysates. DCs are then returned to the host with the goal of driving an immune response to the tumor.[60] As stated earlier, a therapy protocol using DC transfer, Sipuleucel-T (Provenge), has been approved by the FDA to treat prostate cancer after it was shown to improve patient survival.[61] The therapy involves 3 cycles of harvesting DCs via leukopheresis followed by ex vivo exposure of the DCs to PA2024, which is a fusion protein between GM-CSF and prostatic acid phosphatase (PAP), and finally infusion of the activated DCs back into the patient.

Cell-based immunotherapies represent an exciting field of cancer therapy that is under intense investigation. Technical challenges present significant hurdles for evaluation and implementation of these protocols, but technologic advances are allowing these strategies to gain further ground.

Antibody Therapy

The ability to design, purify, and mass produce MoAbs has dramatically altered the landscape of cancer therapeutics during the last 3 decades. Several landmark technological advances have made antibody therapy a reality. First, the use of hybridoma technology allowed continuous production of monospecific antibodies in culture. Hybridomas are created by fusing spleen cells harvested from mice or rabbits injected with a specific antigen, to immortalized myeloma cells. This allows continuous culture of hybrid cells, which are then screened for clones that express the antibody of interest. The selected clones are then expanded, and the antibody can be continually produced in culture.[62]

Most mouse-derived antibodies had several disadvantages, including limited efficacy, short half-lives and development of antibodies to the MoAbs in patients exposed to the murine proteins (often referred to as HAMA—human anti-mouse antibodies).[47] These problems have been overcome as evolving genetic methods have allowed progressive "humanization" of MoAbs. First, chimeric antibodies were created, which replaced portions of the mouse antibody, such as the Fc region, with a human sequence. Later, "fully" humanized antibodies were developed in which the entire antibody except for the complementary determining region (CDR) was replaced with human-specific sequences.[63] It is also possible to "de-immunize" antibodies by altering antigenic sequences resulting in protein that is significantly less immunogenic.[63] The results of these technological advances have led to the development of hundreds of MoAb therapeutics over the last 3 decades that can be used safely and repeatedly in humans, utilizing a myriad of different strategies to treat human disease.

The therapeutic function of a MoAb depends on which proteins are targeted and the result of the protein-antibody interaction. Antibodies that target a surface protein on a cell can lead to an immune response directed at that cell. Bound antibodies can recruit effector cells such as NK cells, neutrophils, cytotoxic T cells, and macrophages to the target, eliciting antibody-dependent cell cytotoxicity (ADCC). The Fc regions of antibodies can also activate complement, thus activating complement-dependent cytotoxicity (CDC) as a means to destroy targeted tumor cells.[47] An example of a MoAb that acts primarily through these mechanisms is the chimeric MoAb rituximab, which targets CD20. CD20 is a surface protein primarily expressed on B cells, and thus rituximab is utilized to treat several B cell malignancies and autoimmune diseases caused largely by B cell dysfunction.

MoAbs can also function via direct killing of targeted cells. In some cases, this is secondary to antibody-induced apoptosis. Alternatively, antibody-drug conjugates (ADCs) are a class of MoAbs that have been created with the goal of direct killing of tumor cells. MoAbs can be chemically linked to a biologically active payload, for example a radioactive particle, toxin, or drug. The goal, therefore, is to selectively deliver these substances to a tumor via the antigen-MoAb interaction.[64] An example of an ADC approved to treat cancer is the drug brentuximab vedotin. This drug is composed of the chimeric MoAb brentuximab, which targets CD30, linked to the antimitotic agent vedotin, or monomethyl auristatin E (MMAE). Brentuximab vedotin is FDA-approved to treat refractory Hodgkin lymphoma and systemic anaplastic large cell lymphoma. CD30 is expressed on these lymphoma cells, and when brentuximab binds CD30 the ADC is internalized, and the bond linking MMAE to the MoAb is specifically cleaved via cathepsin within the cell lysosome. Thus, the MMAE payload is delivered into the tumor cell preferentially.[65]

MoAb therapy can also function by altering key cell signaling pathways that drive tumor proliferation and survival. This is the basis for many drugs currently available to treat cancer. MoAbs can target extracellular signaling molecules.[47] This is the intended mechanism of action for bevacizumab, a humanized MoAb that targets the vascular endothelial growth factor A (VEGF-A). The mechanistic goal of bevacizumab therapy is to bind VEGF-A, inhibiting the interaction between VEGF-A and the VEGF receptor both on tumor cells and cells in the tumor microenvironment, thus decreasing tumor angiogenesis.[66] MoAbs can also target cell surface receptors, blocking signals from the tumor microenvironment. An example of this type of drug is cetuximab, a chimeric MoAb that targets the epidermal growth factor receptor (EGFR). EGFR has been shown to be upregulated and overexpressed in several cancers, and EGF signaling leads to increased proliferation of cancer cells. Cetuximab competitively inhibits EGFR with the goal of diminishing EGFR signaling.[67] MoAb function can also be agonistic, activating pathways with which they interact, such as antibodies that activate the pro-apoptosis TNF-related apoptosis inducing ligand (TRAIL) receptor, but examples are rare and therapeutic advantages not yet realized in the clinical setting.[47] Additionally, MoAbs used to treat cancer often function via multiple mechanisms of action. For example, cetuximab not only blocks EGFR signaling but also induces immune-mediated cell death.[68]

Antibody therapy has thus revolutionized cancer therapy, and the potential utility of MoAbs in cancer is now being realized.

Immune Checkpoint Inhibitors

Immune checkpoints describe the multitude of mechanisms that the immune system has evolved to quell the immune response, largely composed of inhibitory signals that temper the immune reaction in order to maintain self-tolerance and reduce damage to normal healthy tissues while attacking foreign invaders and diseased cells. These checkpoints largely rely on the action of costimulatory and coinhibitory molecules/receptors that coincide with antigen presentation and T-cell receptor (TCR) recognition and activation. Generally, mediators that lead to T-cell activation are not altered in tumor cells or cells in the tumor microenvironment, whereas signaling molecules that lead to T cell inhibition are commonly overexpressed. It appears that tumor cells thus modify immune checkpoint signals as a means of immune evasion.[69] Recently, methods for targeting immune checkpoint signals have resulted in effective cancer therapeutics that ultimately act by enhancing the immune response to tumor cells. The two checkpoint receptors that have been most successfully exploited to date are the cytotoxic T-lymphocyte-associated antigen-4 (CTLA-4) and programmed cell death receptor-1 (PD-1).

CTLA-4 and its important costimulatory receptor (CD28) are generally expressed on T cells and share the same ligands, CD80 and CD86 (also called B7.1, and B7.2, respectively, and commonly referred to collectively as B7 ligands). Antigen presented with CD80 or CD86 drives both activation and inhibitory signals in different classes of T cells. In general, CTLA-4 activation appears to dampen $CD4^+$ T-helper cell response while increasing TReg activity, both of which are advantageous for tumor cell immune evasion. Therefore, selective CTLA-4 inhibition can increase T-cell activation and diminish TReg-mediated suppression of immune activity toward TAAs.[69] The efficacy of this approach has been embodied in the recent development of the drug ipilimumab for the treatment of metastatic melanoma. Ipilimumab is a fully humanized MoAb that binds CTLA-4, thus inhibiting binding of CD80/CD86 and decreasing CTLA-4 coregulatory signaling.[70] Ipilimumab has shown significant efficacy in the treatment of patients with metastatic malignant melanoma[71,72] and is currently approved by the FDA for these patients.

The PD-1 pathway is another immune checkpoint pathway that is under wide evaluation as a therapeutic target in cancer. PD-1 receptors are found broadly on immune cells, including NK, T, and B cells, and the receptor interacts with two ligands, programmed death-ligands 1 and 2 (PD-L1, PD-L2). PD-1 signaling is a crucial mechanism for limiting the immune response in peripheral tissues to combat autoimmunity and tissue damage secondary to inflammation. PD-1 activation appears to inhibit the activity of both T-helper cells and cytotoxic T cells, as well as enhance proliferation of TRegs. PD-1 activation also appears to inhibit NK cells and B cells.[69] Tumor cells appear to use the profound immunosuppressive effect of the PD-1 pathway to an advantage. In general, it has been noted that TILs from solid tumors express high levels of PD-1, while tumor cells commonly express PD-1 ligands.[69] The implication that tumors utilize the PD-1 pathway for immune evasion has led to the development of PD-1 pathway inhibitors as cancer therapeutics. Pembrolizumab (previously named lambrolizumab) is a humanized MoAb that targets the PD-1 receptor. Efficacy of pembrolizumab among patients with advanced cutaneous malignant melanoma has been established, with approximately 38% of patients demonstrating a response, several of whom experienced durable control.[73] A significant number of patients who had tumor progression after previous treatment with ipilimumab demonstrated tumor response to pembrolizumab. These promising results led to the accelerated FDA approval of pembrolizumab for the treatment of patients with unresectable or metastatic melanoma who have progressed after treatment with ipilimumab, and, if positive for BRAF V600E mutation, after treatment with a BRAF inhibitor.

A large host of immune checkpoint mechanisms remain comparatively unexplored,[69] and it is hoped that success in targeting the CTLA-4 and PD-1 pathways to date represents the dawn of significant and efficacious advances in cancer immunotherapy. Figure 14–2 presents a schematic to help describe how the CTLA-4 inhibitor ipilimumab and the PD-1 inhibitor pembrolizumab can promote the immune response.

> Immunotherapy is any treatment that utilizes the immune system. Active immunotherapy approaches are those in which a patient's immune response is generated, whereas passive immunotherapy approaches are those in which immune components are directly administered to a patient. Immunotherapy approaches can also be categorized as "cell based" and "antibody based." Several immunotherapy strategies, with examples, are summarized in Table 14–2.

Immunotherapy Approaches in HNSCC

Patients with HNSCC may have defects in innate and adaptive immunity, and cancer treatments including radiation therapy and cytotoxic chemotherapy can further exacerbate cellular immune deficiencies. Immunotherapy therefore represents a new frontier in cancer therapy, in general, and several promising approaches for HNSCC therapy are under active investigation. Targeting the epidermal growth factor receptor (EGFR) with cetuximab is currently standard (as an example, at least in part, of passive immunotherapy), and various active immunotherapy strategies in HNSCC have demonstrated potential efficacy, warranting further investigation.

Monoclonal Antibodies Targeting the Epidermal Growth Factor Receptor (EGFR)

The EGFR is overexpressed in HNSCC, and EGFR signaling has been implicated in cancer cell survival, proliferation, and angiogenesis. Targeting this cell surface receptor with monoclonal antibodies has been the most clinically effective biological approach to date for the treatment of head and neck cancers.

Cetuximab (Erbitux) is a recombinant, human/mouse chimeric monoclonal antibody with specificity against the extracellular domain of EGFR,

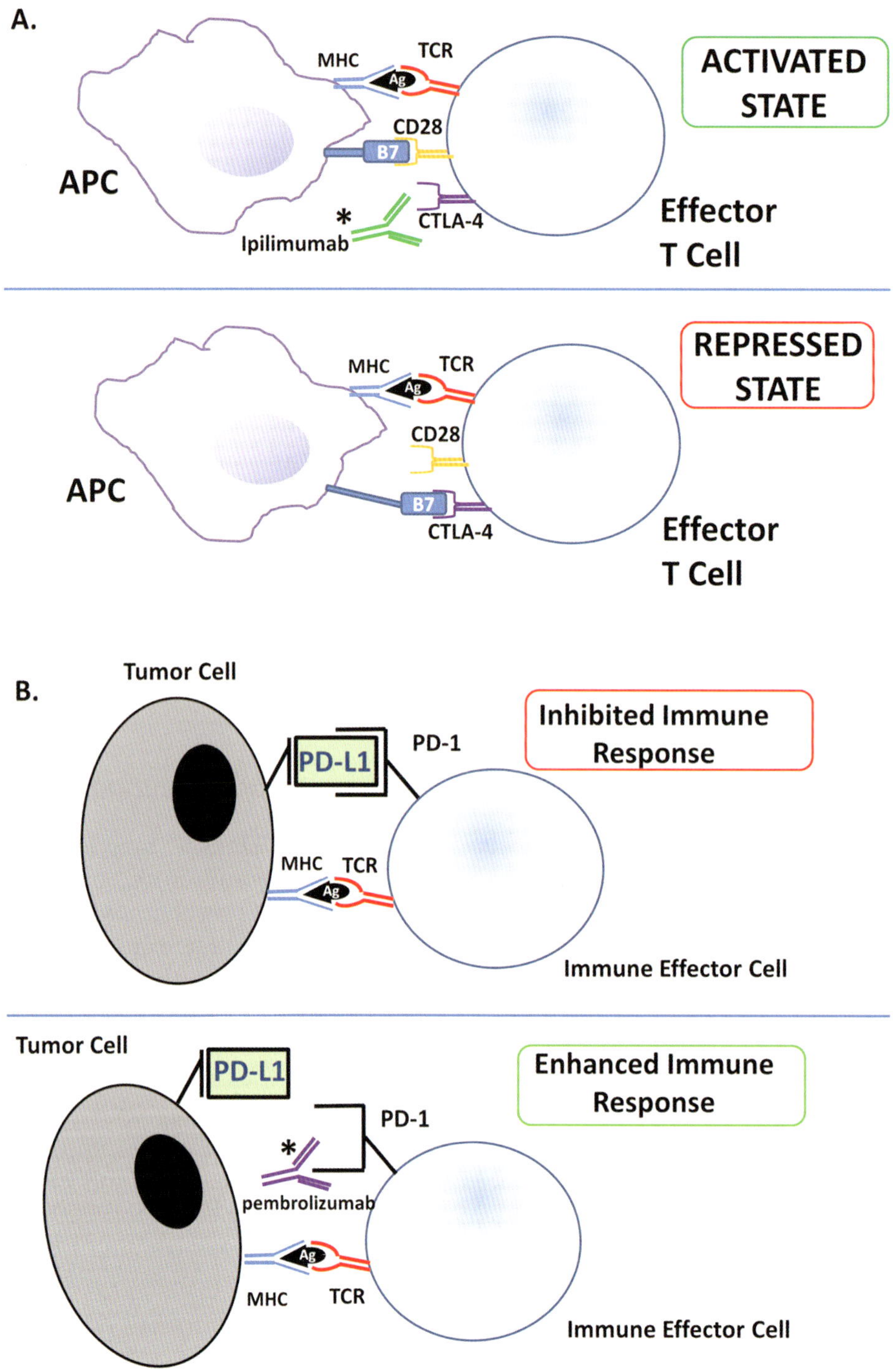

Figure 14-2. Mechanism of action of CTLA-4 and PD-1 checkpoint inhibitors. **A.** Activation of effector T cells requires antigen presentation via the MHC complex to the TCR, along with a costimulation between CD28 and B7 ligands. The CTLA-4 receptor is also stimulated by B7 ligands, and CTLA-4 activation results in inhibition of the T-cell activation, thus providing a competing signal to regulate the immune response. *Ipilimumab inhibits CTLA-4, thus diminishing CTLA-4 costimulation resulting in a greater proportion of activated effector T cells. **B.** Interaction of PD-L1 with the PD-1 receptor on immune effector cells inhibits the immune response. Tumor cells commonly overexpress PD-L1, which leads to general immune suppression in the tumor microenvironment. *Pembrolizumab inhibits the PD-1 receptor, and thus enhances the response of immune effector cells to tumor antigens. (Abbreviations: *APC* = antigen-presenting cell; *Ag* = antigen; MHC, major histocompatability complex; *TCR*= T-cell receptor; *CTLA-4* = cytotoxic T-lymphocyte-associated protein 4; *PD-1* = programmed cell death protein 1; *PD-L1* = programmed death ligand 1.)

competitively inhibiting the binding of epidermal growth factor (EGF) and other ligands, such as transforming growth factor-alpha (TGF-α). Preclinical studies have shown that binding of cetuximab to the EGFR blocks phosphorylation and activation of downstream kinases resulting in inhibition of head and neck squamous cell carcinoma cell growth and induction of apoptosis; it also has radiosensitizing effects. As noted above, cetuximab can also mediate antibody-dependent cellular cytotoxicity (ADCC) and thereby contribute passive immunotherapy.[68]

In patients with locoregionally advanced disease, the addition of cetuximab to radiotherapy resulted in improved overall survival over radiotherapy alone.[74] In patients with incurable disease, cetuximab has demonstrated modest single agent activity[75] but potentiates the effect of platinum-based palliative chemotherapy leading to improved survival outcomes.[76] As a result of these trials, cetuximab is currently FDA approved for 3 indications for patients with HNSCC: (1) in combination with radiation therapy for locoregionally advanced disease; (2) in combination with platinum-based therapy with 5-FU in patients with incurable recurrent or metastatic disease; and (3) as a single agent in patients with disease progression after platinum-based therapy. It is also approved for incurable patients with KRAS wild-type colorectal cancer. Cetuximab, however, did not improve outcomes of HNSCC patients treated with concurrent cisplatin and radiotherapy[77] and should not be administered in this setting.

EGFR is expressed on tumor and normal cells, and the most common toxicity of cetuximab and other EGFR targeted therapies is a papulopustular skin rash, the development of which surprisingly has been associated with favorable clinical outcomes across several studies.[78] The association of cetuximab-induced skin toxicity and favorable cancer outcomes has led to suggestion of as yet undefined effects of the responding tumor on the immune system.[79,80]

HPV Vaccines

The clinically available HPV vaccines (Gardasil and Cervarix) have received FDA approval for prevention of cervical carcinoma and may possibly have preventive effects in other HPV-associated malignancies including head and neck cancers. Both vaccines target the HPV L1 major capsid protein, which can self-assemble into virus-like particles for each HPV type. Gardasil is a quadrivalent HPV6/11/16/18 L1 virus-like particle vaccine. Cervarix is an HPV16/18 L1 virus-like particle vaccine, which unlike Gardasil does not target HPV 6 and 11. The clinical trials of these agents demonstrated high immunogenicity rates in unexposed persons, but no evidence that vaccination altered the course of disease or infection in women with known HPV infection at the time of vaccination; therefore, these vaccines should not be used as a therapeutic intervention to treat preexisting HPV infection and related neoplasia.

There are, however, several therapeutic HPV vaccine strategies in clinical development using viral vectors, peptides, proteins, and plasmid DNA, with a goal to generate an effective immune response against an existing cancer. In the case of cervical cancer, lack of functional HPV-specific T-cell immunity is often associated with HPV persistence and is a contributing factor for carcinogenesis[81]; these therapeutic vaccines target T-cell immune stimulation. Recently, an HPV E6/E7 DNA vaccine successfully targeted HPV antigens to dendritic cells, eliciting significant HPV-specific CD8 T-cell response in patients with cervical intraepithelial neoplasia and was associated with high rates of complete regression of lesions and viral clearance.[82]

Immune Stimulatory Cytokines

Cytokines stimulate a broad-based immune response rather than generate a highly focused response to a specific antigen. Historically, this approach has centered on the use of high-dose IL-2 to stimulate T-cell proliferation in patients with malignant melanoma and renal cell carcinoma, 4% to 6% of whom experience durable complete response to treatment.[83,84] This approach unfortunately has been limited by uncommon responses, life-threatening treatment-associated toxicities and lack of ability to select appropriate patients.

Immunomodulatory cytokines have been employed in clinical trials for HNSCC in an attempt to restore immune homeostasis and induce an immune-mediated tumor response. One of the more recently studied approaches is the IRX-2 regimen (IRX Therapeutics, New York, New York), containing physiological quantities of T-helper type I (Th1) cytokines

(IL-2, IL-1β, γ-interferon, and TNF-α) combined with low-dose immunomodulatory cyclophosphamide, indomethacin, and zinc. This regimen was evaluated in a small trial in HNSCC patients and was found to be tolerable as a 21-day neoadjuvant treatment prior to surgical resection; moreover, 11 of 23 evaluable patients had evidence of minor tumor regression following the neoadjuvant therapy.[85] Additional studies suggested increased lymphocyte infiltration in tumors of patients treated with IRX-2[86] without change in TRegs.[87]

Immune Checkpoint Inhibitors

The CTLA-4 and PD-1 receptor-ligand pathways are negative regulators of T-cell activation that can be used by tumors to avoid immune surveillance, and immune checkpoint inhibitors are a new class of immune stimulatory anticancer agents demonstrating a broad range of anticancer activity in early phase trials. Agents with current FDA approval in patients with malignant melanoma include ipilimumab (Yervoy, recombinant human IgG1κ anti-CTLA-4 monoclonal antibody) and pembrolizumab (Keytruda, MK-3475, humanized IgG4κ anti-PD-1 monoclonal antibody), and several other agents with similar targets are in clinical development.

Initial results from the first phase II trial of pembrolizumab in patients with PD-L1-expressing recurrent/metastatic HPV-associated and non-HPV–associated HNSCC were recently reported.[88] The majority of screened patients (77.9%) were PD-L1 positive, defined as ≥1% of stained cells in the tumor microenvironment. Of 60 patients enrolled in the study and treated with pembrolizumab intravenously at 10 mg/kg every 2 weeks, 23 were HPV positive and 37 were HPV negative. Treatment was well tolerated, with fatigue, pruritus, and nausea as the most common drug-related adverse events. Of 51 evaluable patients, 26 (51%) had some measure of decreased tumor burden, and nearly 20% of patients had evidence of objective response (by RECIST 1.1); one HPV-positive patient had a complete response to therapy. Of note, the response rates were irrespective of HPV status, and responses appeared durable. Interestingly, HPV-positive patients had a markedly higher median progression-free survival (17.2 months, 95% CI: 8 to 41.7) as compared to HPV-negative patients (8.1 months, 95% CI: 7.9 to 15.6).[89] Several phase II and phase III trials of this agent and other agents targeting the immune checkpoint pathways in HNSCC are currently underway or are in planning.

> Cetuximab (Erbitux) targets EGFR in HNSCC, but the ability of the antibody to generate an immune response to tumor cells also contributes to the clinical efficacy of the drug. Vaccination efforts using HPV vaccines (Gardasil and Cervarix) aim to ultimately decrease the incidence of HPV-associated oropharyngeal squamous cell carcinoma. The role of immunomodulatory cytokines has been established for malignant melanoma and is under investigation for HNSCC. Immune checkpoint inhibitors, specifically antibodies targeting CTLA-4 and PD-1/PD-L1, are a promising class of drugs. Ipilimumab (anti-CTLA-4) and Pembrolizumab (anti–PD-1) have been approved for malignant melanoma, and these and other checkpoint inhibitors are actively being studied in HNSCC.

Immunotherapy-Specific Treatment Considerations

The advent of immunomodulatory therapies for cancer, particularly active immunotherapy approaches targeting immune checkpoint pathways, will require some new considerations in treatment, including toxicity management and evaluations of treatment outcomes.

Management of Toxicities

Augmenting the immune system may result in toxicities that differ considerably from more standard cytotoxic chemotherapy. Known toxicities of anti-CTLA4 and anti-PD-1 antibodies include severe inflammatory reactions of any organ system, including immune-mediated enterocolitis, pneumonitis, hepatitis, dermatitis, neuropathies, endocrinopathies, and ocular manifestations. When present, corticosteroid administration is recommended based on the severity of the reaction. Balancing optimal outcomes with patient safety will continue to be a treatment challenge.

Evaluation of Treatment Response and Optimization of Treatment Outcomes

Patients respond differently to immunotherapy than traditional cancer treatments. As opposed to traditional chemotherapies, immunotherapy can produce a delayed but durable response, suggesting that treatment effects may not be observed immediately. Immunotherapy may result in immune cell infiltration of the tumor, suggesting the potential clinical value of treatment beyond traditional (tumor size–based) evidence of disease progression. Immunotherapy may also result in immunologic memory and then boost anticancer immune function long after the treatment has been completed. Though most clinical trials currently focus on efficacy for patients with large volume disease, the optimal utility of immunotherapy for solid tumors, such as HNSCC, may be for the treatment of early-stage cancers, though this remains speculative. Immune-boosting therapy is also postulated to be most effective for patients with normal functioning immune systems, and effects in immunocompromised persons may be limited. Finally, combinations of immunotherapy with other standard treatment modalities (chemotherapy or radiotherapy) or combinations of immunotherapy approaches (eg, anti-PD-1 plus anti-CTLA-4 monoclonal antibodies) may be synergistic, though these strategies require careful preclinical assessment prior to launching clinical investigations due to the potentially dangerous untoward effects.

> Known toxicities of immune checkpoint inhibitors include severe inflammatory reactions of any organ system. Traditional measures of treatment response and outcome may not be adequate to assess a patient's response to new methods of immunotherapy. Responses can be delayed or perhaps more durable as a tumor immune response is established.

SUMMARY

After decades of research in tumor immunology, it seems that now a new horizon of broadly utilizable immunotherapy approaches for cancer patients is being realized. In addition to standard treatment modalities of surgery, radiation therapy, and chemotherapy, early clinical experience with the immune checkpoint inhibitors suggest that immunotherapy may truly represent the 4th treatment modality in the management of head and neck malignancies. Although the immune checkpoint inhibitors were expected to have their best effect in viral-associated cancers, where defects in immune surveillance resulted in persistent infection of oncogenic viruses, early studies have suggested broad range of clinical activity in solid tumors, including both HPV-associated and non-HPV–associated HNSCC. Optimizing this newly identified approach in the current context of cancer care will require many years of dedicated clinical research, and patient participation in these paradigm-changing studies should be strongly encouraged. A better understanding of the interactions between the human immune system and malignancy has led to an exciting and promising era in cancer medicine.

Acknowledgments. This work was funded by the Clinical Core of the Center for AIDS Research at the Albert Einstein College of Medicine and Montefiore Medical Center (NIH AI-51519) and the AIDS Malignancy Consortium grant (U01CA121947).

REFERENCES

1. Hanahan D, Weinberg RA. Hallmarks of cancer: the next generation. *Cell.* Mar 4 2011;144(5):646–674.
2. Cobucci RN, Lima PH, de Souza PC, et al. Assessing the impact of HAART on the incidence of defining and non-defining AIDS cancers among patients with HIV/AIDS: A systematic review. *J Infect Public Health.* 2014;8(1):1–10.
3. Mitsuyasu RT. Non–AIDS-defining malignancies in HIV. *Top HIV Med* Oct–Nov 2008;16(4):117–121.
4. Engels EA, Pfeiffer RM, Fraumeni JF, Jr, et al. Spectrum of cancer risk among US solid organ transplant recipients. *JAMA.* Nov 2 2011;306(17):1891–1901.
5. Wheless L, Jacks S, Mooneyham Potter KA, Leach BC, Cook J. Skin cancer in organ transplant recipients: more than the immune system. *J Am Acad Dermatol.* Aug 2014; 71(2):359–365.
6. Gooden MJ, de Bock GH, Leffers N, Daemen T, Nijman HW. The prognostic influence of tumour-infiltrating lymphocytes in cancer: a systematic review with meta-analysis. *Br J Cancer.* Jun 28 2011;105(1):93–103.
7. Yasunaga M, Tabira Y, Nakano K, et al. Accelerated growth signals and low tumor-infiltrating lymphocyte levels

predict poor outcome in T4 esophageal squamous cell carcinoma. *Ann Thoracic Surg.* Nov 2000;70(5):1634–1640.
8. Reichert TE, Day R, Wagner EM, Whiteside TL. Absent or low expression of the zeta chain in T cells at the tumor site correlates with poor survival in patients with oral carcinoma. *Cancer Res.* Dec 1 1998;58(23):5344–5347.
9. Haanen JB, Baars A, Gomez R, et al. Melanoma-specific tumor-infiltrating lymphocytes but not circulating melanoma-specific T cells may predict survival in resected advanced-stage melanoma patients. *Cancer Immunol Immunother.* Apr 2006;55(4):451–458.
10. Naito Y, Saito K, Shiiba K, et al. CD8+ T cells infiltrated within cancer cell nests as a prognostic factor in human colorectal cancer. *Cancer Res.* Aug 15 1998;58(16):3491–3494.
11. Ishigami S, Natsugoe S, Tokuda K, et al. Prognostic value of intratumoral natural killer cells in gastric carcinoma. *Cancer.* Feb 1 2000;88(3):577–583.
12. Ishigami S, Natsugoe S, Tokuda K, et al. Clinical impact of intratumoral natural killer cell and dendritic cell infiltration in gastric cancer. *Cancer Lett.* Oct 16 2000;159(1):103–108.
13. Kondo E, Koda K, Takiguchi N, et al. Preoperative natural killer cell activity as a prognostic factor for distant metastasis following surgery for colon cancer. *Dig Surg.* 2003;20(5):445–451.
14. Villegas FR, Coca S, Villarrubia VG, et al. Prognostic significance of tumor infiltrating natural killer cells subset CD57 in patients with squamous cell lung cancer. *Lung Cancer.* Jan 2002;35(1):23–28.
15. Kim R, Emi M, Tanabe K. Cancer immunoediting from immune surveillance to immune escape. *Immunology.* May 2007;121(1):1–14.
16. Dranoff G. Experimental mouse tumour models: what can be learnt about human cancer immunology? *Nat Rev Immunol.* Jan 2012;12(1):61–66.
17. Dunn GP, Bruce AT, Ikeda H, Old LJ, Schreiber RD. Cancer immunoediting: from immunosurveillance to tumor escape. *Nat Immunol.* Nov 2002;3(11):991–998.
18. DuPage M, Jacks T. Genetically engineered mouse models of cancer reveal new insights about the antitumor immune response. *Curr Opin Immunol.* Apr 2013;25(2):192–199.
19. Bhatia A, Kumar Y. Cellular and molecular mechanisms in cancer immune escape: a comprehensive review. *Expert Rev Clin Immunol.* Jan 2014;10(1):41–62.
20. DuPage M, Mazumdar C, Schmidt LM, Cheung AF, Jacks T. Expression of tumour-specific antigens underlies cancer immunoediting. *Nature.* Feb 16 2012;482(7385):405–409.
21. Lowe DB, Storkus WJ. Chronic inflammation and immunologic-based constraints in malignant disease. *Immunotherapy.* Oct 2011;3(10):1265–1274.
22. Schafer M, Werner S. Cancer as an overhealing wound: an old hypothesis revisited. *Nat Rev Mol Cell Biol.* Aug 2008;9(8):628–638.
23. Dvorak HF. Tumors: wounds that do not heal. Similarities between tumor stroma generation and wound healing. *N Engl J Med.* Dec 25 1986;315(26):1650–1659.
24. Coussens LM, Werb Z. Inflammation and cancer. *Nature.* Dec 19–26 2002;420(6917):860–867.
25. Dolberg DS, Hollingsworth R, Hertle M, Bissell MJ. Wounding and its role in RSV-mediated tumor formation. *Science.* Nov 8 1985;230(4726):676–678.
26. Martins-Green M, Boudreau N, Bissell MJ. Inflammation is responsible for the development of wound-induced tumors in chickens infected with Rous sarcoma virus. *Cancer Res.* Aug 15 1994;54(16):4334–4341.
27. Schuh AC, Keating SJ, Monteclaro FS, Vogt PK, Breitman ML. Obligatory wounding requirement for tumorigenesis in v-jun transgenic mice. *Nature.* Aug 23 1990;346(6286):756–760.
28. Grivennikov SI, Greten FR, Karin M. Immunity, inflammation, and cancer. *Cell.* Mar 19 2010;140(6):883–899.
29. Qian BZ, Pollard JW. Macrophage diversity enhances tumor progression and metastasis. *Cell.* Apr 2 2010;141(1):39–51.
30. Head and Neck Cancers, Version 2.2014. National Comprehensive Cancer Network.
31. Wang WY, Twu CW, Chen HH, et al. Long-term survival analysis of nasopharyngeal carcinoma by plasma Epstein-Barr virus DNA levels. *Cancer.* Mar 1 2013;119(5):963–970.
32. Koba S, Paulson KG, Nagase K, et al. Diagnostic biopsy does not commonly induce intratumoral CD8 T cell infiltration in Merkel cell carcinoma. *PloS One.* 2012;7(7):e41465.
33. Gillison ML, Koch WM, Capone RB, et al. Evidence for a causal association between human papillomavirus and a subset of head and neck cancers. *J Natl Cancer Inst.* May 3 2000;92(9):709–720.
34. Chaturvedi AK, Engels EA, Anderson WF, Gillison ML. Incidence trends for human papillomavirus-related and -unrelated oral squamous cell carcinomas in the United States. *J Clin Oncol.* Feb 1 2008;26(4):612–619.
35. Chaturvedi AK, Engels EA, Pfeiffer RM, et al. Human papillomavirus and rising oropharyngeal cancer incidence in the United States. *J Clin Oncol.* Nov 10 2011;29(32):4294–4301.
36. D'Souza G, Kreimer AR, Viscidi R, et al. Case-control study of human papillomavirus and oropharyngeal cancer. *N Engl J Med.* May 10 2007;356(19):1944–1956.
37. Westra WH, Taube JM, Poeta ML, Begum S, Sidransky D, Koch WM. Inverse relationship between human papillomavirus-16 infection and disruptive p53 gene mutations in squamous cell carcinoma of the head and neck. *Clin Cancer Res.* Jan 15 2008;14(2):366–369.
38. Fakhry C, Westra WH, Li S, et al. Improved survival of patients with human papillomavirus-positive head and neck squamous cell carcinoma in a prospective clinical trial. *J Natl Cancer Inst.* Feb 20 2008;100(4):261–269.
39. Fakhry C, Zhang Q, Nguyen-Tan PF, et al. Human papillomavirus and overall survival after progression of oropharyngeal squamous cell carcinoma. *J Clin Oncol.* Oct 20 2014;32(30):3365–3373.
40. Ang KK, Harris J, Wheeler R, et al. Human papillomavirus and survival of patients with oropharyngeal cancer. *N Engl J Med.* Jul 1 2010;363(1):24–35.

41. Gillison ML, Broutian T, Pickard RK, et al. Prevalence of oral HPV infection in the United States, 2009–2010. *JAMA.* Feb 15 2012;307(7):693–703.
42. Beachler DC, Abraham AG, Silverberg MJ, et al. Incidence and risk factors of HPV-related and HPV-unrelated head and neck squamous cell carcinoma in HIV-infected individuals. *Oral Oncol.* Dec 2014;50(12):1169–1176.
43. D'Souza G, Carey TE, William WN, Jr, et al. Epidemiology of head and neck squamous cell cancer among HIV-infected patients. *J Acquir Immune Defic Syndr.* Apr 15 2014;65(5):603–610.
44. McLemore MS, Haigentz M, Jr, Smith RV, et al. Head and neck squamous cell carcinomas in HIV-positive patients: a preliminary investigation of viral associations. *Head Neck Pathol.* Jun 2010;4(2):97–105.
45. Shiels MS, Pfeiffer RM, Gail MH, et al. Cancer burden in the HIV-infected population in the United States. *J Natl Cancer Inst.* May 4 2011;103(9):753–762.
46. Schuster M, Nechansky A, Kircheis R. Cancer immunotherapy. *Biotechnol J.* Feb 2006;1(2):138–147.
47. Reichert JM, Valge-Archer VE. Development trends for monoclonal antibody cancer therapeutics. *Nat Rev Drug Discov.* May 2007;6(5):349–356.
48. Patyar S, Joshi R, Byrav DS, Prakash A, Medhi B, Das BK. Bacteria in cancer therapy: a novel experimental strategy. *J Biomed Sci.* 2010;17(1):21.
49. West WH, Tauer KW, Yannelli JR, et al. Constant-infusion recombinant interleukin-2 in adoptive immunotherapy of advanced cancer. *N Engl J Med.* Apr 9 1987; 316(15):898–905.
50. Ilson DH, Motzer RJ, Kradin RL, et al. A phase II trial of interleukin-2 and interferon alfa-2a in patients with advanced renal cell carcinoma. *J Clin Oncol.* Jul 1992; 10(7):1124–1130.
51. Lamm DL, Blumenstein BA, Crawford ED, et al. A randomized trial of intravesical doxorubicin and immunotherapy with bacille Calmette-Guerin for transitional-cell carcinoma of the bladder. *N Engl J Med.* Oct 24 1991;325(17):1205–1209.
52. Lu T, Seto WK, Zhu RX, Lai CL, Yuen MF. Prevention of hepatocellular carcinoma in chronic viral hepatitis B and C infection. *World J Gastroenterol.* Dec 21 2013;19(47): 8887–8894.
53. Bosch FX, Broker TR, Forman D, et al. Comprehensive control of human papillomavirus infections and related diseases. *Vaccine.* Dec 31 2013;31(suppl 7):H1–31.
54. Melero I, Gaudernack G, Gerritsen W, et al. Therapeutic vaccines for cancer: an overview of clinical trials. *Nat Rev Clin Oncol.* Sep 2014;11(9):509–524.
55. Tsoukas CD, Landgraf B, Bentin J, et al. Activation of resting T lymphocytes by anti-CD3 (T3) antibodies in the absence of monocytes. *J Immunol.* Sep 1985;135(3): 1719–1723.
56. Barrett DM, Singh N, Porter DL, Grupp SA, June CH. Chimeric antigen receptor therapy for cancer. *Ann Rev Med.* 2014;65:333–347.
57. Weber J, Atkins M, Hwu P, et al. White paper on adoptive cell therapy for cancer with tumor-infiltrating lymphocytes: a report of the CTEP subcommittee on adoptive cell therapy. *Clin Cancer Res.* Apr 1 2011;17(7):1664–1673.
58. Rosenberg SA, Yang JC, Sherry RM, et al. Durable complete responses in heavily pretreated patients with metastatic melanoma using T-cell transfer immunotherapy. *Clin Cancer Res.* Jul 1 2011;17(13):4550–4557.
59. Maude SL, Frey N, Shaw PA, et al. Chimeric antigen receptor T cells for sustained remissions in leukemia. *N Engl J Med.* Oct 16 2014;371(16):1507–1517.
60. Palucka K, Banchereau J. Cancer immunotherapy via dendritic cells. *Nat Rev.* Apr 2012;12(4):265–277.
61. Kantoff PW, Higano CS, Shore ND, et al. Sipuleucel-T immunotherapy for castration-resistant prostate cancer. *N Engl J Med.* Jul 29 2010;363(5):411–422.
62. Kohler G, Milstein C. Continuous cultures of fused cells secreting antibody of predefined specificity. *Nature.* Aug 7 1975;256(5517):495–497.
63. Presta LG. Engineering of therapeutic antibodies to minimize immunogenicity and optimize function. *Adv Drug Deliv Rev.* Aug 7 2006;58(5–6):640–656.
64. Kovtun YV, Goldmacher VS. Cell killing by antibody-drug conjugates. *Cancer Lett.* Oct 8 2007;255(2):232–240.
65. Francisco JA, Cerveny CG, Meyer DL, et al. cAC10-vcMMAE, an anti-CD30-monomethyl auristatin E conjugate with potent and selective antitumor activity. *Blood.* Aug 15 2003;102(4):1458–1465.
66. Ellis LM. Mechanisms of action of bevacizumab as a component of therapy for metastatic colorectal cancer. *Semin Oncol.* Oct 2006;33(5, suppl 10):S1–7.
67. Graham J, Muhsin M, Kirkpatrick P. Cetuximab. *Nat Rev Drug Discov.* Jul 2004;3(7):549–550.
68. Bleeker WK, Lammerts van Bueren JJ, van Ojik HH, et al. Dual mode of action of a human anti-epidermal growth factor receptor monoclonal antibody for cancer therapy. *J Immunol.* Oct 1 2004;173(7):4699–4707.
69. Pardoll DM. The blockade of immune checkpoints in cancer immunotherapy. *Nat Rev Cancer.* Apr 2012;12(4):252–264.
70. Schaer DA, Hirschhorn-Cymerman D, Wolchok JD. Targeting tumor-necrosis factor receptor pathways for tumor immunotherapy. *J Immunother Cancer.* 2014;2:7.
71. Hodi FS, O'Day SJ, McDermott DF, et al. Improved survival with ipilimumab in patients with metastatic melanoma. *N Engl J Med.* Aug 19 2010;363(8):711–723.
72. Robert C, Thomas L, Bondarenko I, et al. Ipilimumab plus dacarbazine for previously untreated metastatic melanoma. *N Engl J Med.* Jun 30 2011;364(26):2517–2526.
73. Hamid O, Robert C, Daud A, et al. Safety and tumor responses with lambrolizumab (anti-PD-1) in melanoma. *N Engl J Med.* Jul 11 2013;369(2):134–144.
74. Bonner JA, Harari PM, Giralt J, et al. Radiotherapy plus cetuximab for squamous-cell carcinoma of the head and neck. *N Engl J Med.* Feb 9 2006;354(6):567–578.
75. Vermorken JB, Trigo J, Hitt R, et al. Open-label, uncontrolled, multicenter phase II study to evaluate the efficacy and toxicity of cetuximab as a single agent in patients with recurrent and/or metastatic squamous cell carcinoma of the head and neck who failed to respond to platinum-based therapy. *J Clin Oncol.* Jun 1 2007;25(16):2171–2177.

76. Vermorken JB, Mesia R, Rivera F, et al. Platinum-based chemotherapy plus cetuximab in head and neck cancer. *N Engl J Med.* Sep 11 2008;359(11):1116–1127.
77. Ang KK, Zhang Q, Rosenthal DI, et al. Randomized phase III trial of concurrent accelerated radiation plus cisplatin with or without cetuximab for stage III to IV head and neck carcinoma: RTOG 0522. *J Clin Oncol.* 2014 Sep 20;32(27):2940–2950.6.
78. Bonner JA, Harari PM, Giralt J, et al. Radiotherapy plus cetuximab for locoregionally advanced head and neck cancer: 5-year survival data from a phase 3 randomised trial, and relation between cetuximab-induced rash and survival. *Lancet Oncol.* Jan 2010;11(1):21–28.
79. Perez-Soler R, Saltz L. Cutaneous adverse effects with HER1/EGFR-targeted agents: is there a silver lining? *J Clin Oncol.* Aug 1 2005;23(22):5235–5246.
80. Abdullah SE, Haigentz M, Jr, Piperdi B. Dermatologic toxicities from monoclonal antibodies and tyrosine kinase ihibitors against EGFR: pathophysiology and management. *Chemother Res Pract.* 2012;2012:351210.
81. de Vos van Steenwijk PJ, Piersma SJ, Welters MJ, et al. Surgery followed by persistence of high-grade squamous intraepithelial lesions is associated with the induction of a dysfunctional HPV16-specific T-cell response. *Clin Cancer Res.* Nov 15 2008;14(22):7188–7195.
82. Kim TJ, Jin HT, Hur SY, et al. Clearance of persistent HPV infection and cervical lesion by therapeutic DNA vaccine in CIN3 patients. *Nat Commun.* 2014;5:5317.
83. Negrier S, Escudier B, Lasset C, et al. Recombinant human interleukin-2, recombinant human interferon alfa-2a, or both in metastatic renal-cell carcinoma. Groupe Francais d'Immunotherapie. *N Engl J Med.* Apr 30 1998;338(18):1272–1278.
84. Schwartzentruber DJ, Lawson DH, Richards JM, et al. gp100 peptide vaccine and interleukin-2 in patients with advanced melanoma. *N Engl J Med.* Jun 2 2011;364(22): 2119–2127.
85. Wolf GT, Fee WE, Jr, Dolan RW, et al. Novel neoadjuvant immunotherapy regimen safety and survival in head and neck squamous cell cancer. *Head Neck.* Dec 2011;33(12): 1666–1674.
86. Berinstein NL, Wolf GT, Naylor PH, et al. Increased lymphocyte infiltration in patients with head and neck cancer treated with the IRX-2 immunotherapy regimen. *Cancer Immunol Immunother.* Jun 2012;61(6):771–782.
87. Whiteside TL, Butterfield LH, Naylor PH, et al. A short course of neoadjuvant IRX-2 induces changes in peripheral blood lymphocyte subsets of patients with head and neck squamous cell carcinoma. *Cancer Immunol Immunother.* Jun 2012;61(6):783–788.
88. Seiwert TY BB, Weiss J, Gluck I, et al. A phase Ib study of MK-3475 in patients with human papillomavirus (HPV)-associated and non-HPV–associated head and neck (H/N) cancer. *J Clin Oncol.* 2014 32(5s).
89. Chow LQ BB, Weiss J, Berger R, et al. *A phase Ib study of pembrolizumab (Pembro; MK-3475) in patients (Pts) with human papiilloma virus (HPV)-positive and negative head and neck cancer (HNC).* 2014 ESMO meeting; Bilbao, Spain; LBA31.

15

Primary Immunodeficiency

Tatyana Gavrilova and Arye Rubinstein

INTRODUCTION

Primary immunodeficiency (PID) refers to conditions involving nonacquired disorders of the immune system. These disorders can be based on cellular, humoral, or combined immune defects. Forty percent of primary immunodeficiencies are not diagnosed until adulthood. Patients often experience multiple bouts of infections, particularly sinusitis, otitis media, bronchitis, and pneumonia before the diagnosis is finally made. Otolaryngologists are therefore important sentinels in the diagnosis of PID. For instance, antibody deficiencies can be a cause of chronic rhinosinusitis and a frequent reason for referral to otolaryngologists. Otitis media and respiratory tract infections are the most common infections at the time of common variable immunodeficiency (CVID) diagnosis.[1] Although primary immunodeficiencies may present with clinical symptoms at a very early age, it is not uncommon for them to be diagnosed only later in life after repeated bouts of frequent infections resulting in unfortunate sequelae that could have been prevented with early diagnosis and intervention. Seventy percent of patients report being hospitalized prior to diagnosis, with significantly less hospitalizations after appropriate diagnosis and initiation of treatment.[2] Early diagnosis of immunodeficiency can therefore prevent clinical complications, prevent morbidity, and improve a patient's overall quality of life. Otolaryngologists may not only be in the forefront of referrals to immunologists, but early diagnosis may require surgical and nonsurgical ear, nose, and throat (ENT) interventions.

> Early diagnosis of PID is crucial, and otolaryngologists play a key role in this process.

WARNING SIGNS OF IMMUNODEFICIENCY

A constellation of symptoms is often required in order to establish a diagnosis of a primary immunodeficiency. These symptoms will depend on the type of immune defect present; therefore, an understanding of the different aspects of immunity becomes important. Family history can be helpful in establishing a pattern for some PIDs. Additionally, physical exam findings can be suggestive of PID. These include absent or small tonsillar tissue, scarring of the tympanic membranes suggestive of frequent or chronic otitis media, as well as abnormal breath sounds possibly signifying chronic pulmonary infections, such as bronchiectasis.[1] Special mention needs to be made of the importance of tonsillar tissue, which are central organs of immunity in the upper airway and oropharyngeal cavity. Often patients with recurrent upper respiratory tract infections are referred to otolaryngologists for evaluation and possible tonsillectomy. Otolaryngologists can initiate an evaluation of possible underlying disease, including immunodeficiency, prior to proceeding with a tonsillectomy in patients with recurring respiratory tract infections.

A compilation of early warning signs of immunodeficiencies in children has been adopted in order to aid physicians in early diagnosis of immunodeficiency (Table 15–1) [3] Additionally, there are other clinical manifestations of disease that should raise the suspicion of the otolaryngologist (Table 15–2).[4] Clinical suspicion for PID should then prompt a referral to an immunologist and further immune evaluation. Understanding of the underlying mechanisms of PID becomes important for the otolaryngologist who can play a vital role in the initial recognition and diagnosis of PID.

Table 15–1. Early Warning Signs of Immunodeficiencies in Children

1. Four or more ear infections within 1 year
2. Two or more serious sinus infections within 1 year
3. Two or more pneumonias within 1 year
4. Two or more months of antibiotics with little effect
5. Recurrent, deep skin or organ abscesses
6. Persistent oral thrush or cutaneous fungal infections
7. Requiring intravenous antibiotics to clear an infection
8. Two or more deep-seated infections including septicemia
9. Failure of an infant to gain weight or grow normally
10. Family history of primary immunodeficiencies

Table 15–2. Otolaryngologic Manifestations of Immunodeficiencies

1. Oral candidiasis
2. Chronic gingivitis
3. Periodontitis
4. Aphthous stomatitis, aphthous ulcers
5. Mucosal lichen planus
6. Chronic oral herpetic infections
7. Dry mouth, poor salivation.
8. Split uvula, high-arched palate
9. Laryngeal papillomas
10. Chronic nasal polyps
11. Recurrent otitis media

INNATE IMMUNITY

Innate immunity is the body's first line of defense against invading pathogens but is not tailored to specific pathogens or conferring long-term memory for future infections. Although somewhat limited in its scope of action, it is vital to maintaining immune homeostasis as is evidenced by the varied pathology that ensues when a defect of innate immunity is present. In this section we discuss some of the more common defects in innate immunity (Table 15–3).

Defects of Phagocyte Function: Chronic Granulomatous Disease (CGD)

CGD results from a defect in the NADPH oxidase complex of phagocytic (neutrophils, monocytes, and macrophages) cells. The oxidase complex functions to create a respiratory burst necessary to eradicate invading pathogens. In the absence of a properly functioning oxidase system, individuals become vulnerable to bacterial and fungal microorganisms that are usually eliminated via this system. There are 5 gene mutations that can result in a defective NADPH oxidase system, with $gp91^{phox}$ being the only X-linked defect known to date and is associated with the most severe clinical outcomes.[5] Because it is an X-linked mutation, this condition primarily affects males. However, due to skewed X-inactivation, there have been reports of affected females with X-linked CGD. Female carriers are otherwise mosaics.[6] The identified autosomal mutations include $p47^{phox}$, $p67^{phox}$, $p22^{phox}$, and $p40^{phox}$.

Bacterial and fungal infections are prominent in CGD, ranging from skin and other organ abscesses to bacteremia and fungemia. *Staphylococcus aureus*, *Serratia marcescens*, *Nocardia*, and *Burkholderia cepacia* are among the most common offending bacteria seen in patients with CGD. *Candida* and *Aspergillus* can result in particularly invasive and deadly infections.

Table 15-3. Innate Immunodeficiencies

Disease	Hallmark Infectious Organisms
Chronic granulomatous disease (CGD)	*Staphylococcus aureus, Serratia marcescens, Nocardia, Burkholderia cepacia, Candida,* and *Aspergillus*
Chediak-Higashi syndrome (CHS)	*S. aureus* and beta-hemolytic streptococci
C3, Factors H and I deficiency	*Streptococcus pneumoniae, Haemophilus influenzae* type b, and *Neisseria meningitides*
C5 deficiency	Neisseria meningitides
Properdin, factor B, factor D	*Neisseria meningitides* and *Streptococcus pneumoniae*

Patients can present to the otolaryngologist with the complaint of gingivitis, aphthous ulcers, and cervical adenopathy. External ear and mastoid involvement can be rapidly progressive. Superficial and deep-seated abscesses with granuloma formation are one of the clinical hallmarks of this disease. Surgical incision and drainage may become necessary. Culturing these pathogens from a sinus irrigation or cervical adenitis is suggestive of CGD.[1] The current screening test for CGD is the flow cytometric dihydrorhodamine 123 (DHR) assay that measures the neutrophil respiratory burst, a function that is impaired in CGD.[7] Antibacterial (trimethoprim/sulfamethoxazole) and antifungal (itraconazole) prophylaxis have reduced the frequency of infections in CGD.[5] Immunomodulatory therapy with interferon gamma is part of the prophylactic regimen in many centers.[8] Currently the only known cure for CGD is allogeneic hematopoietic cell transplantation, with outcomes strongly associated with the degree of the HLA match.[5]

Staphylococcus aureus, Serratia marcescens, Nocardia, Burkholderia cepacia, Candida, and *Aspergillus* are the more common infectious species identified in CGD patients.

Chediak-Higashi Syndrome (CHS)

CHS is a rare, autosomal recessive disease that presents with severe immunodeficiency often predisposing to recurrent bacterial infections, bleeding diathesis, varying degrees of albinism, and progressive neurologic dysfunction.[9] The degree of oculocutaneous albinism varies, but patients typically have gray or light blonde/white hair (Figure 15–1).[10] The disease is caused by a mutation in the *LYST* gene, which results in defective fusion of intracellular vesicles, impairing neutrophil chemotaxis and degranulation. Severe disease can also result in pancytopenia. Periodontitis and recurrent infections, particularly with *S aureus* and beta-hemolytic streptococci have been described.[4]

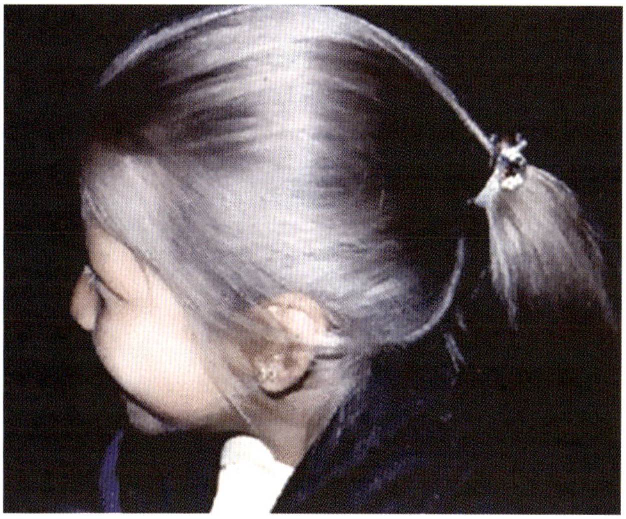

Figure 15-1. Chediak-Higashi syndrome illustrating characteristic hair hypopigmentation.[10] Reprinted with permission from Springer Science and Business Media.

Recurrent bacterial infections, albinism, and progressive neurologic dysfunction are part of the common triad identified with Chediak-Higashi syndrome.

Complement Deficiencies

The complement system is a group of proteins that results in pathogen cell lysis and phagocytosis through opsonization. These proteins are tightly regulated and require activation for proper function. A dysregulation of this system can result in immunodeficiency, as well as autoimmunity[11] (Table 15–4).

The complement system has 3 primary pathways known as the classical, alternative, and mannose-binding lectin (MBL) pathway. Defects in these pathways are known to predispose to infections, autoimmunity, and angioedema. Although some complement deficiencies, such as C1q, mostly predispose to autoimmunity such as systemic lupus erythematosis,[12] others are responsible for severe infectious complications.

C3 activation is the common denominator of the 3 complement pathways. C3 is critical for bacterial opsonization, and C3 deficiency can result in severe, life-threatening infections with encapsulated organisms such as *Streptococcus pneumoniae, Haemophilus influenzae* type b, and *Neisseria meningitides*. Otolaryngologists need to be vigilant of this as recurrent sinus, ear, and pharyngeal infections/abscesses with these organs should prompt a consideration for complement deficiency evaluation. Factors H and I prevent C3 depletion, and absence of these regulatory proteins can also result in C3 deficiency.[13] Deficiency of C2, a classical pathway protein, can result in recurrent pyogenic infections with encapsulated bacteria.[14] Absence of the terminal complement proteins (C5-C9) predisposes individuals to meningeal infections with *Neisseriae*.[15] Alternative pathway deficiencies involving properdin, factor B, and factor D have been implicated in neisserial, meningococcal, and pneumococcal infections. MBL defects have also been associated with a predisposition to encapsulated bacterial infections.[16–18]

Serious or frequent infections with encapsulated bacteria should raise the suspicion of an underlying complement deficiency. The CH50 assay is a useful tool for screening for classical complement activation. Heterozygous protein deficiencies can result in reduced and not completely absent CH50 values. C2, C3, and C4 can be measured individually as well.[11] AH50 is an assay that can be used to screen for alternative pathway deficiency. Complement replacement therapy is not recommended. Vigilance for signs of infection, routine health maintenance, and vaccinations are advised.[19]

Hereditary angioedema (HAE) is a condition that occurs due to C1 esterase inhibitor (C1-inh) deficiency, a protein responsible for inhibition of the complement system and maintenance of its homeostasis. C1-inh deficiency results in uncontrolled complement activation and bradykinin production. The abnormal swelling seen in this condition is due primarily to the effects of excessive bradykinin (reviewed in Chapter 7). Patients can present with oropharyngeal edema and even potentially fatal laryngeal edema that can result in asphyxiation. Patients also experience facial, limb, and abdominal edema. Diagnostic studies usually identify C1 esterase inhibitor decreased function and/or quantitative value in type I and II HAE. A rare subgroup, HAE type III is thought to be related to hormonal aberrancies. It has a predilection for occurring in women in their third decade of life.

Table 15–4. Bacterial Infections Associated With Complement Deficiencies

Complement Factor Deficiency	Disease
C1q	Systemic lupus erythematosus
C3, factor H and I	*Streptococcus pneumoniae, Haemophilus influenzae* type b, and *Neisseria meningitides*
C5-C9	*Streptococcus pneumoniae, Haemophilus influenzae* type b, and *Neisseria meningitides*
Properdin, factors B and D	*Neisseria meningitides* and *Streptococcus pneumoniae*
C1 esterase inhibitor	Hereditary angioedema

Although patients have clinical findings consistent with HAE, laboratory tests reveal normal C1 esterase inhibitor levels and function. Treatment of HAE I and II primarily consists of prophylactic and acute management with C1-esterase inhibitor concentrates (ie, Cinryze, Berinert), anti-kallikrein (ie, ecallantide or Kalbitor) or antibradykinin receptor preparations (ie, icatibant or Firazyr).[20] These agents can be used for treatment of acute HAE attacks. Patients who experience frequent HAE attacks can also receive prophylactic treatment. At this time, C1-esterase inhibitor concentrates are the first-line agents for prophylactic treatment. Steroid derivatives, such as danazol, are second-line agents for treatment of HAE but have significant adverse effects such as weight gain, virilization, and being contraindicated in pregnant women that limit its use.

> Recurrent episodes of facial or upper airway edema may be a hallmark of complement deficiency. Frequent bouts of otolaryngologic infections with encapsulated bacteria can also be a manifestation of this condition.

ADAPTIVE IMMUNITY

The adaptive immune system is required to develop an acquired response to antigen. Its mechanisms are mediated by the cellular and humoral pathways of the immune system. Humoral immunodeficiencies are marked by impaired immunoglobulin responses. These abnormalities can manifest as isolated antibody deficiencies, or in combination with impaired T-lymphocyte function. Patients with these conditions show a predisposition to encapsulated bacterial infections, especially sinopulmonary disease. Additionally, cellular deficiencies can manifest as frequent viral and fungal infections. In this section we address the more common humoral and combined immunodeficiencies that the otolaryngologist should be aware of in clinical practice (Table 15–5).

Common Variable Immunodeficiency (CVID)

CVID is defined as impaired production of IgG, IgM, or IgA antibody classes in the absence of other known primary immunodeficiency defects.[21] Multiple mutations have been identified in patients with CVID. The primary defect appears to be in the B-cell differentiation pathway. The B-cell development and survival are dependent on the survival signaling cytokines BAFF, and APRIL that act on the B-cell activating factor receptor (BAFF-R), tumor necrosis factor receptor superfamily member 13B receptor (TNFRSF13B) also known as transmembrane

Table 15–5. Adaptive Immunodeficiencies

Disease	Hallmark Infectious Organisms
CVID	Encapsulated organisms such as *Streptococcus pneumoniae*, *Haemophilus influenzae* type
SPAD	Same as above
IgA deficiency	Same as above with a predilection for mucosal sites
X-linked agammaglobulinemia (XLA)	*Streptococcus pneumoniae*, *Haemophilus influenzae* type, *Pseudomonas aeruginosa*, echovirus, coxsackie virus, adenovirus, and poliovirus
Hyper-IgM syndrome	*Streptococcus pneumoniae*, *Haemophilus influenzae* type b, and *Neisseria meningitides*
Severe combined immunodeficiency (SCID)	Recurrent viral (ie, HPV), fungal (ie, *Candida*) and encapsulated bacterial infections

activator and CAML interactor receptor (TACI-R), and B-cell maturation antigen receptor (BCMA-R). A mutation resulting in dysregulation of the cytokine-receptor interaction results in impaired B-cell development and the subsequent impaired immunoglobulin production seen in CVID patients.[22]

The clinical spectrum of CVID is very broad, with the usual time of symptom presentation and diagnosis occurring in the second to third decades of life. Patients present with increased infections such as sinusitis, otitis media, bronchitis, and pneumonia caused by encapsulated bacteria. Bronchiectasis is a frequent complication that is often identified prior to the establishment of the diagnosis of CVID. Patients also have a predisposition to autoimmune and lymphoproliferative conditions.

> CVID is most commonly diagnosed in adulthood and can present as frequent sinopulmonary infections. The diagnosis requires evidence of impaired production of IgG accompanied by low levels of IgM or IgA.

Immunoglobulin Replacement

Options for replacement immunoglobulin include intravenous immunoglobulin (IVIG) and subcutaneous immunoglobulin (SCIg). Immunoglobulin is prepared from the plasma of at least 1000 human donors. IVIG is typically administered once every 3 to 4 weeks, usually by a nurse at the patient's home or in an infusion center. Infusions typically take 3 to 4 hours. SCIg is usually patient self-administered on a weekly basis. SCIg is thought to more closely mirror physiologic immunoglobulin peaks and troughs. Its other benefit is its ease of administration, typically into abdominal fat pads, obviating the need for intravenous access. Additionally, there are less systemic side effects associated with this mode of administration. IVIG, however, is dosed less frequently and allows for higher immunoglobulin peak levels, which is sometimes also more helpful in the treatment of the autoimmune complications associated with CVID. However, this route obviously requires venous access, less mobility during infusion and the possibility of more systemic effects such as headache, myalgias, and arthralgias. These side effects can be minimized with the preinfusion administration of antihistamines and systemic corticosteroids. There are multiple commercial sources of IVIG that vary in methods of preparation, immunoglobulin concentrations and levels of IgA. Low IgA preparations are sometimes used in patients with selective IgA deficiency in order to reduce the occurrence of anaphylaxis from the reaction between the patient's own anti-IgA IgG or IgE and IgA in the IVIG preparation.

Specific Polysaccharide Antibody Deficiency (SPAD)

SPAD is marked by an absence or limited response to polysaccharide antigens. Patients with SPAD have normal responses to protein antigens, normal serum levels of immunoglobulins, and normal IgG subclass concentrations. Although the pathophysiologic mechanisms underlying SPAD are not clear, the clinical presentation is similar to other antibody-deficient states. Patients have a predisposition to bacterial sinopulmonary infections and exhibit impaired responses to polysaccharide vaccines, such as pneumococcal or meningococcal.[23] Otolaryngologists should be vigilant and aware of this condition in patients who present with recurrent otitis media and sinus infections with pneumococcus and Hib, despite appropriate vaccination. Patients also need to be closely monitored since SPAD can transition to CVID.

> Patients with SPAD have normal immunoglobulin levels but show impaired responses to specific antigens. This can be clinically demonstrated as a poor response to pneumococcal vaccines.

IgA Deficiency

Selective IgA deficiency is defined as an isolated deficiency in serum IgA in the presence of otherwise normal cellular and humoral immune function. The prevalence is approximately 1:600 with marked ethnic variability.[23] Since the primary function of IgA is in mucosal immunity, patients with IgA deficiency are significantly more predisposed to developing upper and lower respiratory tract infections, having recurrent bouts of sinusitis, otitis media, and bacterial pneumonia. Treatment is limited to monitoring for infections, prompt initiation of appropriate antibiotics and supportive care. There is currently no available IgA replacement therapy for use in standard clinical practice.[24]

Selective IgA deficiency is the most common primary immunodeficiency that predisposes patients to recurrent sinopulmonary infections.

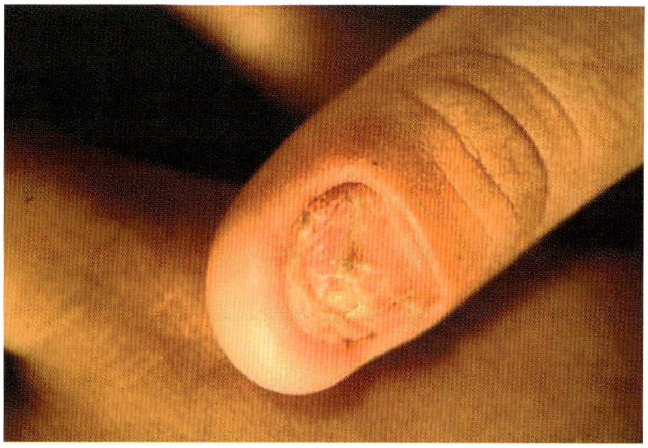

Figure 15–2. Onychomycosis in chronic mucocutaneous candidiasis.

Chronic Mucocutaneous Candidiasis

Certain immunodeficiencies present as a predisposition to recurrent *Candida* infections. Otolaryngologists may be requested to evaluate chronic or frequent oropharyngeal candida infections. Such clinical presentations should generate suspicion about the underlying defects mentioned above and prompt a referral to an immunologist. One such condition is autoimmune polyendocrinopathy candidiasis and ectodermal dystrophy (APECED), a rare autosomal recessive condition that manifests as recurrent *Candida* infections (Figure 15–2), [25] and autoimmune polyendocrinopathies, such as hypoparathyroidism and hypoadrenalism. This disorder is caused by a mutation in the *AIRE* gene that codes for the AIRE protein. A defect in thymic function and AIRE expression results in the autoimmune manifestations seen in APECED, as well as the immunodeficiency predisposing to *Candida* infection.[26] Multiple other mutations have been identified that can lead to the syndrome of chronic mucocutaneous candidiasis. One of the best studied is a mutation in the *STAT1* gene. STAT 1 codes for a transcription factor that is required for the development of Th1 and Th17 cells, as well as subsequent interferon gamma production, a cytokine that is essential for effective antifungal immunity.[27] Treatment and sometimes prophylaxis with antifungal agents is required.

Chronic mucocutaneous candidiasis can be a hallmark of serious immune disease and should be evaluated by an immunologist.

Human Papillomavirus (HPV)

Oropharyngeal HPV infections can be associated with immunodeficiency and can often be identified by otolaryngologists. CD4 T cells and cytotoxic T cells (CTL) are especially important in anti-HPV immunity. Although HIV is a frequent acquired immunodeficiency associated with HPV infections, several PID's are associated with this condition as well. Idiopathic CD4 lymphopenia (ICL) is a condition characterized by an absolute CD4 T lymphocyte count less than 300 cells/mm, or of less than 20% of the total lymphocyte count on more than one occasion without evidence of HIV infection or other known immunodeficiency. ICL can also present with laryngeal papillomatosis.[28]

WHIM syndrome (warts, hypogammaglobulinemia, infections, and myelokathexis) is a rare primary immunodeficiency disorder that occurs due to impaired chemokine CXCR4 signaling. This results in neutrophil and lymphocyte retention in the bone marrow. Of note, these patients have also been reported to have severe recurrent oral and genital herpes infections.[29]

X-Linked Agammaglobulinemia (XLA)

This condition affects males in the first few years of life. The defect is in the expression of Bruton tyrosine kinase (BTK), a protein responsible for transitioning pre-B cells to immature B cells that can then be released from the bone marrow into the periphery. This condition is characterized by severe hypogammaglobulinemia and few or no mature B cells in the blood, as well as the absence of tonsillar tissue.[30] Upper respiratory tract infections are the most common presentation of XLA, with otitis and sinusitis being most frequent. Pneumonia is another common infection, especially due to encapsulated organisms such as pneumococcus, *Haemophilus influenzae* type B (Hib), or *Pseudomonas*. Viral infections also occur, and cases of meningitis and encephalitis secondary to echovirus, coxsackie virus, adenovirus, and poliovirus have been reported. During the first 6 months of life infants are protected by passive immunity from maternally derived IgG antibodies, so serious infections usually occur after the first 6 months of life, and hypogammaglobulinemia is not detected until later in the course of the first year of life. Replacement gammaglobulin therapy is the primary treatment currently available, along with aggressive treatment of infections and supportive care. It is important to note, however, that since IVIG consists of pooled human IgG and contains lower levels of IgM and IgA, patients can still be predisposed to sinopulmonary infections. Prophylactic antibiotics can be considered for such patients.[31]

> Although patients with XLA are identified early in childhood, infectious complications of this condition are a lifelong risk, and otolaryngologists should be aware of its potential clinical manifestations.

Hyper-IgM Syndrome

This group of disorders is characterized by defective class-switch recombination (CSR) of immunoglobulin genes from IgM to IgG, IgA and IgE, resulting in impaired immunoglobulin isotype production. CD40 ligand (CD40L) is a receptor expressed on $CD4^{+}$ follicular helper T cells (Th) that binds to CD40 expressed on B cells. This interaction results in B-cell activation of the NF-kB signaling pathway and subsequent gene expression of proteins required for CSR, such as activation-induced cytidine deaminase (AID) and UNG-encoded uracil-DNA glycosylase (UNG). The most frequent cause of HIGM is the X-linked mutation in the gene encoding CD40L. Patients demonstrate impaired production of antigen-specific IgG and IgA in response to bacterial infections or vaccines.[32] Patients are predisposed to ear and sinopulmonary infections with encapsulated bacteria and demonstrate poor response to vaccines, including pneumococcal and Hib vaccines.

Hyper IgE Syndrome (HIES)

HIES is a rare disorder characterized by extremely elevated serum IgE levels (>2000 IU/mL), eczema, and recurrent skin (particularly staphylococcal) and sinopulmonary infections. The most common mutation identified in this disorder is an autosomal dominant (AD) loss of function *STAT3* mutation. This mutation interferes with the cell growth, division, and inflammation for which the STAT3 protein is normally responsible. The AD-HIES is unique in that it involves connective tissue and skeletal abnormalities. These patients also tend to develop pneumatoceles. Patients with AD-HIES have a high arching palate and characteristic facial appearances that including bulging forehead, deep-set eyes, and a broad nasal bridge.[33]

A mutation in the *DOCK8* gene is responsible for the autosomal recessive (AR) variant of HIES. This disorder is marked by elevated IgE levels, severe atopy that includes anaphylactic food reactions and asthma, cutaneous viral infections, and a notable lack of skeletal and connective tissue involvement. Patients are prone to developing mucocutaneous candidiasis as well as bacterial and viral sinopulmonary infections. Of note, HIES patients are at a long-term higher risk for the development of malignancy.

Patients with the autosomal dominant variant of HIES, have a characteristic retention of deciduous teeth along with ectopic eruption or abnormal growth of permanent teeth. An otolaryngologist might find HIES patients to have a susceptibility to developing caries (Figure 15–3),[34] mucosal fungal infections, and plaques.[35]

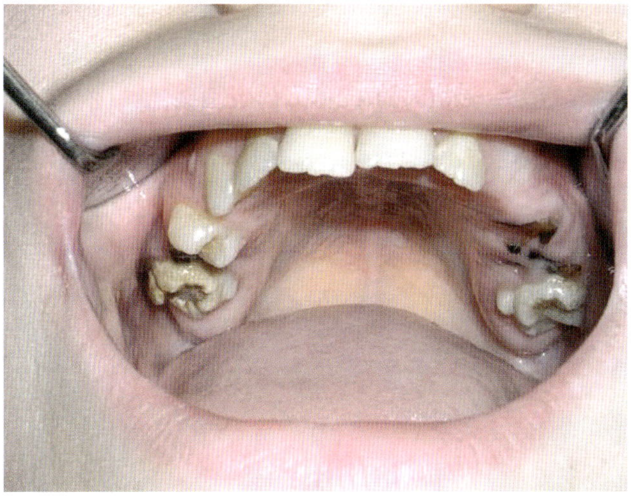

Figure 15–3. Hypereosinophilic syndrome (HIES). Primary and permanent teeth severely damaged by caries.

The definitive treatment of AR-HIES is hematopoietic stem cell transplantation. This treatment, however, is not typically recommended for AD-HIES. Instead, prophylactic treatment with antibiotics and symptomatic treatment is advised.[33]

Severe Combined Immunodeficiency (SCID)

Severe combined immunodeficiency (SCID) is a heterogeneous group of disorders marked by T, B, and/or NK cell defects. Presentation occurs very early in life and is associated with very severe infections, since these conditions result in significant immune impairments. Patients have early onset of failure to thrive, are susceptible to opportunistic infections, and require bone marrow transplantation for survival. Otolaryngologists may therefore not typically encounter these diseases, but some of the more common ones will be mentioned here.

SCID is often due to an absence of proteins required for cellular survival and signaling. The lymphocytic phenotypes are defined as absent T, B, and/or NK cells. Adenosine deaminase (ADA) deficiency, reticular dysgenesis, and methylenetetrahydrofolate dehydrogenase 1 gene (MTHFD1) deficiency result in a particularly severe PID characterized by absent T, B, and NK cells.[36–37] Patients are predisposed to invasive bacterial, viral, and fungal infections. Mutations in the genes responsible for immunoglobulin gene recombination, such as recombinase activating genes 1 and 2 (RAG1, RAG2), artemis, and the DNA protein kinase catalytic subunit (DNA-PK complex), result in the absence of T and B cells.[38–39] Of note, the wide impact of artemis and DNA-PKC deficiencies on other cell types also results in these patients having increased sensitivity to ionizing radiation, and precautionary measures should be taken in order to minimize exposure to imaging radiation.

A subgroup of combined immunodeficiencies is defined by the absence of T and NK cells, but preserved presence and function of B cells. These types of PID are due to impaired production of the specific cytokines, such as IL-2, 4, 7, 9, 15, and 21, that are necessary for T- and NK-cell development and function.[40] Since T and NK cells play critical roles in antiviral and antifungal immunity, these PIDs can present as recurrent viral (HPV as discussed above) and fungal infections. Hematopoietic cell transplantation (HCT) can be curative for SCID.[41] Gene therapy is another new alternative treatment available for SCID, specifically for ADA and (γ_c) deficiencies.[42]

> SCID is the most severe subgroup of immunodeficiencies and can present as bacterial, viral, and fungal infections. Prompt referral to an immunologist and subsequent bone marrow transplant are necessary.

CONCLUSION

PID are comprised of diverse diseases, underlying defects, and a wide range of clinical manifestations. The genetic mutations causing many of these have been identified (Table 15–6). Otolaryngologists serve as important gatekeepers in the early diagnosis and prompt treatment of these conditions. Therefore, these specialists should be aware of the otolaryngologic presentations of these PIDs in order to allow early referral to a clinical immunologist and treatment of the patient, thereby reducing the morbidity and lifelong complications associated with these conditions.

Table 15-6. Genetic Mutations Associated With Primary Immune Deficiencies

Immunodeficiency	Defect
Chronic granulomatous disease	NADPH oxidase complex
Chediak-Higashi syndrome	*LYST* gene
Common variable immunodeficiency	*TACI, BAFF, APRIL* genes
APECED	*AIRE* gene
WHIM	CXCR4 receptor signaling
XLA	Bruton tyrosine kinase
Hyper-IgM syndrome	CD40L (X-linked;majority), CD40 (AR)
HIES	STAT3 (AD); DOCK8 (AR)
SCID: T–B–NK+	RAG1, RAG2, artemis, ligase 4, DNA-PK complex
SCID: T–B+NK–	Common gamma chain receptor (X-linked); JAK3
SCID: T–B–NK–	Adenosine deaminase deficiency
SCID: T–B+NK+	CD3, CD45, IL7 receptor

REFERENCES

1. Wasserman RL, Manning SC. Diagnosis and treatment of primary immunodeficiency disease: the role of the otolaryngologist. *Am J Otolaryngol*. Jul–Aug 2011;32(4):329–337.
2. McCusker C, Warrington R. Primary immunodeficiency. *Allergy Asthma Clin Immunol*. 2011;7(suppl 1):S11.
3. Reda SM, El-Ghoneimy DH, Afifi HM. Clinical predictors of primary immunodeficiency diseases in children. *Allergy Asthma Immunol Res*. Mar 2013;5(2):88–95.
4. De Vincentiis GC, Sitzia E, Bottero S, Giuzio L, Simonetti A, Rossi P. Otolaryngologic manifestations of pediatric immunodeficiency. *Int J Pediatr Otorhinolaryngol*. Dec 2009;73(suppl 1):S42–S48.
5. Kang EM, Marciano BE, DeRavin S, Zarember KA, Holland SM, Malech HL. Chronic granulomatous disease: overview and hematopoietic stem cell transplantation. *J Allergy Clin Immunol*. Jun 2011;127(6):1319–1326; quiz 1317–1318.
6. Lewis EM, Singla M, Sergeant S, Koty PP, McPhail LC. X-linked chronic granulomatous disease secondary to skewed X chromosome inactivation in a female with a novel CYBB mutation and late presentation. *Clin Immunol*. Nov 2008;129(2):372–380.
7. Mauch L, Lun A, O'Gorman MR, et al. Chronic granulomatous disease (CGD) and complete myeloperoxidase deficiency both yield strongly reduced dihydrorhodamine 123 test signals but can be easily discerned in routine testing for CGD. *Clin Chem*. May 2007;53(5):890–896.
8. George PM, Badiger R, Alazawi W, Foster GR, Mitchell JA. Pharmacology and therapeutic potential of interferons. *Pharmacol Ther*. Jul 2012;135(1):44–53.
9. Kaplan J, De Domenico I, Ward DM. Chediak-Higashi syndrome. *Curr Opin Hematol*. Jan 2008;15(1):22–29.
10. Saez-De-Ocariz M, Orozco-Covarrubias L, Duràn-McKinster C, Ruiz-Maldonado R. Silver hair syndromes: Chediak-Higashi syndrome (CHS) and Griscelli syndromes (GS). In: Ruggieri M, Pascual-Castroviejo I, Di Rocco C, eds. *Neurocutaneous Disorders Phakomatoses and Hamartoneoplastic Syndromes*. Vienna, Austria: Springer; 2008:407–426.
11. Costabile M. Measuring the 50% haemolytic complement (CH50) activity of serum. *J Vis Exp*. 2010;(37):1923.
12. Botto M, Dell'Agnola C, Bygrave AE, et al. Homozygous C1q deficiency causes glomerulonephritis associated with multiple apoptotic bodies. *Nat Genet*. May 1998; 19(1):56–59.
13. Miller EC, Chase NM, Densen P, Hintermeyer MK, Casper JT, Atkinson JP. Autoantibody stabilization of the classical pathway C3 convertase leading to C3 deficiency and Neisserial sepsis: C4 nephritic factor revisited. *Clin Immunol*. Dec 2012;145(3):241–250.
14. Jonsson G, Truedsson L, Sturfelt G, Oxelius VA, Braconier JH, Sjoholm AG. Hereditary C2 deficiency in Sweden: frequent occurrence of invasive infection, atherosclerosis, and rheumatic disease. *Medicine*. Jan 2005;84(1):23–34.
15. Zhu Z, Atkinson TP, Hovanky KT, et al. High prevalence of complement component C6 deficiency among African-Americans in the south-eastern USA. *Clin Exp Immunol*. Feb 2000;119(2):305–310.

16. Slade C, Bosco J, Unglik G, Bleasel K, Nagel M, Winship I. Deficiency in complement factor B. *N Engl J Med*. Oct 24 2013;369(17):1667–1669.
17. Stengaard-Pedersen K, Thiel S, Gadjeva M, et al. Inherited deficiency of mannan-binding lectin-associated serine protease 2. *N Engl J Med*. Aug 7 2003;349(6): 554–560.
18. Sprong T, Roos D, Weemaes C, et al. Deficient alternative complement pathway activation due to factor D deficiency by 2 novel mutations in the complement factor D gene in a family with meningococcal infections. *Blood*. Jun 15 2006;107(12):4865–4870.
19. Costa-Carvalho BT, Grumach AS, Franco JL, et al. Attending to warning signs of primary immunodeficiency diseases across the range of clinical practice. *J Clin Immunol*. Jan 2014;34(1):10–22.
20. Bork K, Steffensen I, Machnig T. Treatment with C1-esterase inhibitor concentrate in type I or II hereditary angioedema: a systematic literature review. *Allergy Asthma Proc*. Jul–Aug 2013;34(4):312–327.
21. Cunningham-Rundles C, Bodian C. Common variable immunodeficiency: clinical and immunological features of 248 patients. *Clin Immunol*. Jul 1999;92(1):34–48.
22. Barbosa RR, Silva SL, Silva SP, et al. Reduced BAFF-R and increased TACI expression in common variable immunodeficiency. *J Clin Immunol*. Jul 2014;34(5):573–583.
23. Ocampo CJ, Peters AT. Antibody deficiency in chronic rhinosinusitis: epidemiology and burden of illness. *Am J Rhinol Allergy*. Jan 2013;27(1):34–38.
24. Jorgensen GH, Gardulf A, Sigurdsson MI, et al. Clinical symptoms in adults with selective IgA deficiency: a case-control study. *J Clin Immunol*. May 2013;33(4):742–747.
25. Tay YK, Seow CS. What syndrome is this? Chronic mucocutaneous candidiasis. *Pediatr Dermatol*. Jul–Aug 2001; 18(4):353–355.
26. Perheentupa J. Autoimmune polyendocrinopathy candidiasis-ectodermal dystrophy. *J Clin Endocrinol Metabolism*. Aug 2006;91(8):2843–2850.
27. van de Veerdonk FL, Plantinga TS, Hoischen A, et al. STAT1 mutations in autosomal dominant chronic mucocutaneous candidiasis. *N Engl J Med*. Jul 7 2011;365(1): 54–61.
28. Leiding JW, Holland SM. Warts and all: human papillomavirus in primary immunodeficiencies. *J Allergy Clin Immunol*. Nov 2012;130(5):1030–1048.
29. McDermott DH, Liu Q, Velez D, et al. A phase 1 clinical trial of long-term, low-dose treatment of WHIM syndrome with the CXCR4 antagonist plerixafor. *Blood*. Apr 10 2014;123(15):2308–2316.
30. Kanegane H, Futatani T, Wang Y, et al. Clinical and mutational characteristics of X-linked agammaglobulinemia and its carrier identified by flow cytometric assessment combined with genetic analysis. *J Allergy Clin Immunol*. Dec 2001;108(6):1012–1020.
31. Winkelstein JA, Marino MC, Lederman HM, et al. X-linked agammaglobulinemia: report on a United States registry of 201 patients. *Medicine*. Jul 2006;85(4):193–202.
32. Kracker S, Gardes P, Mazerolles F, Durandy A. Immunoglobulin class switch recombination deficiencies. *Clin Immunol*. May 2010;135(2):193–203.
33. Zhang Q, Su HC. Hyperimmunoglobulin E syndromes in pediatrics. *Curr Opin Pediatr*. Dec 2011;23(6):653–658.
34. Szczawinska-Poplonyk A, Kycler Z, Pietrucha B, Heropolitanska-Pliszka E, Breborowicz A, Gerreth K. The hyperimmunoglobulin E syndrome—clinical manifestation diversity in primary immune deficiency. *Orphanet J Rare Dis*. 2011;6:76.
35. Esposito L, Poletti L, Maspero C, et al. Hyper-IgE syndrome: dental implications. *Oral Surg Oral Med Oral Pathol Oral Radiol*. Aug 2012;114(2):147–153.
36. Keller MD, Ganesh J, Heltzer M, et al. Severe combined immunodeficiency resulting from mutations in MTHFD1. *Pediatrics*. Feb 2013;131(2):e629–e634.
37. Henderson LA, Frugoni F, Hopkins G, et al. First reported case of Omenn syndrome in a patient with reticular dysgenesis. *J Allergy Clin Immunol*. Apr 2013;131(4):1227–1230, 1230.e1221–1223.
38. IJspeert H, Driessen GJ, Moorhouse MJ, et al. Similar recombination-activating gene (RAG) mutations result in similar immunobiological effects but in different clinical phenotypes. *J Allergy Clin Immunol*. Apr 2014;133(4): 1124–1133.
39. van der Burg M, van Dongen JJ, van Gent DC. DNA-PKcs deficiency in human: long predicted, finally found. *Curr Opin Allergy Clin Immunol*. Dec 2009;9(6):503–509.
40. Candotti F, Oakes SA, Johnston JA, et al. Structural and functional basis for JAK3-deficient severe combined immunodeficiency. *Blood*. Nov 15 1997;90(10):3996–4003.
41. Antoine C, Muller S, Cant A, et al. Long-term survival and transplantation of haemopoietic stem cells for immunodeficiencies: report of the European experience 1968–1999. *Lancet*. Feb 15 2003;361(9357):553–560.
42. Kohn DB. Update on gene therapy for immunodeficiencies. *Clin Immunol*. May 2010;135(2):247–254.

16

Acquired Immune Deficiencies

Jasmeen S. Dara, Arye Rubinstein, and Jenny Shliozberg

INTRODUCTION

Secondary immunodeficiencies, or acquired immunodeficiencies, can have a number of different etiologies, including human immunodeficiency virus (HIV) infection, immunosuppressive agents, cancer, malnutrition, nephrotic syndrome, and more rarely autoimmune disease.

Similar to the clinical presentation of primary immunodeficiency disorders, secondary immunodeficiencies often present with recurrent or severe infections or with infections from atypical bacterial or fungal pathogens. Resistant thrush, oral ulcers, periodontitis, recurrent sinusitis, and recurrent pneumonias are frequent sinopulmonary manifestations. Patients may also have failure to thrive, malabsorption, or diarrhea.

HUMAN IMMUNODEFICIENCY VIRUS

Over 30 years after its discovery, HIV remains a global pandemic, particularly in sub-Saharan Africa, southeast Asia, and Latin America. HIV remains one of the world's most significant public health challenges. At the end of 2013, the World Health Organization (WHO) estimated that there were 35 million people living with HIV/AIDS worldwide and 2.1 million new infections were occurring every year.[1] At the end of 2009, the US Centers for Disease Control (CDC) estimated that 1 148 200 persons aged 13 and older were living with HIV infection in the United States, including 207 600 (18.1%) persons whose infections had not yet been diagnosed. The CDC estimates that there will be approximately 50 000 new infections per year in the United States.[2]

Although prevention and treatment of HIV has significantly reduced the incidence of advanced disease and opportunistic infections in the United States, patients are still often impacted by the adverse effects of prolonged viral immune activation and/or medications. Up to 80% of HIV-infected patients eventually develop otolaryngologic manifestations of disease,[3–5] which include infections, malignancy, neuropathies, and atopic disease.

Disease Classification

HIV disease can be categorized according to signs and symptoms of the disease or by CD4 lymphocyte count (Table 16–1). When CD4 lymphocyte counts exceed 500/uL, patients usually exhibit no clinical symptoms of disease.[6] However, when CD4 lymphocytes decrease below 200/uL, patients become susceptible to many infections and that risk continues to increase as the CD4 lymphocyte count decreases below 50/uL. At that point the patient becomes susceptible to rare opportunistic infections.[6] However, there is an important caveat to relying solely on the CD4 lymphocyte count to estimate risk for opportunistic conditions. Patients who have responded to antiretroviral therapy may have had CD4 lymphocyte counts that were previously low

Table 16–1. Classification of HIV Disease

	Clinical Signs/Symptoms	CD4 T Cell	Category
Category CDC-A	Asymptomatic HIV infection	>500/uL	CDC-A1
	Persistent generalized lymphadenopathy	200–499	CDC-A2
	Acute (primary) HIV infection with accompanying illness or history of acute infection	<200	CDC-A3
Category CDC-B	Bacillary angiomatosis	>500/uL	CDC-B1
	Candiasis, oropharyngeal	200–499	CDC-B2
	Candidiasis, vulvovaginal; persistent frequent, or poorly responsive to therapy	<200	CDC-B3
	Cervival dysplasia (moderate or severe)/cervical carcinoma in situ		
	Constitutional symptoms, such as fever or diarrhea, lasting >1 month		
	Hairy leukoplakia, oral		
	Herpes zoster (2 distinct episodes or >1 dermatome)		
	Idiopathic thrombocytopenic purpura		
	Listeriosis		
	Pelvic inflammatory disease		
	Peripheral neuropathy		
Category CDC-C	**Candidiasis of bronchi, trachea, or lungs**	>500/uL	CDC-C1
	Candidiasis, esophageal	200–499	CDC-C2
	Coccidiomycosis, disseminated, or extrapulmonary	<200	CDC-C3
	Cryptococcosis, extrapulmonary		
	Cryptosporidiosis >1 month		
	CMV disease (other than liver/spleen/nodes)		
	CMV retinitis		
	HIV encephalopathy		
	Herpes simplex, chronic ulcers (>1 month)		
	Herpes simples, bronchitis/pneumonitis/esophagitis		
	Histoplasmosis, disseminated, or extrapulmonary		
	Invasive cervical carcinoma		
	Isosporiasis >1 month		
	Kaposi sarcoma		
	Lymphoma		
	***Mycobacterium avium* complex**		
	Mycobacterium tuberculosis		
	***Pneumocystis jirovecii* pneumonia**		
	Progressive multifocal encephalopathy		
	Recurrent pneumonia >2		
	Salmonella sepsis		
	Toxoplasmosis (cerebral)		
	Wasting syndrome—loss >20% of body weight		

Note. Signs/symptoms important for otolaryngologists appear in boldface.

but subsequently increased as a result of therapy. In this scenario, current CD4 lymphocyte counts could mask an underlying immune deficiency; therefore, an individual's risk for opportunistic infections should be based on their lowest CD4 count, not on his or her most recent CD4 count.[7]

Many of the first signs of HIV infection involve the ear, nose, and throat, and early recognition of these signs will allow for HIV treatment to be started before significant immunodeficiency occurs.[7] Additionally, many of the stages of HIV disease classifications are identified in the ear, nose, and throat systems, and recognition of these signs may indicate a failure of the anti-retroviral therapy that the patient is currently receiving and predict impending immunologic deterioration.

Patients are classified as having acquired immune deficiency syndrome (AIDS) when there are one or more diagnoses considered to be consistent with severe immune suppression (see Table 16–1) or have a CD4 lymphocyte count below 200 cells/μL.

Common otolaryngological diagnoses that confirm an AIDS diagnosis include multiple or recurrent bacterial infections, chronic herpes simplex virus ulcers (>1 month's duration), Kaposi sarcoma, lymphoma (Burkitt or immunoblastic), and *Mycobacterium avium* complex, *Mycobacterium kansasii*, or other mycobacterial species with extrapulmonary infection and *Mycobacterium tuberculosis* of any site Table 16–2 lists all CDC AIDS-defining conditions.

Table 16–2. CDC AIDS-Defining Conditions

Bacterial infections, multiple or recurrent[a]
Candidiasis of bronchi, trachea, or lungs
Candidiasis of esophagus[b]
Cervical cancer, invasive[c]
Coccidioidomycosis, disseminate or extrapulmonary
Cryptococcosis, extrapulmonary
Cryptosporidiosis, chronic intestinal (>1 month's duration)
Cytomegalovirus disease (other than liver, spleen, or nodes), onset at age >1 month
Cytomegalovirus retinitis (with loss of vision)
Encephalopathy, HIV related
Herpes simplex: chronic ulcers (>1 month's duration) or bronchitis, pneumonitis, or esophagitis (onset at age >1 month)
Histoplasmosis, disseminated or extrapulmonary
Isosporiasis, chronic intestinal (>1 month's duration)
Kaposi sarcoma
Lymphoid interstitial pneumonia or pulmonary lymphoid hyperplasia complex
Lymphoma, Burkitt
Lymphoma, immunoblastic
Lymphoma, primary or brain
***Mycobacterium avium* complex or *Mycobacterium kansasii*, disseminated or extrapulmonary**
***Mycobacterium tuberculosis* of any site, pulmonary, disseminated, or extrapulmonary**
***Mycobacterium*, other species or unidentified species, disseminated or extrapulmonary**
Pneumocystis jirovecii pneumonia
Pneumonia, recurrent
Progressive multifocal leukoencephalopathy
Salmonella septicemia, recurrent
Toxoplasmosis of brain, onset at age >1 month
Wasting syndrome attributed to HIV

[a]Only among children <13 years.
[b]Condition that might be diagnosed presumptively.
[c]Only among adults and adolescents aged ≥13 years.

Diagnosis of HIV

Testing for HIV should be performed when historical or clinical findings are suspicious for disease. Children older than 18 months of age can be diagnosed by serological testing. If antibody is present by serologic testing, Western blot should be performed for confirmation of the diagnosis. RNA viral load by polymerase chain reaction (PCR) and CD4 counts should be performed to classify the disease stage and severity of immune deficiency. Children under 18 months of age may still have maternal antibody present, so if antibody is present it will be unclear if this is antibody produced by the child or the mother. In this case, a DNA or RNA PCR should be performed to identify childhood infection.[7] Other laboratory testing may suggest HIV infection such as thrombocytopenia, lymphopenia, anemia, low CD4 counts, increased serum amylase, and an increased serum globulin fraction due to increased serum levels of IgG.[7]

> Serologic tests should not be performed to diagnose HIV in children younger than 18 months of age, as a positive test could merely indicate maternal antibody.

Treatment of HIV

In 1987, zidovudine became the first approved treatment for HIV disease. Since that time, more than 30 drugs have been approved to treat HIV/AIDS patients. Since the advent of multidrug antiretroviral therapy regimens, patients with access to treatment and care can live long and healthy lives. HIV-infected patients are usually placed on a regimen of antiretroviral therapy that consists of nucleoside or nucleotide reverse transcriptase inhibitors (NRTIs), nonnucleoside reverse transcriptase inhibitors (NNRTIs), protease inhibitors (PIs), entry/fusion inhibitors, or integrase inhibitors. A multidrug regimen is important for preventing the development of HIV resistance mutations. As a general rule, patients should take 3 different drugs from at least 2 different classes. Adherence to therapy is an important barrier to effective disease treatment and prevention. Poor adherence leads to increased HIV viral load and increased resistance mutations, leading to less therapeutic options. Medication side effects may sometimes contribute to poor adherence to therapy. Common side effects include anemia, diarrhea, dizziness, fatigue, headaches, nausea, vomiting, neuropathies, and rashes. Various antiretroviral therapies may cause inhibition or induction of cytochrome P450 metabolism and can therefore contribute to varying drug concentrations. A list of these interactions can be found in Table 16–3.

Oropharyngeal Manifestations of HIV

Oral Candidiasis

Oral candidiasis is the most common oral manifestation of HIV infection with a prevalence that ranges from 30% to 90% among HIV-infected adult patients.[4,8,9] Candida infection can occur in the oropharynx, hypopharynx, and larynx and causes severe odynophagia. There are three common forms of presentation: pseudomembranous candidiasis, erythematous candidiasis, and angular cheilitis.

Table 16–3. Medication Interactions With Antiretroviral Therapy

ENT Medication	Mechanism of Interaction	Medication Combination	Clinical Effect	Management
Itraconzaole	Inhibition or induction of CYP450 3A4	Darunavir	↑ Darunavir and itraconazole	Do not exceed 200 mg itraconazole daily
		Didanosine (ddl)	↓ Itraconazole	Administer itraconazole >2 hours after ddl
		Efavirenz	↓ Itraconazole	Do not coadminister
		indinavir	↑ Indinavir	Decrease indinavir dose
		Lopinavir/ritonavir	↑ Lopinavir/ritonavir and ↑ Itraconazole	Avoid using high doses of itraconazole
		Ritonavir	↑ Ritonavir	Dose adjustment not established
		Saquinavir	↑ Saquinavir and itraconazole	Reduce itraconazole to 100 mg twice a day

Table 16-3. *continued*

ENT Medication	Mechanism of Interaction	Medication Combination	Clinical Effect	Management
Voriconzaole	Inhibition or induction of CYP450 3A4	Atazanavir/ darunavir	↓ Voriconazole	Do not coadminister
		Etravirine	↑ Etravirine	No dose adjustment necessary
		Lopinavir/ ritonavir	↓ Voriconazole	Do not coadminister
		Ritonavir	↓ Voriconazole	Avoid coadministration
		Efavirenz	↓ Voriconazole	Increase voriconazole to 400 mg twice a day and decrease efavirenz to 300 mg nightly
Fluconazole	Inhibition or induction of CYP450 3A4	Etravirine	↑ Etravirine	No dose adjustment
		Nevirapine	↑ Nevirapine	No dose adjustment
		Saquinavir	↑ Saquinavir	No dose adjustment
		Tipranavir	↑ Tipranavir	No dose adjustment
		Zidovudine	↑ Zidovudine	No dose adjustment
Ketoconazole	Inhibition or induction of CYP450 3A4	Darunavir	↑ Darunavir and ketoconazole	Dose adjustment not established
		Delavirdine	↑ Delavirdine	No dose adjustment
		Didanosine	↓ Didanosine	Administer ketoconazole at least 2 hours prior to didanosine
		Efavirenz	↓ Ketoconazole	Do not coadminister
		Indinavir	↑ Indinavir	Decrease indinavir to 600 mg 3 times a day
		Lopinavir/ ritonavir	↑ Ketoconazole and ↓ Lopinavir/ritonavir	Do not coadminister
		Maraviroc	↑ Miraviroc	Reduce maraviroc dose to 150 mg twice a day
		Nelfinavir	↑ Nelfinavir	No dose adjustment
		Nevirapine	↓ Ketoconazole	Do not coadminister
		Rilpivirine	↓ Ketoconazole	No dose adjustment necessary but should be monitored for failure of antifungal therapy
		Ritonavir/ saquinavir	↑ Ritonavir/saquinavir	Dose adjustment not established

Source: Adapted from Iacovou E, Vlastarakos PV, Papcharalampous G, et al. Diagnosis and treatment of HIV-associated manifestations in otolaryngology. *Infectious Dis Rep*. 2012;4(1):e9.

Oral pseudomembranous candidiasis is the most common presentation of fungal infection in HIV disease and is used as a clinical marker of disease progression to AIDS. It appears as creamy white, curd-like plaques on the buccal mucosa, tongue, and other oral mucosal surfaces (Figure 16–1). If the plaques are removed, a red or bleeding underlying surface is exposed.[10] The most common organism is *Candida albicans*; less commonly *C. glabrata* and *C. dubliniensis* have been reported.[11,12]

Erythematous candidiasis presents as a red, flat lesion on the dorsal surface of the tongue, hard palate, or soft palate (Figure 16–2). The lesion often involves two opposing surfaces. For example, a lesion on the tongue would be matched by a similar lesion on the hard palate. Patients will complain of a burning sensation particularly with spicy or salty foods and will often have more severe odynophagia requiring hospitalization for intravenous antifungal therapy.

Angular cheilitis presents with erythema or fissuring at one or, more commonly, both corners of the mouth (Figure 16–3). The condition may coexist with erythematous or pseudomembranous candidiasis.

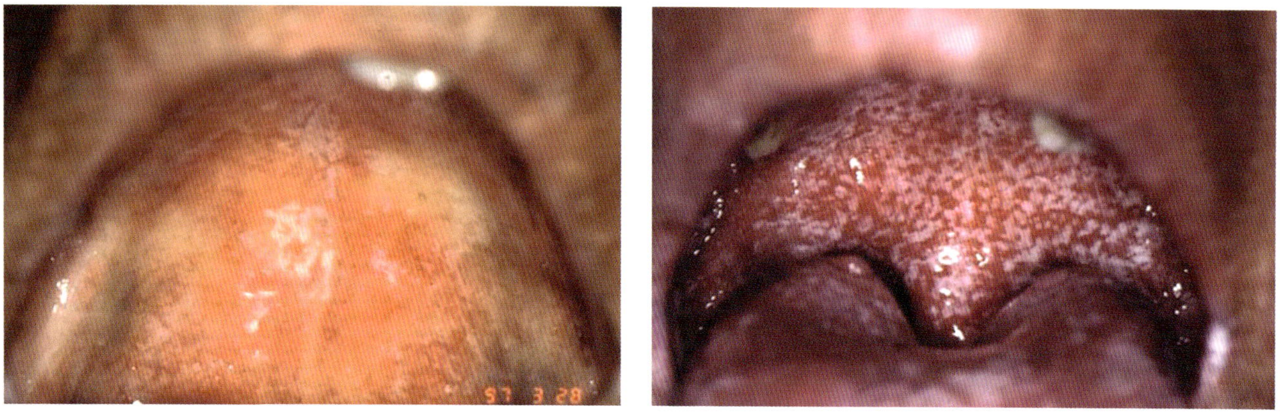

A B

Figure 16–1. Mild to moderate (**A**) and severe (**B**) oral pseudomembranous candidiasis. Reprinted with permission from the International AIDS Society and David A. Reznik, DDS. Reznik DA. Oral manifestations of HIV disease. *Top HIV Med.* 2005;13(5):143–148.

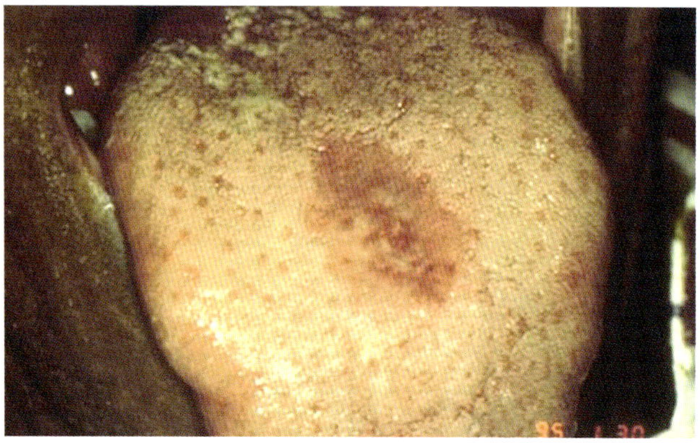

Figure 16–2. Eythematous candidiasis. Reprinted with permission from the International AIDS Society and David A. Reznik, DDS. Reznik DA. Oral manifestations of HIV disease. *Top HIV Med.* 2005;13(5):143–148.

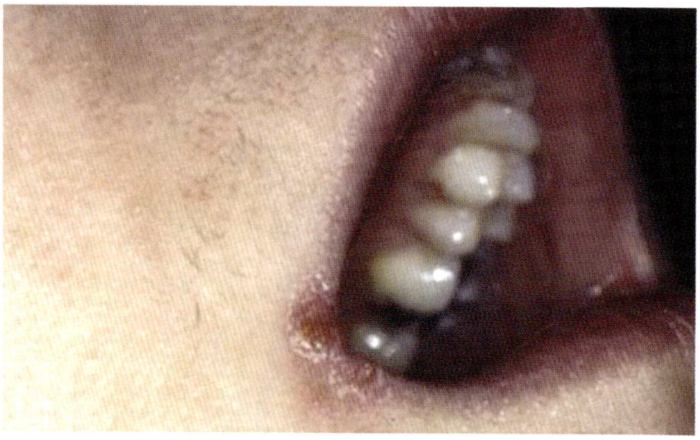

Figure 16–3. Angular cheilitis. Reprinted with permission from the International AIDS Society and David A. Reznik, DDS. Reznik DA. Oral manifestations of HIV disease. *Top HIV Med.* 2005;13(5):143–148.

The diagnosis of oropharyngeal candidiasis is typically made on clinical grounds but refractory or persistent cases can be confirmed by identification of fungal hyphae in a potassium hydroxide (KOH) preparation, and by fungal cultures for species identification and susceptibility testing.[10]

Oral candidiasis can be treated with topical nystatin or systemic fluconazole depending on the extent and persistence of disease. Angular cheilitis treatment involves the use of topical antifungal creams. Systemic antifungals should be used for angular cheilitis with coexistent invasive oral mucosal or pharyngeal candidiasis.

> Oral pseudomembranous candidiasis is the most common presentation of fungal disease in HIV infection.

Periodontal and Gingival Disease

Periodontal and gingival disease can be frequently seen in HIV-infected patients with a prevalence that varies from 0% to 47% in adults[13] and 0% to 20% in children.[14]

Linear gingival erythema presents as a red band of petechia-like patches along the gingival margin, accompanied by occasional bleeding and discomfort, and most frequently occurs on the anterior dentition but can also extend posteriorly (Figure 16–4A). Treatment includes debridement and chlorhexidine mouth rinses twice daily for 2 weeks.[10]

Necrotizing gingivitis and necrotizing periodontitis can result in rapid destruction of soft tissue and hard tissues, respectively (Figure 16–4B). Necrotizing ulcerative periodontitis is a marker of severe immune suppression, characterized by severe pain, loosening of the teeth, bleeding, fetid odor, ulcerated gingival papillae, and rapid loss of bone and soft tissue.[10] Treatment involves debridement and use of topical antiseptic agents such as chlorhexidine gluconate or povidone-iodine lavages. More severe cases should be supplemented by a short course of systemic antimicrobial therapy, usually penicillin, amoxicillin, amoxicillin/clavulanate, clindamycin, or metronidazole.[15]

> The principal treatment of necrotizing gingival or periodontal disease in HIV-infected patients is prompt debridement and the use of topical antiseptic agents.

Other Oral Infections

Herpes Simplex Virus (HSV). Oral herpes simplex virus (HSV) infections occur in up to 9% of adults[4,9] and 1.3% to 2.4% of children[16] with HIV. Oral HSV presents as a cluster of vesicles that produce small painful ulcerations extending onto the adjacent skin and may coalesce to form larger lesions.[10] Lesions

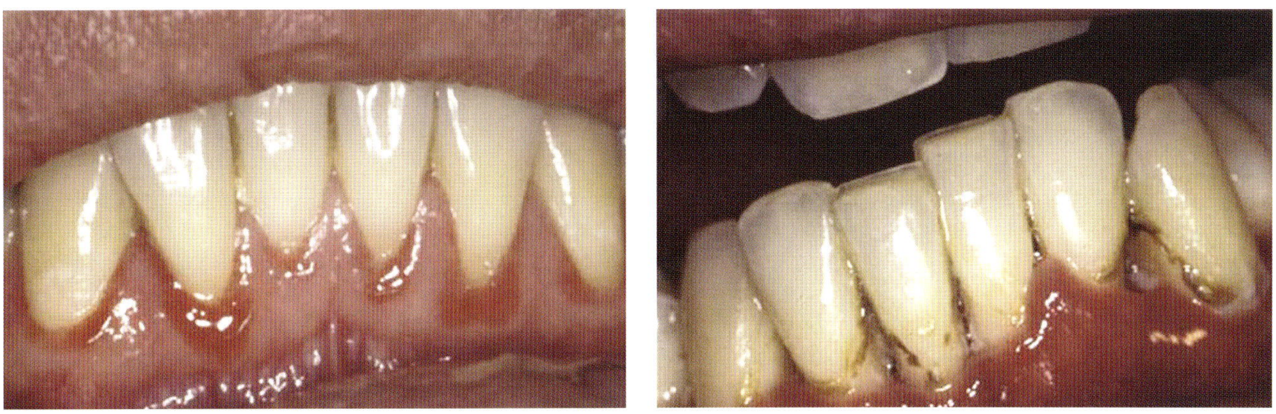

A B

Figure 16-4. **A.** Linear gingival erythema. **B.** Necrotizing ulcerative periodontitis. Reprinted with permission from the International AIDS Society and David A. Reznik, DDS. Reznik DA. Oral manifestations of HIV disease. *Top HIV Med.* 2005;13(5):143–148.

are often larger and recur more frequently in HIV patients as compared to immunocompetent patients. Lesions are typically self-limited, but antiviral treatment with acyclovir, valacyclovir, or famciclovir may be required for severe or persistent disease.[10] Studies have shown that oral valacyclovir has increased bioavailability as compared to oral acyclovir, and upon absorption, near complete conversion to L-valine and acyclovir; therefore, it is preferred over acyclovir in the treatment of herpesvirus infections. Valacyclovir is also the preferred agent for pediatric patients. However, it is not manufactured as a suspension and may therefore be more cumbersome to compound and administer.

> Oral valacyclovir has increased bioavailability as compared to oral acyclovir and is the preferred agent in the treatment of HSV infections.

Epstein-Barr Virus (EBV). Epstein-Barr virus (EBV) may cause thickening of epithelial cells of the tongue[17] or, less frequently, other parts of the oral cavity, causing oral hairy leukoplakia (discussed in more detail in a later section).

Human Papillomavirus (HPV). The incidence of oral human papillomavirus (HPV) infections in HIV-infected patients has been increasing despite the use of highly active antiretroviral therapy (HAART), suggesting a corresponding increase in oral sexual activities.[10] HPV infections present as cauliflower-like, spiked, or raised lesions with a flat surface (Figure 16–5). At least 17 HPV types have been detected in oral mucosal lesions, the more common of which include subtypes 2, 6, 11, 13, 32, and 57.[18] Treatment involves surgery (laser or cryotherapy) and may require repeat therapy due to frequent recurrences.[10] Topical cidofovir has been shown, in one case report, to be effective for treatment of oral HPV in the setting of HIV infection.[19]

Oral Hairy Leukoplakia. Oral hairy leukoplakia is a largely asymptomatic condition of the tongue caused by EBV infection, that is found in approximately 0.42% to 38% of adults with HIV. It presents as a white corrugated lesion on the lateral borders of the tongue that, in contrast to oral candidiasis, cannot be wiped away[17] (Figure 16–6). The condition is seen in the presence of immune deterioration; therefore, patients on antiretroviral therapy who develop oral hairy leukoplakia may be experiencing failure of their current regimen.[20] No treatment is absolutely necessary except for the sake of cosmetic improvement, for which trichloroacetic or glycolic acid,[21] podophyllum resin solution 25%,[22] or oral acyclovir[23] have been shown to be effective.

> Treatment of oral hairy leukoplakia may be desired for cosmetic improvement but is not absolutely necessary.

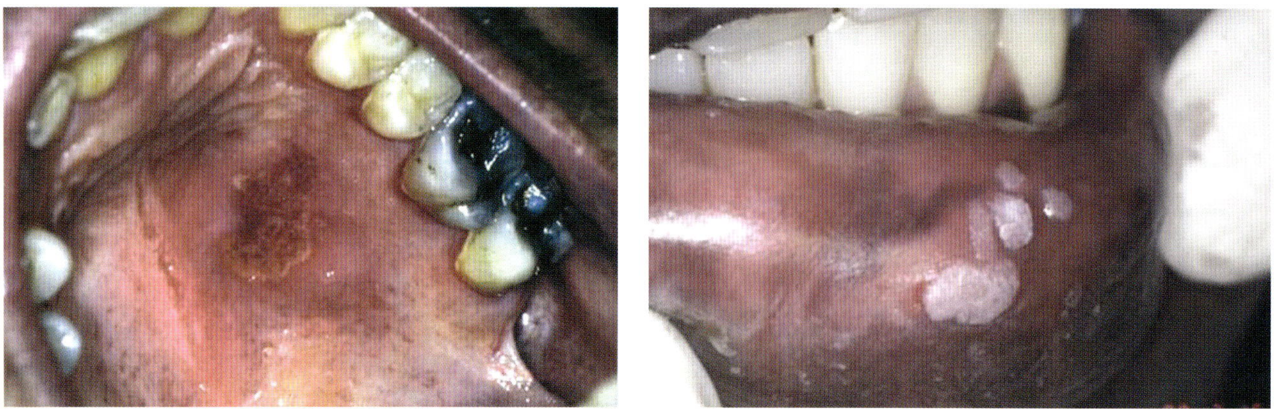

A B

Figure 16–5. A. Oral HSV. **B.** Oral HPV. Reprinted with permission from the International AIDS Society and David A. Reznik, DDS. Reznik DA. Oral manifestations of HIV disease. *Top HIV Med.* 2005;13(5):143–148.

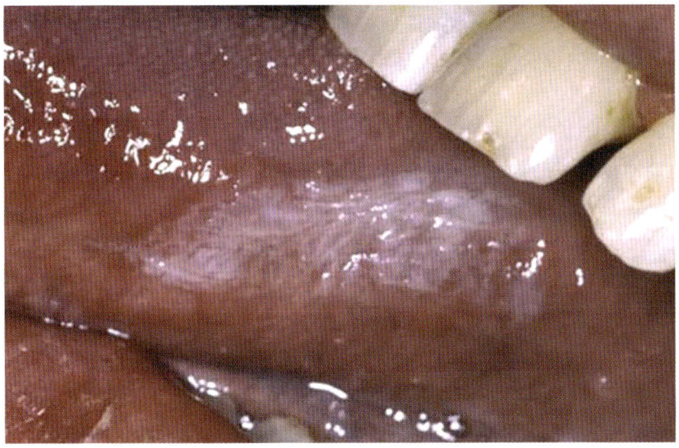

Figure 16-6. Oral hairy leukoplakia. Reprinted with permission from the International AIDS Society and David A. Reznik, DDS. Reznik DA. Oral manifestations of HIV disease. *Top HIV Med.* 2005;13(5):143–148.

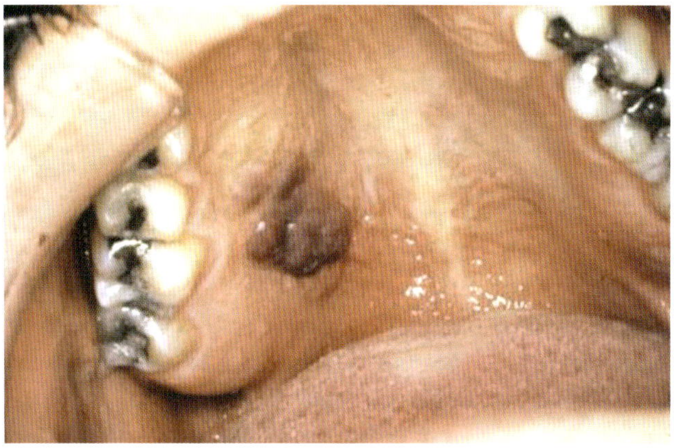

Figure 16-7. Kaposi sarcoma. Reprinted with permission from the International AIDS Society and David A. Reznik, DDS. Reznik DA. Oral manifestations of HIV disease. *Top HIV Med.* 2005;13(5):143–148.

Oral Malignancies

Kaposi Sarcoma. Kaposi sarcoma is the most common oral malignancy seen among patients with HIV, both prior to and during the era of HAART, with a prevalence of 0% to 12% in Africa and 0% to 38% in the United States and Europe.[24,25] The hard palate is most frequently involved, followed by the gingival and buccal mucosa and the dorsum of the tongue.[10] It occurs concomitantly with skin and visceral disease in up to 70% of patients.[24] Lesions in the oral cavity may occur earlier than those on the skin.[17] Kaposi sarcoma can be macular, nodular, or raised and ulcerated with a color that ranges from red to purple (Figure 16–7). As the lesions progress, they may become painful due to trauma or infection. Treatment involves improvement of oral hygiene, local injection of chemotherapeutic agents, surgical excision, laser therapy, cryotherapy, or radiation therapy.[10] Systemic chemotherapy is used for the majority of cases due to concomitant visceral involvement.

Non-Hodgkin Lymphoma. Non-Hodgkin lymphoma is the second most common malignant condition associated with HIV infection. Patients present with fevers, night sweats, and significant weight loss. Lesions present as a focal, ulcerated, soft tissue mass on the palate or gingiva, which may be red, inflamed, or painful. Treatment involves systemic chemotherapy and possible surgical debulking for pain reduction and functional improvement.[10]

> Kaposi sarcoma is the most common oral malignancy seen in patients with HIV and presents with skin and visceral disease in up to 70% of patients.

Neck Manifestations of HIV

Cervical Adenopathy

Cervical adenopathy is the most common manifestation of HIV infection in the neck. HIV lymphadenopathy is defined as the presence of diffuse lymphadenopathy in 2 or more neck sites for longer than 3 months.[26] The enlarged lymph nodes most frequently occur in the posterior cervical triangle and are often symmetrical, ranging from 1 to 5 cm in diameter.[4] This condition can occur in up to 70% of HIV patients within the first few months after seroconversion,[10] so it is one of the earliest clinical signs of HIV infection and a marker of acute disease. In addition to reactive lymphadenitis, cervical lymphadenitis may result from tuberculosis, lymphoma, or Kaposi sarcoma. Fine needle aspiration is necessary in the case of asymmetry, rapidly enlarging lymph nodes, or other suspicious features suggestive of alternative diagnoses.[10]

> Cervical adenopathy is one of the earliest signs of HIV infection, found in the first few months of seroconversion.

Salivary Gland Disease

Salivary gland disease is also a common manifestation of HIV infection. It usually involves the parotid glands, tends to be bilateral, sometimes, cystic, and can be accompanied by generalized lymphadenopathy. Salivary gland enlargement occurs in approximately 3% to 30% of adults[27] and up to 30% of infected children[5] and may often be the earliest clinical sign of HIV infection. Clinical examination should include characteristics of the facial mass and facial nerve function. The hypothesized causes of parotid enlargement in HIV infected patients include reactive hyperplasia of an intraparotid lymph node, benign lymphoepithelial lesions with ductal metaplasia, and benign lymphoepithelial cysts.[7,10] Microscopic examinations reveal 3 types: follicular hyperplasia of the parotid lymph nodes, diffuse lymphocytic infiltration of the gland with mostly $CD8^+$ lymphocytes, or benign lymphoepithelial cysts. Lymphoepithelial cysts are more common in adults than in children. Ultrasound, computed tomography (CT) scan, magnetic resonance imaging (MRI), fine needle aspiration, or biopsy may aid in diagnosis of HIV parotitis.[28,29] Surgical treatment is controversial but may include surgical debulking for cosmetic purposes. Aspiration of cystic lesions can provide temporary benefit. Intralesional tetracycline and doxycycline injections have been shown to be beneficial.[10]

> Clinical evaluation of salivary gland disease should always include examination of facial nerve function.

Otological Manifestations of HIV

Otitis Externa

Otitis externa occurs frequently in HIV-infected patients and is typically caused by *Pseudomonas aeruginosa* and *Candida albicans*.[4,10] Patients usually present with a small furuncle, but with severe pain and local swelling of the ear canal and accompanying posterior auricular lymphadenopathy. Fever is moderate if present at all. Diffuse otitis externa presents similarly but also with pruritic eczematous skin, pain with ear or jaw movement, and thick purulent and sometimes hemorrhagic discharge from the ear canal. Seborrheic dermatitis of the auricular or preauricular regions may sometimes present similarly to otitis externa and must be considered as well. Topical antibiotic treatment with an antipseudomonal or antifungal agent is recommended unless there is extension to the surrounding area with evidence of cellulitis, which then requires systemic treatment. Topical steroids used in conjunction with antibiotic therapy have been shown to be effective in this condition.

Malignant (necrotizing) external otitis also occurs. Patients with this problem tend to be younger,[30] and it is often caused by *Aspergillus fumigatus* or *Pseudomonas aeruginosa* infection. The diagnosis should be considered in any AIDS patient who presents with painful otorrhea that is unresponsive to treatment for bacterial or fungal otitis externa.[4] Treatment involves both oral systemic and topical therapy for suspected or confirmed organisms including *Pseudomonas*, *Candida*, and *Aspergillus* species.

> Malignant external otitis is often caused by *Aspergillus fumigatus* or *Pseudomonas aeruginosa*.

Otitis Media, Otitis Media with Effusion, and Serous Otitis Media

Recurrent acute and chronic sinusitis are common in HIV-infected patients. Infected sinus mucous drainage into the nasopharynx can cause mucosal swelling around the eustachian tube orifice and therefore an increased susceptibility to middle ear infections.[31] Although *Streptococcus pneumoniae* and *Haemophilus influenzae* are the most frequently isolated organisms in both HIV-infected and HIV-uninfected patients, *Staphylococcus aureus* and *Pseudomonas aeruginosa* are more frequently isolated in HIV-infected patients than HIV-uninfected patients. Standard empiric therapy includes amoxicillin or amoxicillin-clavulanate (500 mg, 3 times daily or 875 mg, 2 times daily amoxicillin component). An alternative in patients with penicillin allergy may include oral third-generation cephalosporins (cefdinir, cefuroxime, and cefpodoxime) for patients with a history of only mild to moderate penicillin allergic reaction, or erythromycin, azithromycin or clindamycin for those with a history of a severe penicillin allergy (eg, anaphylaxis). Recurrent acute otitis media often occurs in patients with end-stage HIV disease with severe immunosuppression[10] and may indicate infection with *S. aureus* or *P. aeruginosa*. Otitis media with effusion secondary to nasopharyngeal lymphoid hyperplasia or other nasopharyngeal masses occurs with an increased frequency in HIV patients. Persistent effusion in a patient with end-stage disease should prompt an evaluation for nasopharyngeal Kaposi sarcoma. There have also been several reports of *Pneumocystis jirovecii*–infected aural polyps associated with chronic otitis media and mastoiditis in HIV-infected patients.[4,32]

> Recurrent otitis media in the patient with end-stage HIV disease may indicate infection with *S. aureus* or *P. aeruginosa*.

Acute inflammation of the mastoid air cells can occur with any middle ear infection; however, suppurative mastoiditis, presenting with protrusion of the anterior-inferior external ear, is relatively rare. The infection can cause a subperiosteal abscess of the mastoid air cells or progress with intracranial extension to cause an epidural abscess or temporal lobe abscess. Etiologic organisms include those that typically cause acute otitis media, so the infection usually responds to standard antibacterial therapy; however, unusual organisms may occur, including *M tuberculosis* or *Aspergillus* species. Diagnosis of acute mastoiditis should prompt an evaluation for a cholesteatoma, to prevent recurrent infection. There is no evidence that HIV-infected patients have a higher incidence of complications of otitis media than the general population.

Serous otitis media occurs more frequently in HIV-positive adults than in the general population.[33] Nasopharyngeal examination should be performed for unilateral or recurrent serous otitis media to exclude benign or malignant tumors in this region.[17] Associated symptoms of nasopharyngeal carcinoma might include nasal obstruction, conductive hearing loss, acute otitis media, and recurring otitis media secretoria.[17]

Sensorineural Hearing Loss

Sensorineural hearing loss (SNHL) occurs in approximately 21% to 49% of HIV-infected patients.[10] Hearing loss is typically in the moderate or high-frequency ranges, so speech discrimination is usually not significantly affected. Middle ear disease, prior cerebral infection, and low CD4 cell count have been associated with hearing impairment.[34] Possible etiologies include primary infection by HIV of either the retrocochlear pathways or the cochlear nerve itself.[10,17] Histological examination shows that HIV-infected patients have a normal organ of Corti except for some cystic changes in the spiral ligament and stria vascularis.[35] Other causes of SNHL should also be excluded, such as central nervous system infections, neoplasms, and adverse effects of ototoxic medications.[10,17] Otic herpes zoster should be suspected in the case of sudden unilateral hearing loss.[36]

Vertigo

HIV patients may experience significant disequilibrium or vertigo, often attributed to the central nervous system. This is usually present with a multitude of other neurologic symptoms and is frequently a symptom of subacute encephalitis or HIV disease dementia complex.[33] Inner ear abnormalities have also been reported, such as subepithelial elevation of the neurosensory epithelium of the saccule and utricle and inflammatory endolymphatic precipitations[35]; however, these may be incidental findings and not effects of HIV infection.

Facial and Trigeminal Neuropathies

Facial Nerve Palsy

Unilateral and bilateral facial nerve palsy occurs with a 4.1% frequency in the HIV-infected population—a 100-fold increase from the general population (0.04%).[37–39] Facial nerve palsy may precede the detection of HIV antibodies and can therefore be an early clinical sign of HIV infection. However, facial nerve neuropathy can occur at any stage of HIV disease. Peripheral nerve neuropathy is usually self-limited and may be idiopathic or due to herpes virus infection (Ramsay Hunt syndrome).[40] Treatment of Ramsay Hunt syndrome includes acyclovir 800 mg, 5 times daily for 7 days and administration of prednisone 30 mg once daily for 5 days.[10] Facial nerve palsy also occurs in end-stage disease as a result of involvement of multiple cranial nerves due to central nervous system opportunistic infections or intracranial tumors.[10]

> Facial nerve palsy may be an early clinical sign of HIV infection.

Trigeminal Nerve Disease

Herpes zoster, caused by reactivation of latent varicella zoster virus, can occur along any branch of the trigeminal nerve. Intraoral or extraoral presentation along nerve branches is possible. The intraoral lesion will start as vesicles and progress to larger oral ulcerations. Prodromal symptoms are frequent and include headaches, malaise, photophobia, and infrequently fever. Cutaneous lesions are usually present as well. Otic zoster should be suspected in the case of sudden unilateral hearing loss.[36]

Rhinosinusitis

Rhinosinusitis has been reported to occur with a frequency of 11% to 70% in HIV-infected patients.[41–44] Impaired mucociliary clearance is reported in HIV-infected individuals and may contribute to the increased prevalence of rhinosinusitis. The typical bacterial pathogens are the same as the general population and include *Streptococcus pneumoniae*, *Haemophilus influenzae*, *Moraxella catarrhalis*, and *Streptococcus viridans* in acute infection and *Staphylococcus aureus*, *Staphylococcus epidermidis*, and anaerobes in subacute and chronic infections. Atypical organisms may also be seen particularly in patients with severely compromised immune systems. These organisms include *Alternaria alternata*, *Aspergillus*, *Pseudallescheria boydii*, *Cryptococcus*, *Candida albicans*, *Acanthamoeba castellani*, *Microsporidia*, and *Legionella pneumophila*.[44,45] Oral antibiotics, such as high-dose amoxicillin or high-dose amoxicillin/clavulanate, should be used for a total of 14 days or 7 days after resolution of symptoms. Treatment course should be extended to 4 to 6 weeks and broadened to include coverage for *Pseudomonas* and *Staphylococcus* spp. in patients with CD4 counts less than 200 cells/uL[46] or with chronic sinusitis.[47] Surgical management is often required in cases of persistent disease despite maximal medical therapy and for cases of invasive fungal sinusitis, which require debridement of infected bone and tissue.[48] Table 16–4 provides a summary of treatment, alternative agents, and alternatives in children.

Allergic Disease

Allergic Rhinosinusitis

There are reports of up to a 2-fold increase in the incidence of allergic symptoms in HIV-infected men[49] which may include perennial thick nasal rhinorrhea and nasal congestion. Rhinitis, characterized by symptoms of sneezing, nasal blockage, rhinorrhea, and itching, is the result of both humoral and cellular immune reactions to airborne allergens. There is a release of inflammatory mediators from IgE-dependent mast cells in the nasal mucosa.[50] Rhinitis may be allergic (IgE-mediated) or nonallergic (non-IgE-mediated) in origin. In HIV-infected patients, chronic nasal symptoms are common. It is often difficult to differentiate between allergic rhinitis and rhinitis from other nonallergic conditions.[51,52]

Possible etiologies of allergic disease in HIV-infected patients include a secondary polyclonal B-cell activation which produces increased circulating immune complexes with increased production of IgA, IgG, and IgE.[17] Serum IgE levels are increased in HIV-infected women, as compared to men.[53] Increased serum IgE has been associated with HIV-infected patients with increased disease progression and were strongly correlated with sinusitis severity.[53,54] Additionally, pediatric HIV-infected patients have increased serum IgE very early after HIV infection and levels continued to increase if there is HIV-associated systemic disease.[55] HIV-infected patients and atopic patients display a similar cytokine profile. Both demonstrate a Th2 cytokine profile with elevated IgE levels, increased eosinophils, and increased interleukins-4 and 5.[56]

Table 16-4. Treatment of Otolaryngological Manifestations of HIV

HIV Manifestation	Preferred Agent	Alternative Agent(s)	Alternative in Children
Oral candidiasis	Topical nystatin oral suspension or fluconazole (100 mg orally daily for 7 to 14 days)	Topical clotrimazole troches Itraconazole oral suspension	Topical nystatin oral suspension or fluconazole (3–6 mg/kg orally daily for 7 to 14 days)
Angular chelitis	Miconazole cream daily for 14 days ketoconazole cream daily for 14 days	—	—
Necrotizing periodontitis	Amoxicillin (500 mg, 3 times daily or 875 mg, 2 times daily for 14 days)	Metronidazole Clindamycin	Amoxicillin (40–45 mg/kg twice daily for 14 days)
Oral HSV	Valacyclovir[a] (1 g orally twice daily for 5 days) or acyclovir (400 mg orally, 3 times daily for 5 to 10 days)	—	Valacyclovir (for patients ≥12 years of age, dosing same as adults)
Sinusitis	CD4 >200 cells/μL Amoxicillin (500 mg, 3 times daily; or 875 mg, 2 times daily for 14 days or 7 days after resolution of symptoms) CD4 <200 cells/μL or treatment failure fluoroquinolone plus clindamycin or metronidazole	CD4 >200 cells/μL Amoxicillin-clavulante	Amoxicillin (80–90 mg/kg/day divided in 2 doses) Amoxicillin-clavulanate (90 mg/kg/day of amoxicillin, 6.4 mg/kg/day of clavulanate divided in 2 doses)

[a]Valacyclovir has been shown to have greater oral bioavailability than acyclovir.

Source: Adapted from Iacovou E, et al. Diagnosis and treatment of HIV-associated manifestations in otolaryngology. *Infectious Dis Rep.* 2012;4(1):e9.

Clinical evaluation of rhinitis includes a thorough history for allergen exposure and physical examination, with findings of pale, swollen nasal turbinates and thin, clear nasal secretions. A nasal smear may be normal or show eosinophilia. Associated clinical features may include infraorbital "shiners," scleral or conjunctival inflammation, otitis media, sinusitis, or nasal polyps. Skin-prick or allergen-specific IgE testing are a sensitive and useful means to diagnose allergy. Treatment of allergic rhinitis in HIV-infected patients is the same as in HIV-uninfected individuals. Allergen avoidance, oral and intranasal antihistamines, leukotriene antagonists, and intranasal corticosteroids are the usual forms of therapy. Drug interactions must be considered in any patient on antiretroviral therapy. Risks of treatment with intranasal corticosteroids include iatrogenic Cushing syndrome in HIV-infected patients on protease inhibitor-containing regimens.[57] Budesonide is preferred over fluticasone due to its shorter half-life.[49] Leukotriene antagonists and H1-antihistamines can be safely used.[49,58,59]

> HIV-infected patients on protease inhibitors should not be started on intranasal corticosteroids due to risk of iatrogenic Cushing syndrome.

Atopic Dermatitis

Atopic dermatitis is characterized by erythematous scaling plaques with associated pruritus. There may also be secondary lichenification or hyperpigmentation with excessive excoriations and secondary bacterial infection.[56] Alternative diagnoses such as psoriasis, cutaneous T-cell lymphoma, scabies, tinea corporis, and drug eruptions, should be considered in an HIV-infected patient with suspected atopic dermatitis. Atopic dermatitis may be confirmed with histologic evidence of epidermal hyperplasia with perivascular infiltrates of eosinophils and lymphocytes, and may be associated with elevated serum IgE levels and peripheral eosinophilia. Treatment includes avoidance of irritants, the use of emollients, topical corticosteroids, and oral antihistamines. Antiretroviral therapy also reduces the severity of the condition.[60]

The use of allergen immunotherapy (AIT) in HIV-infected patients is controversial in that there is a concern over decreased efficacy and potential for causing progression of HIV disease. Theoretically, AIT should be a safe and efficacious method of controlling atopy in HIV-infected patients.[61]

OTHER ACQUIRED IMMUNE DEFICIENCIES

Hematopoietic Stem Cell and Solid-Organ Transplantation

Patients undergoing stem cell transplantation and solid-organ transplantation require periods of extensive immunosuppression; however, they differ in the magnitude and duration of immune compromise.[62] Hematopoietic stem cell transplantation may include transfusion of stem cells derived from bone marrow, peripheral blood, or umbilical cord. Stem cell transplant recipients experience a brief period of total to near-total bone marrow ablation and complete vulnerability to infections before and during engraftment of stem cells.[62] Solid organ transplant recipients receive induction and maintenance immune suppression which varies based on the type of organ transplant.

Stem cell transplant recipients receive immunosuppressive therapy that targets cell-mediated immunity to prevent graft rejection. Patients receive these agents with varying intensity and duration depending on the type of transplantation and risk of graft-versus-host disease.[62] Therapy may include agents such as mycophenolate mofetil, calcineurin inhibitors (tacrolimus or cyclosporine), sirolimus, or corticosteroids. The degree of immune compromise depends on the types of agents being used and the time that has elapsed since transplantation. In the first month after transplantation, infections generally occur at the same sites and with the same organisms seen in immunocompetent patients, although the infections may be more severe. From 1 to 6 months after transplantation, the recipient is particularly susceptible to viral infections with EBV and CMV, as well as sinusitis, tuberculosis, listeriosis, and *P. jirvecii*. After 6 months, most patients who have not experienced graft rejection can be tapered to safer doses of immunosuppressive drugs and for the most part experience infections similar to those of immunocompetent hosts. Graft rejection, however, requires higher doses of immunosuppressive agents and can result in severe and prolonged immunocompromise.[62]

> Stem cell transplant recipients are particularly susceptible to severe bacterial and opportunistic infections, from 1 to 6 months after transplantation.

Stem cell transplant recipients are particularly susceptible to bacterial and fungal sinusitis with a reported incidence of 30%.[63] The incidence of bacterial and fungal sinusitis is lower in solid-organ transplant recipients than stem cell transplant recipients. Sinusitis may present paradoxically with only mild symptomatology due to a deficient inflammatory response; however, disease can progress rapidly to severe and invasive.[62] One study of 18 adult bone marrow transplant recipients with sinusitis revealed that the associated organism was a Gram-negative bacteria in 57% of patients, a Gram-positive bacteria in 27%, and a fungus in 17%.[64] Treatment of bacterial sinusitis should initially include coverage for all Gram-positive and Gram-negative organisms, including *Pseudomonas* and anaerobic organisms. Failure to improve after several days of antibiotic treatment should prompt evaluation for fungal sinusitis. Although the incidence of invasive fungal sinusitis is only 0.5% to 4%, the mortality can be as high as 50% to 90%.[65–67] The most common cause of fungal sinusitis is *Aspergillus fumigatus*.[62] Fulminant invasive fungal sinusitis may progress relentlessly over a course of hours to days; therefore, a high index of suspicion must be maintained, and immediate diagnostic and therapeutic management must be initiated.[62] Fungal sinus cultures are not sensitive for diagnosis, and tissue biopsy with endoscopic guidance is required. Treatment of invasive fungal sinusitis always involves aggressive medical and surgical therapy. Radical excision of all involved tissue is usually not necessary, instead surgical debridement to decrease the infectious load and eliminate anatomic barriers to sinus drainage is more likely to provide effective recovery. Treatment also involves the use of amphotericin B and immunologic restoration, such as decreasing maintenance immunosuppression or promoting neutrophil restoration with granulocyte colony-simulating factor (GCSF) or granulocyte transfusions.[62]

> First-line therapy for bacterial sinusitis in stem cell transplant recipients should include coverage for *Pseudomonas* and anaerobic organisms.

Other infections that can occur after stem cell or solid organ transplantation may include oral mucositis and candidiasis,[68] necrotizing external otitis media and brain abscess,[69] tuberculous cervical adenopathy,[70] and more rarely, pituitary abscess.[71] Hairy leukoplakia, discussed in a previous section, also develops in these other forms of immunosuppression, such as transplant recipients or after chronic corticosteroid therapy.[17] It is rare in immunocompetent patients.

Posttransplant Lymphoproliferative Disease (PTLD)

PTLD occurs with a frequency of approximately 1.2% in North America[72] and varies based on the type of transplant, stem cells compared to solid organ, and degree of cytoreductive and maintenance immunotherapy. PTLD is caused by uncontrolled EBV infection and can manifest as tonsillitis, lymphadenitis, otitis media, or sinusitis and may progress to airway obstruction. Management involves definitive diagnosis by biopsy of oral lesions or adenotonsillar tissues, antiviral therapy, and reduction of the immunosuppressive regimen.[73,74]

> Upper airway obstruction caused by tonsillitis may be a presenting symptom of posttransplant lymphoproliferative disease, which is caused by uncontrolled EBV infection.

Graft-Versus-Host Disease (GVHD)

GVHD is the process in which donor stem cells attack host tissues. This process may result in accumulation of leukocytes in the mucocutaneous tissues of the head and neck and may present as nonspecific masses or lesions on physical exam or CT scan.[73] GVHD can be mild, moderate, or severe, and can be acute or chronic. Symptoms may include rashes, blistering, nausea, vomiting, abdominal cramps, diarrhea, loss of appetite, jaundice, ulceration of the mouth and throat, or dryness of other mucosal membranes. Treatment involves the use of immunomodulatory agents such glucocorticoids, antithymocyte globulin, mycophenolate mofetil, calcineurin inhibitors, or monoclonal antibodies such as daclizumab, infliximab, or rarely alemtuzumab.

Radiation and Chemotherapy

Radiation therapy and cytotoxic chemotherapy cause increased susceptibility to infection by disrupting the normal mucosal barriers to colonization and by direct effects on immune cells.[62] Particular attention must be given to oral hygiene and treatment of seemingly minor infections, and there should be a low threshold for biopsy of suspicious lesions in patients receiving radiation and/or chemotherapy.

Head and neck irradiation causes a number of immune aberrations including decreased CD8 and CD4 lymphocyte counts, impaired lymphocyte response to mitogens, and decreased delayed skin-test reactivity to antigens.[75–77] These deficiencies typically normalize after cessation of radiotherapy.[75,76] Patients are particularly susceptible to varying degrees of stomatitis. Organisms that may contribute to worsening stomatitis include both candida and herpes simplex virus.[68,78,79]

Chemotherapy also asserts direct effects on immune cells and disruption of mucosal barriers to infection. Stomatitis during and after cytotoxic chemotherapy is common. Postchemotherapy neutropenia below 100 cells/uL is associated with an even greater risk of infection. Severe and prolonged neutropenia is associated with an increased risk of fungal infections particularly *Candida* and *Aspergillus* species.[80] *Candida* species may cause significant oropharyngeal infections, while *Aspergillus* species, particularly *Aspergillus fumigatus* and *Aspergillus flavus*, cause infections of the sinopulmonary tract.[81] Other fungal pathogens (*Mucor*, *Rhizopus*, *Malassezia furfur*) may cause invasive sinonasal disease. Aggressive therapy is required for suspected fungal sinusitis in the setting of severe neutropenia. Management includes early imaging to define the severity and location of disease, tissue sampling for culture and sensitivity, reversing of the underlying neutropenia, intravenous amphotericin B, and local debridement.[62]

> Severe, prolonged neutropenia is a risk factor for oropharyngeal and sinopulmonary fungal infections.

Corticosteroids and Other Immunomodulatory Agents

Corticosteroids

Corticosteroids cause immune suppression of the innate and adaptive immune systems through their effects on phagocyte migration and activation, and on T-lymphocyte function.[82] Corticosteroids also reduce inflammation by inhibiting prostaglandin synthesis.[62] Despite the wide range of effects on the immune system, corticosteroid-related immune suppression depends greatly on the dose and duration of therapy. Significant immunosuppression is seen with doses of 40 mg per day or 2 mg/kg per day for longer than 14 days, generally used during management of rheumatologic disease or posttransplantation regimens. Shorter durations of therapy, such as pulse corticosteroids for allergic nasal polyps or asthma exacerbations, do not usually cause a significant risk of infectious complications in most patients. Use of intranasal corticosteroids has not been associated with infectious complications[83]; however, inhaled corticosteroids used for maintenance of persistent asthma have been associated with oropharyngeal candidiasis and are infrequently associated with infectious complications.[84–86]

> Short courses of oral corticosteroids used for nasal polyps or asthma exacerbations are not a risk factor for immunologic dysfunction and subsequent infectious complications.

Other Immunomodulatory Drugs

Transplant recipients and patients with rheumatologic diseases may also receive other immunomodulatory agents including methotrexate, cyclophosphamide, azathioprine, and mycophenolate. Although these agents have different mechanisms of action, they are all antiproliferative agents that interfere with the synthesis of immunologically essential macromolecules in active and dividing B and T lymphocytes. Tacrolimus (FK506) and cyclosporine are calcineurin inhibitors that interfere with the intracellular signal transduction pathways important to T-lymphocyte function and are therefore relatively more specific for cell-mediated immunity. Although sirolimus (rapamycin) is not a calcineurin inhibitor, it acts similarly through the mTOR pathway to suppress T-lymphocyte proliferation. Antilymphocyte globulin (ATG) promotes complement-mediated clearance of lymphocytes from the circulation. Intravenous immunoglobulin can be used in the management of rheumatologic diseases to decrease immunoglobulin production through Fc receptor-mediated endocytosis by phagocytes.[62]

Increasingly, biologic agents are being used in the immune modulation of autoimmune disease. These agents include monoclonal antibodies directed against cytokines, cytokine receptors, or even specific cell surface markers. History of or current use of these agents should be considered in the evaluation of patients with rheumatologic problems who experience recurrent infections.

REFERENCES

1. World Health Organization website. http://www.who.int. Accessed September 20, 2014.
2. Centers for Disease Control and Prevention website. http://www.cdc.gov. Accessed September 20, 2014.
3. Baccaglini L, Atkinson JC, Patton LL, et al. Management of oral lesions in HIV-positive patients. *Oral Surg Oral Med Oral Pathol Oral Radiol Endod*. 2007;103(suppl):S50, e51–23.
4. Prasad HK, Bhojwani KM, Shenoy V, et al. HIV manifestations in otolaryngology. *Am J Otolaryngol*. 2006;27(3): 179–185.
5. Williams MA. Head and neck findings in pediatric acquired immune deficiency syndrome. *Laryngoscope*. 1987;97(6):713–716.
6. Dodd CL, Greenspan D, Schiodt M, et al. Unusual oral presentation of non-Hodgkin's lymphoma in association with HIV infection. *Oral Surg Oral Med Oral Pathol*. 1992;73(5):603–608.
7. De Vincentiis GC, Sitzia E, Bottero S, et al. Otolaryngologic manifestations of pediatric immunodeficiency. *Int J Pediatr Otorhinolaryngol*. 2009;73(suppl 1):S42–S48.
8. Phelan JA, Saltzman BR, Friedland GH, et al. Oral findings in patients with acquired immunodeficiency syndrome. *Oral Surg Oral Med Oral Pathol*. 1987;64(1):50–56.
9. Silverman S, Jr., Migliorati CA, Lozada-Nur F, et al. Oral findings in people with or at high risk for AIDS: a study of 375 homosexual males. *J Am Dent Assoc*. 1986;112(2): 187–192.
10. Iacovou E, Vlastarakos PV, Papacharalampous G, et al. Diagnosis and treatment of HIV-associated manifestations in otolaryngology. *Infect Dis Rep*. 2012;4(1):e9.
11. Johnson NW. The mouth in HIV/AIDS: markers of disease status and management challenges for the dental profession. *Aust Dent J*. 2010;55(suppl 1):85–102.
12. Pienaar ED YT, Holmes H. Interventions for the prevention and mangement of oropharyngeal candidiasis associated with HIV infections in adults and children. Cochrane Library. 2007; *Cochrane Review*, Oxford (3).
13. Ranganathan K, Reddy BV, Kumarasamy N, et al. Oral lesions and conditions associated with human immunodeficiency virus infection in 300 south Indian patients. *Oral Dis*. 2000;6(3):152–157.
14. Flaitz C, Wullbrandt B, Sexton J, et al. Prevalence of orodental findings in HIV-infected Romanian children. *Pediatr Dent*. 2001;23(1):44–50.
15. Winkler JR, Robertson PB. Periodontal disease associated with HIV infection. *Oral Surg Oral Med Oral Pathol*. 1992; 73(2):145–150.
16. Flaitz CM, Hicks MJ, Carter AB, et al. Saliva collection technique for cytologic, microbiologic and viral evaluation in pediatric HIV infection. *ASDC J Dent Child*. 1998; 65(5):318–324, 355.
17. Rzewnicki I, Olszewska E, Rogowska-Szadkowska D. HIV infections in otolaryngology. *Med Sci Monit*. 2012; 18(3):RA17–RA21.
18. Cherry-Peppers G, Daniels CO, Meeks V, et al. Oral manifestations in the era of HAART. *J Natl Med Assoc*. 2003; 95(2, suppl 2):21S–32S.
19. DeRossi SS, Laudenbach J. The management of oral human *Papillomavirus* with topical cidofovir: a case report. *Cutis*. 2004;73(3):191–193.
20. Reznik DA. Oral manifestations of HIV disease. *Top HIV Med*. 2005;13(5):143–148.
21. Nishio CE PV, Narahashi E. *Oral hairy leukoplakia: topical use of trichloracetic and glycolic acids*. 10th International Conference of AIDS, Yokohama, Japan. 1994.
22. Gowdey G, Lee RK, Carpenter WM. Treatment of HIV-related hairy leukoplakia with podophyllum resin 25% solution. *Oral Surg Oral Med Oral Pathol Oral Radiol Endod*. 1995;79(1):64–67.
23. Bartlett. *The Johns Hopkins Hospital Guide to Medical Care of Patients with HIV Infection*. 4th ed., 1994. Baltimore, MD: Williams & Wilkins.
24. Leao JC, Ribeiro CM, Carvalho AA, et al. Oral complications of HIV disease. *Clinics (Sao Paulo, Brazil)*. 2009; 64(5):459–470.
25. Tappuni AR, Fleming GJ. The effect of antiretroviral therapy on the prevalence of oral manifestations in HIV-infected patients: a UK study. *Oral Surg Oral Med Oral Pathol Oral Radiol Endod*. 2001;92(6):623–628.
26. Lee KC CC. Evaluation of the neck mass in human immunodeficiency virus-infected patients. *Otolaryngol Clin North Am*. 1992(25):1287–1305.
27. Patton LL. Sensitivity, specificity, and positive predictive value of oral opportunistic infections in adults with HIV/AIDS as markers of immune suppression and viral burden. *Oral Surg Oral Med Oral Pathol Oral Radiol Endod*. 2000;90(2):182–188.
28. Beitler JJ, Vikram B, Silver CE, et al. Low-dose radiotherapy for multicystic benign lymphoepithelial lesions of the parotid gland in HIV-positive patients: long-term results. *Head Neck*. 1995;17(1):31–35.
29. Mandel L, Surattanont F. Regression of HIV parotid swellings after antiviral therapy: case reports with computed tomographic scan evidence. *Oral Surg Oral Med Oral Pathol Oral Radiol Endod*. 2002;94(4):454–459.
30. Rubin Grandis J, Branstetter BFt, Yu VL. The changing face of malignant (necrotising) external otitis: clinical,

radiological, and anatomic correlations. *Lancet Infect Dis.* 2004;4(1):34–39.
31. Church JA. Human immunodeficiency virus (HIV) infections at Children's Hospital of Los Angeles: recurrent otitis media or chrocni sinusitis as the presenting process in pediatric AIDS. *Immunol Allergy Pract.* 1987;9:51–58.
32. Moazzez AH, Alvi A. Head and neck manifestations of AIDS in adults. *Am Fam Physician.* 1998;57(8):1813–1822.
33. Lalwani AKSCD. Otologic and neurotologic manifestations of acquired immunodeficiency syndrome. *Otolaryngol Clin North Am.* 1992;25:1183–1189.
34. Chao CK, Czechowicz JA, Messner AH, et al. High prevalence of hearing impairment in HIV-infected Peruvian children. *Otolaryngol Head Neck Surg.* 2012;146(2):259–265.
35. Chandrasekhar SS, Siverls V, Sekhar HK. Histopathologic and ultrastructural changes in the temporal bones of HIV-infected human adults. *Am J Otol.* 1992;13(3):207–214.
36. Gnann JW, Jr, Whitley RJ. Clinical practice. Herpes zoster. *N Engl J Med.* 2002;347(5):340–346.
37. Anders KH, Guerra WF, Tomiyasu U, et al. The neuropathology of AIDS. UCLA experience and review. *Am J Pathol.* 1986;124(3):537–558.
38. Belec L, Georges AJ, Vuillecard E, et al. Peripheral facial paralysis indicating HIV infection. *Lancet.* 1988;2(8625):1421–1422.
39. Kim MS, Yoon HJ, Kim HJ, et al. Bilateral peripheral facial palsy in a patient with Human Immunodeficiency Virus (HIV) infection. *Yonsei Med J.* 2006;47(5):745–747.
40. Chand V, Sweeney C, Agger WA. Mental neuropathy in patients with AIDS-associated malignant lymphoma. *Clin Infect Dis.* 1997; 24(3): 521–522.
41. Campanini A, Marani M, Mastroianni A, et al. Human immunodeficiency virus infection: personal experience in changes in head and neck manifestations due to recent antiretroviral therapies. *Acta Otorhinolaryngol Ital.* 2005;25(1):30–35.
42. Miziara ID, Araujo Filho BC, La Cortina RC, et al. Chronic rhinosinusitis in HIV-infected patients: radiological and clinical evaluation. *Braz J Otorhinolaryngol.* 2005;71(5):604–608.
43. Sanjar FA, Queiroz BE, Miziara ID. Otolaryngologic manifestations in HIV disease—clinical aspects and treatment. *Braz J Otorhinolaryngol.* 2011;77(3):391–400.
44. Tami TA, Wawrose S. Diseases of the nose and paranasal sinus in the acquired immunodeficiency virus-infected population. *Otolaryngol Clin North Am.* 1992;25:1199–1210.
45. Milgrim LM, Rubin JS, Rosenstreich DL, et al. Sinusitis in human immunodeficiency virus infection: typical and atypical organisms. *J Otolaryngol.* 1994;23(6):450–453.
46. Sinus and Allergy Health Partnership. Antimicrobial treatment guidelines for acute bacterial rhinosinusitis. *Otolaryngol Head Neck Surg.* 2004;130:1–45.
47. Gurney TA, Lee KC, Murr AH. Contemporary issues in rhinosinusitis and HIV infection. *Curr Opin Otolaryngol Head Neck Surg.* 2003;11(1):45–48.
48. Anon JB, Jacobs MR, Poole MD, et al. Antimicrobial treatment guidelines for acute bacterial rhinosinusitis. *Otolaryngol Head Neck Surg.* 2004;130(1, suppl):1–45.
49. Sample S, Chernoff DN, Lenahan GA, et al. Elevated serum concentrations of IgE antibodies to environmental antigens in HIV-seropositive male homosexuals. *J Allergy Clin Immunol.* 1990;86(6, pt 1):876–880.
50. Gentile DA SG, Skoner DP. Allergic rhinitis. In: Leung DYM, Sampson HA, Geha RS, et al., eds. *Pediatric Allergy Principles and Practice.* St. Louis, MO: Mosby; 2003:291–300.
51. Paul ME SW. Human immunodeficiency virus and allergic disease. In: Adkinson NF, Bochner BS, Burks AW, et al., eds. *Middleton's Allergy: Principles and Practice.* London, UK: Mosby; 2014:1175–1186.
52. Therattil JFM. Allergic rhinitis in HIV infected patients. *Immunol Allergy Clin N Am.* 1997;17:291–301.
53. Small CB, McGowan JP, Klein RS, et al. Serum IgE levels in patients with human immunodeficiency virus infection. *Ann Allergy Asthma Immunol.* 1998;81(1):75–80.
54. Small CB, Kaufman A, Armenaka M, et al. Sinusitis and atopy in human immunodeficiency virus infection. *J Infect Dis.* 1993;167(2):283–290.
55. Ellaurie M, Rubinstein A, Rosenstreich DL. IgE levels in pediatric HIV-1 infection. *Ann Allergy Asthma Immunol.* 1995;75(4):332–336.
56. Dlova NC, Mosam A. Inflammatory noninfectious dermatoses of HIV. *Dermatol Clin.* 2006;24(4):439–448, vi.
57. Kedem E, Shahar E, Hassoun G, et al. Iatrogenic Cushing's syndrome due to coadministration of ritonavir and inhaled budesonide in an asthmatic human immunodeficiency virus infected patient. *J Asthma.* 2010;47(7):830–831.
58. Been-Tiktak AM, Boucher CA, Brun-Vezinet F, et al. Efficacy and safety of combination therapy with delavirdine and zidovudine: a European/Australian phase II trial. *Int J Antimicrob Agents.* 1999;11(1):13–21.
59. Van Heeswijk RP, Bourbeau M, Campbell P, et al. Time-dependent interaction between lopinavir/ritonavir and fexofenadine. *J Clin Pharmacol.* 2006;46(7):758–767.
60. Vanker ADR. Human immunodeficiency virus and allergic disease. *Curr Allergy Clin Immunol.* 2009;22(4):168–172.
61. Marshall GD. Allergen immunotherapy in HIV infected patients. *Immunol Allergy Clin N Am.* 1997;17:303–317.
62. Sikora AG, Lee KC. Otolaryngologic manifestations of immunodeficiency. *Otolaryngol Clin North Am.* 2003;36:647–672.
63. Kennedy CA Adams GI, Neglia JP, Giebink GS. Impact of surgical treatment on paranasal fungal infections in bone marrow transplant patients. *Otolaryngol Head Neck Surg.* 1997;116:610–616.
64. Drakos PE, Nagler A, Or R, et al. Invasive fungal sinusitis in patients undergoing bone marrow transplantation. *Bone Marrow Transplant.* 1993;12(3):203–208.
65. Billings KR, Lowe LH, Aquino VM, et al. Screening sinus CT scans in pediatric bone marrow transplant patients. *Int J Pediatr Otorhinolaryngol.* 2000;52(3):253–260.
66. Choi SS, Milmoe GJ, Dinndorf PA, et al. Invasive *Aspergillus* sinusitis in pediatric bone marrow transplant patients. Evaluation and management. *Arch Otolaryngol Head Neck Surg.* 1995;121(10):1188–1192.

67. Savage DG, Taylor P, Blackwell J, et al. Paranasal sinusitis following allogeneic bone marrow transplant. *Bone Marrow Transplant*. 1997;19(1):55–59.
68. Tezcan I, Tuncer AM, Yenicesu I, et al. Necrotizing otitis externa, otitis media, peripheral facial paralysis, and brain abscess in a thalassemic child after allogeneic BMT. *Pediatr Hematol Oncol*. 1998;15(5):459–462.
69. Posey LA, Kerschner JE, Conley SF. Posttransplantation lymphoproliferative disease in children: otolaryngologic manifestations and management. *South Med J*. 1999; 92(11):1079–1082.
70. Medina JE, Frame R, Toth B, et al. Head and neck manifestations of the chronic graft vs. host disease. *Laryngoscope*. 1984;94(9):1145–1151.
71. George B, Mathews V, Srivastava V, et al. Tuberculosis among allogeneic bone marrow transplant recipients in India. *Bone Marrow Transplant*. 2001;27(9):973–975.
72. Dharnidharka VR, Tejani AH, Ho PL, et al. Post-transplant lymphoproliferative disorder in the United States: young Caucasian males are at highest risk. *Am J Transplant*. 2002;2(10):993–998.
73. Patel R, Portela D, Badley AD, et al. Risk factors of invasive *Candida* and non-*Candida* fungal infections after liver transplantation. *Transplantation*. 1996;62(7):926–934.
74. Slater JM, Ngo E, Lau BH. Effect of therapeutic irradiation on the immune responses. *AJR Am J Roentgenol*. 1976; 126(2):313–320.
75. Maca RD, Panje WR. Indomethacin sensitive suppressor cell activity in head and neck cancer patients pre- and postirradiation therapy. *Cancer*. 1982;50(3):483–489.
76. Maier H, Daniel V, Heimlich F, et al. [Cellular immune defect caused by postoperative irradiation in patients with squamous epithelial carcinomas of the upper aerodigestive tract]. *HNO*. 1995;43(6):364–370.
77. Redding SW, Gordon SM. Oral herpes simplex virus infection with cardiac transplantation. *Spec Care Dentist*. 1990;10(6):196–199.
78. Sneller M CH. Infections in the immunocompromised host. In: Rich RR, Fleisher TA, Shearer WT, et al. eds. *Clinical Immunology Principles and Practices*. London, UK: Mosby; 2008:477–491.
79. Wagner W, Alfrink M, Haus U, et al. Treatment of irradiation-induced mucositis with growth factors (rhGM-CSF) in patients with head and neck cancer. *Anticancer Res*. 1999;19(1B):799–803.
80. Rombaux P, Bertrand B, Eloy P. Sinusitis in the immunocompromised host. *Acta Otorhinolaryngol Belg*. 1997;51(4): 305–313.
81. Lueg EA, Ballagh RH, Forte V. Analysis of the recent cluster of invasive fungal sinusitis at the Toronto Hospital for Sick Children. *J Otolaryngol*. 1996;25(6):366–370.
82. Horn R, Wong B, Kiehn TE, et al. Fungemia in a cancer hospital: changing frequency, earlier onset, and results of therapy. *Rev Infect Dis*. 1985;7(5):646–655.
83. Parikh A, Scadding GK, Darby Y, et al. Topical corticosteroids in chronic rhinosinusitis: a randomized, double-blind, placebo-controlled trial using fluticasone propionate aqueous nasal spray. *Rhinology*. 2001;39(2): 75–79.
84. Babu S, Samuel P. The effect of inhaled steroids on the upper respiratory tract. *J Laryngol Otol*. 1988;102(7): 592–594.
85. Peter E, Bakri F, Ball DM, et al. Invasive pulmonary filamentous fungal infection in a patient receiving inhaled corticosteroid therapy. *Clin Infect Dis*. 2002;35(5):e54–e56.
86. Sahay JN, Chatterjee SS, Stanbridge TN. Inhaled corticosteroid aerosols and candidiasis. *Br J Dis Chest*. 1979; 73(2):164–168.

17

Allergen Immunotherapy

Ma. Lourdes B. de Asis and William R. Reisacher

DEFINITION

Allergen immunotherapy is a disease-modifying therapy that involves the repeated administration of specific allergen vaccines to patients with IgE-mediated diseases such as allergic rhinitis, asthma, and stinging insect hypersensitivity. It provides long-term relief of allergic symptoms and protection against inflammatory reactions related to exposure to specific allergens. Other terms for allergen immunotherapy include allergen-specific desensitization, hyposensitization, and the lay terms "allergy shots or allergy injections."[1,2]

> Allergen immunotherapy involves the repeated administration of specific allergen vaccines for long-term relief of IgE-mediated diseases such as allergic rhinitis, asthma, and stinging insect hypersensitivity.

MECHANISMS OF ACTION

Successful allergen immunotherapy induces immunologic tolerance, which is defined as a decrease in immediate and delayed allergen-specific responsiveness and sensitivity of end organs such as the skin, nasal and conjunctival mucosa, and bronchi[3–6] with associated humoral and cellular immune changes such as increases in $CD4^+$ $CD25^+$ regulatory T lymphocytes that release cytokines interleukin-10 and TGF beta;[7,8] and decreased recruitment and activation of mast cells, basophils, and eosinophils.[9]

Cytokines are the hormonal messengers secreted by T-cell lymphocytes, which produce either pro-inflammatory or anti-inflammatory/allergic responses. T-helper lymphocytes, a subset of T lymphocytes, are further subdivided into Th1 and Th2 cells. Th1 cells produce Th1-type cytokines that are proinflammatory and are responsible for killing intracellular parasites and promoting autoimmune responses. Th2 cells produce Th2-type cytokines that counteract the Th1-mediated microbicidal action and are associated with the promotion of IgE and eosinophilic responses in an allergic reaction, as well as interleukin-10 which is anti-inflammatory.[10]

Among the various types of allergen immunotherapy, the immunologic changes associated with subcutaneous immunotherapy have been best studied in the literature. These changes begin with the generation of allergen-specific regulatory T lymphocytes (T regs) that suppress both Th1 and Th2 responses followed by a shift from a Th2 to a Th1 allergen-specific immune response.[11,12]

Patients beginning subcutaneous immunotherapy are noted to have an increase in specific IgE antibody levels with a subsequent progressive decline to baseline and then to below baseline. However, changes in specific IgE levels have not been associated with clinical response.[13] Levels of specific IgA, IgG1, and IgG4 also increase during the course of allergen immunotherapy but have not been correlated with clinical improvement.[14,15]

Similar immunologic responses have been observed in patients who receive sublingual immunotherapy.[16] Experimental animals treated with local intranasal immunotherapy show increased production of interleukin 10 in the local mucosa but do not develop systemic immunologic changes such as the increase in specific IgG4 antibodies that is seen in subcutaneous allergen immunotherapy.[17,18]

> Allergen immunotherapy induces immunologic tolerance with associated humoral and cellular immune changes involving T lymphocytes, cytokines, mast cells, basophils, and eosinophils.

CLINICAL EFFICACY AND LONG-TERM BENEFITS

Numerous double-blind, placebo-controlled studies have demonstrated the efficacy of subcutaneous and sublingual allergen immunotherapy in adults and children for the treatment of allergic rhinitis with and without ocular symptoms[19,20] and allergic asthma.[21,22] Subcutaneous allergen immunotherapy is also efficacious in stinging insect hypersensitivity.[23,24] Subcutaneous allergen immunotherapy with aeroallergens such as pollens, animal allergens, dust mites, cockroach, and fungi have demonstrated efficacy.[25–29] Clinical efficacy has been demonstrated with outcome measures such as significant reduction in symptom and medication scores, significant improvement in quality of life scores,[30] and support by meta-analyses.[31,32] Documented long-term benefits of allergen immunotherapy include reduction in the development of new allergen sensitivities,[33] reduced risk for developing asthma in patients with allergic rhinitis,[34] and sustained disease-modifying effects as measured by symptom reduction and improved quality of life after discontinuation.[35–38]

Subcutaneous venom immunotherapy has been shown to be the most effective therapy for the treatment and prevention of Hymenoptera sting-induced anaphylaxis.[39,40]

> Allergen immunotherapy has demonstrated long-term clinical efficacy. This includes reduction in symptoms and medication use; reduced development of new allergen sensitivities; improved quality of life; and prevention of Hymenoptera sting–induced anaphylaxis.

INDICATIONS/CONTRAINDICATIONS TO ALLERGEN IMMUNOTHERAPY

Strong Indications

Allergic Rhinitis/Rhinoconjunctivitis and Allergic Asthma

As discussed previously, allergen immunotherapy has been shown to be clinically efficacious and has long-term benefits in patients with allergic rhinitis, rhinoconjunctivitis, and allergic asthma. It should be considered in these patients if they have specific IgE antibodies to clinically relevant allergens (Table 17–1). Other factors such as patient preference, adherence, medication requirements, response to allergen avoidance measures, adverse reactions to medications, and presence of comorbidities such as asthma and allergic rhinitis should be considered in the selection of patients who would benefit from allergen immunotherapy. Allergic patients with increased medication requirements, whose symptoms are not adequately controlled with medications and allergen avoidance measures and/or who have adverse reactions to medications, particularly those who have coexistent allergic rhinitis and stable asthma, would be appropriate candidates for allergen immunotherapy.[1]

Systemic Reactions to Hymenoptera Insect Sting and Flying/Imported Fire Ant Sting

Immunotherapy is indicated for patients with a history of a systemic reaction with associated respiratory and/or cardiovascular symptoms, and evidence of specific IgE to Hymenoptera venom or fire ants.[41,42] Adults and patients older than 16 years

Table 17-1. Indications for Allergen Immunotherapy

In patients with allergic rhinitis, allergic conjunctivitis, or asthma	Allergen immunotherapy should be considered for patients who have demonstrable evidence of specific IgE antibodies to clinically relevant allergens. Coexisting allergic rhinitis and asthma; and possible prevention of asthma in patients with allergic rhinitis.
Potential indication	Atopic dermatitis, if associated with aeroallergen sensitivity
Indications for allergen immunotherapy in patients with reactions to Hymenoptera stings	Patients with a history of a systemic reaction to a Hymenoptera sting (especially if such a reaction is associated with respiratory symptoms, cardiovascular symptoms, or both) and demonstrable evidence of clinically relevant specific IgE antibodies;
	Patients older than 16 years with a history of a systemic reaction limited to the skin and demonstrable evidence of clinically relevant specific IgE antibodies (patients ≤16 years of age who present with a history of only cutaneous symptoms to Hymenoptera stings usually do not require immunotherapy); and
	Adults and children with a history of a systemic reaction to imported fire ant and demonstrable evidence of clinically relevant specific IgE antibodies.
Potential indication	For large local reactions in patients who have frequent and disabling large local reactions, particularly if related to occupational exposure

Source: Reprinted with permission from Elsevier. Cox L, Nelson H, Lockey R, et al. Joint Task Force on Practice Parameters. Allergen immunotherapy: a practice parameter third update. *J Allergy Clin Immunol.* 2011;127(1, suppl 1):1–53.

old with systemic reactions to insect stings limited to the skin are also candidates for immunotherapy, but in patients younger than 16 years old with systemic reactions limited to the skin, venom immunotherapy is not always indicated.[43]

> Allergen immunotherapy should be strongly considered in patients with rhinitis, rhinoconjunctivitis, and/or asthma with demonstrable specific IgE to clinically relevant aeroallergens and are inadequately controlled with avoidance or medications, or have adverse reactions to medications. It is strongly indicated in patients with a history of anaphylaxis associated with Hymenoptera insect or fire ant sting and specific IgE to Hymenoptera insect or fire ant venom.

Relative Indications

Decreased symptom scores and medication use have been shown in patients with atopic dermatitis and aeroallergen sensitivity treated with allergen immunotherapy to a relevant aeroallergen such as house dust mites.[44,45]

Venom immunotherapy has also been shown to reduce size and duration of large local reactions to insect stings and may be considered in patients with significant disabling local reactions, particularly if related to occupational exposure.[46]

Immunotherapy Not Indicated

Allergen immunotherapy has not been shown to be beneficial in chronic urticaria and/or angioedema and is not indicated for these conditions.[1]

Subcutaneous allergen immunotherapy has also not been shown to be efficacious for food hypersensitivity. However, oral and sublingual immunotherapy for food hypersensitivity is currently being investigated and has shown some benefit.[47,48]

Contraindications

Due to the low but significant risk of severe systemic allergic reactions associated with allergen immunotherapy, alternatives should be considered in patients with medical conditions that may reduce their ability to survive a systemic allergic reaction. Examples of these medical conditions include, but are not limited to, severe or uncontrolled asthma, markedly compromised lung function, uncontrolled hypertension, and significant cardiovascular disease.[1]

> Allergen immunotherapy is currently not shown to be of benefit in chronic urticaria/angioedema and food hypersensitivity. It is contraindicated in patients with medical conditions that reduce their ability to survive an anaphylactic episode such as uncontrolled asthma.

TYPES OF ALLERGEN IMMUNOTHERAPY

Subcutaneous Immunotherapy (SCIT)

Delivery of allergen immunotherapy has traditionally been by subcutaneous injection. Conventional subcutaneous immunotherapy treatment schedules entail two phases: a buildup phase and a maintenance phase. During the buildup phase, there is a gradual increase in the allergen content of injections, usually involving 1 or 2 injections per week over a 3- to 6-month period to minimize the risk of adverse reactions in sensitized patients. Once the specified target maintenance treatment dose has been achieved, or the maximum tolerated dose for any given patient attained, treatment continues with this maintenance dose at regular intervals, usually every 4 weeks, for the duration of therapy. The maximum tolerated dose varies between individual patients and may be lower than the target therapeutic dose.[49] SCIT is currently approved by the US Food and Drug Administration for the treatment of allergic rhinoconjunctivitis and asthma in patients with pollen, pet and animal dander, cockroach, mold spores, and dust mite allergies, and in patients with stinging insect hypersensitivity.

Sublingual Immunotherapy (SLIT)

Sublingual immunotherapy involves placement of allergen extract in the form of drops or tablets under the tongue for 1 and 2 minutes which is then swallowed. This is repeated on a regular schedule varying from daily to 3 times a week over a prescribed treatment period. Compared with subcutaneous immunotherapy, sublingual immunotherapy has a significantly lower risk of systemic reactions and may be administered at home, does not require direct medical supervision or monitoring during administration of the allergen extract, and does not involve administration of injections.[50] In the United States, sublingual immunotherapy is currently FDA approved for the treatment of allergic rhinitis/asthma patients with grass and ragweed sensitization. SLIT for dust mite allergy treatment is currently undergoing clinical trials.

Other Routes

Oral Immunotherapy

Oral immunotherapy is currently in the investigational phase for the treatment of peanut, egg, and milk allergy. It involves ingestion of the concentrated food mixed in a vehicle and ingested in gradually increasing doses in a controlled setting.[51] It is not FDA approved at this time.

> Subcutaneous and sublingual immunotherapy are currently the FDA-approved forms of allergen immunotherapy in the United States. Subcutaneous immunotherapy is approved for the treatment of allergic rhinitis/asthma in patients with pollen, animal dander, cockroach, mold spores, and dust mite allergies and in patients with stinging insect hypersensitivity. Sublingual immunotherapy is approved in patients with grass and ragweed allergy.

ADVERSE REACTIONS/SAFETY

Allergen immunotherapy is generally safe and well tolerated when used in appropriately selected patients. The prevalence of severe systemic reactions with conventional subcutaneous allergen immunotherapy has been reported to be less than 1%,[52] and the rate of systemic reactions per injection with conventional SCIT schedules is 0.2%.[53] However, life-threatening, possibly fatal reactions can occur in spite of the low risk of severe systemic reactions. Severe systemic reactions have been found to occur generally within 30 minutes after an allergy injection. It is therefore recommended that patients be observed for at least 30 minutes or even longer In the physician's office/clinic after receiving an injection, and those considered at increased risk of a serious systemic reaction should carry injectable epinephrine.[54]

Risk factors for severe systemic/fatal reactions include extremely high degrees of allergen sensitivity, injections coincident with seasonal allergen exposure, a history of previous systemic reactions, and, the presence of asthma, particularly labile or severe asthma.[55,56] Other risk factors that have been identified include concomitant use of beta-blockers (and ACE inhibitors in venom immunotherapy patients), injections from new vials, and dosing errors.[57]

Large local reactions (LLRs) at the injection site are the most common adverse reaction to subcutaneous allergen immunotherapy and have generally not been found to be predictive of systemic reactions.[58] Local reactions to sublingual immunotherapy (SLIT) commonly consist of mild to moderate oral pruritus and mouth edema which usually resolve with continued treatment. No fatalities have been reported, but systemic reactions including anaphylaxis have been reported with SLIT.[59] However, eosinophilic esophagitis was reported in one patient after starting SLIT that resolved after SLIT was discontinued. SLIT is contraindicated in patients with preexisting eosinophilic esophagitis.[60]

> Allergen immunotherapy is generally safe and well tolerated, with a low risk of severe systemic reactions when used appropriately. However, severe systemic and possibly life-threatening reactions can occur, and appropriate precautions are recommended to minimize this risk.

MANAGEMENT OF ADVERSE REACTIONS/ANAPHYLAXIS

Prior to starting a course of allergen immunotherapy, informed consent should be obtained after a discussion of the benefits and risks, and possible adverse reactions of immunotherapy, with the patient consent documented in the medical record[61] (Figure 17–1).

In order to reduce the risk of systemic reactions or anaphylactic episodes, a preinjection evaluation administered prior to each allergy injection is recommended to determine whether any health changes are present that might necessitate withholding or modifying a patient's immunotherapy treatment. The preinjection evaluation should include questions related to asthma control (with peak flow measurement), beta blocker use, change in health status such as pregnancy or concurrent illness, and adverse reaction to previously administered allergy injection. Allergy injections should be held for patients with uncontrolled asthma or significant systemic illnesses such as sinusitis, pneumonia, or viral syndromes with fever and malaise.[1]

Local Reactions

Local reactions, such as redness or itching at the injection site, are the most common adverse reactions to allergy injections. These are usually managed with local treatment such as cold compresses or topical corticosteroids or oral antihistamines.[62]

Systemic Reactions and Anaphylaxis

Systemic reactions associated with allergen immunotherapy can be mild to severe. The most severe reaction is anaphylaxis. It is therefore recommended that allergen immunotherapy be administered only in a setting where physicians and health-care professionals are trained to promptly recognize and treat the early symptoms and signs of anaphylaxis and administer emergency treatment, and have policies and procedures in place that minimize the risk of anaphylaxis[1] (Table 17–2).

It is important to note that the signs and symptoms of anaphylaxis may vary from patient to patient. Epinephrine is the first-line treatment for anaphylaxis[62] and should be given early in the treatment course. There is no absolute contraindication to its administration in anaphylaxis patients. Fatalities from anaphylaxis are usually related to delayed administration of epinephrine resulting in severe respiratory and/or cardiovascular morbidity.[63] For

<Prescribing allergist/practice letterhead>

ALLERGEN IMMUNOTHERAPY PATIENT CONSENT FORM

Immunotherapy, hyposensitization, or allergy injections should be administered at a medical facility with a medical physician present since occasional reactions may require immediate therapy. These reactions may consist of any or all the following symptoms: itchy eyes, nose, or throat; nasal congestion; runny nose; tightness in the throat or chest; coughing; increased wheezing; lightheadedness; faintness; nausea and vomiting; hives; generalized itching; and shock, the last under extreme conditions. Reactions, even though unusual, can be serious and rarely, fatal. You are required to wait in the medical facility in which you receive the injections for 30 minutes after each injection. If the patient is 17 years of age or younger, a parent or legal guardian must be present during the waiting period. I verify that I (or patient) am not taking beta blocker medications or that if I am, I have discussed the risks/benefits of doing so with my physician (see information sheet).

I have read (if new patient) or re-read (if established patient) the patient information sheet on immunotherapy and understand it. The opportunity has been provided for me to ask questions regarding the potential side effects of immunotherapy and these questions have been answered to my satisfaction. I understand that every precaution consistent with the best medical practice will be carried out to protect me against such reactions. I also agree that if I have an allergic reaction to the injections that the physician-in-charge has permission to treat said reaction.

I acknowledge the fact with my signature that I am authorizing the office to bill for allergen vaccines, even if, for any reason, I decide not to initiate the allergen immunotherapy program after the vaccine has been made. Vaccines may be prepared up to 1½ weeks prior to my appointment. I agree to obtain prior authorization, if needed, from my insurance plan.

PATIENT____ DATE _______________

PARENT or LEGAL GUARDIAN_______________________ DATE _______________

As parent or legal guardian, I understand that I must accompany my child throughout the entire 30-minute wait.

WITNESS____ DATE________________

Figure 17-1. Sample Allergen Immunotherapy Patient Consent Form. Reprinted with permission from the American Academy of Allergy, Asthma, and Immunology.

Table 17-2. Actions to Reduce Immunotherapy Risk

Assess the patient's general medical condition at the time of injection (eg, recent asthma exacerbation and increased asthma symptoms).
In addition to assessing asthma symptoms, consider obtaining a peak expiratory flow rate (PEFR) for patients with a history of asthma before administration of the injection.
The intention of assessing PEFR is to alert the provider to the need for a more in-depth assessment of asthma control. If the PEFR is substantially reduced compared with the patient's baseline value, the clinical condition of the patient should be evaluated before administration of the injection.
The patient should not receive his or her immunotherapy injection if his or her asthma is poorly controlled.
Adjust the immunotherapy dose or injection frequency if symptoms of anaphylaxis occur and immunotherapy is continued.
Use appropriately diluted initial allergen immunotherapy extract in patients who appear to have increased sensitivity on the basis of history or tests for specific IgE antibodies.
Instruct patients to wait in the physician's office/medical facility for 30 minutes after an immunotherapy injection. Patients at greater risk of reaction from allergen immunotherapy (eg, patients who have previously had a systemic reaction) might need to wait longer.
Educate the patient on signs and symptoms of systemic reactions and instruct them to report symptoms immediately if in the office/medical facility or to report to his or her physician any delayed systemic reactions. The physician will then advise the patient to take antihistamines or rescue albuterol or seek further medical care if indicated.
Ensure procedures to avoid clerical or nursing errors (eg, careful checking of patient identification).
Recognize that dosage adjustments downward are usually necessary with a newly prepared allergen immunotherapy extract or a patient who has had a significant interruption in the immunotherapy schedule.

Source: Reprinted with permission from Elsevier. Cox L, Nelson H, Lockey R, et al. Joint Task Force on Practice Parameters. Allergen immunotherapy: a practice parameter third update. *J Allergy Clin Immunol.* 2011;127(1, suppl 1):1–53.

further discussion on the treatment of anaphylaxis, see Chapter 9. Because some postimmunotherapy reactions may occur when patients have left the medical facility, it is essential that all patients have easy access to antihistamines to treat any allergic symptoms, and patients should be instructed to take them at the first sign of any allergic reaction. Asthmatic patients should also have easy access to bronchodilator inhalers.

> Due to the low but significant risk of systemic reactions and possible anaphylaxis associated with allergen immunotherapy, it is recommended that measures be taken to minimize risk. These include patient education on the signs and symptoms of anaphylaxis, administration of SCIT or initiation of SLIT in an appropriate health-care setting, monitoring of the patient's reactions while on allergen immunotherapy, and early treatment with epinephrine if anaphylaxis occurs.

ADHERENCE WITH IMMUNOTHERAPY

Successful allergy immunotherapy relies heavily on the consistent administration of allergen extracts over 3 to 5 years, and this is often challenging for the patient. Adding to this challenge, the patient may not see a clear improvement for the first several months of therapy. Published adherence rates for subcutaneous immunotherapy (SCIT) vary widely, ranging from a low of 13%[64] to a high of 89%.[65] The inconvenience of weekly injections is most commonly cited as the primary reason for discontinuing SCIT.[66] Other common reasons include unaffordable cost,[67] adverse systemic reactions,[68] medical comorbidities,[69] symptom resolution,[70] and perceived ineffectiveness.[71]

Published adherence rates for sublingual immunotherapy (SLIT) vary between 30%[72] and 85%[73] over a period of 2 to 3 years. Because SLIT involves a nonroutine, self-administered activity performed at home, it may be more easily forgotten, and physicians lose the ability to monitor the proper dosing of extract. Sales data provided by two large Italian SLIT manufacturers suggest that real-world adherence may be even lower than described in published trials, with fewer than 50% of patients renewing their prescriptions after 1 year and nearly 90% discontinuing treatment by the third year.[74] Local side effects from SLIT, including oral cavity itching and swelling, were cited in multiple studies as the most common reason for missed doses or discontinuation of therapy.[75,76] Other reasons included perceived ineffectiveness,[73] difficulty following dosing instructions,[77] unaffordable cost,[78] and unpleasant taste.[79]

THE FUTURE OF IMMUNOTHERAPY

Even though SCIT remains in practice worldwide, the use of SLIT has been steadily increasing. In Europe, approximately 45% of allergists are prescribing SLIT, and in many regions, such as Scandinavia and France, it represents the majority of new immunotherapy prescriptions and is reimbursed at the highest rate.[80] In the United States, the rate of SLIT use among general allergists rose from 5.9% in 2007 to 11.4% in 2011.[81] The most common barriers to prescribing SLIT in this group included the lack of FDA approval (90.2%), the lack of established practice parameters (66.9%), and the lack of knowledge concerning the most effective dose (63.4%). However, in 2014, FDA approval was obtained for allergy immunotherapy tablets (AIT) containing either grass or ragweed allergen. The past several years have also seen some promising research in the areas of antigen modifications and alternative routes of delivery for immunotherapy.

Peptide immunotherapy, using synthetic peptides containing the B-cell or T-cell epitopes, but without IgE-binding epitopes, has been investigated. In vitro studies have shown that regulatory antigen-specific T cells (Tregs) suppress antigen-specific T-cell proliferation, induced by IL-10, which down-regulates the Th2 response to allergens.[82,83] Clinical trials have demonstrated benefits for patients treated with peptide immunotherapy for both cat and ragweed allergies.[84,85] Peptides may also be coupled to immunostimulatory adjuvants, such as viral carrier proteins or toll-like receptor agonists, which stimulate Th1 and Tregs, and suppress the Th2 response.[86] Recombinant proteins, made from allergen-encoded DNA, may be produced as either wild-type or hypoallergens by mutating the IgE binding sites. Clinical trials are underway for recombinant birch pollen (Bet v 1) using both SCIT as well as SLIT.[87,88] Like synthetic peptides, recombinant allergens can be produced in a standardized fashion, ensuring quality, consistency, and a reliable supply of antigens.[89]

Alternate routes for the delivery of allergenic proteins have also been suggested. Intralymphatic injection for antigen-specific immunotherapy (ILIT) has the potential benefits of enhanced immunogenicity, decreased systemic side effects, reduction in the treatment dose, and a decrease in the overall length of therapy.[90] In an open-label study of 165 patients with grass pollen–induced rhinoconjunctivitis, ILIT was found to induce allergen tolerance faster than SCIT (4 months versus 1 year) and was found to cause fewer allergic side effects.[91] Epicutaneous immunotherapy (EPIT) utilizes the repeated application of adhesive skin patches to effectively strip the skin of the stratum corneum, allowing penetration of the allergen into the epidermis and stimulating the release of pro-inflammatory cytokines by keratinocytes.[92,93] Oral mucosal immunotherapy (OMIT), using a toothpaste vehicle, is another promising delivery method because of the higher density of Langerhans cells in the vestibule and gingival tissues, compared to the sublingual mucosa.[94] In their 2013 position paper, the World Allergy Organization (WAO) stated that targeting the vestibule has the potential to induce enhanced immune tolerance, possibly with a lower potential for mast cell–related local side effects.[95]

SPECIFIC IMMUNOTHERAPY TECHNIQUES

Following skin prick testing (SPT), intradermal testing is often performed. This can be used after a negative SPT when suspicion remains, to determine a safe starting point for SCIT or as a vial test prior to giving an injection from a treatment vial (Figure 17–2). Intradermal testing is only done using dilutions of the concentrated extract, either 1:5 or 1:10. Blended techniques, such as modified quantitative testing (MQT), use one skin prick and one intradermal test to determine the "endpoint," or the dilution of extract at which it is appropriate to begin SCIT.[96] Intradermal dilutional testing (IDT) is another method that can be used to determine a safe starting point for SCIT.[97] This method uses six 5-fold dilutions of a concentrated extract on a standard testing board. Starting with the weakest dilution (which is referred to as the #6 dilution), progressively stronger dilutions are placed at 10 minute intervals. The first positive wheal (generally 7 mm in diameter) which initiates progressive whealing (2 mm greater in diameter than the one before) signifies the endpoint for that antigen. (See Chapter 3 for details of skin testing methods.)

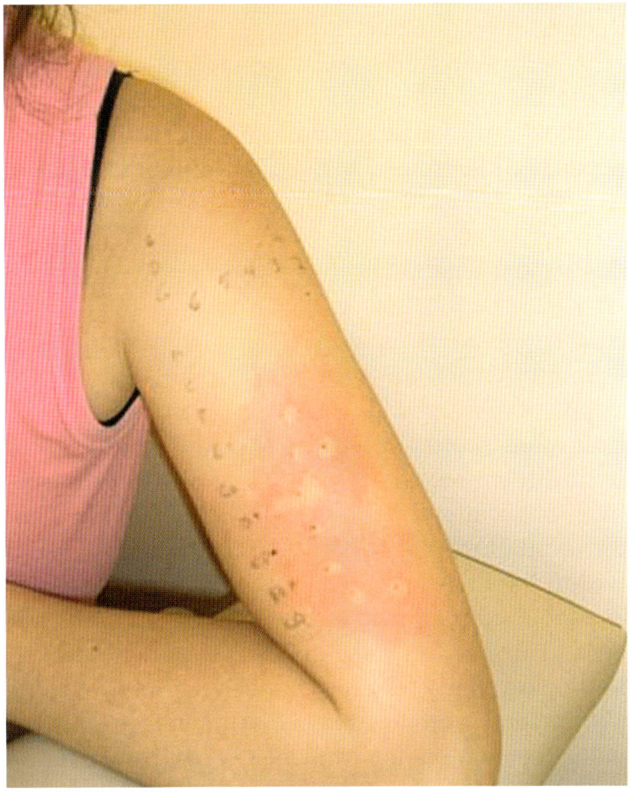

Figure 17–2. Quantitative intradermal skin testing.

As mentioned above, for subcutaneous allergy immunotherapy visits, a preinjection evaluation should be made at each visit to determine whether the patient can receive his or her allergy shot. The patient should be well, without severe asthma symptoms, illness, fever, or other recent immunization. The time interval since the last injection and any delayed local or systemic reactions following the previous injection and treatment of the reaction should be documented in the medical record. Injectable epinephrine, antihistamines, and other medications to treat acute local and systemic reactions, and anaphylaxis should be easily available and a protocol in place for treatment of early signs and symptoms of anaphylaxis.[2]

For asthmatic patients, the peak flow rate should be recorded before (and possibly after) injections. After review of the preinjection evaluation, time interval since last injection, and previous local or systemic reactions following the previous injection; the dose of immunotherapy is selected and double checked. Dosage is reduced according to established office guidelines in relation to previous systemic or local reactions, during periods of increased allergen exposure, and if there is an extended time interval since the previous injections. A record should be made of the date, dose, and volume of allergen vaccine given. Injections are given subcutaneously in the upper outer surface of the arm with sterile technique. Any immediate (0 to 30 minutes) local or systemic reactions should be recorded.

Dosing with SLIT tablets is on a daily basis, while for liquid SLIT, dosing can range from daily to weekly.[98] However, in a recent review of SLIT randomized clinical trials, daily dosing was found to be the most common schedule.[99] Although escalation periods are not universally used, a randomized, controlled open study of 43 patients receiving 3 different induction schedules (8 days, 15 days, and 20 days) demonstrated no difference in adverse events.[100] Even though preseasonal and coseasonal SLIT therapy have been found to be effective, patients receiving continual therapy for 4 to 5 years have been found to achieve long-term relief.[101] As the therapeutic window for SLIT dosing is relatively large, the monthly maintenance dose for SLIT generally ranges between 5 and 45 times the dose given for SCIT.[102]

Concentrated allergenic extracts from antigen manufacturers, typically sold in a 1:20 weight-to-volume solution, are used for liquid SLIT. These extracts are often mixed in a 10 or 15 mL glass dropper vial, but actuator pumps or small TB syringes without the needle may also be used to deliver the dose (Figure 17–3). For patients beginning sublingual immunotherapy, it is important to give the first dose in the office setting and review the home instructions very carefully with them. Tingling, itching, or swelling is very common during the first few weeks of therapy, and the escalation period may be extended for those patients who experience these symptoms. If possible, it is desirable to keep the liquid drops in the refrigerator, but if this becomes a barrier to therapy adherence, the drops may be kept outside the refrigerator away from intense heat or direct sunlight. Patients on sublingual immunotherapy should be monitored for progress and adverse events by regular office visits as well as periodic phone calls as needed.

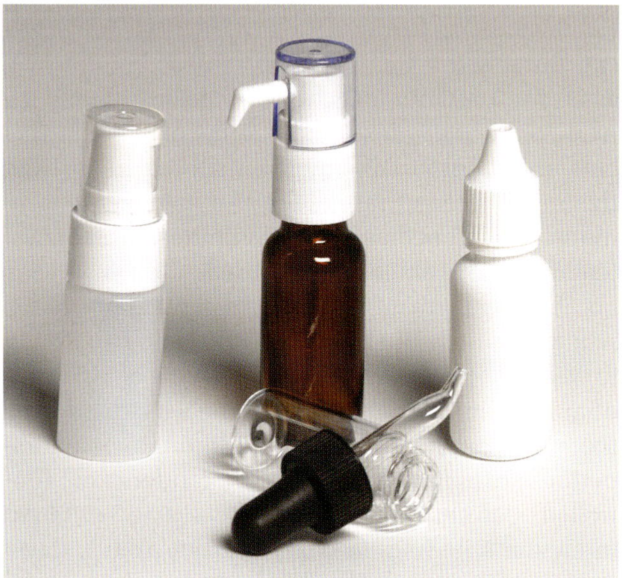

Figure 17–3. Devices for delivering allergens for sublingual immunotherapy.

PRACTICAL ASPECTS OF IMMUNOTHERAPY

Practitioner Qualifications

Supervising physicians are responsible for the competency and general oversight of the staff preparing and administering allergen immunotherapy. Because allergen immunotherapy has a small but significant risk for life-threatening anaphylaxis, competency training is required for both nursing and supervising physician personnel. State laws vary with regard to the licensure of personnel who may give injections. The various ways in which to obtain training in allergen immunotherapy preparation and administration include on-the-job training or apprenticeship with a qualified coworker or supervisor, AAOA (American Academy of Otolaryngic Allergy), AAAAI (American Academy of Allergy, Asthma, and Immunology), or ACAAI (American College of Allergy, Asthma, and Immunology), courses, workshops and seminars, and the use of references such as the "Allergen Immunotherapy: A practice parameter third update" published by the (JCAAI) Joint Council of Allergy, Asthma, and Immunology.[1] Standard operating procedures, competency standards, and forms should be developed that meet the specific needs of different practice settings and practitioners.

Allergen Extracts

Allergen extracts used for allergy skin testing and immunotherapy are complex liquid solutions consisting of dissolved allergenic proteins from pollens, dust mites, molds, animal dander, and insects mixed with diluents or solvents, additives, and preservatives. Stock allergen extracts are licensed by the Center for Biologics Evaluation and Research (CBER) within the FDA in the United States. Commercially available stock extracts are supplied by manufacturers and are used to mix individual treatment sets and to prepare allergy skin test panels (Figure 17–4).[103]

Several commonly used extracts (cat hair and pelt, dust mite, short ragweed, grass, and Hymenoptera venoms) have been standardized such that allergen content and biologic activity are consistent

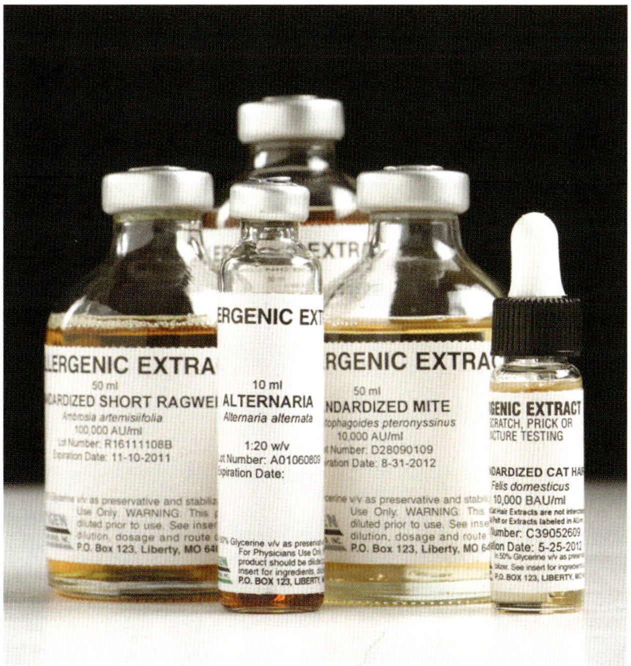

Figure 17–4. Standard stock allergen extracts.

between manufacturers and between lots made from the same manufacturer, thus reducing extract potency variability and the risk of possible adverse reactions. It is recommended that standardized allergen extracts be used to prepare immunotherapy treatment sets whenever possible. Standardization of extracts is a 2-step process that involves the selection of a reference extract and use of a quantitative skin test method to compare the manufactured extract with the reference extract. Units of potency applied to standardized extracts include bioequivalent allergy unit/mL (BAU/mL), allergy unit/mL (AU/mL), microgram protein/mL (μg/mL), or weight per volume (wt/vol).

Most allergen extracts are not yet standardized and are labeled as weight per volume (gram/mL) or protein nitrogen units (PNUs). Nonstandardized extracts can have a wide range of potencies and biologic activity regardless of particular weight/volume or PNU designation and should not be considered as equipotent.[1]

Diluents are used to keep the allergens in suspension and prevent adherence to the glass vials. Commonly used diluents include glycerin (with or without phenol) which acts as a preservative and a stabilizer, phenol which is a preservative, and HSA (human serum albumin) which acts as a stabilizer. Glycerin is bacteriostatic at concentrations greater than 20% and also inhibits proteases found in some allergen extracts. It is irritating to the skin at higher concentrations, but its preservative and stabilizing properties are diminished at lower concentrations.[103]

Allergen Immunotherapy Prescriptions

Allergen immunotherapy prescriptions specify the contents of individualized patient immunotherapy treatment sets. Table 17–3 contains recommended formulas for calculating allergen immunotherapy extract dilutions.

Standardized allergen immunotherapy prescription forms, as seen in Figure 17–5, facilitate the prescribing physician and allergen immunotherapy solution preparer to identify and focus on key elements of an optimal individualized immunotherapy prescription such as the use of effective doses of relevant allergens for each patient and avoidance of allergen combinations that may decrease overall potency. Prescription forms should contain at least 2 patient identifiers (an updated picture for the file is recommended); patient contact information; name of prescriber, date of prescription; allergen information (name, concentration, and volume); schedule of administration; and special measures such as preinjection peak flow measurements for asthmatics.[103]

Allergen Immunotherapy Solution Preparation

The supervising physician is responsible for general oversight of allergen immunotherapy solution preparation and ensuring that the immunotherapy solution preparers or compounders are trained in, and adhere to recommended allergen extract preparation guidelines (Table 17–4), the revised USP 797 pharmaceutical compounding guidelines (Table 17–5),[104] or both.[1] Both guidelines require compounding personnel to pass a written test and a media-fill test which assesses aseptic technique.

Table 17-3. Allergen Immunotherapy Extract Dilution Calculations

All dilutions can be calculated by using the following formula:	V1 × C1 = V2 × C2	
Where	V1 = Final volume you want to prepare C1 = Concentration (wt/vol or PNU) of extract you want to prepare V2 = Volume of extract you will need for dilution C2 = Concentration of extract you will use.	
Example	Solve for V2; (V1 × C1)/C2 = V2.	
To determine the concentration of an item in a mixture	1. Determine which formula you need to use. 2. Choose the numbers/fractions that will be inserted into the formula for V1, C1, V2, and C2. 3. Change all wt/vol fractions to a decimal number and insert into the formula (see below). 4. Multiply first and then divide to get the answer.	
To express concentration as a percentage	1:10 wt/vol 1/10 = 0.1 × 100 = 10% solution 1:20 wt/vol 1/20 = 0.05 × 100 = 5% solution 1:40 wt/vol 1/40 = 0.025 × 100 = 2.5% solution	
Example	V1 = 5 mL	Final volume you want to prepare
	C1 = 1:200	Concentration you want to prepare
	V2 = Unknown	Volume of extract you will need for dilution
	C2 = 1:10	Concentration of extract you will use
Add values into formula	V1 × C1 = V2 × C2	5 × (1/200) = V2 × (1/10) 5 × (0.005) = V2 × (0.1)
	V2 = (V1 × C1)/C2	V2 = 0.025/0.1 = 0.25
To determine amount of diluent needed	V1 – V2	5 – 0.25 = 4.75 mL

Source: Adapted from the Greer Allergy Compendium. Lenoir, NC: Greer Laboratories; 2005.

Example of a Completed Allergen Immunotherapy Prescription

Patient Name: Jerry Cleanex
Patient Number: 23456
Birth Date: 05/05/90
Telephone: 645-345-0987

Prescribing Physician: Dr. Ah Choo
Address: 665 Rosebud Lane
Hollywood, Fl. 33424
Telephone: 645-123-4444
Fax: 645-123-4567

Allergen Extract Content: C, R, G, T, W

Maintenance Concentrate Prescription Form

Bottle Name Abbreviations

Tree: T	Mold: M
Grass: G	Cat: C
Weed: W	Dog: D
Ragweed: R	Cockroach: Cr
Mixture: Mx	Dust Mite: Dm

Prepared by: Mary Lancet Date Prepared: 6/10/15

* **Components of mixes listed on a separate sheet**

Antigen Number	Extract Name Allergen or Diluent (Common name or Genus/species)*	Concentration and Type Manufacturer's Extract (AU, BAU, W/V, PNU)/ (50% G, Aq, Ly, AP)	Volume of Manufacturer's Extract to Add¶	Extract Manufacturer	Lot Number	Expiration Date
1	Short ragweed	1:10 w/v G (350 mcg Amb a1)	0.25 ml	Greer	12345	1/01/10
2	*D. farinae*	10,000 AU/ml G	0.5 ml	Allermed	5765	2/06/10
3	*D. Pteronyssinus*	10,000 AU/ml G	0.5 ml	Antigen labs	4222	3/24/08
4	Cat hair	10,000 BAU/ml G	2 ml	Hollister–Stier	9898	2/27/10
5	Timothy grass	100,000 BAU/ml G	0.4 ml	ALK	56789	7/09/09
6						
7						
8						
9						
10						
Diluent	HSA		1.35 ml	ALK	68597	12/12/11
Total Volume			5 ml			6/09/09

¶ **Assumes 0.5 ml injection as target maintenance dose**

$$\text{Volume to add} \quad \frac{\text{Maintenance Concentration}}{\text{Conc. Of Manufacturer's}} \quad \text{x Total Volume}$$

Maintenance concentration and subsequent dilutions reported as volume/volume (v/v) dilutions with maintenance concentration=1:1 v/v

BAU = Bioeqivalent Allergy Unit, AU =Allergy Unit
PNU=Protein Nitrogen Unit
W/V=Weight per Volume Ratio
G= 50 % Glycerinated
Aq=Aqueous, Ly=Lyophilized
AL= Alum precipitated, AP= Acetone precipitated

Figure 17–5. Sample allergen extract patient prescription. Reprinted with permission from the American Academy of Allergy, Asthma, and Immunology.

Table 17-4. Recommended Allergen Immunotherapy Extract Preparation Guidelines

1. Qualifications of extract preparation personnel	Compounding personnel must pass a written test on aseptic technique and extract preparation. Compounding personnel must be trained in preparation of allergenic products. Compounding personnel must annually pass a media-fill test, as described in Addendum A. Compounding personnel who fail written or media-fill tests would be reinstructed and reevaluated. Compounding personnel must be able to demonstrate understanding of antiseptic hand cleaning and disinfection of mixing surfaces. Compounding personnel must be able to correctly identify, measure, and mix ingredients. Compounding personnel should be appropriately trained health professionals, including, but not limited to, registered nurses, licensed practical nurses, medical technicians, medical assistants, physicians' assistants, advanced practice nurses, and physicians.
2. Physician responsibility	A physician with training and expertise in allergen immunotherapy is responsible for ensuring that compounding personnel are instructed and trained in preparation of immunotherapy with aseptic techniques as defined below and that they meet the requirements of these guidelines. Evidence of such compliance shall be documented and maintained in personnel files. The physician is responsible for providing general oversight and supervision of compounding.
3. Bacteriostasis	Allergen extract dilutions must be bacteriostatic, meaning that they must contain phenol concentrations of at least 0.25%, or if the phenol concentration is less than 0.25%, the extract must have a glycerin concentration of at least 20%.
4. Dilutions prepared in accordance with manufacturer's instructions	Allergen extracts must be diluted in accordance with the antigen manufacturer's instructions.
5. Potency	The manufacturer's expiration dates must be followed. Beyond-use dates for allergy extract dilutions should be based on the best available clinical data.
6. Mixing of extracts with high and low proteolytic enzymes	Cross-reactivity of antigens. Separation of aqueous extracts with high proteolytic enzyme activities from other extracts is recommended.
7. Storage	Extracts should be stored at 48°C to reduce the rate of potency loss or according to the manufacturer's directions. Extracts beyond the expiration date of the manufacturer are to be discarded. Storage must be in a designated refrigerator for medications and not used for food or specimens.
8. Subcutaneous injection	Allergen extracts can only be administered intradermally or through subcutaneous injection unless FDA-approved package inserts or accepted standards of clinical practice permit another route of administration.
9. Aseptic technique	Preparation of allergy immunotherapy follows aseptic manipulations defined as follows.
10. Labeling	Immunotherapy vials are to be clearly labeled with the patient's name and the beyond-use date of the vial.
11. Mixing log	A mixing log is to be kept with information on the patient's name, extract used for mixing, mixing date, and expiration date and lot numbers.
12. Policy and procedure manual	Practices preparing allergy extracts must maintain a policy and procedure manual for the procedures to be followed in mixing, diluting, or reconstituting of sterile products and for the training of personnel in the standards described above.

Table 17-4. *continued*

Addendum A. Example of a media-fill test procedure	This or an equivalent test is performed at least annually by each person authorized to compound allergen immunotherapy extracts under conditions that closely simulate the most challenging or stressful conditions encountered during compounding of allergen immunotherapy extracts. Once begun, this test is completed without interruption. A double-concentrated medium, such as from Valiteq, is transferred in ten 0.5-mL increments with a sterile syringe to a sterile 10-mL vial. Five milliliters of sterile water (preservative free) is added. This is the "concentrate." The vial is incubated within a range of 208°C to 358°C for 14 days. Failure is indicated by visible turbidity in the medium on or before 14 days.

Source: Reprinted with permission from Elsevier. Cox L, Nelson H, Lockey R, et al. Joint Task Force on Practice Parameters. Allergen immunotherapy: a practice parameter third update. *J Allergy Clin Immunol.* 2011;127(1, suppl 1):1–53.

Table 17-5. USP Chapter 797 Sterile Compounding Standards for Allergy Vaccine Preparation

1. Before beginning compounding activities, personnel perform a thorough hand cleansing procedure by removing debris from under fingernails (using a nail cleaner under running warm water), followed by vigorous hand and arm washing to the elbows for at least 30 seconds with either nonantimicrobial or antimicrobial soap and water.
2. Compounding personnel wear hair covers, facial hair covers, gowns, and face masks.
3. Compounding personnel perform antiseptic hand cleansing with an alcohol-based surgical hand scrub with persistent activity.
4. Compounding personnel wear powder-free sterile gloves that are compatible with sterile 70% isopropyl alcohol before beginning compounding manipulations.
5. Compounding personnel disinfect their gloves intermittently with sterile 70% isopropyl alcohol when preparing multiple allergenic extract as CSPs.
6. Ampule necks and vial stoppers on packages of manufactured sterile ingredients are disinfected by careful wiping with sterile 70% isopropyl alcohol swabs to ensure that the critical sites are wet for at least 10 seconds and allowed to dry before they are used to compound allergen extract as CSPs.
7. The label of each multidose vial of allergen extract as CSPs lists the name of one specific patient, a beyond-use date, and a storage temperature range that is assigned based on the manufacturer's recommendations or peer-reviewed publications.
8. Single-dose allergen extract as CSPs should not be stored for subsequent additional use.

Source: Adapted from the United States Pharmacopeil Convention. USP 797 guidebook to pharmaceutical compounding—sterile preparations, 2008. http://www.usp.org/products/797Guidebook/. Accessed March 21, 2010. NR.

It is recommended that individual patient allergen extract treatment vials and vial sets be used, particularly when allergen mixing is required. Giving allergy injections "off the board" or mixing of antigens in a syringe is not recommended due to the risk of cross-contamination of allergen extracts and an increased risk of medication errors. Stinging insect and aeroallergen extracts should not be mixed. High protease extracts (molds and cockroaches) should not be mixed with pollens. Initial treatment sets consist of a maintenance vial and a series of 10-fold dilutions. Vials should be labeled in accordance with the patient's individual prescription and should include (1) patient name and second identifier, (2) concentration of vial, (3) antigens, and (4) expiration date. Verifications of accurate prescription, labels, and color coding are required to prevent errors. Quality assurance checks throughout the preparation process are highly recommended.[103]

Allergen Immunotherapy Schedule and Dosage Regimens

Allergen immunotherapy administration involves the initial buildup phase, which may take several months, followed by the maintenance phase which lasts several years. During the initial buildup phase, the patient starts at a diluted dose of the maintenance concentrate based on the individual's allergy history and skin test reactivity. If the starting dose is too concentrated, there is an increased risk of a systemic reaction, whereas starting at too dilute a dose delays the patient from reaching the effective dose in the shortest possible time. The most commonly used schedule during the buildup phase is 1 injection, 1 to 3 times a week, as recommended in most allergen extract package inserts, with at least a 1 day interval between allergy injections. The volume of doses is increased depending on the patient's reactivity to the specific allergen extract, history of prior local or systemic reactions, and the concentration of the dose administered at that time. When the patient reaches a therapeutically effective dose of the allergen extract (Table 17–6) during the maintenance phase, this dose is repeated and the interval between immunotherapy doses can be increased from 2 to 4 weeks, or up to 8 weeks in the case of Hymenoptera venom immunotherapy.[1]

Allergen immunotherapy doses should be decreased after a systemic reaction to immunotherapy, usually to a dose that the patient had previously tolerated or even lower. Immunotherapy doses are also customarily reduced when the interval between injections is longer than recommended and may be considered during periods of increased exposure to an allergen to which the patient is highly sensitive such as the pollen season.

Cluster and Rush Immunotherapy Schedules

Cluster and rush immunotherapy schedules have accelerated buildup phases, compared to conventional immunotherapy, and are designed to enable the patient to reach the maintenance phase in a shorter period of time. Cluster schedules consist of 2 or more injections of the relevant allergen per visit given at least 30 minutes apart, and visits are 1 to 2 times a week on nonconsecutive days. This schedule allows the patient to reach a maintenance dose in 4 weeks, compared to 3 to 6 months with conventional immunotherapy. Rush schedules are even more accelerated than cluster schedules, with some schedules administered in hospitalized patients, allowing patients to reach a maintenance dose within a few days or less for aeroallergen immunotherapy,[105] and 4 hours for venom immunotherapy.[106] Patients who reached maintenance doses using cluster and rush immunotherapy schedules were shown to have symptomatic improvement. However, cluster and rush aeroallergen immunotherapy protocols are associated with a similar or an increased frequency of systemic reactions which may be reduced with antihistamine premedication. Systemic reactions with rush immunotherapy protocol were reported up to 2 hours after the final injection, and it is recommended that patients be monitored for 3 hours during rush immunotherapy with aeroallergens. However, rush immunotherapy protocols with Hymenoptera venom were not shown to have increased frequency of systemic reactions compared to conventional immunotherapy protocols.[1]

Duration of Treatment

Patients on allergen immunotherapy should be seen by their physician at least every 6 to 12 months to evaluate compliance and response to immunotherapy and monitor adverse reactions and reinforce safe administration. Patients on conventional aeroallergen immunotherapy schedules may consider discontinuing immunotherapy after a period of 3 to 5 years of treatment, but some may continue immunotherapy beyond this period. The decision to continue or discontinue effective immunotherapy must be

Table 17-6. Probable Effective Dose Range for Standardized and Nonstandardized US- Licensed Allergen Extracts

Allergenic Extract	Labeled Potency or Concentration	Probable Effective Dose Range	Range of Estimated Major Allergen Content in US-Licensed Extracts
Dust mites: *Dermatophagoides farinae* and *D pteronyssinus*	3000, 5000, 10 000, and 30 000 AU/mL	500–2000 AU	10 000 AU/mL; 20–160 mg/mL Der p 1, Der f 1[a]; 2–180 mg/mL Der p 2, Der f 2[a]; 78–206 mg/mL Der p 1, Der f 1[b]; 13–147 mg/mL Der p 2, Der f 2[b]
Cat hair	5000 and 10 000 BAU/mL	1000–4000 BAU	10 000 BAU/mL; 20–50 mg/mL Fel d 1[ac]; 30–100 mg/mL cat albumin[d]
Cat pelt	5000–10 000 BAU/mL	1000–4000 BAU	10 000 BAU/mL; 20–50 mg/mL Fel d 1[ac]; 400–2000 mg/mL cat albumin[d]
Grass, standardized	100 000 BAU/mL	1000–4000 BAU	100 000 BAU/mL; 425–1100 mg/mL Phl p 5[a]; 506–2346 mg/mL group 1[e]
Bermuda	10 000 BAU/mL	300–1500 BAU	10 000 BAU/mL; 141–422 Cyn d 1 mg/mL[a]
Short ragweed	1:10, 1:20 wt/vol, 100 000 AU/mL	6–12 mg of Amb a 1 or 1000–4000 AU	1:10 wt/vol 300 mg/mL Amb a 1[c]; concentration of Amb a 1 is on the label of wt/vol extracts
Nonstandardized AP Dog	1:100 wt/vol	15 mg of Can f 1	80–400 mg/mL Can f1 10–20 mg/mL dog albumin[f]
Nonstandardized extract, dog	1:10 and 1:20 wt/vol	15 mg of Can f 1	0.5–10 mg/mL Can f 1[b]; <12–1500 mg/mL dog albumin[f]
Allergenic extract	Labeled potency or concentration	Probable effective dose range	Range of estimated major allergen content in US-licensed extracts
Nonstandardized extracts, pollen	1:10 to 1:40 wt/vol or 10 000–40 000 PNU/mL	0.5 mL of 1:100 or 1:200 wt/vol	NA
Nonstandardized extracts: mold/fungi, cockroach	1:10 to 1:40 wt/vol or 10 000–40 000 PNU/mL	Highest tolerated dose	NA
Hymenoptera venom	100 mg/mL single venom; 300 mg/mL in mixed vespid extract	50–200 mg of each venom	100–300 mg/mL of venom protein
Imported fire ant	1:10 to 1:20 wt/vol whole-body extract	0.5 mL of a 1:100 wt/vol to 0.5 mL of a 1:10 wt/vol extract	NA

Note. *NA* = Information not available.

[a]ALK-Abello ELISA.

[b]Indoor Biotechnology ELISA.

[c]FDA radial immunodiffusion assay.

[d]Greer Radial Immunodiffusion assay.

[e]Greer ELISA.

[f]Hollister-Stier ELISA using Innovative Research, Inc, reagents.

Source: Cox L, Nelson H, Lockey R, et al. Joint Task Force on Practice Parameters. Allergen immunotherapy: a practice parameter third update. *J Allergy Clin Immunol.* 2011;127(1, suppl 1):1–53. Reprinted with permission from Elsevier Inc tailored to the individual patient because some patients have sustained clinical remission after discontinuing immunotherapy, and others may relapse. Factors to consider in the decision to discontinue immunotherapy include severity of disease, treatment benefits, and convenience. The decision to continue or discontinue immunotherapy must be reached after a thorough discussion between the physician and patient of these factors and the risks and benefits of continuing or discontinuing immunotherapy.[1]

In contrast to conventional aeroallergen immunotherapy, it is recommended that patients receive stinging insect/Hymenoptera venom immunotherapy for at least 5 years or more. Patients at high risk of relapse after discontinuing venom immunotherapy include those with severe systemic sting reactions, increased baseline serum tryptase levels, a history of a systemic reaction to venom immunotherapy, and honeybee venom allergy. There are currently no specific tests available that identify patients at risk of relapsing after discontinuing venom immunotherapy. As with aeroallergen immunotherapy, the decision to continue or discontinue venom immunotherapy should be made after a discussion of the risks and benefits between the patient and prescribing physician.[1]

Use of Premedication and Omalizumab with Allergen Immunotherapy

Premedication with antihistamines may reduce the frequency of systemic reactions associated with conventional SCIT; however, there are concerns that antihistamines taken before an immunotherapy injection may mask the warning signs of an impending systemic reaction and thus delay appropriate treatment. It should therefore be noted in the chart whether a patient did or did not take an antihistamine on the day of his or her immunotherapy injection, and patients should be instructed to either consistently take their prescribed antihistamine or avoid it on the day of their immunotherapy injections. The addition of epinephrine or corticosteroids to allergen immunotherapy extracts is not recommended because these may delay the onset of a systemic reaction beyond the usual 30 minute observation period in the physician's office. The use of oral antihistamines alone has been shown to reduce local and systemic reactions in rush venom immunotherapy protocols.[1]

Omalizumab is a recombinant, DNA-derived, humanized monoclonal antibody that binds IgE and is approved for the treatment of asthma and chronic urticaria. When used as a pretreatment prior to cluster and rush immunotherapy protocols, omalizumab has been shown to improve asthma and allergic rhinitis symptoms and significantly reduce risk of anaphylaxis. There is also evidence that it may improve tolerability of immunotherapy in high-risk patients such as those with systemic mastocytosis or those who are very sensitive to bee venom.[1]

Special Populations

Allergen immunotherapy is not usually initiated in pregnant patients due to concerns about the risk of systemic reactions to immunotherapy and the effects of resultant treatment for systemic reactions on the mother and the fetus. An exception may be considered in case of a high-risk condition such as anaphylaxis due to Hymenoptera hypersensitivity. Allergen immunotherapy maintenance doses may be continued during pregnancy. When a patient on immunotherapy reports she is pregnant, the immunotherapy dose is not usually increased till after delivery.[1]

Allergen immunotherapy is not contraindicated in patients with immunodeficiency and autoimmune disorders. Benefits and risks must be considered for these patients on an individual basis. Aeroallergen immunotherapy may be considered in patients with early to middle HIV disease (CD4 count >400 cells/ mL, no plasma HIV viremia, and no history of opportunistic infections or other AIDS-associated pathology).[107]

Figure 17–6 summarizes the various important steps in evaluating, starting, and maintaining a patient on a successful allergen immunotherapy program.

SUMMARY

Allergy immunotherapy is an effective, disease-modifying therapy that involves the repeated administration of specific allergen vaccines to patients with

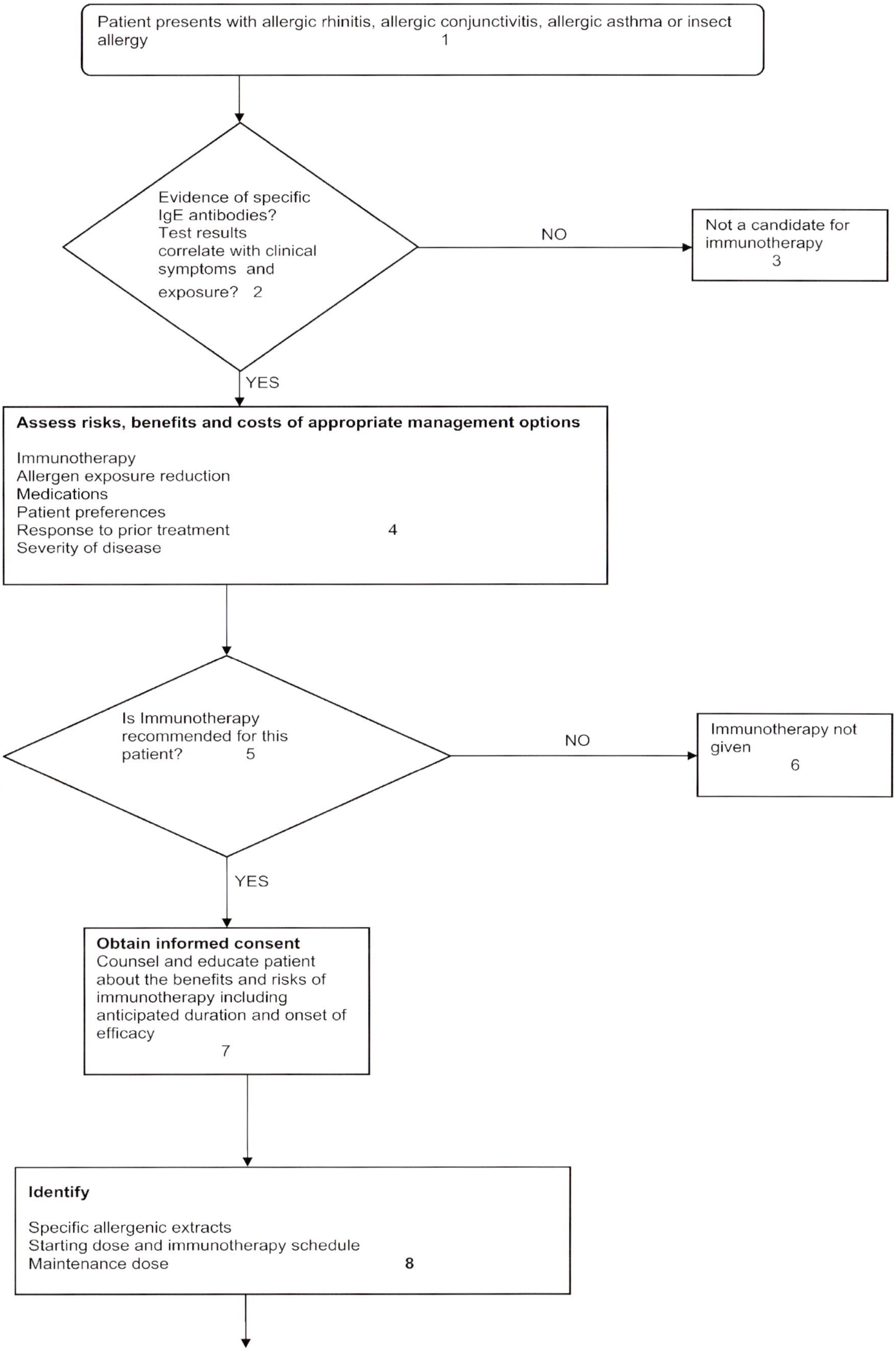

Figure 17-6. Algorithm for immunotherapy patient selection, allergen administration and patient monitoring. *continues*

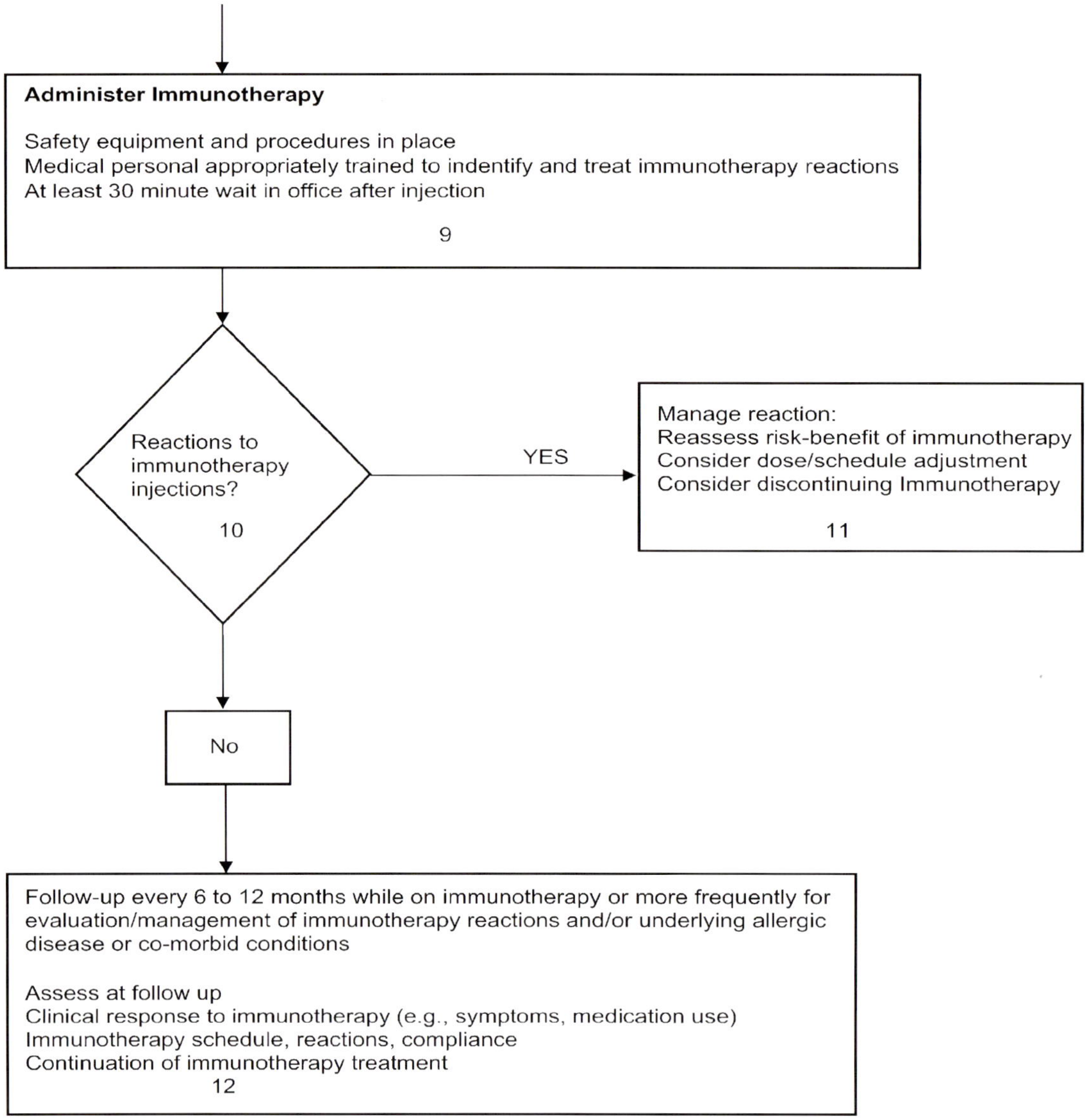

Figure 17–6. *continued* Reprinted with permission from Elsevier. Cox L, Nelson H, Lockey R, et al. Joint Task Force on Practice Parameters. Allergen immunotherapy: a practice parameter third update. *J Allergy Clin Immunol.* 2011;127(1, suppl 1):1–53.

IgE-mediated diseases. It is indicated in allergic rhinitis-conjunctivitis, allergic asthma, and stinging insect hypersensitivity.

It is currently FDA approved to be administered via subcutaneous injection or sublingually.

Allergen immunotherapy is safe and well tolerated in appropriately selected patients, but severe systemic, possibly fatal reactions may still occur. It is therefore recommended that allergy immunotherapy be administered by physicians and healthcare professionals trained to promptly recognize and treat the early symptoms and signs of anaphylaxis and administer emergency treatment, and have policies and procedures in place that minimize the risk of severe systemic reactions. Patients should be educated on the signs and symptoms of systemic reactions and instructed to report symptoms immediately to their physician.

REFERENCES

1. Cox L, Nelson H, Lockey R, et al. Joint Task Force on Practice Parameters. Allergen immunotherapy: a practice parameter third update. *J Allergy Clin Immunol*. 2011; 127(1, suppl 1):1–53.
2. Canonica GW, Durham SR. Allergen immunotherapy: a synopsis. World Allergy Organization Allergy Diseases Resource Center. August 2004. http://www.worldallergy.org/professional/allergic_diseases_center/immunotherapy/immunotherapysynopsis.php. Accessed January 11, 2015.
3. Bousquet J, Maasch H, Martinot B, Hejjaoui A, Wahl R, Michel FB. Double-blind, placebo-controlled immunotherapy with mixed grass-pollen allergoids. II. Comparison between parameters assessing the efficacy of immunotherapy. *J Allergy Clin Immunol*. 1988;82(3, pt 1): 439–446.
4. Van Bever HP, Bosmans J, De Clerck LS, Stevens WJ. Modification of the late asthmatic reaction by hyposensitization in asthmatic children allergic to house dust mite (*Dermatophagoides pteronyssinus*) or grass pollen. *Allergy*. 1988;43(5):378–385.
5. Iliopoulos O, Proud D, Adkinson NF Jr, et al. Effects of immunotherapy on the early, late, and rechallenge nasal reaction to provocation with allergen: changes in inflammatory mediators and cells. *J Allergy Clin Immunol*. 1991;87(4):855–866.
6. Nish WA, Charlesworth EN, Davis TL, et al. The effect of immunotherapy on the cutaneous late phase response to antigen. *J Allergy Clin Immunol*. 1994;93(2):484–493.
7. Francis JN, Till SJ, Durham SR. Induction of IL-101CD41CD251 T cells by grass pollen immunotherapy. *J Allergy Clin Immunol*. 2003;111(6):1255–1261.
8. Jutel M, Akdis M, Budak F, et al. IL-10 and TGF-beta cooperate in the regulatory T cell response to mucosal allergens in normal immunity and specific immunotherapy. *Eur J Immunol*. 2003;33(5):1205–1214.
9. Till SJ, Francis JN, Nouri-Aria K, Durham SR. Mechanisms of immunotherapy review. *J Allergy Clin Immunol*. 2004;113(6):1025–1034.
10. Berger A. TH1 and TH2 responses: what are they? *BMJ*. 321(7258):424.
11. Till SJ, Durham SR. Immunological responses to allergen immunotherapy. *Clin Allergy Immunol*. 2004;18:85–104.
12. Hamid QA, Schotman E, Jacobson MR, Walker SM, Durham SR. Increases in IL-12 messenger RNA1 cells accompany inhibition of allergen-induced late skin responses after successful grass pollen immunotherapy. *J Allergy Clin Immunol*. 1997;99(2):254–260.
13. Bousquet J, Braquemond P, Feinberg J, Guerin B, Maasch H, Michel FB. Specific IgE response before and after rush immunotherapy with a standardized allergen or allergoid in grass pollen allergy. *Ann Allergy*. 1986;56(6):456–459,
14. Jutel M, Akdis M, Budak F, et al. IL-10 and TGF-beta cooperate in the regulatory T cell response to mucosal allergens in normal immunity and specific immunotherapy. *Eur J Immunol*. 2003;33(5):1205–1214.
15. Ewan PW, Deighton J, Wilson AB, Lachmann PJ. Venom-specific IgG antibodies in bee and wasp allergy: lack of correlation with protection from stings. *Clin Exp Allergy*. 1993;(8);23:647–660.
16. Canonica GW, Cox L, Pawankar R, et al. Sublingual immunotherapy World Allergy Organization position paper 2013 update. *World Allergy Organ J*. 2014;7(1):6. doi:10.1186/1939-4551-7-6.
17. Barbey C, Donatelli-Dufour N, Batard P, et al. Intranasal treatment with ovalbumin but not the major T cell epitope ovalbumin 323-339 generates interleukin-10 secreting T cells and results in the induction of allergen systemic tolerance. *Clin Exp Allergy*. 2004;34(4):654–662.
18. Giannarini L, Maggi E. Decrease of allergen specific T cell response induced by nasal immunotherapy. *Clin Exp Allergy*. 1998;28:404–412.
19. Ross RN, Nelson HS, Finegold I. Effectiveness of specific immunotherapy in the treatment of allergic rhinitis: an analysis of randomized, prospective, single- or double-blind, placebo-controlled studies. *Clin Ther*. 2000;22(3): 342–345.
20. Lowell FC, Franklin W. A double-blind study of the effectiveness and specificity of injection therapy in ragweed hay fever. *N Engl J Med*. 1965;273(13):675–679.
21. Ross RN, Nelson HS, Finegold I. Effectiveness of specific immunotherapy in the treatment of asthma: a meta-analysis of prospective, randomized, double-blind, placebo-controlled studies. *Clin Ther*. 2000;22(3):329–341.
22. Abramson MJ, Puy RM, Weiner JM. Allergen immunotherapy for asthma. *Cochrane Database Syst Rev*. 2003;4: CD001186.
23. Ross RN, Nelson HS, Finegold I. Effectiveness of specific immunotherapy in the treatment of hymenoptera venom hypersensitivity: a meta-analysis. *Clin Ther*. 2000; 22(3):351–358.
24. Hunt KJ, Valentine MD, Sobotka AK, Benton AW, Amodio FJ, Lichtenstein LM. A controlled trial of immunotherapy in insect hypersensitivity. *N Engl J Med*. 1978; 299(4):157–161.
25. Ortolani C, Pastorello EA, Incorvaia C, et al. A double-blind, placebo-controlled study of immunotherapy with an alginate-conjugated extract of *Parietaria judaica* in patients with *Parietaria* hay fever. *Allergy*. 1994;49(1): 13–21.
26. Horst M, Hejjaoui A, Horst V, Michel FB, Bousquet J. Double-blind, placebo-controlled rush immunotherapy with a standardized *Alternaria* extract. *J Allergy Clin Immunol*. 1990;85(2):460–472.
27. Haugaard L, Dahl R. Immunotherapy in patients allergic to cat and dog dander. I. Clinical results. *Allergy*. 1992;47(3):249–245.
28. Tabar AI, Echechipia S, Garcia BE, et al. Double-blind comparative study of cluster and conventional immunotherapy schedules with *Dermatophagoides pteronyinus*. *J Allergy Clin Immunol*. 2005;116(1):109–118.

29. Kang BC, Johnson J, Morgan C, Chang JL. The role of immunotherapy in cockroach asthma. *J Asthma.* 1988; 25(4):205–218.
30. Ross RN, Nelson HS, Finegold I. Effectiveness of specific immunotherapy in the treatment of allergic rhinitis: an analysis. *Clin Ther.* 2000;22(3):342–350.
31. Ross RN, Nelson HS, Finegold I. Effectiveness of specific immunotherapy in the treatment of asthma: a meta-analysis of prospective, randomized, double-blind, placebo-controlled studies. *Clin Ther.* 2000;22(3):329–341.
32. Abramson MJ, Puy RM, Weiner JM. Injection allergen immunotherapy for asthma. *Cochrane Database Syst Rev.* 2010;8:CD001186.
33. Inal A, Altintas DU, Yilmaz M, Karakoc GB, Kendirli SG, Sertdemir Y. Prevention of new sensitizations by specific immunotherapy in children with rhinitis and/or asthma monosensitized to house dust mite. *J Investig Allergol Clin Immunol.* 2007;17(2):85–91.
34. Pajno GB, Barberio G, De Luca F, Morabito L, Parmiani S. Prevention of new sensitizations in asthmatic children monosensitized to house dust mite by specific immunotherapy. A six-year follow-up study. *Clin Exp Allergy.* 2001;31(7):1392–1397.
35. Durham SR, Walker SM, Varga EM, et al. Long-term clinical efficacy of grass-pollen immunotherapy. *N Engl J Med.* 1999;341(7):468–475,
36. Eng PA, Borer-Reinhold M, Heijnen IAFM, Gnehm HPE. Twelve-year follow-up after discontinuation of preseasonal grass pollen immunotherapy in childhood. *Allergy.* 2006;61(2):198–201.
37. Jacobsen L, Nuchel Petersen B, Wihl JA, Lowenstein H, Ipsen H. Immunotherapy with partially purified and standardized tree pollen extracts. IV. Results from long-term (6-year) follow-up. *Allergy.* 1997;52(9):914–920.
38. Eifan AO, Shamji MH, Durham SR. Long-term clinical and immunological effects of allergen immunotherapy. *Curr Opin Allergy Clin Immunol.* 2011 Dec;11(6):586–593.
39. Bonifazi F, Jutel M, Bilò BM, et al. The EAACI Interest Group on Insect Venom Hypersensitivity: prevention and treatment of hymenoptera venom allergy: guidelines for clinical practice. *Allergy.* 2005;60(12):1459–1470.
40. Ross RN, Nelson HS, Finegold I. Effectiveness of specific immunotherapy in the treatment of hymenoptera venom hypersensitivity: a meta-analysis. *Clin Ther.* 2000;22(3):351–358.
41. Reisman RE. Insect stings. *N Engl J Med.* 1994;331(8): 523–527.
42. Valentine MD. Allergy to stinging insects. *Ann Allergy.* 1993;70(6):427–432.
43. Valentine MD, Schuberth KC, Kagey-Sobotka A, et al. The value of immunotherapy with venom in children with allergy to insect stings. *N Engl J Med.* 1990;323(23): 1601–1603.
44. Werfel T, Breuer K, Rueff F, et al. Usefulness of specific immunotherapy in patients with atopic dermatitis and allergic sensitization to house dust mites: a multi-centre, randomized, dose-response study. *Allergy.* 2006;61(2): 202–205.
45. Novak N. Allergen specific immunotherapy for atopic dermatitis. *Curr Opin Allergy Clin Immunol.* 2007;7(6): 542–546.
46. Golden DB, Kelly D, Hamilton RG, Craig TJ. Venom immunotherapy reduces large local reactions to insect stings. *J Allergy Clin Immunol.* 2009;123(6):1371–1375.
47. Enrique E, Malek T, Pineda F, et al. Sublingual immunotherapy for hazelnut food allergy: a follow-up study. *Ann Allergy Asthma Immunol.* 2008;100(3):283–284.
48. Jones SM, Pons L, Roberts JL, et al. Clinical efficacy and immune regulation with peanut oral immunotherapy. *J Allergy Clin Immunol.* 2009;124(2):292–300. 300.e1-97. doi:10.1016/j.jaci.2009.05.022.
49. Fitzhugh DJ, Lockey RF. History of immunotherapy: the first 100 years. *Immunol Allergy Clin North Am.* 2011; 31(2):149–157.
50. Lin SY, Erekosima N, Kim JM, et al. Sublingual immunotherapy for the treatment of allergic rhinoconjunctivitis and asthma: systematic review. *JAMA.* 2013;309(12): 1278–1288.
51. Nowak-Wegrzyn A, Fiocchi A. Is oral immunotherapy the cure for food allergies? *Current Opin All Clin Immunol.* 2010;10(3):214–219. doi: 10.1097/ACI.0b013e32833 99404.
52. Bernstein DI, Epstein T, Murphy-Berendts K, Liss GM. Surveillance of systemic reactions to subcutaneous immunotherapy injections: year 1 outcomes of the ACAAI and AAAAI collaborative study. *Ann Allergy Asthma Immunol.* 2010;104(6):530–535. doi:10.1016/j.anai .2010.04.008.
53. Cox L, Larenas-Linnemann D, Lockey RF, Passalacqua G. Speaking the same language: the World Allergy Organization Subcutaneous Immunotherapy Systemic Reaction Grading System. *J Allergy Clin Immunol.* 2010; 125(3):569–574. doi: 10.1016/j.jaci.2009.10.060.
54. DaVeiga SP, Caruso K, Golubski S, Lang DM. A retrospective survey of systemic reaction from allergen immunotherapy. *J Allergy Clin Immunol.* 2008;121(suppl): S124.
55. Reid MJ, Lockey RF, Turkeltaub PC, Platts-Mills TAE. Survey of fatalities from skin testing and immunotherapy 1985-1998. *J Allergy Clin Immunol.* 1993;92(1, pt 1): 6–15.
56. Amin HS, Liss GM, Bernstein DI. Evaluation of near-fatal reactions to allergen immunotherapy injections. *J Allergy Clin Immunol.* 2006;1170(1):169–175.
57. Allergen immunotherapy: therapeutic vaccines for allergic diseases. Geneva: January 27–29, 1997. *Allergy.* 1998; 53(44, suppl):1–42.
58. Kelso JM. The rate of systemic reactions to immunotherapy injections is the same whether or not the dose is reduced after a local reaction. *Ann Allergy Asthma Immunol.* 2004;92(2):225–227.
59. Lombardi C, Incorvaia C, Braga M, Senna G, Canonica GW, Passalacqua G. Administration regimens for sublingual immunotherapy to pollen allergens: what do we know? *Allergy.* 2009; 64(6):849–854. doi: 10.1111/j.1398-9995.2009.02063.x.

60. Miehlke S, Alpan O, Schroder S, Straumann A. Induction of eosinophilic esophagitis by sublingual pollen immunotherapy. *Case Rep Gastroenterol.* 2013;7(3):363–368.
61. American Academy of Allergy, Asthma, and Immunology. Immunotherapy Consent and Instruction 2011. http://www.aaaai.org/Aaaai/media/MediaLibrary/PDF%20Documents/Immunotherapy%20Forms/Immunotherapy%20Consent%20and%20Instruction/5a-2011-patient-consent-for-immunotherapy.pdf. Accessed January 11, 2015.
62. Frew AJ. Allergen immunotherapy. *J Allergy Clin Immunol.* 2010;125(2, suppl 2):S306–S313. doi: 10.1016/j.jaci.2009.10.064.
63. Kemp SF, Lockey RF, Simons FE. Epinephrine: the drug of choice for anaphylaxis. A statement of the World Allergy Organization. *Allergy.* 2008;63:1061–1070, IV.
64. Donahue JG, Greineder DK, Connor-Lacke L, et al. Utilization and cost of immunotherapy for allergic asthma and rhinitis. *Ann Allergy Asthma Immunol.* 1999;82:339–347.
65. Tinkelman D, Smith F, Cole WQ, 3rd, et al. Compliance with an allergen immunotherapy regime. *Ann Allergy Asthma Immunol.* 1995;74:241–246.
66. Hsu NM, Reisacher WR. A comparison of attrition rates in patients undergoing sublingual immunotherapy vs subcutaneous immunotherapy. *Int Forum Allergy Rhinol.* 2012;2:280–284.
67. Pajno GB, Vita D, Caminiti L, et al. Children's compliance with allergen immunotherapy according to administration routes. *J Allergy Clin Immunol.* 2005;116:1380–1381.
68. Rhodes BJ. Patient dropouts before completion of optimal dose, multiple allergen immunotherapy. *Ann Allergy Asthma Immunol.* 1999;82:281–286.
69. More DR, Hagan LL. Factors affecting compliance with allergen immunotherapy at a military medical center. *Ann Allergy Asthma Immunol.* 2002;88:391–394.
70. Ruiz FJ, Jimenez A, Cocoletzi J, et al. [Compliance with and abandonment of immunotherapy]. *Rev Alerg Mex.* 1997;44:42–44.
71. Lower T, Henry J, Mandik L, et al. Compliance with allergen immunotherapy. *Ann Allergy.* 1993;70:480–482.
72. Vita D, Caminiti L, Ruggeri P, et al. Sublingual immunotherapy: adherence based on timing and monitoring control visits. *Allergy.* 2010;65:668–669.
73. Marogna M, Spadolini I, Massolo A, et al. Randomized controlled open study of sublingual immunotherapy for respiratory allergy in real-life: clinical efficacy and more. *Allergy.* 2004;59:1205–1210.
74. Senna G, Lombardi C, Canonica GW, et al. How adherent to sublingual immunotherapy prescriptions are patients? The manufacturers' viewpoint. *J Allergy Clin Immunol.* 2010;126:668–669.
75. Roder E, Berger MY, de Groot H, et al. Sublingual immunotherapy in youngsters: adherence in a randomized clinical trial. *Clin Exp Allergy.* 2008;38:1659–1667.
76. Chang H, Han DH, Mo JH, et al. Early compliance and efficacy of sublingual immunotherapy in patients with allergic rhinitis for house dust mites. *Clin Exp Otorhinolaryngol.* 2009;2:136–140.
77. Lombardi C, Gani F, Landi M, et al. Quantitative assessment of the adherence to sublingual immunotherapy. *J Allergy Clin Immunol.* 2004;113:1219–1220.
78. Passalacqua G, Musarra A, Pecora S, et al. Quantitative assessment of the compliance with once-daily sublingual immunotherapy in children (EASY project: evaluation of a novel SLIT formulation during a year). *Pediatr Allergy Immunol.* 2007;18:58–62.
79. Pajno GB, Caminiti L, Crisafulli G, et al. Adherence to sublingual immunotherapy in preschool children. *Pediatr Allergy Immunol.* 2012;23:688–689.
80. Cox L, Jacobsen L. Comparison of allergen immunotherapy practice patterns in the United States and Europe. *Ann Allergy Asthma Immunol.* 2009;103:451–460.
81. Sikora JM, Tankersley MS. Perception and practice of sublingual immunotherapy among practicing allergists in the United States: a follow-up study. *Ann Allergy Asthma Immunol.* 2013;110:194–197.
82. Tanabe S. Epitope peptides and immunotherapy. *Curr Protein Pept Sci.* 2007;8:109–118.
83. Moldaver D, Larche M. Immunotherapy with peptides. *Allergy.* 2011;66:784–791.
84. Patel D, Couroux P, Hickey P, et al. Fel d 1-derived peptide antigen desensitization shows a persistent treatment effect 1 year after the start of dosing: a randomized, placebo-controlled study [published online September 13, 2012]. *J Allergy Clin Immunol.* 2013 Jan;131(1):103–109. e1-7. doi:10.1016/j.jaci.2012.07.028.
85. Creticos PS, Schroeder JT, Hamilton RG, et al. Immunotherapy with a ragweed-toll-like receptor 9 agonist for vaccine for allergic rhinitis. *N Engl J Med.* 2006;355: 1445–1455.
86. Fonseca DE, Kline JN. Use of CpG oligonucleotides in treatment of asthma and allergic disease. *Adv Drug Deliv Rev.* 2009;61:256–262.
87. Pauli G, Larsen TH, Rak S, et al. Efficacy of recombinant birch pollen vaccine for the treatment of birch-allergic rhinoconjunctivitis. *J Allergy Clin Immunol.* 2008;122: 951–960.
88. Larenas-Linnemann D. Oralair Birch, a recombinant major birch pollen allergen tablet for sublingual immunotherapy of allergic rhinitis caused by birch pollen. *Curr Opin Investig Drugs.* 2010;11:586–596.
89. Larche, M. T Cell epitope-based allergy vaccines. *Curr Top Microbiol Immunol.* 2011;352:107–119.
90. Von Moos S, Kundig TM, Senti G. Novel administration routes for allergen-specific immunotherapy: a review of intralymphatic and epicutaneous allergen-specific immunotherapy. *Immunol Allergy Clin N Am.* 2011;31: 391–406.
91. Senti G, Prinz Vavricka BM, Erdmann I, et al. Intralymphatic allergen administration renders specific immunotherapy faster and safer: a randomized controlled trial. *Proc Natl Acad Sci USA.* 2008;105:17908–17912.
92. Dickel H, Goulioumis A, Gambichler T, et al. Standardized tape stripping: a practical and reproducible protocol to uniformly reduce the stratum corneum. *Skin Pharmacol Physiol.* 2010;23:239–265.

93. Nickoloff BJ, Naidu Y. Perturbation of epidermal barrier function correlates with initiation of cytokine cascade in human skin. *J Am Acad Dermatol.* 1994;30:535–546.
94. Allam JP, Stojanovski G, Friedrichs N, et al. Distribution of Langerhans cells and mast cells within the human oral mucosa: new application sites of allergens in sublingual immunotherapy? *Allergy.* 2008;63:720–727.
95. World Allergy Organization (WAO). Position paper 2013; http://www.waojournal.org/content/7/1/6#B19. Accessed October 2014.
96. King HC, Mabry RI, Mabry CS, et al. Interaction with the patient. In: *Allergy in ENT Practice: The Basic Guide.* 2nd ed. New York, NY: Thieme Medical Publishers; 2005:67–104.
97. Krouse JH, Krouse HJ. Modulation of immune mediators with MQT-based immunotherapy. *Otolaryngol Head Neck Surg.* 2006;134:746–750.
98. Cox LS, Linnemann KI, Nolte H, et al. Sublingual immunotherapy: a comprehensive review. *J Allergy Clin Immunol.* 2006;117:1021–1035.
99. Lin SY, Sublingual immunotherapy: current concepts for the U.S. practitioner. *Int Forum Allergy Rhinol.* 2014; 4:S55–S59.
100. Samburago R, Puccinelli P, Burastero SE, et al. The efficacy of subligual immunotherapy for respiratory allergy is not affected by different dosage regimens in the induction phase. *Allergol Immunopathol (Madr).* 2003; 31:329–337.
101. Marogna M, Spadolini J, Massolo A, et al. Long-lasting effect of sublingual immunotherapy according to its duration: a 15 year prospective study. *J Allergy Clin Immunol.* 2010;126:9675–9699.
102. Larenas-Linnemann D, Cox LS. European allergen extract units and potency: review of available information. Immunotherapy and Allergy Diagnostics Committee of the American Academy of Allergy, Asthma and Immunology. *Ann Allergy Asthma Immunol.* 2008;100:137–145.
103. Nelson MR, Cox L, *Allergen Immunotherapy Extract Preparation Manual.* American Academy of Allergy, Asthma & Immunology; 2012.
104. USP 797 guidebook to pharmaceutical compounding —sterile preparations, 2008. http://www.usp.org/products/797Guidebook/. Accessed March 21, 2010.
105. Sharkey P, Portnoy J. Rush immunotherapy: experience with a one-day schedule. *Ann Allergy Asthma Immunol.* 1996;76:175–180.
106. Roll A, Hofbauer G, Ballmer-Weber BK, Schmid-Grendelmeier P. Safety of specific immunotherapy using a four-hour ultra-rush induction scheme in bee and wasp allergy. *J Investig Allergol Clin Immunol.* 2006;16:79–85.
107. Marshall GD Jr. AIDS, HIV-positive patients, and allergies. *Allergy Asthma Proc.* 1999;20:301–304.

18

Immunomodulator Therapies: Monoclonal Antibodies, Fusion Proteins, and Immunoglobulins

Anna Rossovsky Smith and Larry Borish

INTRODUCTION

Immunology involves an array of interactions between host defense mechanisms targeted against antigens that are seen as foreign. Evolutionarily, it developed as a means of protection from pathogens and a way of maintaining equilibrium. It can be divided into 2 immunologic response systems, the innate and adaptive. Innate immunity is composed of pattern recognition receptors (PRRs), molecules that are either secreted or located transmembrane, which identify microbial ligands, also known as pathogen-associated molecular patterns (PAMPs), and other danger signals. The ligation of these molecules results in a cascade of events that leads to defense mechanisms which include other actions of innate immunity such as activation of complement, opsonization, chemoattractant release, phagocytosis by mononuclear phagocytes and granulocytes, activation of other innate immune cells such as natural killer (NK) cells, and, ultimately, target lysis.

The adaptive immune system is a more refined system of identification of specific antigens that are deemed foreign and includes B cell–mediated humoral immune and T cell–mediated cellular immune responses. The interaction between the innate and adaptive systems is essential in ensuring that an appropriate fortress of protection exists to defend the host.

LYMPHOCYTES: T EFFECTOR CELLS, T HELPER SUBTYPES, AND TH2 IMMUNE DEVIATION

$CD4^+$ T cells that have been activated by antigens can differentiate into 4 subtypes of effector (Teff) cells, Th1, Th2, or Th17 as well as immune suppressive regulatory (Treg) cells (Figure 18–1). Th1 cells facilitate cell-mediated responses, specifically by macrophages, that aid in the elimination of intracellular pathogens, primarily producing the cytokines, interferon (IFN-γ), and tumor necrosis factor (TNF-β). Th17 cells activate neutrophils through their production of their defining cytokine interleukin (IL)-17 and promote immune defense mechanism at mucosal surfaces including against extracellular Gram-negative organisms, staphylococci, and fungi (*Candida*). Th2 cells activate the humoral system, particularly IgE, as well as stimulate eosinophils. They produce IL-4, IL-5, IL-9, and IL-13. Allergic responses are primarily Th2-mediated disease

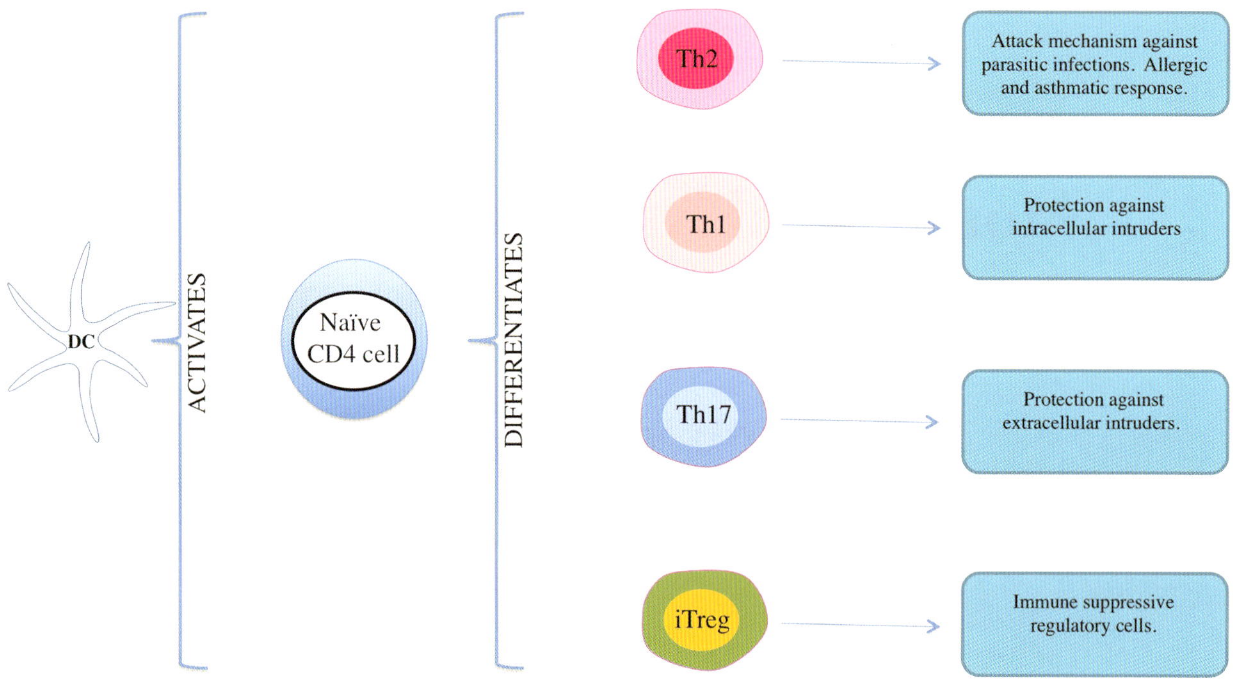

Figure 18–1. T-helper lymphocyte families.

processes. Numerous studies have established the involvement of Th2 immune responses in allergic rhinitis.[1] The focus of this chapter is on Th2 mechanisms since they contribute to the allergic response and to sinus disease pathology.

The initial trigger driving Th2 immune deviation includes signals derived at mucosal surfaces (eg, in response to helminths but, pathologically in allergic diseases, to otherwise innocuous aeroallergens). As discussed later in this chapter, these signals include those derived from the cytokines IL-25, Il-33, and TSLP (thymic stromal lymphopoietin). However, once these (and other Th2-promoting processes) are engaged, IL-4 becomes the main cytokine establishing the Th2 pathway.

Th2 activation, proliferation, and differentiation occur in secondary lymphoid tissues over a period of 4 or more days. During this time, chemokines and other receptors develop on the cell surface which allow both for selective and immediate recruitment back to the site of inflammation (such as the nose and sinuses) and also for the production of memory cells that will be available in the future for activation without the need for receptor engagement. These chemokine receptors are unique to the type of $CD4^+$ effector T cell. For example, Th2 cells express receptors, such as CCR4 and CCR8 to allow for a customized, unique ligand-mediated chemotactic and activation response that is specific to allergic inflammation.

IMMUNE MECHANISMS OF CHRONIC RHINOSINUSITIS (CRS)–CRS WITH NASAL POLYPOSIS AS A TH2 DISEASE

Early and Late-Phase Responses

Upon exposure of the nasal mucosa to allergens, antigen-presenting cells take up these molecules after which they process and present them to helper T lymphocytes. These activated T cells then produce IL-4 and IL-13 that stimulate the B-cell isotype switch to synthesize allergen-specific IgE. The IgE then binds with high affinity to IgE receptors located on mast cells, which, on future exposure to those allergens, results in mast cell degranulation that rapidly releases mediators such as histamine, tryptase, leukotrienes, and prostaglandins that drive the immediate response.[2]

The late-phase response generally occurs 4 to 6 hours after exposure to the allergen. It is a cell-mediated response composed of T lymphocytes, eosinophils, and newly recruited basophils. These basophils also release histamine, prostaglandins, and leukotrienes. In addition to their production of potent bioactive allergic mediators, a large number of different cytokines are produced, which in turn recruit more cells to the site, which then release their proinflammatory mediators. This phase of the response in an allergen challenge will last about 18 to 24 or more hours and is the cause of symptoms such as nasal congestion, rhinorrhea, and sneezing.[2] On natural chronic exposures, this late-phase response becomes the predominent source of symptoms.[3]

Innate Cytokine and Chemokine Mechanisms of Eosinophilic Sinusitis

The innate system represents evolutionarily generated immunity that is embedded in our phenotypic makeup. It is the frontline in host defense; generally composed of a less-specific system of attack against molecules that are identified as different from self. Within the sinuses there are numerous anatomic structures that contribute to the innate defense system.

The sinus epithelium is an essential barrier to microbe entrance into the subepithelial layer of mucosa. It does this by promoting mucosal hydration, which, combined with healthy mucociliary function, drives microbial clearance out the sinus ostia. Intact epithelial tight junctions preclude penetration of foreign particles. And while no pathogenic primary defect has been described in tight junctions in patients with chronic rhinosinusitis or nasal polyposis, the evolution of mucosal inflammatory disease results in a decreased and irregular pattern of expression of these proteins.[4] Similarly, chronic rhinosinusitis (CRS) is associated with an acquired deficiency in mucociliary transport.[4]

Toll-like receptors, a type of PRR, are present on sinus epithelium and their binding of microbial-derived components such as lipoproteins, peptidoglycans, lipopolysaccharides, flagella, and bacterial (CpG) DNA, leads to the activation of innate antimicrobial peptides and cytokines as well as chemokines that initiate and augment innate responses but also stimulate activation of the adaptive immune system.

In addition to epithelial cells, macrophages present in the respiratory mucosa are activated as part of the innate immune responses. These cells primarily produce the cytokines IL-1, IL-6, and TNF-a, when exposed to allergens. In addition to their own pro-inflammatory effects, these cytokines stimulate epithelial cells to release a "second wave" of cytokines and chemokines, including GM-CSF, IL-8, eotaxins (CCL11, CCL24, and CCL26), and RANTES (regulated on activation, normal T cell expressed and secreted; CCL5) that stimulate eosinophils to aggregate and activate at the site of allergen exposure. These cytokines also synergize with GM-CSF, IL-3, and IL-5 to facilitate the differentiation and mobilization of eosinophils. Even though these latter cytokines are products of Th2 cells, they are also produced by many cells of the innate immune system including mast cells, basophils, and innate lymphoid type 2 cells. In addition, once recruited, eosinophil inflammation becomes a self-propagating process because eosinophils are also able to produce IL-3 and GM-CSF.

GM-CSF is a pro-inflammatory cytokine that facilitates eosinophil activation and tissue damage as well as promotes release of cysteinyl leukotrienes, molecules identified in asthmatics and patients with allergic rhinitis that contribute to bronchospasm, mucus production, tissue edema, and inflammation. IL-3 and IL-5 also activate eosinophils, and more specifically, IL-5 is currently the only cytokine known to differentiate eosinophils from hematopoietic progenitors. RANTES (CCL5), along with the eotaxins (CCL11, 24, and 26), are chemokines that serve as chemoattractants for eosinophils and also activate them.

Recent evidence has identified other epithelial cytokines that play essential roles in airway inflammation, especially through their ability to initiate the drive to Th2 immune deviation (Figure 18–2). As noted, TSLP, IL-33, and IL-25 are particularly relevant in regard to their roles in asthma and CRS with

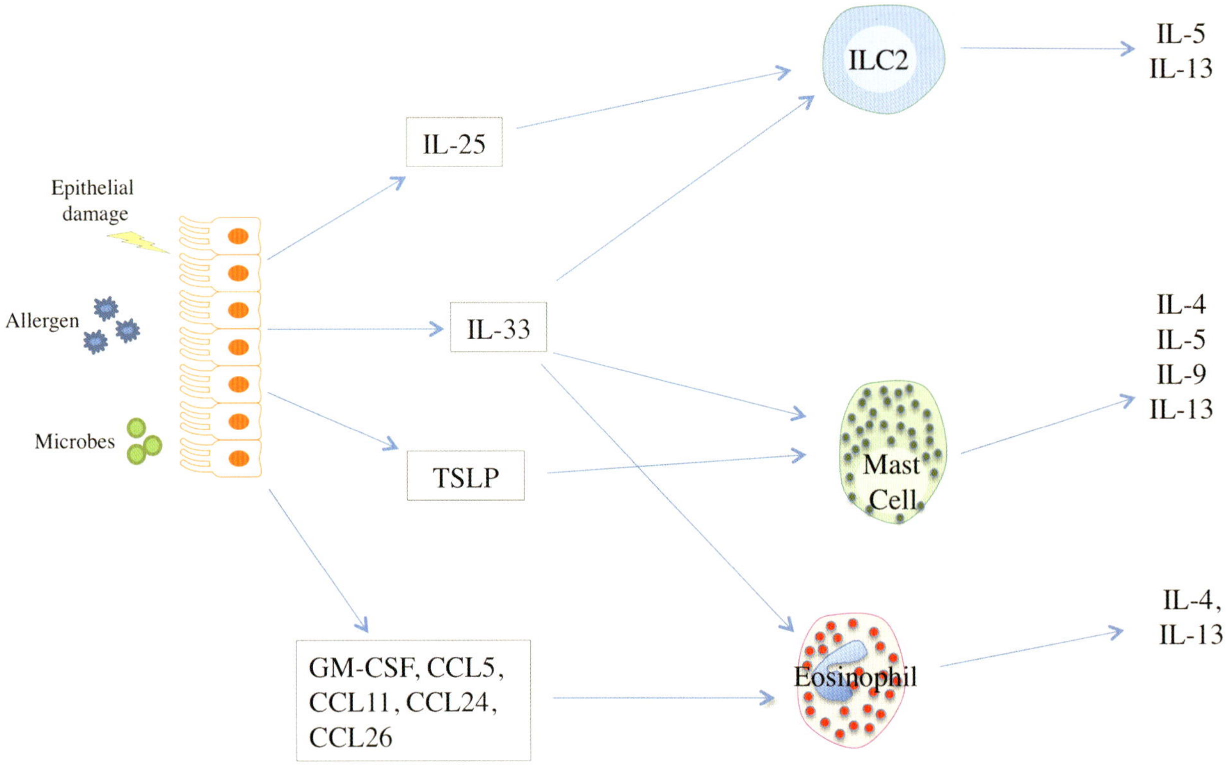

Figure 18–2. Innate immune mechanisms in allergic inflammation. Innate immune mechanisms include epithelial cell-derived cytokines that promote Th2 inflammation, including IL-25, IL-33, and TSLP as well as other chemokines and cytokines that recruit and activate eosinophils. In addition, many innate cells including eosinophils themselves but also ILC2 and mast cells produce cytokines associated with the Th2 "signature."

nasal polyposis.[5] IL-25 and IL-33 provide an initial signal driving naïve T cells to differentiate into Th2-like cells, while TSLP acts primarily on antigen (allergen)-presenting dendritic cells to direct them to promote a Th2 response.

Adaptive (Th2) Mechanisms: IgE, IL-4, IL-5, IL-9, IL-13

Mechanisms of Immune Modulation

Allergen-exacerbated asthma and allergic rhinitis are predominantly Th2-mediated disease processes. Although corticosteroids have generally been the mainstay of therapy, this therapeutic modality has numerous untoward side effects, particularly with long-term use, and many patients demonstrate various degrees of corticosteroid resistance, thereby limiting their efficacy. An understanding of the mechanism of action of Th2 lymphocyte activation provides us with the opportunity to focus on specific immune-targeting therapies in the treatment and management of this disorder. Biologic agents can facilitate immune modulation via many different mechanisms. Examples of these include antibodies, soluble receptors, antireceptors, and small molecule signaling antagonists (Figure 18–3).

Monoclonal Antibodies. Monoclonal antibodies are proteins that are generated to target a specific antigen, in this case, specifically, a mediator of allergic inflammation. There are several ways to produce these antibodies. Murine, chimeric, and even "humanized" murine antibodies have been used in human recipients. They work by neutralizing the biological effectiveness of the antibody. However, because of their varying degrees of nonhuman characteristics, they are able to cause hypersensitivity reactions. More recently, an increasingly popu-

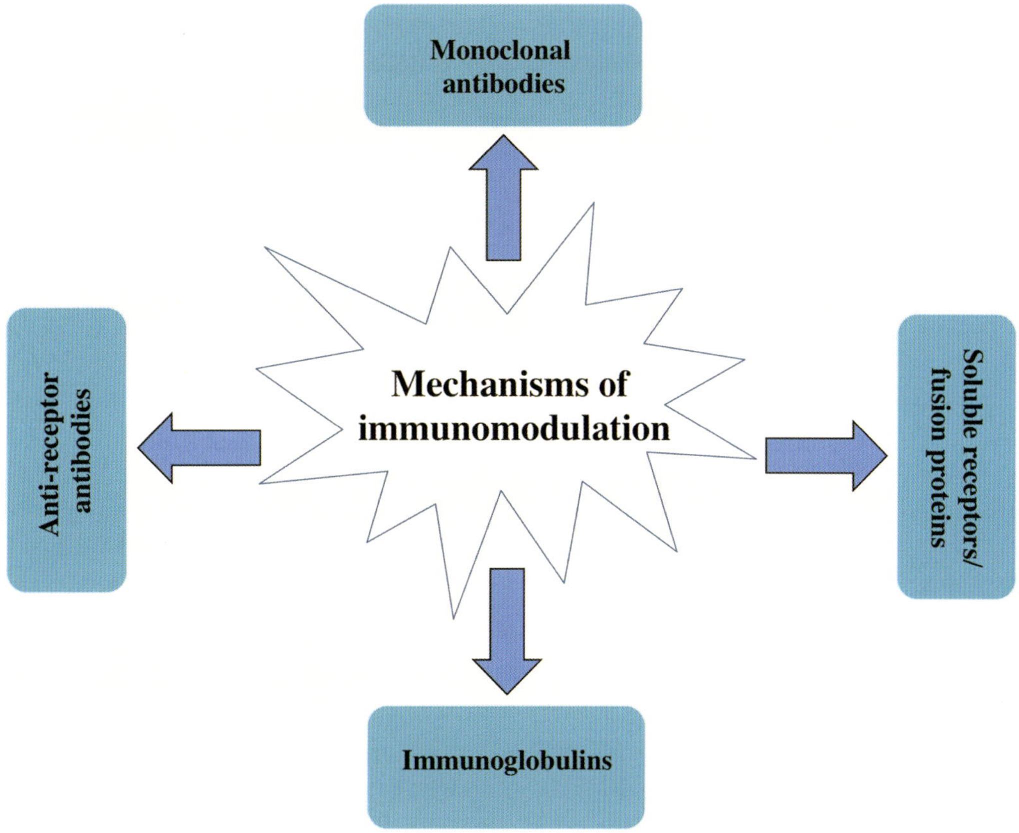

Figure 18–3. Mechanisms of immune modulators.

lar approach is to utilize human/severe combined immunodeficient mouse chimeras. These are mice in which the murine immune system, and in particular the antibody-coding domains, are replaced with the human genes, and can thereby be utilized to generate fully "human" antibodies. The benefit of these molecules is that they are less immunogenic since they are completely human. The naming of these molecules is generally determined by several factors. The last 4 or 5 letters of the name are based upon the source of the molecule with –zumab meaning "humanized," –omab indicating "murine," –ximab for "chimeric molecules," and umab for "human." The central part of the name reflects the disease indication of therapy, and the first 3 or 4 letters are chosen by the developing organization (Table 18–1).[6] For example, omalizumab is a humanized antibody ("zumab") targeting the immune system ("li," specifically IgE), whereas tralokinumab is a fully human antibody ("umab") that targets an interleukin ("ki," specifically IL-13).

Soluble Receptors and Fusion Proteins. Soluble receptors, or fusion proteins (consisting of cytokine receptors covalently linked to a *multivalent* carrier protein [multivalent to increase avidity]), are composed of the extracellular domain of the transmembrane receptor. Soluble receptors are made through alternative mRNA splicing or by proteolytic cleavage of the extracellular portion of the transmembrane domain where they are natural mediators of immune modulation. They have several mechanisms of action that depend upon the relationship of the ligand to the receptor. In general, these actions include receptor downregulation, competitive binding inhibition, or alternatively acting as serum binding proteins to prevent ligand degradation.[7]

Table 18-1. Nomenclature for Monoclonal Antibodies

Antibody Source	Nomenclature	Example	Function
Mouse	"omab"	Muromomab	Anti-CD3 (T cell)
Chimeric (human/mouse)	"ximab"	Infliximab	Anti-TNFα
Humanized	"zumab"	Omalizumab	Anti-IgE
Fully human	"umab"	Dupilumab	Anti-Il-4/Il-13R

Antireceptor antibodies are agents that inhibit cytokines by binding their receptors on the cell membranes, thereby blocking ligand binding and receptor activation.

Immunoglobulins. Immunoglobulins are another therapeutic form of immunomodulation. These are delivered as a concentrate composed of a pool of plasma obtained from thousands of individual donors. Immunoglobulin can be administered either intravenously (IVIG) or subcutaneously (SCIG). The mechanisms of action of immunoglobulin replacement therapy is not well understood but includes downregulation of generation of autoantibodies. At present immunoglobulin replacement therapy is approved for use in primary humoral immunodeficiency, multifocal motor neuropathy, B-cell chronic lymphocytic leukemia, immune thrombocytopenic purpura (ITP), Kawasaki syndrome, or chronic inflammatory demyelinating polyneuropathy.[6] However, immunoglobulin replacement has been used successfully in asthma and, by extension, could theoretically be useful in CRS, were it not cost prohibitive.[8]

IMMUNOMODULATOR THERAPY IN ASTHMA AND CRS WITH NASAL POLYPOSIS

In the management of asthma, one of the most frequently used medications is corticosteroids (CCS). It is important to emphasize the long-term complications of chronic oral corticosteroid use, such as osteoporosis and development of glaucoma. However, CCS, even if they were to be given systemically, are not universally effective in ameliorating allergic inflammation and, indeed, many patients are refractory to CCS, driving much of the current unmet medical need in these disorders. In addition, while CCS suppress the expression of Th2 cytokines, they are more of a "patch" rather than true disease-modifying agents, and as such, do not produce any long-term benefit once they are discontinued. Immunomodulator therapy has thus become attractive as a treatment modality that can truly alter the disease's natural history. As it relates to asthma (and perhaps CRS), to the extent that these are diseases reflecting T-cell responses to allergen (and perhaps other antigens), T-cell immunomodulation therapy offers the promise of direct disease modification.

Innate Immune Targeting

Anti-TNF Therapy

Tumor necrosis factor, or TNF, is a homotrimer composed of 3 17-kD molecules. It is primarily produced by activated monocytes, macrophages, and lymphocytes. One TNF molecule must bind to 2 or more TNF-receptors on a target cell to trigger signal transduction. Once activated, the vascular endothelial cell will express cell surface adhesion molecules such as ICAM and VCAM, which will subsequently help recruit leukocytes to the inflammatory site. It also plays a key role in promoting smooth muscle cell and fibroblast hyperplasia, which are prominent components of airway remodeling in asthma. Currently, TNF-inhibitors are indicated for the treatment of rheumatologic disorders and inflammatory bowel disease. Common TNF-inhibitor therapies are the monoclonal antibodies, infliximab and adalimumab, and the soluble receptor, etanercept. Less commonly encountered, but approved as well, are certolizumab pegol and golimumab. Adverse events are generally related to immunosuppression. Patients are at increased risk of infectious complications, in particular, to *Mycobacterium tuberculosis*. Other concerns are their ability to cause hepatotoxicity and demyelinating disease. A 2006 study investigating TNF-α blockade in patients with severe persistent asthma was discontinued prematurely after safety evaluation identified an increased tendency toward serious adverse events in patients receiving the study drug when compared to placebo. The most common reported events were asthma exacerbations and infectious complications. Also, the study group had more malignancies reported.[9]

Anti-IL-1 Therapy

Interleukin-1 is a superfamily composed of 11 cytokines. The most studied members of this group are IL-1α, IL-1β, and IL-1 receptor antagonist (IL-1Ra). In general, this cytokine is released in its inactive precursor state and is then activated by the converting enzyme caspase 1. After activation, it acts as a pro-inflammatory cytokine in conditions such as sepsis or rheumatoid arthritis. The competitive IL-1R antagonist (anakinra), the fusion IL-1 receptor protein (rilonacept), and monoclonal anti-IL-1β antibody (canakinumab), are IL-1 inhibitors that are presently in clinical use. Anakinra is approved for use in rheumatoid arthritis and cryopyrin-associated periodic syndrome (CAPS) patients. It is a recombinant IL-Ra that differs by one amino acid from the naturally occurring IL-1Ra. Rilonacept is a type of fusion protein consisting of 2 soluble IL-1 receptors linked to the Fc region of human IgG1, that strongly binds to IL-1α and IL-1β and both it and canakinumab have been approved for the treatment of CAPS.[6,10,11] At present, no interleukin-1 antagonists are approved for the treatment of allergic disease.

IL-25/IL-33/TSLP

As noted, current research has established the importance of epithelial-secreted cytokines in airway inflammatory processes, specifically in asthma and CRS with nasal polyposis. Through the mechanisms of activation of pathogen-associated pattern recognition receptors, identification of other "danger" signals including those generated via tissue injury, or by direct allergen activation (such as through protease-activated receptors), sinonasal epithelial cells release IL-25, IL-33, and TSLP [see Figure 18–2]). As noted, IL-25 and IL-33 provide an initial signal directly driving the differentiation of naïve T cells into Th2-like cells, whereas TSLP acts primarily on antigen (allergen)-presenting dendritic cells to direct them to support a Th2 response. In addition, IL-25 facilitates Th2 activation by promoting the activity of TLSP.[5,12] TSLP blockade was recently shown to have efficacy in allergen-induced asthmatic responses supporting potential future applications in CRS.[13]

Eosinophilic Chemokines (Eotaxin (CCL11, 24, and 26), RANTES (CCL5))

Chemokines play a central role in the recruitment of inflammatory cells to a specific site. More than 40 chemokines have been identified; however, in CRS the focus is on eosinophilic chemokines, specifically the eotaxins (CCL11, 24, and 26), and RANTES (CCL5), and their interaction with chemokine receptors, CCR3 and CCR5. RANTES (CCL5) facilitates the release of inflammatory molecules from eosinophils. In addition to its actions on eosinophils, RANTES (CCL5) promotes basophil histamine release and is among the most potent molecules to do so.[14] Antagonism of CCR3 is a proposed therapeutic approach in the management of eosinophil-predominant disease states. In a study of murine allergic airway inflammation by Wegmann et al, CCR3 antagonists produced a decrease in eosinophils in the airway epithelium along with subsequent reduction in airway hyperresponsiveness and reduced goblet cell hyperplasia.[15]

Adaptive (Th2) Targeting

Anti-IgE Therapy

Allergen exposure in atopic individuals results in the production of specific IgE antibodies. This immunoglobulin then binds to high-affinity FcεRI receptors, predominantly expressed on mast cells and basophils. Future reexposure to that same allergen results in cross-linking of IgE receptors, causing cell degranulation. As such, IgE is essential to the immediate allergic response, particularly in allergic rhinitis and asthma.[16] Omalizumab is a monoclonal antibody against IgE. It functions by both decreasing the concentration of free IgE as well as by the downregulation of the FcεRI receptor.[17] It binds to the part of the IgE molecule (the Ce3 domain), which is the binding site for FceRI. As a result, when IgE is bound to its receptor, this binding site is no longer accessible and omalizumab cannot inadvertently cause mast cell or basophil activation. A study by Gevaert et al., investigating the use of omalizumab in patients with chronic rhinosinusitis with nasal polyposis found that there was a statistically significant decrease in total nasal polyps and improvement in overall quality of life and symptoms (Figure 18–4).[18] It is approved for use in the United States in patients 12 years and older, with moderate to severe asthma, who have positive skin or blood tests to a perennial allergen, and who are not responsive to inhaled corticosteroids.[19] It is also approved for use in patients with refractory chronic urticaria.

Anti-IL-4 Therapy

Interleukin-4 has many essential functions in driving the allergic response, including inducing the IgE isotype switch, stimulating IgE secretion from B lymphocytes, and enhancing the production of IgE receptors on mast cells.[20] It also promotes VCAM-1 expression on endothelial cells, which when bound to VLA-4, helps attract eosinophils, basophils, monocytes, and lymphocytes to sites of inflammation. IL-4 also augments the secretion of eotaxins (CCL11, 24, and 26) (Figure 18–5).[21] It plays a key role in the inhibition of apoptosis of Th2 lymphocytes along with promoting their differentiation. IL-4 has been found in elevated concentrations in allergic patients in bronchoalveolar fluid as well as serum. With the extensive role that IL-4 plays in the allergic response, it is an attractive target in the field of therapeutics. Early studies in asthma (phases I and II) utilizing soluble IL-4 receptor (altrakincept) were promising, showing improved quality of life, decreased responsiveness to methacholine challenge testing, decreased reliance on glucocorticoid inhalers, and minimal adverse events.[22] However, phase III trials failed to show efficacy in treatment of asthma.[23] Similarly, studies with monoclonal anti-IL-4 antibodies and IL-4 receptor inhibitors were stopped due to lack of consistent efficacy.[24] In contrast, as discussed below, dual IL-4/IL-13 antagonists have shown promise in asthma, consistent with the redundant roles of these cytokines.

Anti-IL-5 Therapy

The association of interleukin 5 with eosinophilic inflammation makes it a cytokine that is particularly active in the allergic response and attractive as a therapeutic target. This cytokine is secreted by many different cells including basophils, $CD34^+$ progenitors, Th2-like lymphocytes, mast cells, and innate lymphoid type 2 (ILC2) cells. It works in synergy with eotaxins and other chemokines to potentiate the expansion of eosinophils. It has a significant role in the development of mature eosinophils in the bone marrow, which subsequently translocate to sites of allergic inflammation. It also is important in the prevention of apoptosis of eosinophils thereby propagating the allergic response. Stimulation of basophils by IL-5 potentiates their release of leukotrienes. Eosinophilic inflammation is associated with the development of increased mucous production as well as airway hyperresponsiveness. In mouse models, increased expression of IL-5 in lung epithelium induces pathologic findings similar to asthma. Elevated levels of IL-5 have been identified in bronchial biopsies of patients with asthma.[25,26] Mepolizumab and reslizumab, humanized monoclonal antibodies to IL-5, are the leading therapeutic agents under investigation in the management of asthma (and other eosinophil-mediated diseases). Mepolizumab is effective in treatment of severe eosinophilic asthma producing a reduction in exacerbations and an improvement in quality of life. Studies evaluating reslizumab have identified similar findings, noting a reduction in eosinophil count in sputum as well as improvement in FEV_1.[27] However, with both of these agents, it is important to emphasize that these benefits were only found in patients screened for having asthma associated with eosinophilic inflammation.[28] Interestingly, in the reslizumab study, efficacy was most prominent in patients with concomitant nasal polyposis.[27] Nasal polyps may merely have served as a "biomarker" for eosinophilic asthma, but this study may support efficacy in CRS. A study of

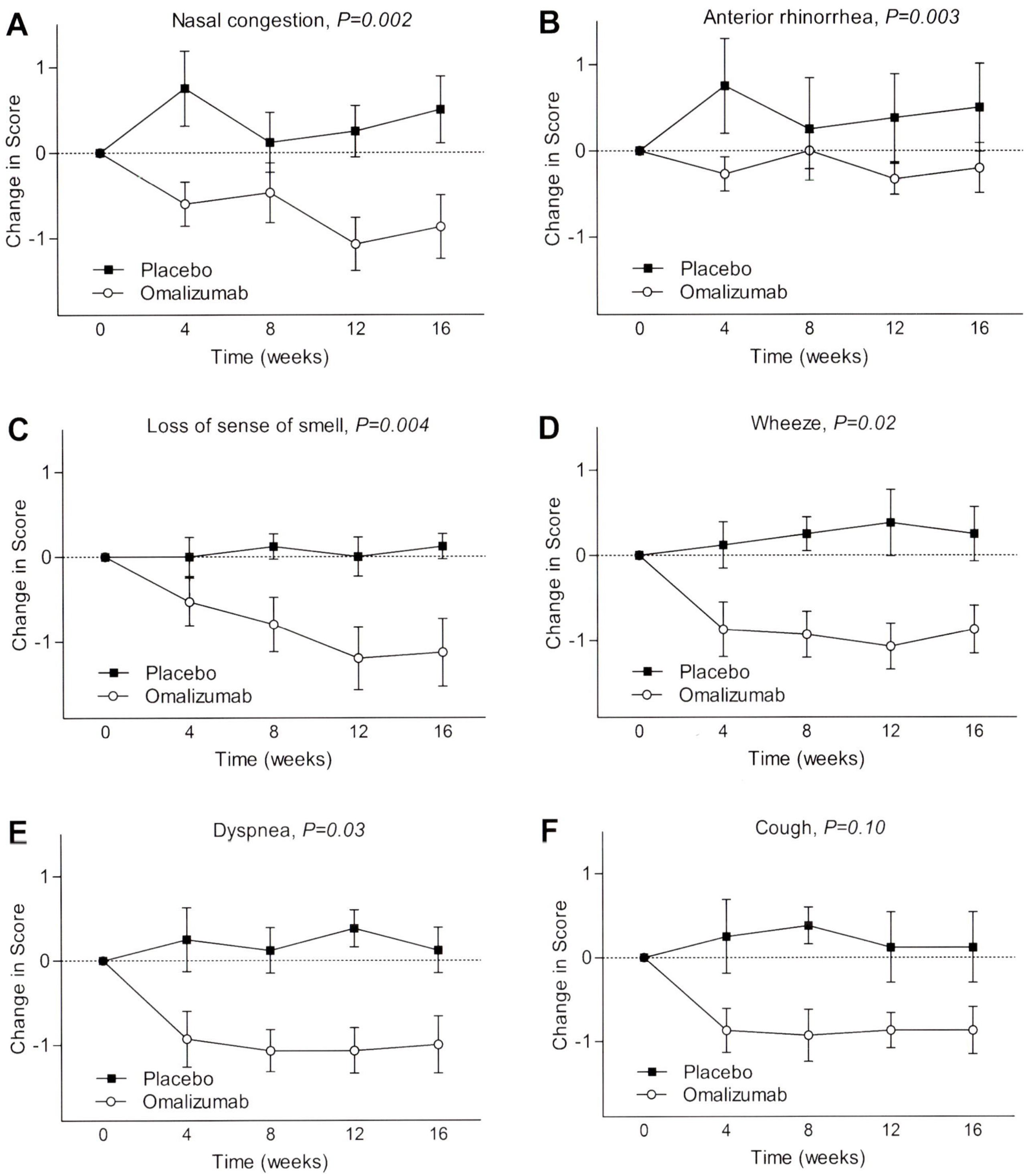

Figure 18-4. Omalizumab in CRS. Change from baseline in nasal congestion (**A**), anterior rhinorrhea (**B**), sense of smell (**C**), wheezing (**D**), dyspnea (**E**), and cough (**F**) in the omalizumab-treated (*open circles*) and placebo-treated (*solid squares*) groups. *P* values represent the change from baseline after 16 weeks of treatment. Error bars indicate 95% CIs of the mean based on normal approximation. Reprinted with permission from Elsevier. Gevaert P, Calus L, Van Zele T, et al. Omalizumab is effective in allergic and nonallergic patients with nasal polyps and asthma. *J Allergy Clin Immunol.* 2013;131(1):110–116 e111.

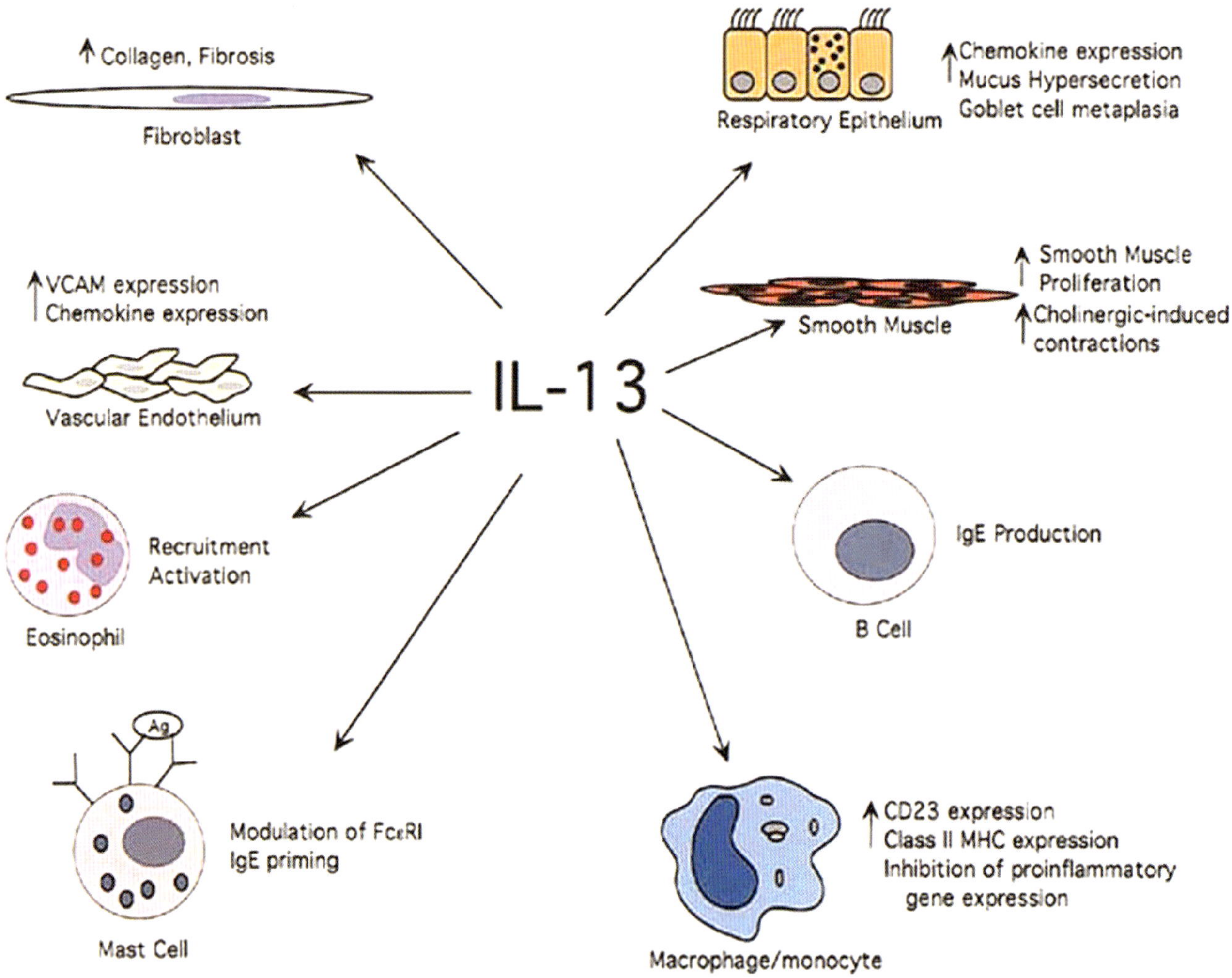

Figure 18–5. Biological effects of IL-4 and IL-13. Reprinted with permission from Elsevier. Hershey GK. IL-13 receptors and signaling pathways: an evolving web. *J Allergy Clin Immunol.* 2003;111(4):677–690; quiz 691.

mepolizumab by Bachert et al found that that there was a statistically significant reduction in total polyp score when compared to placebo and the authors suggested that if the study were further prolonged this difference may become even greater.[29]

Benralizumab is a monoclonal humanized antibody targeting IL-5Ra (CD125). A phase I study identified a reduction in sputum, peripheral, and bone marrow eosinophil counts[30] again lending support to its potential use in eosinophilic forms of sinusitis.

Anti-IL-9 Therapy

IL-9 is a Th2 (and the related Th9) lymphocyte-derived cytokine that has a significant role in the allergic response.[31,32] Another important source of this cytokine is the mast cell. IL-9 receptors are expressed primarily on Th2 and Th17 cells. In asthma, this receptor has also been found on polymorphonuclear cells and mast cells in the lung parenchyma. Its functional capabilities include promoting growth and cytokine production by Th2 cells and stimulating the production of IgE and IgG by B cells. Also, it has a role in the production of mast cells and in increasing airway inflammation. Finally, IL-9 has a role in directly stimulating mucus gene expression.

Transgenic mice that overexpress IL-9 in the lung show increased mucous production, airway hyperresponsiveness, infiltration by eosinophils and lymphocytes, and collagen deposition.[33] In a mouse model using IL-9 monoclonal antibodies, long-term inhibition showed decreases in mucous cell hyperplasia, airway hyperresponsiveness, and fibrotic changes.[34] However, at present, no agent specifically targeting IL-9 is under investigation in humans.

Anti-IL-13 Therapy

IL-13 is an additional cytokine associated with the Th2 "signature" that activates macrophages and eosinophils, and promotes isotype switching in B cells to IgE (Figure 18–5).[35] IL-13 is also secreted by ILC2s. ILC2 release of IL-13 (and IL-5) occurs as a result of the release of IL-25 and IL-33 from the respiratory epithelium, something that can occur in response to viral infection, allergen exposure, or other innate signaling pathways (see Figure 18–2).[35]

The secretion of IL-13 results in the establishment of many of the processes that are responsible for the phenotypic characteristics of allergic asthma. These include mobilization of eosinophils and conversion of respiratory fibroblasts to myofibroblasts, which are essential for collagen deposition and subsequently fibrosis.[35] Also, IL-13 drives the metaplastic transformation of epithelial cells into goblet cells, enhances mucous secretion, and stimulates macrophages.[35] Importantly, it is one of the most essential factors in generating airway hyperresponsiveness. Lebrikizumab and tralokinumab are monoclonal antibodies to IL-13 that are under investigation. In a recent study of lebrikizumab in subjects with mild asthma, there was no statistical difference identified in late asthma responses, as measured by FEV_1. However, exploratory analyses did find that patients with higher baseline levels of IgE and peripheral eosinophils tended to respond better to this treatment.[36]

IL-4/IL-13 Dual Antagonists

IL-4 and IL-13 are cytokines that bind to specific receptor subunits that dimerize to initiate their signaling cascades. IL-4 binds to the IL-4Rα subunit which in turn dimerizes with either the common γ chain (γc) cytokine receptor, or to the IL-13Rα subunit.[35] In contrast, IL-13 binds directly to the IL-13Rα subunit which then recruits IL-4Rα.[37] Since both forms of the IL-4 receptor (IL-4Rα/γc and IL-4Rα/IL-13Rα) and the IL-13 receptor (IL-13Rα/IL-4Rα) utilize IL-4Rα, then competitive inhibitors that bind and block this chain are capable of acting as dual IL-4 and IL-13 antagonists.

Pitrakinra is an interleukin 4 variant molecule that competitively inhibits the IL-4Rα complex.[24,38] In clinical trials of asthma, pitrakinra produced a decreased reduction in FEV_1 following allergen exposure. However, this effect was not statistically significant and no impact on airway hyperresponsiveness was observed,[24] so studies with this agent were subsequently discontinued.

In contrast, dupilumab is a monoclonal antibody against the IL-4Rα that blocks both IL-4 and IL-13 signaling, and this agent has shown significant therapeutic promise.[20] In patients with moderate to severe asthma, it was found to improve FEV_1 and quality of life while decreasing reliance on β-agonist therapy. Biomarkers of asthma also decreased.[39] Along with IL-5 antagonists this agent has the most potential to advance in clinical practice where its efficacy in CRS can be further explored.

CONCLUSION

The intricate choreography of the immune system allows it to function effectively in its protection of the host. However, at times the response can be more bothersome than the initial insult, for example, in the generation of allergic inflammation. Fortunately, the numerous pathways involved in this activation result in a system with several portals of potential therapeutic intervention. As summarized in Table 18–2, many biologics are under investigation to help attenuate the body's responses in allergic inflammatory responses that drive the development of CRS.

Table 18-2. Immunomodulatory Monoclonal Antibodies and Soluble Receptors Available or in Development for Allergic Inflammatory Diseases

Target	Agent	Mechanism	Clinical Applications[a]
IgE	Omalizumab	Humanized monoclonal antibody	Asthma[a] Chronic idiopathic urticaria[a] Allergic rhinitis Chronic rhinosinusitis Food allergy
IL-4	Altrakincept	Soluble receptor	Asthma
IL-5	Mepolizumab	Humanized anti-IL-5 antibody	Asthma Chronic rhinosinusitis
	Reslizumab	Humanized anti-IL-5 antibody	Asthma
	Benralizumab	Humanized anti-IL-5Rα antibody	Asthma
IL-13	Lebrikizumab	Humanized anti-IL-13 antibody	Asthma
	Tralokinumab	Human anti-IL-13 antibody	Asthma
IL-4/IL-13	Pitrakinra	Receptor antagonist	Asthma
	Dupilumab	Human anti-receptor antibody	Asthma Atopic dermatitis
TSLP	AMG 157	Human anti-TSLP antibody	Asthma

[a]FDA-approved indications.

REFERENCES

1. Broide DH. Allergic rhinitis: Pathophysiology. *Allergy Asthma Proc.* 2010;31(5):370–374.
2. Pawankar R. Inflammatory mechanisms in allergic rhinitis. *Curr Opin Allergy Clin Immunol.* 2007;7(1):1–4.
3. Pipkorn U, Karlsson G, Enerback L. The cellular response of the human allergic mucosa to natural allergen exposure. *J Allergy Clin Immunol.* 1988;82(6):1046–1054.
4. Hamilos DL. Host-microbial interactions in patients with chronic rhinosinusitis. *J Allergy Clin Immunol.* 2014;133(3):640–653, e644.
5. Scadding G. Cytokine profiles in allergic rhinitis. *Curr Allergy Asthma Rep.* 2014;14(5):435.
6. Lee SJ, Chinen J, Kavanaugh A. Immunomodulator therapy: monoclonal antibodies, fusion proteins, cytokines, and immunoglobulins. *J Allergy Clin Immunol.* 2010;125(2, suppl 2):S314–S323.
7. Heaney ML, Golde DW. Soluble receptors in human disease. *J Leukocyte Biol.* 1998;64(2):135–146.
8. Orange JS, Hossny EM, Weiler CR, et al. Use of intravenous immunoglobulin in human disease: a review of evidence by members of the Primary Immunodeficiency Committee of the American Academy of Allergy, Asthma and Immunology. *J Allergy Clin Immunol.* 2006;117(4, suppl):S525–S553.
9. Wenzel SE, Barnes PJ, Bleecker ER, et al. A randomized, double-blind, placebo-controlled study of tumor necrosis factor-alpha blockade in severe persistent asthma. *Am J Respir Crit Care Med.* 2009;179(7):549–558.
10. Hoffman HM, Throne ML, Amar NJ, et al. Efficacy and safety of rilonacept (interleukin-1 Trap) in patients with cryopyrin-associated periodic syndromes: results from two sequential placebo-controlled studies. *Arthritis Rheumatism.* 2008;58(8):2443–2452.
11. Kanariou M, Tantou S, Varela I, et al. Successful management of cryopyrin-associated periodic syndrome

with canakinumab in infancy. *Pediatrics.* 2014;134(5): e1468–e1473.
12. Chin D, Harvey RJ. Nasal polyposis: an inflammatory condition requiring effective anti-inflammatory treatment. *Curr Opin Otolaryngol Head Neck Surg.* 2013;21(1):23–30.
13. Gauvreau GM, O'Byrne PM, Boulet LP, et al. Effects of an anti-TSLP antibody on allergen-induced asthmatic responses. *N Engl J Med.* 2014;370(22):2102–2110.
14. Alam R. Chemokines in allergic inflammation. *J Allergy Clin Immunol.* 1997;99(3):273–277.
15. Wegmann M, Goggel R, Sel S, et al. Effects of a low-molecular-weight CCR-3 antagonist on chronic experimental asthma. *Am J Respir Cell Mol Biol.* 2007;36(1):61–67.
16. Gould HJ, Sutton BJ. IgE in allergy and asthma today. *Nat Rev Immunol.* 2008;8(3):205–217.
17. McKeage K. Omalizumab: a review of its use in patients with severe persistent allergic asthma. *Drugs.* 2013;73(11): 1197–1212.
18. Gevaert P, Calus L, Van Zele T, et al. Omalizumab is effective in allergic and nonallergic patients with nasal polyps and asthma. *J Allergy Clin Immunol.* 2013;131(1):110–116, e111.
19. Sandstrom T. Omalizumab in the management of patients with allergic (IgE-mediated) asthma. *J Asthma Allergy.* 2009;2:49–62.
20. Vatrella A, Fabozzi I, Calabrese C, Maselli R, Pelaia G. Dupilumab: a novel treatment for asthma. *J Asthma Allergy.* 2014;7:123–130.
21. Hershey GK. IL-13 receptors and signaling pathways: an evolving web. *J Allergy Clin Immunol.* 2003;111(4):677–690; quiz 691.
22. Steinke JW, Borish L. Th2 cytokines and asthma. Interleukin-4: its role in the pathogenesis of asthma, and targeting it for asthma treatment with interleukin-4 receptor antagonists. *Respir Res.* 2001;2(2):66–70.
23. Holgate ST, Polosa R. Treatment strategies for allergy and asthma. *Nat Rev Immunol.* 2008;8(3):218–230.
24. Wenzel S, Wilbraham D, Fuller R, Getz EB, Longphre M. Effect of an interleukin-4 variant on late phase asthmatic response to allergen challenge in asthmatic patients: results of two phase 2a studies. *Lancet.* 2007;370(9596):1422–1431.
25. Ying S, Durham SR, Corrigan CJ, Hamid Q, Kay AB. Phenotype of cells expressing mRNA for TH2-type (interleukin 4 and interleukin 5) and TH1-type (interleukin 2 and interferon gamma) cytokines in bronchoalveolar lavage and bronchial biopsies from atopic asthmatic and normal control subjects. *Am J Respir Cell Mol Biol.* 1995;12(5): 477–487.
26. Molfino NA, Gossage D, Kolbeck R, Parker JM, Geba GP. Molecular and clinical rationale for therapeutic targeting of interleukin-5 and its receptor. *Clin Exper Allergy.* 2012;42(5):712–737.
27. Castro M, Mathur S, Hargreave F, et al. Reslizumab for poorly controlled, eosinophilic asthma: a randomized, placebo-controlled study. *Am J Respir Crit Care Med.* 2011;184(10):1125–1132.
28. Ortega HG, Liu MC, Pavord ID, et al. Mepolizumab treatment in patients with severe eosinophilic asthma. *N Engl J Med.* 2014;371(13):1198–1207.
29. Gevaert P, Van Bruaene N, Cattaert T, et al. Mepolizumab, a humanized anti-IL-5 mAb, as a treatment option for severe nasal polyposis. *J Allergy Clin Immunol.* 2011; 128(5):989–995, e981–988.
30. Laviolette M, Gossage DL, Gauvreau G, et al. Effects of benralizumab on airway eosinophils in asthmatic patients with sputum eosinophilia. *J Allergy Clin Immunol.* 2013;132(5):1086–1096, e1085.
31. Dardalhon V, Awasthi A, Kwon H, et al. IL-4 inhibits TGF-beta-induced Foxp3+ T cells and, together with TGF-beta, generates IL-9+ IL-10+ Foxp3(-) effector T cells. *Nat Immunol.* 2008;9(12):1347–1355.
32. Goswami R, Kaplan MH. A brief history of IL-9. *J Immunol.* 2011;186(6):3283–3288.
33. McLane MP, Haczku A, van de Rijn M, et al. Interleukin-9 promotes allergen-induced eosinophilic inflammation and airway hyperresponsiveness in transgenic mice. *Am J Respir Cell Mol Biol.* 1998;19(5):713–720.
34. Kearley J, Erjefalt JS, Andersson C, et al. IL-9 governs allergen-induced mast cell numbers in the lung and chronic remodeling of the airways. *Am J Respir Crit Care Med.* 2011;183(7):865–875.
35. Ingram JL, Kraft M. IL-13 in asthma and allergic disease: asthma phenotypes and targeted therapies. *J Allergy Clin Immunol.* 2012;130(4):829–842; quiz 843–844.
36. Scheerens H, Arron J, Zheng Y, et al. The effects of lebrikizumab in patients with mild asthma following whole lung allergen challenge. *Clin Exper Allergy.* 2014;44(1):38–46.
37. Romeo MJ, Agrawal R, Pomes A, Woodfolk JA. A molecular perspective on TH2-promoting cytokine receptors in patients with allergic disease. *J Allergy Clin Immunol.* 2014;133(4):952–960.
38. Nguyen TH, Casale TB. Immune modulation for treatment of allergic disease. *Immunol Rev.* 2011;242(1):258–271.
39. Wenzel S, Ford L, Pearlman D, et al. Dupilumab in persistent asthma with elevated eosinophil levels. *N Engl J Med.* 2013;368(26):2455–2466.

Index

Note: Page numbers in **bold** reference non-text material.

B

C

D

E

F

G

H

I

N

O

P

Q

R

S

T

X

Z